Unless you fix the trauma,
the hole in the soul where the wounds started,
you're working at the wrong thing.

Nadine Burke Harris, MD, MPH
California Surgeon General

Also by Rae Lewis-Thornton
Amazing Grace: Letters Along My Journey
The Politics of Respectability

UNPROTECTED

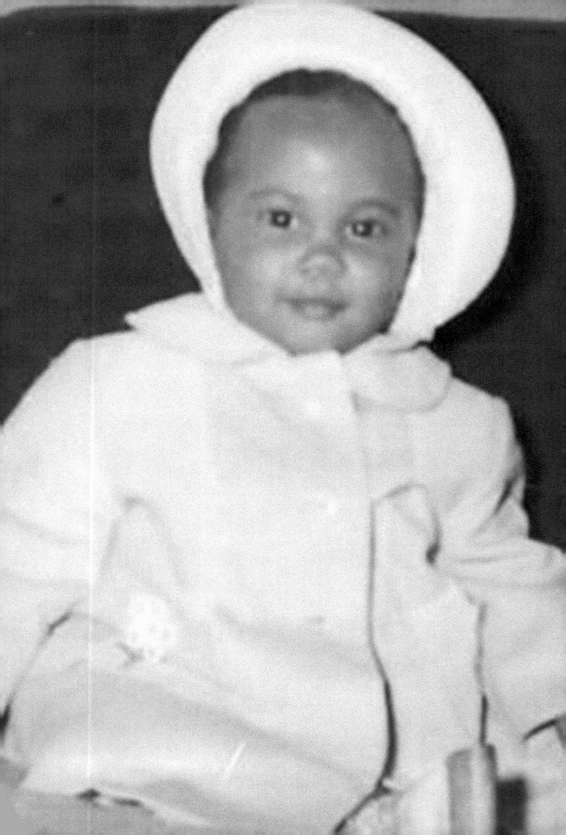

UNPROTECTED

A MEMOIR

RAE
LEWIS-THORNTON

FOREWORD BY SHERYL LEE RALPH

Library of Congress Control Number:
2022907305

First Edition
ISBN 978-1-7378912-0-8
Cover and Interior: Relana Johnson
Editor: Vivian Feggans
Publisher: Rae Lewis-Thornton
www.raelewisthornton.com

ORDERING INFORMATION
Quantity sales: Special discounts are available on quantity purchases by corporations, associations, and others.
Email info@unprotectedamemoir.com
Distributed by Ingramsparks
Printed in the United States of America

CONTACT INFORMATION
Rev. Rae Lewis-Thornton, MDiv: rae@raelewisthornton.com
Website: www.raelewisthornton.com
RLT Collection Hand crafted accessories by Rae Lewis-Thornton: www.rltcollection.com
Diva Living With AIDS Blog: www.divalivingwithaids.com
Information on Unprotected: A Memoir - www.unprotectedamemoir.com
Twitter & Instagram: @RaeLT
Facebook: www.facebook.com/RLTdivawithaids

Jacket design: Relana Johnson
Front Jacket photo: Kirsten Miccoli
Photo Stylist: Brandon Frein and Arlene Matthews @Kitthis
Photo Make-up Artist: Tia Dantzler
Photo Hair Stylist: Trayce Madre
Jacket Dress: Alice and Olivia provided by Bloomingdales, Magnificent Mile Chicago
Back Jacket photo: Kip Meyer for Essence Magazine

For
Jane Clara Lee Lewis
1915-Unknown

My paternal grandmother who left behind an untold story of trauma. I lift up your courage and I will continue to carry your strength with me as long there is breath in my body.

and

All the women and girls who were left unprotected
by the people who should have loved and protected them.
You Matter!

Seeking

I was hot... A girl on fire
A hot girl, simmering into womanhood.
Seeking love anywhere... everywhere
Until...
I lost myself
In a world of cold criticism and judgment
My heat dissipates, the more I seek, the more I hide...
From everyone.
Even myself I begin to question.
Until...
I remembered...
I am Purposed
I am Favored
I am... Ablaze

~LaToya Renae Porter & Rae Lewis-Thornton~

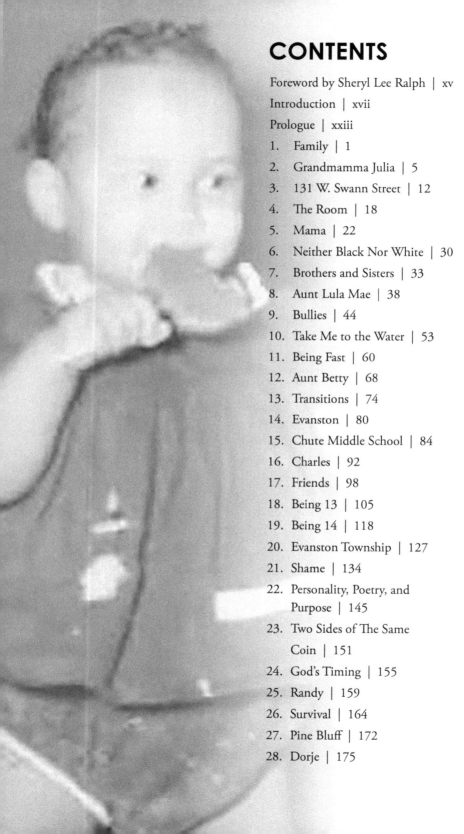

CONTENTS

FOREWORD

Rae Lewis-Thornton is one of the most Divinely Inspired Victoriously Audacious (D.I.V.A.) women I have ever known. As an Emmy Award-winning AIDS activist, she is an internationally known advocate for social justice. Still, most of all, she's my sister, my soror, and my friend.

I often think of how the universe brought us together as sisters, finding our voices in different spaces and colliding in destiny. My journey started in the eighties, the most pivotal, exciting, and beautifully ugly rollercoaster I have ever been on. December 20, 1981, I made my Broadway debut in what has become the iconic musical of the '80s, "Dreamgirls." Picture it…big hair, bright lights, and the magic of Broadway! There I was, a young starlet amongst her peers shining brightly. We were all young, beautiful, and highly talented with our entire lives ahead of us — or so we thought. AIDS had begun to sweep through America, New York City, and Broadway. The bright marquee lights went dim, and the hair went flat. The Broadway that I knew and loved had become a ghost of the talented people we lost. Death and silence went hand-in-hand, and, silently, that 'mysterious' disease blew out the flame of life on Broadway like one does candles on a birthday cake. There was funeral after funeral, memorial after memorial, and THE DEADLY SILENCE. I decided that I couldn't be quiet. Someone had to speak up for my friends, who were marginalized and stigmatized while fighting for their lives. I found my voice and founded The D.I.V.A. (Divinely Inspired and Victoriously Aware) Foundation in 1990 to break the silence and erase the stigma connected to the virus. One year later, I created an annual HIV/AIDS benefit, "DIVAS Simply Singing!" to serve as a living memorial to the many friends I had lost to AIDS. For the past 30+ years, DIVAS worldwide have come together to raise their voices in solidarity to increase awareness about HIV/AIDS and other life-threatening conditions.

Looking back at the start of the epidemic, I was especially concerned about the threat that HIV/AIDS had posed for women and children. Gay men and black South Africans were the initial focus of the conversation. We saw how they were marginalized and stigmatized for having the condition. I felt that behind these disparaged groups of people was another disparaged group, and it was black women. I had so many questions. What about us? What about the black women who were being affected by HIV/AIDS? Where were our stories? Who will be our strength when we desperately need it? I was determined to find answers.

Then, like a divinely placed gift, in December of 1994, my issue of ESSENCE came in the mail, and I was captured by the gaze of a striking black woman on the cover. The cover read "Facing AIDS." I knew right away that everything I thought I knew about HIV/AIDS was about to change because this young, educated, and drug-free black woman who was dying of AIDS was breaking open the conversation no one was having. Rae Lewis-Thornton stared into my soul from that cover. She was regal, poised, and beautiful, with sincerity and severity in her eyes. She was on a mission to educate, and I knew in my soul that our paths would cross one day. For several years, I traveled throughout the country speaking out, raising awareness, building community with my foundation, and producing benefit concerts. In 2006, I finally met Rae Lewis-Thornton at the NAACP Convention, where we both spoke on a women's health panel. Rae shared her deeply personal HIV/AIDS journey. She openly revealed the challenges she faced during diagnosis and treatment, including the medicinal side effects of extreme weight loss, lipodystrophy, and peripheral neuropathy, which left her with a painful stinging sensation in her hands and feet. I was blown away by her transparency and her tone of confidence and conviction. Her audacity and boldness captivated everyone in that room. She was raw! She was real! She was FABULOUS! I later learned that Rae sometimes felt that the world wasn't ready to hear her voice during her early days of activism. She did her work and has become a voice to many voiceless women. In a recent interview I did with Rae, she began with these words that shook my foundation to the core, "HIV can take everything away from me, but I will never let it take my dignity!"

Rae has dedicated her life to informing others about HIV/AIDS and helping shape the difficult conversation women need to have to help protect themselves. She boldly stood face to face with the stigma of AIDS, sharing her truth with the world. Rae changed what people think a person with AIDS looks like, empowering women to stand up for themselves and LIVE, while they are alive.

In 2007, I created and wrote a one-woman show, "Sometimes I Cry Monologues," inspired by Rae's story. I toured the production to audiences of women across the globe. There was never a dry eye whenever I performed the monologue of Miss Chanel, the character inspired by Rae. Her story has inspired tens of thousands of women and men to protect themselves and find the power within to defy the odds. A few years later, I partnered with MAC Cosmetics to launch "Sisters Circle: South Africa," a program of The D.I.V.A. Foundation which brought together 200 women in South Africa living with HIV/AIDS and 25 African American women to share their experiences, exchange ideas, erase stigma, and build bridges to stem the tide of HIV infections in their lives and in the lives of those they loved. Rae shared her stories with the women there, and they returned their own stories, and we were all able to laugh, cry, and share emotions as sisters. The impact of one's story is never small. You never know how your one experience can change a life and how someone else's one experience can change yours. Rae's presence and participation brought healing to many women. Rae has also presented and spoken at DIVAS Simply Singing! on numerous occasions. When I pick up the phone and call to ask for assistance, Rae is always the first to say yes.

In all these years, Rae has been a steadfast, truth-telling, warrior woman of the first order. Many turned their backs on her because they were not ready for her brand of raw truths. She empowered herself to be the bodacious, gracious, graceful, outspoken woman she is still becoming. Rae has learned that every life experience the good, the bad, and even the difficult, ugly ones challenge her to continue growing and evolving.

As you read *Unprotected: A Memoir*, please know that Rae wants to help people, through her story, to break the destructive cycles in their lives and get to a better place. This isn't just a story about HIV/AIDS. This is a story about growing to love oneself unconditionally and paying attention to one's physical and mental health. Rae and I often speak about how wounded girls are often in danger of becoming broken women. People aren't usually aware of how the effects of their experiences manifest into illness. Knowledge and self-awareness are both a part of the process of healing.

Rae is turning 60, and that's a modern-day miracle for a woman who's been told too many times to count that she would die sooner than later. For years, Rae has been pouring her soul onto paper to create this memoir, and I am so happy and excited for its completion and release. It has required deep soul searching to expose the many layers of her personal truth. Despite the difficulties, there have been rich experiences woven into her life and Rae has kept the faith. I'm so proud, and excited for her. All these years later, Rae Lewis-Thornton is not dying of AIDS she has survived AIDS and is THRIVING. She has survived the terror of rape and the childhood trauma of molestation. She has beaten the odds by living out loud, refusing to become a silent statistic, and challenging others to learn more about themselves and HIV/AIDS. Rae Lewis-Thornton has turned her pain into power and passion.

So, make yourself a hot cup of tea and sit. You may shed a few tears, but you will also laugh, and you will be forever inspired and enlightened. Thank you to my friend Rae Lewis-Thornton for being an example to us all and strutting each day victoriously in her high heels with her face towards the sun, with optimism, grace, and poise.

SHERYL LEE RALPH

INTRODUCTION

The journey of writing and publishing *Unprotected: A Memoir* first began fourteen years ago with a book deal at an A-list publishing house. The deal went to hell in a handbasket the same week I met with the publishers, although I wouldn't know it for another six months.

In 2010, two years after I lost the book deal, I was determined to rewrite this memoir. I made this big announcement on social media. I even got thirteen pre-sales. After three chapters, I realized the problem wasn't that I couldn't write as the editor at the publisher's had said. *(The crazy stuff people say about us that we believe – SMH; I was working on my Ph.D. at the time of the book deal. Of course, I could write.)* The problem was the emotional barrier I couldn't break to write the story that needed to be told. Then, around November of 2018 after reading Cookie Johnson's memoir, *Believing in Magic,* I started writing again. Her authenticity touched me profoundly and I knew in my gut that it was time.

I went on a writing retreat to Bali, Indonesia in January of 2019, made possible by many of you who contributed to the Go Fund Me, and my girlfriend Veronica Slater now retired from the airlines who gave me travel passes. Yep, that retreat. (You will read about my friendship with Veronica and others in this memoir, too.) In Bali, I literally pulled the old manuscript apart paragraph by paragraph, so I could envision a new direction and I didn't stop until this memoir was done. Of course, when I started, I had no idea it would take me this long, but then I hadn't realized that I would have to relive the traumatic events of my life to get my story out of me onto paper; that is, not until I was in knee-deep.

My book title hasn't changed from what I proposed to the publishing house in 2008 *Unprotected: A Memoir.* What has changed is the focus of the story in order to make it mine. The publishers wanted a book about a little Black girl who had a horrible childhood and fucked around in the name of looking for love and got HIV, but in the end, made good on her life. However, the story God wanted me to write is about how unprotected I was as a child and how that shaped the trajectory of my life. Plainly stated, this book is about the cycle of trauma and how it impacted my life not just my sex life all areas of my life: my education, my self-esteem, how I viewed the world, and everyone who crossed my path. I recognize today what God already knew, that I could not have written this book fourteen years ago. I was not emotionally or mentally ready and that's why the universe did not cooperate the first time around.

This book is deeply rooted in my gift for storytelling. It is written in my authentic voice and from my memory. However, I went to great lengths to fact-check myself. Stylistically, citations are more about preference when it comes to memoirs and autobiographies, but the scholar in me wouldn't let it rest. As a result, I've added a comprehensive bibliography documenting every article and publication that is mentioned. Additionally, I added a reading list on the topics that intersected with my life as they unfolded in this book. Finally, I've thought carefully about who should be in this book. My final decision rested on one thing: a person or event would land on these pages if the intersection of my life with them helped to tell my story.

My story begins on the South Side of Chicago at the age of six with the death of my grandfather, after which darkness descends over my life like the sky before a storm. I have only one memory of being a happy little girl. That is, sitting on my paternal grandfather's knee in the auto shop garage next door to our home on Swann Street sipping an orange Fanta soda. His death changed my world as I knew it and left me unprotected. In the care of his third wife, the woman I call Mama, trauma becomes a way of life and my new normal.

I introduce Mama and our complicated relationship in the Prologue. In chapters one through twelve you will meet Little Rae and see how she creates a parallel world of resilience while living in abuse. I should warn you, there will be many triggers for those who have survived trauma. It is the darkest part of my story with both sexual and physical violence, and it was the most difficult for me to write. You will have a front-row seat to sexual grooming, manipulation, and rape. You will see how Little Rae tries to make sense of what is happening to her with no name for sex; only an understanding that this is *being fast*. The word *fast* as used in this book is a pejorative term that has been used among generations of Black women as a way to contain Black girls. You will see Little Rae trying to make sense of Mama's frequent use of "*fast*" while navigating the sexual violence all at the same time. You will also meet the first angels God places in Little Rae's path to serve as a buffer a reprieve from the trauma. You will meet Mama's boyfriend, his children, and the family we created. Little Rae is remarkable in that she never gives up. Not after beatings, rapes, or tongue lashings.

In chapters thirteen through twenty-four, my pre-teen and teenage years, you will journey with me as I mature and navigate dating and friendships. At the beginning of the seventh grade, we move from Englewood to Evanston, a suburb on Chicago's North Shore. My exposure to a different cultural and educational environment became a game-changer in my life. I could see fundamental differences from the world in which I had lived in Englewood, and that inspired me to reimagine a life different from the one I lived with Mama. As a result, I latched onto every good thing: my friends and their mothers, my middle schoolteachers, Harlem Renaissance-era books, my new pastor, and church programs influenced by Black Liberation Theology. Again, God placed angels in my life who acted as buffers and helped me to reimagine a life full of love. You will meet Mama's new husband, and bear witness as he makes my life a living hell. Period. It is during this time I start to believe that God has a plan for my suffering, and I appropriate my faith as one of my survival tools. This became the biggest *aha moment* of my life. I would hold on to it until my purpose was manifested years later. What I latched onto in those middle years saved me from total self-destruction, but it was not enough. By the age of seventeen and homeless, I go through another dark period.

In chapters twenty-four to around thirty-one, you will see me lost and trying to survive the best way I could. Moving into my young adult years with low self-esteem clinging to me like a monkey on my back, I go from a victim of abuse to self-abuse. You will have a front row seat to my own missteps and dysfunction. Again, there may be triggers in this section for some of you. In fact, intermittently throughout the book are scenes that may be a trigger. As you read my story take some breaks; have a cup of tea; be kind to yourself.

In the last twenty chapters you witness a turning point in my life. In college, I find my purpose in social justice work. I begin by organizing college students for Harold Washington's mayoral campaign. From there I accept an internship at Operation PUSH which catapults me into the national political landscape. You will meet the people that helped shape me as a young woman and develop me intellectually. Still, there are missteps, and my tumultuous relationship with Mama is never-ending.

Four years later, when I am twenty-four years old and had finally turned my life around, I learn that I have HIV. Unbeknownst to me then, I had been infected four years earlier just after my twenty-first birthday. These chapters will illuminate how I navigated my HIV diagnosis at the darkest period of the AIDS pandemic where there was no treatment and no hope. Facing death, I stepped into the space where I believe God ultimately intended for me to be.

I leaned heavily on the research around the impact of childhood trauma to center my story. Throughout the book, I interweave the terms *toxic stress*, *long-term trauma*, and *continuous cycle of trauma* that are defined by Dr. Nadine Burke-Harris in her book, *The Deepest Well,* as: "...when a child experiences strong and frequent and/or prolonged adversity such as physical or emotional abuse, neglect, caregiver substance abuse, or mental illness."

I was introduced to this topic by watching Dr. Burke-Harris' TED Talk, *How Childhood Trauma Affects Health Across a Lifetime.* (Dr. Burke-Harris is the first Surgeon General of California, and a pediatrician who has dedicated her life to understanding childhood trauma.) In those twelve short minutes she rewired my brain. I had always understood that trauma has a psychological impact, but I was blown away to learn that a cycle of trauma during the developmental stages of a child can change the biology of their body and brain and put them at an increased risk for substance abuse, mental illness, heart disease, cancer, high blood pressure and a host of other illnesses.

Dr. Burke-Harris' starting point was the *Adverse Childhood Experiences (ACEs)* Study, which was conducted by the Centers for Disease Control and Kaiser Permanente and published in 1998 in the *American Journal of Preventive Medicine.* This study looked at ten types of adversities in three categories: neglect, abuse, and household. In so doing, it showed the relationship of childhood abuse and household dysfunction to many of the leading causes of death and dysfunction in adults. (See Figures 2 and 3 in the Appendix.) I rushed to the internet to find the ACEs questionnaire and took the test. An ACEs score is a person's total number of adverse childhood experiences. I scored an 8 out of a possible 10. The higher your score, the greater your chances of health disparities as an adult. Since the original study there have been more than two thousand related studies that substantiate the original study.

Dr. Burke-Harris and other experts argue that a cycle of childhood trauma can lead to an overactive stress response system, which they call "deregulation, a disruption of the normal cortisol pattern." Let me explain. Cortisol is the long-term stress hormone that is designed to activate when there is a threat. It increases your blood pressure, blood sugar, inflammation, makes a person more aggressive, and conserves belly fat. This is commonly referred to as "fight, flight, or freeze." When the threat is over, cortisol turns itself off and the body goes back to normal. However, high doses of trauma cause the stress response to go haywire (i.e., deregulation). Basically, the stress response system has been activated so often it does not turn off even when there is no threat, or it is activated more frequently for the simplest of things. A child who experiences toxic stress caused by a cycle of trauma is likely to develop poor health and social outcomes that follow through adulthood.

Around the same time, I stumbled upon Dr. Bruce Perry, renown clinical child psychiatrist and author of *The Boy Who Was Raised as a Dog,* and his latest book coauthored with Oprah Winfrey, *What Happened to You?* His research illuminates some of the same points as Dr. Burke-Harris and other scholars on the topic of childhood trauma but adds a rich understanding of how the brain works. His research was particularly enlightening and helped me to understand the lack of my impulse control and reasoning ability—or lack thereof—which you will read about in this book. His starting point is the Hierarchical Brain Chart illustrated as an upside-down triangle. The top of the triangle, the cortex, is the smartest part of the brain. It is where we learn and where our values and beliefs are created. The bottom of the triangle, the brainstem, is the regulatory part of the brain; it controls our blood pressure and heart rate, and it happens to be the least intelligent part of the brain. Once the bottom is activated, the cortex shuts down. This was another *aha moment* for me. You will see me going into situations not thinking, triggered, and reactionary—often making mountains out of molehills.

In spite of how life played out in real time, I always had a knowing inside of me that this was not how God intended for me to be. It kept pricking at me like a woodpecker on a tree, steady and constant, *rat-a-tat, tat-tat, rat-a-tat-tat-tat!* I became a broken record, asking myself every single time I did something that hurt me, *What's wrong with you, girl?!* My missteps sometimes felt like an out-of-body experience. I could see me working against myself, but I didn't know how to stop. My soul screamed affirmations. *This is not you! You are better than this! This is not right! This doesn't feel good! No, not again!* But it was me who made the bad choices, who had the destructive impulses, and toted a complicated personality with me every place I went. It was me who was constantly looking for validation. *Pick me! Choose me!* No matter how loudly my soul screamed *rat-a-tat-tat-tat, THIS IS NOT YOU!* my brain was persistent in steering the wheels of my life. Had it not been for that pesky *rat-a-tat-tat-tat* pricking away at me, I would never have done the grueling work of deconstructing my life to rebuild something whole and healthy. I have done the self-work to find a new normal. I have painfully picked apart the old paradigms piece by piece, asking hard questions and trying to understand how to stop the pain and find peace. Over the years there were different stages of growth with different therapists. My hardest work was with Dr. Rebecca G., Dr. Greg G., Dr. Charles A., Dr. Kesha B., and Dr. Crystal C. Once I learned the science, there was even more to pick apart.

Through a new lens I am closer to understanding the toll that living in trauma had on my life. It was a wonderful feeling to learn that nothing was wrong with me. My body and mind responded to the trauma as it was designed to do. It's just that it was never turned off. I was always on high alert, anticipating a beating or dealing with the aftermath of a beating or being cursed out. My life was unpredictable, and I never knew if down meant up or up meant down. I can't recall a period in my life as a child through my young adult years where I wasn't on high alert. Even today, I'm easily triggered, but I understand better what is happening to me. I now have tools to help me address triggers in a positive way. I saw a meme that said, "Trauma is what happens inside of you as a result of what happened to you," and it hit the nail on the head. With this understanding, I work hard to break the cycle of being hot-wired all the time.

It goes without saying, but I will say it anyway: I believe everyone should take the ACEs test, but only when you are ready. (The ACEs test is Figure 1 in the Appendix.) If you take the test, I suggest utilizing the resources available for you on my website www.raelewisthornton.com. I am a strong advocate for trauma informed training for social workers, teachers, doctors, nurses, police officers, correctional officers, and it should be an absolute requirement for foster parents. I also concur with Dr. Burke-Harris, children should be given the ACEs test to identify the trauma in their lives as an intervention tool. Too often we write a child off as problematic—slow, bad, *fast*, hyper, won't pay attention, talks too much—when the problem is not the child but rather the symptoms of trauma showing up in a child's life.

In the pages of this book, I present my life as an example of what trauma can look like in the life of a child. I think often about girls that grow up to be wounded women like myself. Equally important are girls that are currently living in trauma. For instance, Ma'Khia Bryant's tragic death left me gutted. She was a 16-year-old Black girl in Columbus, Ohio who was killed by the police in front of her foster home fighting off teen girls and an adult woman. I think about how different her story could have been with proper intervention. Her death was one of those triggers that stopped my writing. I cried for a week after Ma'Khia's death. Thank God for *GirlTrek's* podcast; they got me back on track, but I wonder about all the girls who are still vulnerable and unprotected. I pray for Ma'Khia's little sister, who tried to get them help, but in the end witnessed her murder.

I cannot erase the experiences that you will read about in these pages, but I don't have to be stuck. I continue to work on myself. The hardest of all was writing this memoir. Yes, it was cathartic. My therapist and psychiatrist held my hand during the writing of this book. They forced me to take breaks. In fact, about a year into writing I had a really bad trigger, and was unable to write for over a month, and then, only in increments. I added additional therapy sessions and medications to help with anxiety while writing this book. This is another reason it has taken so long to complete. With each trigger I had to process what happened to me rather than push it back and leave it unresolved, no matter how painful it was. In every single chapter, I shed another piece of the old me, which brought me closer to who God intended for me to be.

No matter how painful it was to relive my life I forged ahead. Thank God for my editor, Vivian Feggans, who was patient through this entire process; and a process it was. I had to put in place tools to help me along the way. I didn't watch streaming specials that could trigger me. I only made it through one episode of *Surviving R. Kelly,* and then I quit. I missed all three documentaries on my one and only girl, Whitney Houston. I read mindless mysteries rather than books that could be a trigger, unless it was related to research for this book, and I knitted hundreds of bookmarks. I prayed, I cried, and I ate myself twenty pounds worth of fat. I wrote through a ton of health issues. I wrote through George Floyd's murder and the protests demanding justice that followed. I wrote through the COVID-19 pandemic, and an inept president. I wrote through images of the COVID-19 body bags. I wrote through the crippling isolation I endured in my one-bedroom apartment, and the loss of my livelihood as a result of COVID-19, with no speaking engagements for forty-six months and counting. (It's hard to concentrate when you don't know where your next meal is coming from.) I wrote through the bitter elections, and the insurrection that ensued at the U.S. Capitol on January 6, 2021. I wrote through the death of one of my oldest friends, Keith Jennings, and the death of my mentee, Tiara Williams, at the age of twenty-seven— not from COVID-19—but God, there was so much death during that period, it felt like it.

Like Little Rae, I forged ahead, thanks be to God. My hope and prayer are that my story will make you laugh, cry, give you many *aha moments,* and ultimately, that you will take whatever you need from my life to help enrich your own. Namaste.

PROLOGUE

Everyone knew I had AIDS but Mama—and that was fine with me. If I could have figured out a way to be on the cover of *Essence* magazine without her knowledge my life as an AIDS activist would have been complete. Over the years I had thought about telling her, but I could hear her saying, "See, bitch. I told you." That dreaded thought stopped me in my tracks. Now time was almost up. In a matter of weeks, subscribers to *Essence* would receive the December 1994 issue with me on the cover. I toiled and toiled over how to tell her. I even thought about not telling her. The thought that Mama couldn't read well enough to tackle an entire article entered my mind. However, there was nothing wrong with her eyes, and I didn't know how to get around my face sitting at the grocery store checkout counter looking at Mama.

I had known my HIV status since March 1987 and had been speaking in Chicago high schools for about a year. Thankfully, she and I moved in different circles and lived in different areas of Chicago. Now, the entire world was about to learn I had AIDS. It wasn't right to let her hear this from someone else. It was time to face the music. So, I put on my big-girl-panties and called my childhood girlfriend Coré to ask her to go with me. She was one of my closest friends, and I needed her support. Also, Mama really liked Coré. I figured that with her by my side, just maybe, Mama wouldn't show her ass.

That cold November night Coré and I sat in Mama's living room side by side on the sofa, and Mama sat on the loveseat opposite us.

"What kind of bullshit y'all trying to pull?" she chuckled, looking from me to Coré.

"I have something serious to tell you," I said. Again, she looked expectantly from me and then back to Coré. My heart was racing. I felt like that little girl again, uncertain, and afraid that what I had to say could be the death of me. In that moment I was more afraid of Mama's opinion than I was of AIDS. I knew I had to get it over with before I lost my nerve, so I burst out with it.

"I have AIDS."

"You got what?" she asked. Shame and self-loathing gripped me. I had yet to come to the place of self-forgiveness. Sitting in front of Mama, in an instant, I became the whore she had proclaimed me to be. For the last seven years, I held onto the guilt of becoming infected, which fostered even more shame sitting there facing Mama. She hadn't said anything else, and her silence scared me. Mama always had something to say, and I couldn't read her face. I needed a hint of what to say next, but nothing came.

"Mama, I'm sick. I have AIDS," I said, breaking the awkward silence.

Mama looked from me to Coré then back at me.

"You don't look sick," she said finally. I felt an uneasy relief: What needed to be said had been said.

"I know, Mama, but I am."

"Ain't that the thing those gay men get?"

"Yes, Mama, but women can get it, too." My stomach fell to my feet. I felt hopelessly unprepared. I was so busy worrying about her response to me that I never thought about how this would impact her. I felt bad about it. How could I explain HIV/AIDS to my mother who had a third-grade education and received most of her information from television and her drinking buddies? It occurred to me that here I was—her daughter—sitting in front of her saying I was dying like those White men whom she had seen on television. None of it made an ounce of sense to her, and I had no idea what to say to change that fact. She looked at Coré, "Is she telling the truth, Coco?"

"Yes, Mama Georgia," Coré said.

I jumped in to explain my activism as a way of explaining the disease. I wanted her to understand that even though I was sick I had dedicated the rest of my life to educating people about the dangers of HIV/AIDS. I wanted her to understand that I didn't want another person to become infected with this deadly disease. I was seeking her approval for the direction my life had taken. I was going to be on the cover of a prominent magazine to help other women. That was a big deal and I wanted her to be proud of me. She sat and listened. I finished explaining myself and we sat in an uncomfortable silence. Mama seemed lost and guilt flooded me like a tsunami. I needed to get the hell up out of there. I didn't know what else to say neither did I have a solution to ease her pain. She had never been a comfort to me, and I didn't know the words to comfort her. Any attempts to ease her pain were futile. That day was no different than any other day. No tears. No hugs. We each processed that moment in our own way.

"Well, Mama," I said as I stood up. "I just wanted you to know before the magazine came out."

Coré and I made our way to the door. Mama asked, almost in a whisper, "Maybe – could the doctors be wrong?"

"No, Mama. I wish they were." I opened the door to leave, and Mama spoke up again.

"If I can help you in any way let me know," and she added, "You really don't look sick." That would be the only reassurance she would ever give to me. I knew that Mama loved me in her own way. It's just that her brand of love had always been dysfunctional on one end and outright toxic on the other. The fact remained that I was her only child and there was a strong possibility she would have to bury me. No matter the type of relationship we had, no parent should have to bury a child.

Driving home, all the shame I had around HIV consumed me, canceling all the good that I was doing. In a matter of weeks, I would make history becoming the first African American woman to appear in a featured cover story about living with HIV/AIDS. Having told Mama, I now felt like a failure.

In 1994, HIV/AIDS was one of the worst diseases a person could have. With no cure on the horizon, it was plagued with stigmas and judgment around respectability, the one topic that fueled my chaotic relationship with Mama. I felt as if I had failed her by bringing home the greatest taboo of my lifetime. In hindsight, I never considered that the *Essence* cover story would disrupt her world right along with mine. Undoubtedly her friends would call wanting to know the scoop. I knew Mama's response would flow whichever way the wind was blowing. In those first weeks after I told her, the wind went straight to the gutter and Mama made sure I knew. She called. As soon as I answered the phone, she lit into me like a firecracker.

"What I want to tell you is this," she said. I braced myself; I knew her disapproving tone.

"I'm sorry you got that shit, but if you hadn't been fucking around with all those men you wouldn't have it." A part of me wanted to go tit for tat; instead, I listened to her for as long as I could.

"It's your own fault you got that shit!" She hollered. I stood in the kitchen with the phone to my ear as she assessed my life through her lens. Tears flowed down my face reminiscent of my childhood. For a fleeting moment, I drifted away as she blamed me, accused me, and ultimately made me feel like shit. It was all-consuming. I had HIV inside my body destroying my T cells, and AIDS-related infections trying to claim my life—and then, Mama. How hard our relationship had been all these years. I felt tired and weighed down. I wanted to sit on my kitchen floor and cry. Or maybe, even die. But my inner voice said, "You bet' the fuck not!" History had taught me that fighting with Mama was an endless battle. Something had to give, and since HIV was rooted inside every part of me — my blood, my brain, and all my organs — it had to be Mama.

"You ain't nothin' but a fuckin' whore!" she yelled.

"MAMA!" I yelled. I had come to the place of NO MORE. I knew I didn't have enough in me to fight her *and* AIDS. Regaining my composure, I gathered enough nerve to say what I had to say.

"Mama, I've been fighting with you all my life and I'm tired. I'm dying."

To my surprise she got quiet, and I spoke as calmly as I could.

"You have two choices. You can live in my life peacefully for the time that I have left, or you can get the hell out of my life."

"Bitch!" she spat. "Who the fuck do you think you're talking to?" I softly placed the phone on the receiver. I had a lot to do, and according to the science of AIDS in 1994, very little time to do it. Death was working hard to take me out. I understood that God had called me to do advocacy work at this time and place in my life. Rising to the occasion, I felt as if I had to tell my story to as many people as possible before death claimed me. Mama was Mama, and she would always be the only mother she knew how to be. She had not been capable of nurturing or loving me at any point in my life. Why should I have expected it in dying? I knew in my heart she was not going to change. Her brand of love had left me unprotected.

One

FAMILY

"Each unhappy family is unhappy in its own way."
—Leo Tolstoy

My grandfather was my protector. I wasn't used to him not being around. One day, I was sitting on his lap and the next day he was gone. In my six-year-old mind, I couldn't imagine where he was. It was as if he had disappeared into thin air. Mama was no help in solving the mystery. Each time I asked she just gave me the look that said, "Bitch, if you don't go sit your ass down...." I'm not sure what scared me the most: my grandfather's absence or being alone with Mama. This was the first time that I was left solely in her care. My paternal grandfather—Alfred Henry Lewis Sr., who I affectionately called Granddaddy—was the center of my universe. He was a decorated war veteran who assumed the responsibility of raising his son's only child: me. For as long as I could remember, my life started on Swann Street with Granddaddy. Now, there was no Granddaddy.

I don't remember who told me but by six years old, I knew that Mama wasn't my biological mother. She was, however, the only mother figure I had ever known. She was pretty in an ordinary kind of way: tall, with a broad back and a broad nose with high cheekbones, like Janet Jackson. Her skin was dark and smooth, like melted bittersweet chocolate. She started her day with Christian Brothers chased with water and smoked Winston cigarettes as if her life depended on them. She spoke her mind and cursed like a sailor and didn't give a damn who heard what she had to say. My grandfather's third wife, Mama was thirty-two years old when she married him. He was fifty-two. I was four. I was told my paternal grandmother, Jane Clara Lee Lewis, whom I'm named for, died in her thirties.

My life began in Buffalo, New York with my biological parents. I have no memory of life with them, but I believe, in my subconscious that I sucked in their chaotic lifestyle like second-hand smoke. I never knew my father, but I would meet my mother as I was approaching womanhood. My maternal great-aunt Lula Mae told me my father, Alfred Jr. met my mother in Buffalo while he was visiting her sister, Geraldine.

From the few pictures I've seen, my father was dark as coal, with a hint of honey that gave him a glow. My mother Judith was a pale white woman with an air of Victorian elegance. I was born prematurely on May 22, 1962, in Sisters of Charity Hospital forty-six days before my mother and father were married. They were an imperfect couple trying to make a family work against the odds. Born at thirty-six weeks, I weighed three pounds and four ounces. I stayed in an incubator for one month. My mother swore to me that my premature birth was not due to her drug use, but to a life-threatening medical condition. At twenty-one, her being pregnant with me was a deterrent to drugs; however, my birth wasn't enough to hold her together. Two decades after my parents let me go, my mother confirmed they gave me to my grandfather because raising a child and struggling with addiction was a combination designed for failure. My mother told me she and my father believed I would be better off with my grandfather. I never learned the exact age I went to live with him, just that it was after my first birthday and at least a year before my father's death, when I was three.

Over the years of knowing my birth mother, she almost never spoke about her life with my father or her addiction because it was too painful to revisit. On one rare occasion while sitting in her living room in Boulder, Colorado, she gave me a brief glimpse into their life. There was a peacefulness that flooded the living room that day. Her husband, Michael was at work, and we had the day to ourselves. The sun beamed through their picture window with the Rocky Mountains in the near distance. I loved how those mountains emanated a calmness that settled in the middle of the living room. Being there with my mother was a distinct contrast from my life with Mama. Mama and I had never stayed in a room together longer than thirty minutes unless it were required. That day my mother sat in the wingback chair with her legs folded into her thighs, a book in her lap and a cup of tea on the side table. I was curled up in the matching chair with a cup of tea and a book. Our shared love for books and tea was our way of bonding. I was deep into Langston Hughes' *Not Without Laughter* when she broke the silence.

"It was a big fucking mess."

I looked up. "Huh?"

"Me and Al were a big fucking mess," she repeated. "We were an interracial couple living in Buffalo, New York, in the early sixties and strung out on drugs with our Black baby," she said, shaking her head as she explained. I laid my book in my lap and swirled the chair so that I was facing her. She had my full attention.

"It was some crazy shit," she chuckled. "I don't know what would have happened if you had stayed with us," she added. Our life was plain old crazy. We loved you Rae, but we were so unable to take care of you."

I hung onto every word. I was hungry for anything she was willing to give me to help me understand what about their life had affected the path of mine. This new information was giving me a new outlook on their life.

"When you were a newborn, the police chief busted into our apartment and put a gun to Al's head."

"Really?" I asked, eagerly.

"Yes," my mother said, "He told Al to get the hell out of town with his nigger baby." *Nigger* hung in the air like thick fog. She gave me time to digest what she said. After another sip of tea, she said, matter-of-factly, "Al would have been murdered for being a Black man with a white woman if he had stayed in Buffalo."

I was horrified, but not surprised. By then I had a remote understanding of Buffalo as a white racist city. It was a generalization that included most of upstate New York. She now confirmed what I had believed. Years later, my research on Buffalo would also confirm, that like in most cities in the sixties, racial discrimination was an impediment to advancement for most African Americans. My father would likely have been killed, or jobless. Just seven months after I was born, the Congress of Racial Equality (CORE)—most famous for conducting the Freedom Rides in 1961—started organizing for racial equality in Buffalo. Ironically, as politically minded as I am, I had not considered race as a barrier to us remaining a family as much as I had drugs. Talking with my mother that day it was clear that my parents had not escaped hate and discrimination, or the heroin use that was rampant in the early sixties. Failure was knocking at their front door.

My father was murdered in Pontiac, Michigan on Valentine's Day of 1966. I was three years old. He turned thirty-one thirteen days earlier. Mama said he was shot in the back of his head by his first cousin as he walked away from an argument over drugs and a woman. It would be my truth until I was fifty-seven years old.

I learned what really happened from reading the police report. My father was shot in a car that his friend Alfonso Amoriella was driving. They were coming from Alfonso's house in Detroit after partying. My father was sitting in the front seat. Our twenty-year-old cousin, Ronald William Newcomb, was sitting behind my father with his girlfriend, Dorothy Wellons, who was seventeen. The gun, a .32-caliber automatic pistol, allegedly belonged to my father, and he'd asked Ronald to keep it in Dorothy's purse because he didn't want it on him. The report said, as they neared Pontiac, my father raised his right hand over his shoulder and said, "Hand me the gun." Ronald reached over his girlfriend with his left hand and took the gun out of her purse. As he was transferring the gun to his right hand to give it to my father, it discharged and fell to the floor. In Dorothy's statement, she indicated that she'd asked Ronald if the gun's safety latch was on. According to her, they were checking the safety when the gun went off.

"Where'd that shot go?" Ronald asked. Dorothy looked around and pointed to my father's head.

"I shot him! Man, go to the hospital!" Ronald said to Alfonso, still screaming, "I shot my cousin!" The driver looked over and realized that my father was slumped over, and he drove to the police station. They were then escorted to the hospital. Unfortunately, my father died one minute after the bullet reached his brain.

Ronald was arrested. His statement was filled with confusion and remorse. The police report said that he [Ronald] was "very upset" and they "could smell a strong odor of alcoholic beverages about him." It said further, "When he went before the judge," that, "Ronald was mute." The judge ordered a psychiatric evaluation.

I can't stop thinking about the trauma caused by Ronald accidentally killing my father or what it must have been like for this seventeen-year-old young woman to witness such a horrific incident. Then of all the luck, Alfonso was sent back to prison for parole violation just by being in the car with the gun although his fingerprints weren't on it. I have no idea what happened to Dorothy. In the end, my father's death was ruled, "[killed] by careless, reckless or negligent discharge of firearms." Ronald pled guilty and was given "two years' probation, $150 cost at $10 per month, 2 days credit to serve 20 more days in the county jail." What an absolute tragedy.

Now that I've learned the truth about my father's death, I can only speculate that Granddaddy's maternal side absence from my life after his death had something to do with the drama around my father's death. Through research I learned Granddaddy had six siblings from his mother's second marriage. His father, Richard Lewis carries the Dixon/Lewis/Bowden bloodline, that has a rich history of which I'm still learning. I believe the connection to this side of my family is due to death and migration. That my great-grandmother Mable disappeared boggles my mind; especially, because my father was living with her in Michigan when he died.

I could depend on my grandfather just like I could the stars coming out at night and the sun coming up in the morning. His absence was unsettling. While Mama was at work, I was down the street at Ms. Rachel's. She was the neighborhood matriarch and a good friend of my grandfather. Once home, I sat in front of our big picture window and watched for him to come home until Mama told me to go to bed. I continued to ask Mama when my grandfather was coming home and she continued to give me that certain kind of look, and I'd go to my room. Days turned into weeks, and I asked the same question over and over: "When's Granddaddy coming home?" Then one day out of the blue, Mama told me that she was taking me to see him in the hospital. I had no idea what that meant. I was simply excited that I would get to see him.

I remember that visit like it was yesterday. The ride to Hines Veterans Hospital, forty miles outside of Chicago, seemed like the longest car ride I had ever taken in my short life. When we walked into the hospital, I was fascinated by the shiny endless hallways. I eagerly turned my head from side to side looking for Granddaddy, but he was not within eyesight. I wanted to ask where he was, but I was afraid of Mama. She sat me in the lobby because children weren't allowed in the rooms. I kept looking around, soaking up the environment and hoping that he would emerge from one of those rooms I saw people going in and out of. Still, no Granddaddy. I couldn't wait to see him with his arms open wide for me. I kept getting out of my seat and peeping down each hall while trying not to get caught. I finally saw Mama's dark round face. She was walking next to a white nurse coming down the hallway pushing my grandfather in a wheelchair.

"Granddaddy!" I jumped up from the chair. He was wearing a green hospital gown and a white blanket lay over his lap. White fuzz had taken over his smooth caramel face. He didn't look like himself, but I didn't care. As soon as he got close enough, I hopped on his knee and put my arms around his neck. For that moment, we were just as always. Me on his lap; happiness in his eyes.

I looked him over trying to make sense of the physical changes that I was seeing. I was concerned and scared at the same time.

"Granddaddy, what's wrong with your mouth?" He mumbled an answer I couldn't understand.

"He had a stroke," the nurse said.

"What's a stroke?" I asked.

"Why can't he move his arm?"

"Why is his mouth like this?" I took my hands and twisted my mouth just like Granddaddy's to show them what I meant. My questions were endless, and no one answered. Tears welled up in my eyes, and Granddaddy tried to speak but whatever he said sounded like mumbo-jumbo. Mama sat silently and watched. I leaned my body into my grandfather's chest as my tears fell. He hugged me with his good arm, and I buried my head in his chest, sobbing. "I love you, Granddaddy." He affectionately squeezed my arm. The nurse interrupted our special moment to take him back to his room. As she was wheeling Granddaddy away, I frantically hollered down the hall, "Granddaddy, when are you coming home?!" He said something I couldn't understand. I never saw him again.

Granddaddy died on November 18, 1968, at fifty-five years old. I was six years old. His death was the beginning of the end of my peaceful, love-filled life. Family, as I knew it, would never be the same.

Two
GRANDMAMMA JULIA

> **"** Train up a child in the way that he should go:
> And when he is old, he will not depart from it. **"**
> —Proverbs 22:6

My life changed drastically after my grandfather's death. Mama and I moved in with her mother, Julia Roberts, and stepfather, Clayton Roberts. They lived in a large two-bedroom apartment in the 4500 block of South Michigan Avenue about a ten-minute walk from my grandfather's house. There was never a dull moment at Grandmamma Julia's. Looking back, it was as if I had been dropped smack-dab in the middle of a modern-day reality show. If it weren't my reality, I could've gotten some popcorn and live-tweeted the drama as it unfolded.

Grandmamma was the star of the show and the rest of us were her co-stars. She was a God-fearing woman who didn't drink or smoke. She was a big woman easily weighing two hundred pounds, and her skin was the color of a caramel apple. She had a way about her that screamed old-school respectability. She was a proud woman and she reminded me of the gospel singer, Mahalia Jackson in style, demeanor, and voice. Mama was as different from Grandmamma as night is from day. Mama crafted her own brand of respectability and lived by those rules. Grandmamma began each day with prayer, Mama with whatever hard liquor she had in rotation. From my six-year-old lens, it wasn't the differences that caused most of the commotion, but that they didn't like each other very much.

Grandmamma and Grandpapa's relationship was a whole other story. Married for roughly five years they brought life to the saying that opposites attract. Grandmamma ruled by way of the Bible, but Grandpapa didn't give a hoot about her rules. He thought the church was full of hypocrites who were going to hell in a handbasket, and he expressed that opinion every chance he got. He smoked cigars and drank liquor no matter how much Grandmamma complained. I never saw Grandpapa take a sip of liquor. I couldn't even tell you what brand he drank, but by dinner time, he was in his bedroom sleeping it off. Mama and Grandpapa were both functional alcoholics, but they did not drink together. They each claimed their own hiding place away from Grandmamma's watchful eye. Drunk or not, Grandpapa was one cool dude. He was laidback and easygoing, and that was reflected in how he treated me. I can't remember a time in my life when he hollered at me, cursed at me or disciplined me. His swagger was in everything from the way he held his cigar in his mouth to his choice of clothing. He was always impeccably dressed. If he didn't wear a suit, he wore slacks and a beautiful sweater with slick dress shoes and silk socks every day. Grandpapa's tall slim frame, his smooth high-yellow skin tone and black curly hair, which he wore slicked back, reminded me of a light-skinned version of Billy Dee Williams straight out of the movie *Lady Sings the Blues*. I liked him because he was never afraid to speak his mind. He let Grandmamma run her mouth, but she sure wasn't going to "run him." I came to love Grandpapa even though the sum total of our relationship was his physical presence in the home. My love for him was not the same as the love and affection I had for my grandfather. Grandpapa Clayton was like the Star of David shining brightly as I moved through the darkness that settled over me in the aftermath of Granddaddy's death. He went to bat for me against Grandmamma like a mama bear protecting her cubs.

All the changes and constant drama were overwhelming. Adjusting to Mama without my grandfather was hard enough, but Grandmamma was a strict disciplinarian that made all the rules, and that was the epicenter of the drama. She was intimidating in her frame, her voice, and her demands, and I was always afraid. In Grandmamma's world, children were seen and not heard. Living in that two-bedroom apartment, I was isolated and cramped with more energy than three children put together. It was a direct opposite of my life with my grandfather. At our home on Swann Street, I had a backyard and front yard to play with neighborhood friends. My grandfather was an easygoing man and his rules accounted for my age and energy. Maybe he overindulged me because of the circumstances. I remember only that I felt loved in his presence. He would even stop Mama from disciplining me, harshly saying, "Georgia, she's just a child." With Grandmamma Julia, being a child could get you into serious trouble.

The bickering between Mama and Grandmamma was constant. Their relationship was complicated at best, and it dominated the house dynamics—that is, when Mama was home. Mama's greatest form of protest was avoidance by way of absenteeism.

The way the story goes, Grandmamma had Mama when she was fifteen. Unprepared to raise a child, her immediate family assumed the parenting role. Grandmamma left rural Alabama and Mama for a better life in Chicago. Their rocky relationship didn't begin until Mama migrated to Chicago as a young adult. They were always at odds. It seemed to me that Mama was never good enough for Grandmamma and she abhorred her lifestyle. Mama resented Grandmamma for abandoning her and that anger was fueled by Grandmamma's relationship with Grandpapa Clayton's three daughters from his first wife: Remona, Pamela and Carmen. They were a good ten to fifteen years younger than Mama. They were slim, stylish, and light skinned with long hair in an era when those physical traits were celebrated over and above a dark-skinned, size fourteen, wig-wearing woman. You could see the depth of Mama's jealousy if you simply followed her eyes and mannerisms the moment any of them entered the room, especially Aunt Pam. Mama resented Grandmamma's easy relationship with them and never missed an opportunity to express her feelings about the double standard she felt Grandmamma thrust upon her. I will admit that Grandmamma was totally different with Grandpapa's daughters. She treated them with a kindness and respect that I never saw her do with Mama.

I liked all of them, but I idolized Aunt Pam. I felt connected to her as if she should have been my mother. This was not only because we looked more alike than Mama and me, but she was more loving toward me than Mama. As a little girl, I followed her around like a lap dog. As I moved through my childhood and adolescence, she became my first role model. She had grace and style like a supermodel, always elegant with her long legs, sassy style, and beautiful smile. She dressed like she was rich and famous, and lived in some of the most fabulous areas of Chicago. I soaked her up like a sponge every chance I got. I also had to walk a thin line in front of Mama when it came to Pam. Mama's jealousy ran deep, and her wrath ran even deeper. Pam's presence at Grandmamma's home was my comfort in the middle of chaos. When she was around even Grandmamma was mellow.

It didn't matter to Grandmamma that no one except me valued her rules and opinions. Even Pam stood her ground and often told Grandmamma to leave her father alone. But Grandmamma didn't change one thing about her values. She simply put on her boxing gloves and came out swinging. She fussed at me because I was hyper and talked too much. She fussed at Mama for running the streets and drinking instead of taking care of me. She fussed at Grandpapa because the sun was shining. In her opinion, he was a heathen who needed Jesus and she told him that every chance she got. Grandmamma's mouth was her weapon. She would talk about Mama every single night, often saying, "That Georgia's out in those streets hell-raising when she should be taking care of you." And she was right. In the middle of the night, Mama would crawl into the sofa bed beside me smelling like cigarettes and liquor. Her cold body and scent would wake me, and I would scoot close and doze back to sleep content that she had finally made it home. She was all I had left to connect me to Granddaddy. On the rare nights when Mama came straight home after work, I tried my best to get her attention. I would sit next to her on the sofa like I used to with my grandfather. She would never pull me close. She just looked down and ask me, "Girl, what you want all up under me?"

"I'm glad you're home, Mama," I said cautiously. My efforts were futile. She never returned my affection. She just shrugged her shoulders.

Grandmamma would shake her head in disapproval of Mama. I often felt like I was between a rock and a hard place with the two of them. Grandmamma wasn't affectionate either. Her persistence about respectability was the paradigm that ruled our relationship. Everything seemed hopeless and Grandmamma always had the upper hand. I couldn't do anything right in her eyes:

"Rae, stop running in my house."

"Rae, sit your butt down somewhere."

"Girl, you talk too much!" Thank God for Grandpapa coming to my defense.

"Leave that child alone, Julia! You always fucking with her," he would say.

"This is *my* grandbaby!" she would snap.

"Go sit your tail down somewhere man—and get out of my face." And their argument about me would end as quickly as it began. I give Grandpapa credit for always having the last word. As he headed to the bedroom, he said to himself but in earshot of Grandmamma, "Damn NIGGA-woman. Always FUCKING with that child." After Grandpapa left the room Grandmamma would give me a brief reprieve. I tried to do as Grandmamma asked but it was really hard. I had always been a hyper child and Granddaddy never paid it any attention. Grandmamma's insistence that I not run, sit down and be still, was contrary to my being. Change didn't come easy. It was a hard adjustment and even a harder lesson to learn. One evening Grandmamma called me for dinner. I ran from the living room and bounced down into a kitchen chair.

She yelled, "Didn't I tell you to stop running in my house?!" I put my head down. I knew I was in trouble; I just didn't know how much. I thought maybe I could win her over at dinner if I did everything the way she did. After Grandpapa sat down, Grandmamma bowed her head to pray, and I did the same. Praying aloud she said, "Thank you Lord for the food that we are about to receive. And bless it for the nourishment of our bodies. Amen."

"Amen." I smiled.

"Jesus wept," Grandpapa smirked.

Grandmamma rolled her eyes then took her cornbread in one hand and crumbled it over her collard greens. She started mixing it together with her fingers. She then grabbed the mixture between her fingers and started eating. I put my fork down and did the same. While mixing the cornbread and greens her husky voice stopped me in my tracks.

"Girl, what you doin'?!" And she snatched my hands away from my plate. The cornbread and greens slipped from my hand. I was scared out of my wits.

"You don't eat with your fingers!" she snarled.

"But you do, Grandmamma," I whispered. Tears welled in my eyes. I had messed up yet again.

"You don't do everything you see me do!"

"Julia, leave that child alone!" Grandpapa wailed. She dropped my hands and turned to him. Before she could get a word in, he snapped, "You stop eating like a nigga woman!"

Grandmamma lost her momentum.

"How you expect that child to know any better?" He asked, and added, "Goddammit! That child can't have no peace."

Grandmamma regained herself, "Stay out of this, Clayton, before I go upside your head!" Grandpapa countered, "You always talking about hitting somebody, church woman! You ain't gonna do shit!"

Within a flash, Grandmamma raised her hand toward Grandpapa like she was going to hit him. He raised his arms over his head to catch the blow, but she didn't swing. She just turned to me yelling, "Go wash your hands!" When I came back to the table Grandpapa was gone, and so was my plate. I knew not to ask. I walked as slowly as I could to the living room and sat on the sofa. I didn't know what to expect. Grandmamma had never hit me, but Lord, she could fuss all night. I heard a noise across the floor and looked up. Grandmamma was dragging one of the kitchen chairs into the middle of the living room. "You gonna learn to do as I say!"

"Get yo' butt over here and sit in this chair!" I walked slowly to the chair and sat down. I was scared shitless. She stood over the chair with one hand on her hip and the other one she waved in the air as she made her demands.

"Now fold your hands in your lap and you bet' not move!"

"And don't you talk!"

Tears fell onto my folded hands. I was too afraid to even wipe my face. I sat motionless with silent tears. Grandmamma sat reading her Bible. This was by far the lowest I had felt since my grandfather's death. That night I crawled into a ball in the middle of the sofa bed hugging a pillow. "Why you go, Granddaddy?" I whispered. It all seemed hopeless. My grandfather was dead, and he couldn't save me from my new life. The next day, Grandmamma did the same thing and every day after. Like clockwork at three o'clock in the afternoon she went into the kitchen, got a chair from the table, brought it into the living room and placed it in the middle of the floor. She would then say, "Sit down and don't you move!" That one hour each day was torture. I felt like I was bound and gagged with a gun to my head with Grandmamma sitting there with her Bible on her lap, watching. I didn't move or talk, but Lord knows I cried until I was red in the face. No matter how hard I cried she continued to read her Bible. If my discomfort was what it took to get me to behave the way she believed was best for me then so be it. She saw it as her duty and her right to train me up like the Bible said. She believed if she did her job right while I was young that as an adult, I would live my life within the boundaries of respectability unlike her own daughter had done.

While Grandmamma's values were rooted in Christian rhetoric, they also trickled down from the post-slavery belief among many African Americans that any infraction by one person reflected the entire race. As Jim Crow laws and Black Codes emerged in Southern states after Reconstruction, there was an urgency among African Americans to prove to White America that they, too, knew how to be civilized. Black church women were the gatekeepers of the community, and they took that role seriously from how one dressed to how one behaved in public. In *Righteous Discontent*, a book about Black Baptist church women in the post-Reconstruction era, Harvard professor and historian Evelyn Brooks Higginbotham explains it this way:

> *Duty-bound to teach the value of religion, education and hard work, the women of the Black Baptist Movement church adhered to the politics of respectability that equated public behavior with individual self-respect with the advancement of African Americans as a group. They felt certain that "respectable" behavior in public would earn their measure of esteem from White America.*

The church was the center of her life, and my training began at home. Grandmamma was a respected gospel singer in Chicago, often appearing at churches as a guest soloist. Her worldview was clear. She was not going to have me embarrass her in public, so she dealt harshly with my behavior, which she believed was unacceptable. I was a free-spirited little girl coping as best as I could with the traumatic life changes that I had undergone in one month. I was lonely and seeking the love lost by my grandfather's death. I believe Grandmamma meant no harm.

Her goal was to break me of unacceptable behavior; instead, she broke my spirit. Minute by minute, hour by hour, and day by day what joy I had left started to seep out of me. I sank deeper and deeper into misery. Yet, something inside of me instinctively knew that my survival depended on the shift that Grandmamma wanted me to make. I was growing up fast. Instead of playing with teddy bears, my six-year-old mind was working on strategies to protect myself from those who should have been protecting me. Living with Grandmamma was the death of my childhood. My innocence had been lifted right out of my body and buried right along with Granddaddy. Discipline didn't make me better; it made me vulnerable. The little girl that Granddaddy nurtured started to grasp for anything that resembled goodness, no matter what mixed messages it sent. I couldn't spot danger until it was too late. By the time I left Grandmamma's house, I wanted to please everyone because I wanted everyone to love me. I was starving for validation. Anything, no matter how little it resembled the love that my grandfather gave to me, became acceptable.

Mama continued to fail me through both her indifference and her absence. When she was around her interaction with Grandmamma was combative at best. There was never a night free of arguing. The moment Mama walked into the apartment; Grandmamma lit in.

"Georgia, when you gonna keep your tail home with your baby?" Mama looked at Grandmamma out the side of her eye and kept walking. She ignored Grandmamma until she couldn't, and then, it was on.

"Julia, I don't want to hear that bullshit every time I walk through the door!"

"You can't raise that gal in the streets!" Grandmamma pleaded.

"I do what the fuck I please! I'm grown!" Mama yelled. Grandmamma was relentless.

"You may be grown but you need some order in your life! You don't stay put long enough to even give her a bath." All the hollering back and forth frightened me, but the core of the argument scared me even more. I knew what Grandmamma was saying was true. Mama wasn't taking care of me the way she had when my grandfather was alive, but I sure didn't want to be given away. During those arguments, I silently rooted for Mama because there wasn't a day that went by when Grandmamma didn't ask her to give me to her, like passing the bread and butter at the dinner table. She rode Mama's back like it was a rodeo horse.

"You should give her to me," Grandmamma would say. "Let me raise her right!"

"How the hell you gonna tell me how to raise my baby and you didn't raise me?" Whenever Mama responded, "You didn't raise me," Grandmamma shut up, but she watched Mama's every move with contempt.

One night after one of their stormy arguments about who was more fit to raise me Grandmamma was steaming mad. Mama slammed the front door and Grandmamma kept fussing. "It's a shame! She won't stay still long enough to give her child a bath. Georgia don't need no darn child."

A few minutes later Grandmamma called me into the bathroom. I slow-walked out of protest. I had just taken a bath the night before and didn't understand why I had to have two in a row.

"Girl, get them clothes off and get in this tub like I asked."

I took my clothes off and put them on the toilet lid like she had taught me and climbed into the tub. The water was hotter than usual, but I had learned that Grandmamma didn't respond to complaints. She knelt on the floor next to the tub. Even on her knees, Grandmamma loomed over me like a giant.

"Look at that neck! Just black!" she said. She reached for my bath towel and then the bar of soap. She lathered the towel and started washing me. She washed my little arms awkwardly taking them one at a time into her big hands. I liked the smell of the Ivory soap and that helped to calm me. My protest melted away and I settled into my bath.

Grandmamma kept talking, "Look at this! Georgia don't know how to take care of no baby!"

"Look at this neck!" she said, shaking her head side to side. She reached over to the other side of the tub and got the can of *Comet* cleanser. My eyes popped. I didn't understand why she was using the stuff she used to clean the tub on me, but I was too afraid to ask. She methodically laced every inch of my back and neck. I could feel the droplets of *Comet* as they landed on my wet back. At first, it felt like sprinkles of baby powder, but within seconds, the abrasive substance turned pasty and began to sting. Tears formed in my eyes.

"Grandmamma that burns," I said in a low voice. She didn't respond. I felt the weight of her hand again on my back.

"Just dirty," she mumbled, "I'll show Georgia how to clean a child." She rubbed harder, up and down my back then around my neck over and again. It felt like my entire body was on fire. Up and down, she went around my neck and down my back washing me like an old rusty pot. My defiance was to match my tears with her wipes. When she finally stopped scrubbing, I was relieved, but only for the time it took her to dip the towel into the tub of water and began rinsing my back.

"Noooooo, Grandmamma, that hurts!" I screamed. The sting of the water splashing against my raw back sent shock waves through my body. I cried harder. Grandmamma kept to her task. She finished rinsing me, then reached for a bath towel and laid it on top of my clothes on the toilet. Resting one hand on the tub, she pulled herself up from the floor.

"Dry off and get ready for bed," she commanded, leaving the bathroom.

I got out of the pasty water and grabbed the towel to dry off. The touch of the towel on my back felt like sawdust. I gently dried off the best I could. I wanted to see what Grandmamma had done to me. I pushed my clothes onto the floor and climbed on top of the toilet, adjusting my body so I could reach the mirror hanging over the sink. I balanced and positioned myself so that I could see and not fall. My back was bright red with cracks of broken skin that looked like a maze. I sat on the toilet and wept.

I walked into her bedroom naked with my clothes covering my private parts the way she had taught me. She was sitting on the side of the bed reading her Bible. I could feel her eyes watching me as I went to get my pajamas out of my drawer. Tears welled up in my eyes again. I was so sore that I could barely raise my arms. The weight of my pajamas resting on my raw back only added more misery. I went into the living room, climbed in the sleeper sofa, and cried myself to sleep. I was confused and hurt. I missed my grandfather and everything he meant to me. I missed my life on Swann Street. Each night when I went to bed, I asked, "Why you leave Granddaddy?" Then one night he came to me in my sleep. The dream was so real it was as if his love for me was so powerful that he transcended the grave to comfort me. Granddaddy sat on the side of the sleeper sofa.

"Don't be afraid," he said. I sat up in the middle of the bed. I reached for him, and it was like reaching for air.

"I want you to tell Georgia to go back home. I won't bother her." He kissed me on my forehead, like he used to do.

"It's going to be okay," he said, "I'll be watching you." He disappeared, and I touched my forehead and went back to sleep with a peace that I hadn't felt since before his death. The next morning, I couldn't wait to tell Mama—only she hadn't made it home. So, I told Grandmamma with a level of excitement I hadn't exhibited in days. My words came out jumbled.

"Granddaddy came to me last night and he said Mama ain't gotta be scared no more. We can go back home." Grandmamma looked at me like I had lost my mind.

"What are you talking about, girl?"

"Granddaddy came to me last night and told me to tell Mama we can go back home." Grandmamma studied my face then said with a smirk, "I want you to tell your mama just what he said when she brings her tail home."

I met Mama at the door that evening.

"Mama, Mama! Granddaddy said we can go home!"

"Al's dead, girl," she said, looking puzzled.

"But Mama, he came to me last night in my sleep."

"He told me to tell you that you ain't got to be scared no more." She froze at the door with her coat on. I had no idea what she feared. I just repeated what my grandfather told me. I learned later through neighborhood rumors that Mama and Granddaddy had been arguing and she hit him over the head with a radio causing his stroke. I never got the nerve to ask Mama if it was true, but she sure was afraid of that house on Swann Street right after Granddaddy died.

"We're fine right where we at."

"No, Mama!" I pulled her coattail.

"Granddaddy said it's okay!"

Grandmamma interjected, "See Georgia, you have nothing to fear; Al's dead." Mama didn't respond. The next thing I knew we were headed back to 131 W. Swann Street.

Three
❧ ∼ ❧
131 W. SWANN STREET

"Speak to your children as if they are the wisest, kindest,
most beautiful and magical humans on the earth,
for what they believe is what they will become.**"**
—Brooke Hampton

My return to Swann Street was bittersweet. I was happy to be among the things that reminded me of my life before my grandfather's death. Each time I walked past his Buick sitting in front of our house I smiled. I was glad that Mama didn't know how to drive, and it sat like a monument to his life. At the same time, it made his death final. Each night, I lay in bed hoping that he would magically appear in my sleep like he had done at Grandmamma's, but he never did.

Mama never mentioned Granddaddy in the days immediately after our return to Swann Street. Al was dead, and that's where she was going to leave him. The first day back she moved into the small room in the rear of the house off the kitchen and left my grandfather's clothes in the closet in the room they shared together. I was moved into their room in the middle of the house off the kitchen. I didn't want to move. I loved my bedroom up front. It sat off from the living room and had my pretty, ornate dresser. But objecting to Mama's plans was not an option. So, I did as I was told and helped Mama to move my clothes and toys to the dresser drawers she once shared with Granddaddy.

That first week we settled into a routine. In the morning Mama put on a stylish ensemble, and then dressed me. She never wore her maid uniform in public. She resented that conformity and claimed her own identity outside of her profession. She loved clothes and would transfer that quality to me. She dropped me off at Ms. Rachel's and headed to work. Granddaddy and Ms. Rachel's houses were the two most popular ones on the block. Our house sat at one end of Swann Street that led to the adjoining alley of another street. Ms. Rachel's house sat on the opposite side at the end. These one-block streets were cut off by the Dan Ryan Expressway on the west end of the street. Our block insulated us from the rest of the world, and I felt safe. After my grandfather's death, Ms. Rachel's house became the epicenter on the block.

Ms. Rachel King was a character. She dipped snuff and drank Hamm's Beer with the best of them. She was pretty, with deep caramel skin and long black wavy hair that she often wore in a bun. She was short and robust, and her gold-capped teeth shone just like her personality. All the young people affectionately called her Madea and so did I. Ms. Rachel was pleasant and cool headed. She didn't fuss or curse at her grandchildren or at me the way Mama did. She was genuine and she treated me with respect for the little human being who I was. It was a relief to be around her and her family; they made me feel loved.

She had two daughters, Helen, and Minnie, whom we called Peaches. They were both around Mama's age and they all socialized together. Loretta, Helen's daughter, was a year older than me and my best playmate. Her sister Rachel, whom we called Poochie, was four years older than me. They both lived with Ms. Rachel. Peaches' daughter, Vicki, who was also a year older than me was also my friend, but I would only see her whenever she was visiting Ms. Rachel.

My most impressive memories of my grandfather came from Ms. Rachel. She was more loyal to him in death than she was to Mama in life. Even after we moved from Swann Street, Ms. Rachel kept my grandfather's memory alive. She was a godsend who made sure I understood the parts of my life that had to do with my grandfather. Mama tried to spin the narrative that she had been around since the day I came to live with my grandfather, but Ms. Rachel wasn't having it. She told me more than once, "You came to your grandfather in diapers and Georgia was nowhere around." She didn't take crap from anybody; most notably, not from Mama, and I loved her for it.

I dreaded leaving the peace at Ms. Rachel's every evening to go into the war zone that was now my way of life at 131. By the time I arrived home, Mama had already settled in for the evening. She had taken off her wig to let her soft black curly hair breathe and changed into one of those flowered house dresses working-class women in my neighborhood wore back in the day. She then went about the business of making my dinner from scratch. She was a fantastic cook of southern style recipes and dinner was always a treat. I often sat at the kitchen table and watched her cook. I'm not sure *why* she allowed me to sit and watch her, but she did. Being in the kitchen with her was the only space at home we ever shared.

In those *kitchen moments,* she didn't engage me in conversation or ask me to help. She just went about the business of making a meal. Her hands were magical to me, and I really was mesmerized with how all those ingredients became a delicious meal. Those times in the kitchen, while Mama was focused on the meal, I was focused on her. I watched the movements of her body in sync with the task of cooking like a surfer with waves. I watched her hands as she beat the cornbread. My eyes followed the flip of each Johnny Cake and the turning of every pork chop. I studied how much flour she put in the hot skillet to make the gravy. Her hands were magical to me. I was fascinated by how those mixtures became my meal. Now and then, Mama would stop in the middle of pouring or flipping or turning and ask, "Girl, why you watchin' me so much?" I shrugged my shoulders.

In retrospect, I was trying to understand the contradiction in Mama's treatment of me. The duality confused me. I wondered how she could make magic for me every night and then turn around and beat the shit out of me. She was like two people contained in one body. Her unpredictability perplexed me. Every day she used her hands to make scrumptious comfort food only to turn around and use those same hands to make welts on my body. So, in those *kitchen moments,* I sat and watched, mesmerized. I watched her hands slice onions until my eyes stung with tears. I watched her hands wipe down the stove as the grease popped and the corn sizzled. I tried to make sense of her, but I never did. I also hoped my intimate proximity to her would help ease the pain and loneliness of missing my grandfather. I sat at the table like a hungry dog watching and waiting. I would have accepted any small gesture: a hug, a warm kiss, an "I love you." I yearned for some display of love that was recognizable to my six-year-old self. Without question, the *kitchen moments* are the best memories I have about life with Mama. Maybe, in the end, a good meal was all the love she had inside of her to give.

After Mama set my plate on the table, she'd go into the living room and blast some Johnny Taylor or B. B. King on the turntable stereo and sit on the sofa with a cigarette hanging out the side of her mouth. She always had two glasses sitting on the cocktail table in front of her. One was filled with Christian Brothers and the other with water she used to chase each sip of liquor, another thing she had never done when my grandfather was alive. I would go to my bedroom and play with my toys until I was told to go to bed. It was difficult falling asleep with the music blasting. I learned quickly not to approach Mama about anything that pertained to her behavior even if it adversely affected the quality of my life.

We arrived back at Swann Street a couple of weeks before Christmas. It seemed as if we had been at Grandmamma Julia's for months, but it had only been those first few weeks after Grandaddy died.

One evening when I arrived from Ms. Rachel's there was a big box sitting by the front door. Mama opened it after dinner, and lo and behold, a Christmas tree emerged. You talking about one excited kid? That was me. My grandfather always put up a tree with lots of presents and this was the first thing Mama had done that remotely resembled our life before his death. She allowed me to sit on the sofa as she assembled the tree. I watched her hands make the artificial tree come to life. When she finished placing each limb perfectly, she carefully strung the blinking color lights around and around the tree all the way to the top. When she reached to open the box of Christmas ornaments, she looked over at my wide eyes and said, "You can help if you want to." I jumped up as she instructed me to take my time and not be fast. I slowly picked up the shiny red, gold, and silver ornaments one at a time and carefully placed them on the parts of the tree that I could reach. After we had finished hanging ornaments Mama opened the little boxes of icicles.

"Here," she said, taking some out of the box, and handing them to me. "Do it like this," she illustrated by swinging her hands in the air like she was waving. The shiny strings hit the tree, and I went at it. I waved those beautiful icicles in the air like a fairy godmother waving her magic wand. Mama sat on the sofa, lit a cigarette, and watched, sipping on her drink, and shaking her head to the music and getting a kick out of me with a big smile on her face. In retrospect, it felt like a true mother-daughter moment one of the few we would ever have.

Mama rocked to the music as I finished decorating the tree. The little girl in me came alive. I twirled and twirled those shiny icicles in my hand and through the air and they landed on each branch. Mama was always over the top, and she had purchased icicles galore. When I had finished, I stepped back to examine my work. That Christmas tree shined brighter than the Star of David within my heart. I ran over to Mama, grabbed her neck, and almost knocked the cigarette out of her mouth. She grinned from ear to ear. She grabbed her cigarette with one hand and my hand that was hugging her neck with the other, mumbling, "Go on, now."

"Thank you, Mama," I said, and released her neck. I wanted to kiss her on the cheek, but I was too afraid.

A few days later Mama hadn't put any gifts under the tree. I couldn't fathom why, and I began to get a sick feeling smack in the middle of my tummy. Another day or so passed and there were still no presents, and I finally gathered enough nerve to ask why. I peeped into Mama's bedroom where she was sitting on the side of the bed in her nightgown smoking a cigarette. "Mama, ain't no gifts under the tree." She never looked my way.

"You don't get no presents," she said in her exacting, no-nonsense, don't-fuck-with-me tone. I backed out of her doorway.

"Now take yo' ass to bed!" She demanded. I went to my bedroom and sulked. It had all started out so beautifully, and now it was getting uglier each day. Decorating the tree had given me false hope, and the letdown felt like a head-on collision that left my heart in critical condition. Since my grandfather's death, Mama kept me off balance. She was erratic. She would tell me to do one thing and turn around and scold me for the thing she asked of me. Mama had a short fuse and that made me conscious of my every move. I had moments of what seemed like normalcy. I would even have moments of what felt like love, like the night decorating the tree. Peace overtook the chaos, but it was fleeting. Sooner or later enough all hell broke loose, and the cycle began all over.

Those couple of weeks before Christmas I watched the tree in disappointment. After dinner each night I would peek in the living room before bed to see if she had put any gifts under the tree while I was in my room playing. She would look up from the sofa and say something mean to me. One time she told me, "You don't deserve shit with your hard-headed ass." Another night, she said, "Get out of my face. You don't get any gifts." And often, she told me, "Bitch go sit your *fast* ass down somewhere." The name-calling was foreign to me. My grandfather never called me out of my name and didn't allow Mama to do it either. I didn't know what these words, *fast* and *bitch* meant, but her delivery of them was hurtful. In the initial moments of Mama's taunts I sunk deep into despair. Then I pushed the ugly back as a way to cope. My grandfather's absence was still fresh, and I was young enough to hope that Mama would turn back into the mother that she was before his death. Therefore, I dismissed the ugly so that I could keep on hoping.

After Mama's insults I went back to my room. Sometimes I cried myself to sleep and other times I played with my dolls until I was instructed to go to bed. Christmas Eve, I got up enough nerve to ask her again about my Christmas presents. (I had some big ass balls.) I think my desperation to reclaim my life as a child before my grandfather's death trumped Mama's cruelty. The music was blasting, and Mama was sitting on the sofa, as usual, with a cigarette in her mouth. One hand rested on her head, which was hanging low, and she was deep into whatever song was playing. I stepped into the doorway of the living room, but I stayed on the kitchen side of the floor, so it didn't appear that I was challenging her. I took a deep breath.

"Mama, do I get any gifts for Christmas?" I waited, wringing my hands, but she didn't say one word. Her silence was killing me. I felt like I was going to pee my pants, so I crossed my legs to hold it in. She finally lifted her head and took a sip of her liquor and chased it with the water.

"Girl, if you don't get the fuck out of my face…." I went back to my bedroom and put the pillow over my head so Mama wouldn't hear me sobbing.

Christmas morning, I heard Mama's voice calling me out of my sleep. "Rae!" I thought I was dreaming. "Rae, get up!" She hollered toward my room. I sat up in bed to gather myself and assess her tone.

"Come here!" She exclaimed with excitement. I was relieved that it didn't sound like trouble. I climbed down from my bed and followed her voice. When I made it to the doorway of the living room, I saw piles and piles of toys and clothes surrounding the tree and taking up most of the living room floor.

"Mama!" I called out and ran straight to her sitting on the sofa and threw my arms around her neck nearly knocking the cigarette out of her mouth. "Thank you, Mama! I knew you was gonna get me presents!" I exclaimed.

"You didn't know shit," she chuckled.

Mama was right. I didn't know, but I sure hoped like hell. I let her neck go and plopped down to my toys. Sitting in the center of all that joy I forgot my misery. I was glad that she had changed her mind. I told myself that getting me all those toys, she must have loved me after all. What I didn't know on that Christmas morning sitting with my toys was that her brand of love would soon take me so far from my grandfather's love that it would take years to conjure up his goodness in my memory. Her way of life was volatile and unpredictable, and it became my new normal.

I began half-day kindergarten in January 1969 at Beethoven Elementary School on 47th Street, and I walked the few blocks to school. Mama had showed me the way to go. Beethoven was a massive building divided into the colors of blue, white, and yellow. It sat in front of the Robert Taylor Homes public housing project, and many of the kids who lived there attended Beethoven. I loved everything about school, and I embraced it wholeheartedly. My grandfather always called me his big girl, and I really felt like a big girl going to that big building every day with the other kids from Swann Street. After school I walked home with Loretta, who was in first grade, and we played until Mama came home from work.

I loved the coloring, letters, shapes, and interactive projects at school. It was all so stimulating. But the best memory I have of my years at Beethoven was the smell of those infamous Chicago Public School big round butter cookies baking. They were an everyday treat, and I couldn't wait to make it to the lunchroom. At school I felt as if I was truly free to be me. I was a handful, running everywhere I went, but the teachers didn't fuss at me for being hyper. They just called me a busy little bee. I tried to stay in my seat the way Grandmamma Julia had commanded me to do, but all my efforts were futile. My attention span was short, but I was incredibly inquisitive. I wanted to learn, and I also wanted to please everyone that crossed my path. All my report cards said that I wouldn't stay in my seat, and I talked too much, no surprises there!

My tendency for hyperactive behavior followed me throughout my early years of education. The school must have requested that Mama have me tested. I have a distant memory of her taking me to Michael Reese Hospital to assess me for hyperactivity when I was in the first grade. Mama dressed me up nice; she even straightened my hair, which she reserved for special occasions. At the hospital, I recall laying on an exam table while the doctors put something like gray putty on my forehead and in my hair and connected wires to it. I don't remember feeling anything and they gave no narrative explanations. Nothing I can remember became of it at school. Later, I would hear Mama talking about me being "fucked up" because of my biological mother's drug use. But being called a bitch every day at age 6, didn't help either.

One evening my father's half-brother, Michael, appeared from out of nowhere and assumed my after-school care until Mama came home from work. I have no memory of him while Granddaddy was alive. Michael was Granddaddy's son by his second wife, Earlean. They were married in 1943 and divorced in 1957, and had two children, Michael and his sister, Sharon. I didn't know their ages except that they were young adults by the time Granddaddy died. Michael was slim and lanky with big imposing lips. My only resemblance to him was his high-yellow skin tone. He didn't talk much, but his big smile was endearing. His presence made me feel wanted.

I loved going to Ms. Rachel's, but my uncle gave me all his attention, and I latched onto him immediately. As I saw it, Michael's presence proved Mama wrong. Since we arrived back on Swann Street, she had told me often that no one in my family wanted me except her, and she wore it as a badge of honor. It wouldn't have been so bad if she didn't use it against me as if she had done me a favor. Nonetheless, my uncle gave me hope for a better life and it started to rise in me like the sun in the east. In the mornings, I continued to go to Ms. Rachel's. After school my uncle picked me up at my classroom door.

When we arrived at home Michael would make me a sandwich with a glass of milk and sit at the kitchen table as I told him about my day at school. After I finished eating, he allowed me to play with my toys for a while, then he set up a makeshift school in the living room. It had a school desk and a mini blackboard, and we would do my homework of learning the alphabets. Learning the ABC Song was easy because we were also learning it at school, and I mostly knew it. He sang first, and I followed. Then we doubled back and sang it together smiling and waving our hands in the air to the imaginary tune of the song. He praised me for my ability, and I felt smart because that part came easy.

The hard part came next. Michael began teaching me to recognize each alphabet letter. I understood what he wanted from me. It probably was a simple assignment in his mind. However, to identify the twenty-six letters of the alphabet in a short period was difficult for me. Michael would identify an alphabet and I would repeat it with all smiles. But after a few letters, he'd double back and ask me to identify the previous one. That was like asking me to repeat the Preamble to the United States Constitution.

My attention span was extremely short, and so was the shift in my uncle's disposition. He became a drill sergeant and there was nothing lovable about him when I missed a letter. Those free-flowing afternoons began to feel like Grandmamma Julia's prison. It was hard and frustrating, and I felt trapped behind my little desk. He would let me take a break only after I had remembered a group of letters. Each day after school I pleaded with him to give me a day off, but he wasn't having it. After my snack we went straight to the alphabets. His rail thin body was quiet and unassuming, but he was a drill master as we practiced the alphabets. He shifted his chair from my side to face my desk. It was intimidating with him sitting in front of me with a ruler between his legs. When I missed a letter, his big lips would protrude as he said, "Hold out your hand."

WHACK!

He smacked the wooden ruler across the middle of my hand. I was desperate to get it right. I tried hard to remember the letters, but if I paused too long, with a smile across his face and his big lips aimed at me like a monster's, he'd again say, "Hold out your hand."

WHACK!

I didn't understand the change in him, and it hurt deeply. With every whack, my dreams of a happy family dissolved again. The hope I had when he first came settled in the west like the sun at the end of each day, and it never, ever, rose again. The worst of all was that I was afraid: afraid of him and afraid to tell Mama. I understood by then that in her view of the world grown folks were always right. I believed telling would get me a beating. The way I saw it, Uncle Michael's whacks were better than one of Mama's beatings. With Mama's, and now, Michael's cruelty added to the equation, life on Swann Street without Granddaddy had become the hardest thing ever. At that point, the only safe place for me on Swann Street was Ms. Rachel's house.

Four

THE ROOM

"I lost myself somewhere in the darkness."
—Unknown

Each time I walked inside my old bedroom with my uncle, an overwhelming darkness invaded me. I had once loved this room, with its full-size bed, ornate headboard, and matching dresser. Now, I didn't even want to walk past it. From the first time my uncle took me inside, it was no longer my old bedroom; it had become The Room. My young mind couldn't process the danger, yet I knew something in The Room was waiting to descend upon me like a dark cloud smothering me. I even asked myself, *"Why does he let the darkness in The Room hurt me?"*

The Room sat to the right of the living room, so I even hated going in there for any reason. Whenever I could, I quickly shut the door to The Room so it would stop plotting against me. It may sound crazy but walking out of the house felt like the kiss of death because I had to pass by The Room to get to the front door. I walked-ran past it—even if the door was closed. The worst of it was sitting in the living room with Uncle Michael during my alphabet lessons and watching The Room in absolute fear of being taken into its darkness. Concentrating on the lessons became harder because all I could think about was The Room. My survival instincts kicked in. I hoped, if I got my letters right, maybe he wouldn't take me into The Room. I developed a strategy that has stayed with me. As I learned to recognize each letter, I would apply it to the alphabet song and sing the entire song in my head before answering. Even today, while I can identify each letter, I cannot tell you what comes after A-B-C-D-E-F without first singing the song in my head. This strategy helped prevent me from getting whacked, but learning the letters only protected me from some of the trauma at my uncle's hands. Nothing saved me from The Room.

"Please don't take me into the room," I cried. But when Uncle Michael looked down at me, I immediately got quiet. I didn't want to make matters worse for myself. More than anything, I didn't want him to stop loving me. He was the only family I knew until Aunt Lula Mae started picking me up and I didn't want to lose him. In the end, Mama hurt me, too, so what was the point of losing him? I believed if I protested too hard, he would stop spending time with me. I was starving for attention and Uncle Michael was willing to oblige. My futile outcry was the only instinctive device I had to try to protect and stand up for myself as well as continue to love my uncle at the same time.

I wanted to tell Mama about the whacks and the darkness in The Room, but I knew that telling on grown folks could get me into more trouble. To tell the truth, when it came to The Room, I wouldn't know what to tell Mama. All I could really say was that Michael took me into the darkness of the room. I couldn't explain how he hurt me because I didn't understand it myself. I just knew that there was no fear to match what I felt about The Room. It was the devil with big red ears and a long-ass tail. And I, for one, avoided his path every which way I could—that is, until Mama put me smack dab in the middle of it.

One Saturday morning she woke up in a cleaning frenzy. Saturday was our cleaning day, and I wanted to do my part. Mama had shown me how to clean, and I did my best to make her proud. I could smell the bacon as I crawled out of bed. I went to the bathroom, brushed my teeth, and sat at the kitchen table watching her finish making my breakfast. After I started eating, she went into my bedroom. When she walked out with a bunch of my grandfather's clothes in her arms, I didn't know what the heck was going on. I kept my mouth closed and continued to eat breakfast while glancing at her from the corner of my eye as she made trip after trip with my grandfather's clothes and plopped them onto the living room sofa. She startled me out of my trance with barking orders.

"When you finish eating, I want you to take your clothes out of those drawers and put them in the front room."

"In the living room, Mama?" I asked hoping she wasn't talking about my old bedroom.

"Naw, girl. Put them back in your old room up front," she said. I didn't respond. I continued eating, holding my head down as close to the plate as possible. I wanted to disappear to avoid the task.

"Did you hear me, girl?" she hollered, as she returned with another round of clothes.

"Can I just clean the bathroom?" I asked.

"Girl, do what I told you." She was getting impatient with me. I knew her *do-as-I-say-or-get-your-ass-beat* tone.

"Okay, Mama." I was defeated. To delay the inevitable, I asked for more food. Mama never begrudged me a big meal, and I ate until I was about to bust. On one of her trips back through the kitchen, she looked over me and told me, "Girl stop playing with that food and do what I told you to do." I put my plate in the sink like I had been taught and reluctantly made my way into The Room. I grabbed a handful of my clothes from my grandfather's side of the dresser and dropped them into the drawer in my old bedroom. I made that trip over and over as quickly as I could while Mama was loading Grandaddy's clothes into big black garbage bags. It wasn't too bad because Mama was up front with me, but the moment she disappeared I headed back into the kitchen. I sat at the table while she started taking her clothes from the back room and placing them in the closet she had shared with Grandaddy.

The house was clean, and all the clothes were moved. Mama started making dinner. I sat at the table, watching her cook, and dreading my new move. After dinner I bathed, and Mama told me to go to bed. Fear gripped me.

"Mama, but I don't want to sleep in that room," I whispered. She gave me that certain look and told me to get my butt in there. I wouldn't go without a fight. I would have taken an ass-beating if it meant not sleeping in that room.

"Mama, can I sleep in the back room since you sleep in your old room?" I asked.

She chuckled, "Girl, didn't I say to get your butt in that room? Don't let me have to tell you again."

Fear ruled my mind. "Mama!" I screamed as she walked away. She turned around and asked, "Bitch, who the fuck is you hollering at?"

"It's gonna," I said, sniffling through tears and snot, "It's gonna get me!"

She relaxed her body and stared at me for what seemed like forever.

"Why are you raising all this Cain, girl?" she finally asked.

"Please, Mama! Don't make me sleep in there." I was determined.

"What's gonna get you?" Mama asked. I shrugged my shoulders and looked at my hands. I had no way to explain my fear of the room.

"It's dark, Mama." Trying to explain my fear was hopeless.

"Girl, take your ass to sleep! Come on here," she said. She walked me to the bedroom and watched me crawl into the middle of the bed and pull the covers all the way up. As Mama turned to go back out, I pleaded through my tears, "Please, Mama, don't turn off the lights." She left the light on and walked to the door.

"No, Mama," I wailed, as her hand hit the doorknob.

"It's gonna get me!" She turned around and asked why I was afraid. And again, I had no answer, sitting in the bed with the covers all the way to my neck. I just looked down. Mama stood in the doorway looking at me with one hand on her hip trying to figure it out. She opened the closet door, looked in, closed it, and walked back toward the door.

"Girl, ain't nothin' in this room but you."

"But Mama," I demanded, in tears.

"You're getting on my nerves now. Take your ass to sleep, and I mean it." Her patience ran out and she walked out of the room. I cried harder and harder. I jumped out of bed and opened the closet door and my dresser drawers. I believed if I could see it coming, I could get away. I pulled the covers over my head and finally fell asleep. I did this ritual every night in the months that followed until my living arrangements changed yet again.

I couldn't articulate my fear. I had no name for what I didn't know. I only knew danger was lurking in The Room. The words "monsters" and "boogeyman" were my language, and fear was my emotion. And I don't have any specific memories I can recall about the time I spent in The Room with Uncle Michael. I buried the trauma of what occurred there. My memory falls short of reminding my body of any physical pain inflicted on me. What I know for sure are the fear and emotional stress that began there remain in parts of my life today. Somewhere in my subconscious existence I'm still holding this trauma at a safe distance, and the little girl is holding onto her shield of protection for dear life. I have come to respect her distance. Over the years, whenever I searched my memory of being inside The Room with Michael, I have an out-of-body experience like what happened in the old '50s horror movie *The Blob*. The monster devoured a person's body, consuming it into its own, until nothing not even a trace was left of the person.

I have only one other distinct memory about Swann Street and my Uncle Michael. One day I was playing in my backyard. The trees were bare, the ground was hard, and the sun was warming the cold. One of my uncle's friends, who lived in the house that faced the alley, was walking toward his house. He stopped when he saw me in my yard. He came up to the fence and called me over to him. I ran to him, all happy-go-lucky, to see what he wanted. He leaned into the fence, gaining access to my personal space. He whispered smoothly to me like he was macking to a woman and not talking to a child.

"Your Uncle Michael told me what you two do after school," he said.

I took a step backward. I knew I was facing danger.

"You should come over to my house, so we can do the same thing." He was licking his lip like a playa-playa.

I opened my mouth to speak, but nothing came out. My mind said, "Run!" But my little feet were stuck. Then suddenly something dinged inside me, and I took off running into the house and straight to my bedroom into the darkness of my closet until Mama called me to dinner. I ran away from him that day, but I internalized his words: *we can do the same thing.* Those words are carved deep inside of me. I never played in my backyard again.

After Michael stopped coming around, I blocked him out of my life. I forgot he existed until about seven years later. I mean, I erased him THE FUCK OUT. Everything about him, right down to him picking me up from school to the alphabet lessons, and especially The Room. I had even forgotten about Michael's friend, until therapy helped me unleash bits of information about that period. The mind is an interesting being. Even though I had forgotten about Michael's friend, the backyard and alley continued to trigger a fear in me for years to come. After Michael's friend moved away, Ms. Rachel's daughter, Peaches, and her children moved into the house behind us. I still wouldn't go into the backyard or visit Vicki, even after Mama and I moved from the neighborhood. I would visit Loretta at Ms. Rachel's place, but I was still too afraid to go visit Vicki.

Trying to unpack The Room and Michael in therapy has been difficult. I always get stuck in the darkness that first surrounds me, and then, devours me. Fear and anxiety take charge, and I become that vulnerable little girl again. At this stage in my journey, I'm entirely okay not knowing what I don't know. What I do know has placed me on the road to healing. What I also know for sure is that after my uncle's disappearance, I started mimicking sexual acts. I became a different girl and lost myself in the darkness.

Five

MAMA

"For the beauty of the rose, we also water the thorns.**"**
—African Proverb

Mama had a way about herself that commanded attention. She was a free spirit and the life of the party. I loved to see her smile, with her high cheeks glowing. I'm not sure what I enjoyed most about her: the way she threw her head back as if she did not have a care in the world, or how easy it was for her to say what she wanted without caring about retribution.

On Swann Street, Mama was in her element, sitting in Ms. Rachel's kitchen with the other grown folks drinking, laughing, and talking shit. Loretta and I would be in her bedroom playing with our dolls. Sometimes, Poochie played with us and, being the oldest, was the one in charge. On summer days, Helen would blast music from her porch across the street. I'd sit on Ms. Rachel's porch with the other children and watch Mama in amazement as she grooved to the beat. She'd raise her arms high, holding a drink in one hand and snapping her fingers with the other. Her size-fourteen hips swaying in sync to the rhythm of the music mesmerized me. I could never get the beat, no matter how hard I tried.

I loved Mama with all my heart, and I was loyal to her. I figured, if I loved her enough and kept her commandments—no matter how confusing they were—maybe one day she would reciprocate my feelings. When she was happy, I was delighted. Mama's happiness could mean a good day for me, and she was the happiest when she was hanging out and drinking with her friends. At home, she was an entirely different person—short-fused and, it seemed, weary. I would come to understand that making beds and cleaning toilets were not dream jobs for any woman. She was like many Black migrant women from the South who were unskilled with a minimal education. Cleaning toilets is all she would ever do in her lifetime. It was a bleak future, but she had an incredible work ethic. Mama drank her liquor every single morning, but she never missed a day of work, as far as I knew. In the evening after making my dinner, she withdrew into a bottle of Christian Brothers and put music on the turntable.

To Mama's credit, I never saw men lurking around. Sometimes I would go over Grandmamma Julia's on Saturday and go to church with her on Sunday. I assume these were the times she went on dates. Then one Saturday evening, Mama dressed me up and took me with her. She held my hand as we walked together down 47th Street. That was an incredible feeling for me because Mama never took me anywhere and she had never held my hand—and that night, she did both. I felt like I really was her little girl as we walked hand in hand. I didn't let go. "Mama, where we going?" I asked. She looked down at me and shrugged. I dropped any expectation of an answer as we turned into an alleyway and went into what I believe was some transitory boarding house. It was dingy, and the odors in the long dark hallway were in stiff competition with one of Mama's favorite Avon fragrances. I was a little scared and squeezed Mama's hand tightly. She looked down at me and asked, "Girl what's wrong with you?" I was not about to let my mouth get me into trouble, so I shrugged in response.

We stopped at a door, and Mama knocked. A man I had never seen before opened the door, and we entered a clean but even darker room. It had a bed that let out from the wall. There were a small table with two chairs and a small sink on one side of the bed, and a big chair in the corner on the other side. Mama sat me in the big chair, and she sat beside her friend on the bed. He made her a drink and turned on the radio. They talked and laughed and drank. I sat awkwardly with my eyes toward the floor. Mama always told me, *stay out of grown folks' faces,* but this environment was a set-up for failure, mine. Lord knows I did not want to get into trouble. I tried to make myself as invisible as I could, but I was fidgety, and so damn-freaking nosey! Mama was sitting on the man's lap with her arms around his neck, smiling like an alley cat. I had never seen her sit on my grandfather's lap. In fact, I don't remember much about their interactions. It was me who always sat with him on the sofa, and Mama would shake her head at his affection toward me. "Al, you got that gal spoiled," she'd say, and he'd just pull me closer to him. Her interaction with this man was intriguing and I kept sneaking a look. I was glad when Mama got up and made me a pallet on the floor with the blanket from the bed. This way, my curiosity would not get me in trouble. My eyes followed Mama as she undressed down to her slip. She saw me looking, "Take your ass to sleep," she demanded. That did it for me.

The room turned pitch black, and I settled into a nap. Then a banging on the floor startled me out of my sleep. The bed was moving up and down and those metal box springs were hitting the floor like the bed was going to fall through it. I peeked up to see what was happening. I had to focus really hard in the dark to see the man's naked body on top of Mama. To my six-year-old mind, it looked like he had devoured Mama into himself. Something came over me like I was hypnotized. I pulled my dress off over my head and laid it neatly next to me. Still wearing my cotton slip, panties, and big-girl tights, I drifted back to sleep.

"Where the fuck is your dress?" Mama hollered, waking me out of my sleep.

"Bitch, where is your dress?" She asked again, leaning over the side of the bed, and looking down on me. The light was on, but I was still in a daze, half-awake, trying to adjust and compose myself. I looked down at myself, and I was in my slip. My mind was racing, trying to make sense of what was going on. I remembered that I had taken my dress off, but I didn't know why. Something inside had triggered me to undress because I thought it was what I was supposed to do. I didn't know how to articulate what I didn't understand.

"Mama I-" and, before I could continue, she swung her fist down and hit me up beside my head. I raised my hands to catch the blow.

"You little hoe!" Mama screeched. Through my tears, I could only see the outline of her body and her bra. Nevertheless, I felt her fist hit my head repeatedly. WHAM! WHAM!

"Mama. Please, Mama," I pleaded.

"What did I do wrong?" I covered my head with my hands and forearms trying to shield it from the blows.

"You better stop this shit, and I mean it!" she demanded. She kept screaming and beating, repeatedly striking me.

"What did I do wrong?" I asked

"I'm sorry, Mama," I sobbed. Snot ran onto my lips.

WHAM! Her swings were chaotic.

"Please stop, Mama," I begged.

"What did I do wrong?"

All of a sudden, she stopped hitting me and snatched me up by my arm with one hand and threw my dress at me.

"Put it on, bitch!" I pulled my dress on and stood on the pallet sobbing, dumbfounded. Her friend spoke up for the first time, saying, "Georgia, let it go. It's hot in here. Maybe she was hot." She turned to him.

"Stay out of this, muthafucker! This my baby," she said. "This bitch is going to learn!" He didn't say another word. I continued to stand on the pallet, heaving. Mama ignored me, got up from the bed and dressed. We walked home in silence. The cool air helped to settle me, but I was scared out of my mind and confused. Grandmamma was teaching me to pray, and I whispered, "Please God don't let me get a whopping." To my surprise, my prayer worked. When we arrived home, Mama told me to go to bed. As scared as I was of my room, I took my clothes off with a quickness and put the covers over my head. Mama never mentioned the incident again to me or anyone else. This was unusual because she often shared my transgressions with anyone who would listen. I've often wondered if her silence was because she was ashamed of taking me with her that night.

As it started to get warm, my uncle stopped picking me up after school and I was back down at Ms. Rachel's place. Being back in my safe space, playing with Loretta would become the beginning of wiping what happened to me under my uncle's care out of my memory. Taking off my clothes, however, and playing house became my new thing—and I would get into even more trouble.

I don't remember the little boy's name, but I can see his dark chocolate face and deep-set eyes as clear as day. I remember asking him if he wanted to play house with me and him nodding and following me under someone's front porch on Swann Street. I took a plastic tarp that was balled up in the corner, made us a bed and started giving him instructions.

"Pull your pants off and lay down," I said. He reached for his shorts, then paused for a moment.

"Don't you wanna play house with me?" I asked sassily with my hands on my hips. He pulled his shorts down.

"Them, too," I pointed at his drawers.

After they were off, I instructed him to lay down on the tarp; I pulled my shorts and panties down and laid on top of him.

"Move like this," I instructed as I ground my body into his, showing him what to do. I felt his little erection growing on my belly. We were going at it rolling on top of each other, like we were really having sex, when I heard Mama holler to me.

"Bitch! What the fuck are you doing?" I jumped off my playmate at lightning speed. I scrambled to pull up my panties and shorts from around my ankles. I knew that I was in trouble. I crawled from under the porch, leaving him stuck in the moment. As soon as my feet landed on the sidewalk, Mama started beating me across my back with her hand, and yelling, "Get your ass home, you little whore!" I took off running. She entered the house and beat me with a switch until she was too tired to continue.

The shame I felt hit me in the gut like a 1-2-3 sucker-punch from Muhammad Ali. Someone had spotted us under the porch and went to get Mama. The story spread like wildfire up and down Swann Street. At seven years old, I became the neighborhood harlot. Like with taking off my dress in the room with Mama and that man, I didn't know what I had done wrong. Mama never explained anything about sex, nor had she asked the most important question of all: Who had taught me this behavior at such a young age? In retrospect, the easiest way for her to reconcile my behavior was to believe that I was trying to be grown. She saw me mimicking sexual behavior as no different than her actual sexual behavior. Instead of trying to understand what was happening to me, she settled for blaming me.

Being caught under the porch and undressing in that room with Mama would solidify her belief that I was *fast*. She had begun calling me *fast* the moment we walked back into my grandfather's house. It never failed: When I walked through the house Mama would say, *"Go sit your fast ass down somewhere."* At six, I agreed with her that I was *fast*. I walked *fast*, I talked *fast*—and those factors always brought me attention through no effort of my own. I wanted to rectify these characteristics but like with Grandmamma Julia, they were contrary to who I was. The difference between Grandmamma Julia and Mama was that Grandmamma never called me *fast* in the way that Mama did; rather, she said specifically that I walked too *fast* or talked too *fast*. Even from the beginning I sensed a difference in how they each used the word. There was something sinister in Mama's delivery, unlike Grandmamma. And I was correct. *Fast* is a pejorative term often pronounced *fass* and used almost exclusively among older Black women as the barometer to both assess and judge young Black girls' outward behavior. I would begin to equate *fast* with *acting* grown—like a woman—which is unacceptable behavior for a Black girl child. For some Black women, *being fast* could be the way a Black girl child walked—if she swayed her hips, how her clothes fit her body, whether her breasts were showing, or if pants hugged her thigh or butt a little too tight. And girls whose bodies matured quickly were judged more harshly. Even being forward-thinking or asking too many questions could deem you as *fast*. While the incident of me mimicking sex acts confirmed for Mama that I was *fast*, I would also internalize this word and equate it with sexual behavior, like Mama did, even with no understanding of sex. That would have the most profound consequences for me as I aged.

I have no idea what happened to that man in the boarding house, but I looked up one day and another man had moved into our house. Mama had switched the bedrooms that Saturday preparing for her beau, Esker Lee Tobler. I spent my time with my mouth closed and eyes peeled. Tobie, as he was called, was an entrepreneur with a bricklaying business. He was a handsome man who stood about six feet tall. He was prematurely bald with a round, light-caramel-colored face, and a teddy bear kind of build where muscle and fat met in the middle. He was thirty-eight years old, but he came across older than he was. The old folks would have said that he had an old soul. He was an alpha male who fit the most common stereotypes: leader, fearless, decisive, and in control of his emotions, whether privately or publicly. Tobie became the center of Mama's universe. She served him dinner and fetched his beer with a smile. Living with Tobie created a duality in me that was like grabbing a rose from a stem of thorns. His presence was a beautiful gift surrounded by pain. I was starving for the love and nurturing my grandfather had provided, and the attention she gave to him created an even bigger gap between the two of us. By the same token, the more attention she gave to him, the less time she had to pick on me. In this way, Tobie's presence created space between Mama and me that rendered me a respite from her badgering. Calm descended over our house like a cool breeze on a warm summer day. Mama morphed into a different woman. The loud music stopped, and the bottle of Christian Brothers never set on the cocktail table in the living room again. No more cooking with a drink in her hand. No more cursing and fussing about nothing. Tobie was not about the drama. He squashed it all. Whenever he said, *"Enough, Georgia,"* Mama shut the heck up.

Tobie was a light drinker. He had a couple cans of beer—no more than three each night while watching television after dinner. He didn't have drinking buddies that I knew of. He didn't have male friends in and out of our house. He was predictable and strait-laced: he went to work, came home, chilled, and then started another day. He never went down to Ms. Rachel's to hang out. In fact, the entire time they were together, he never hung out with Mama and her drinking buddies. The most entertainment I can recall during those years was when his cousin Johnny returned home from the Army, and when his cousin E.K. and his wife Chris were visiting. He told Mama straight up that she drank too much. "You ain't seen me drink shit!" was her comeback. Actually, I spotted Mama going into the pantry with an empty glass on more than one occasion. One time I got the nerve to peep in and see what she was doing. She moved the bag of flour to one side, pulled out a fifth of Christian Brothers, poured some into her glass and took a sip. She always chased her liquor with water, so if you didn't see her in the pantry but saw her at the sink getting a quick sip of water, then you'd know she had just gotten her a taste. Honestly, I don't know who she thought she was fooling. There was never a time that I can recall where I couldn't smell the alcohol on Mama's breath.

As the summer was coming to an end, the three of us—Mama, Tobie and me— took a road trip somewhere down South. To my surprise, Tobie had seven children who had been living with his aunt since the death of his wife (and the children's mother). His children were stair-steps in age. Kathy was the oldest, at fourteen, and Dorothy was next to her. Esker Lee Jr., who we called Junior, and Patricia, who we called Pat, where the middle children. Ethel was eight—a year older than me. Allen was seven months younger than me and Juan two years younger than me. All the younger kids came back to Chicago with us, and the older ones arrived right before school began in the fall. We became a family in every sense of the word. We settled into this new life in my grandfather's house, and, like most big families, we paired off by age and gender. The younger children were in the care of the older ones when Mama and Tobie were at work. All the elementary school-age children and I walked to and from Beethoven school together each day.

At thirty-five years old, Mama became the mother of eight instantly, and we both had immediate and major life changes. I had never thought about having siblings, and now I had seven. No one explained to me what was happening. It was like when Tobie moved in, it just was. I must hand it to Mama flaws and all: She courageously took on the role of raising eight children to whom she had not given birth. Not many women would have hooked-up with a man with seven children who didn't offer her a wedding ring. She was either brave or in love, or maybe, both.

Nearly every corner of the house was occupied. Ethel became my roommate and the fear of my bedroom—The Room—disappeared. We even used rollaway beds in the kitchen. There was no place to breathe without someone else breathing your air. Prior to this time, the physical space away from Mama's gaze was mine to do as I pleased. I could breathe without the fear of being reprimanded. However, with ten people living in a three-bedroom, one-bathroom house, there was no place or space available to me for solitude. On most days, even the bathroom had someone in there.

The fact is, I liked spending time with myself. It was my way of life. Having instant playmates intruded upon my rituals; yet, at the same time, the isolation I felt living with only Mama started to disappear. I felt the same duality with my new siblings that I had felt with Mama and Tobie. The African proverb "For the beauty of the rose, we also water the thorns," became my reality. While I embraced this new life because it took the weight of Mama's wrath off me, it also demoted my importance in her life. This was especially true because Mama latched on to Dorothy, and a part of me felt replaced. Not only did I feel like I was losing Mama, but I also felt like I was losing the things that were important to me—even the dysfunctional simplicity I had become accustomed to. My daily routine had to be shared with eight other people and I sometimes hated that fact. Even my ritual of watching Mama cook vanished like a magic trick right before my eyes. She was frazzled when cooking for ten. Once she told me to *get the fuck out of her face*, I knew that any attempt to hang onto those special moments was futile, if not dangerous, and I never watched her cook again at the house on Swann. Being the only child was easy because everything was within my reach. Now I had to wait even to use the bathroom. I was an only child through and through, and I sometimes had difficulty sharing. Looking back,

I think some of my selfishness was more about trying to maintain my place in Mama's life and in My (with a capital "M") grandfather's house. It felt like my world had been invaded and I started to show my ass in subtle ways. That never ends well.

The most vivid memory of my selfishness happened one night while playing with my paper dolls. That night, Mama and Tobie were entertaining Tobie's cousin in the front room, and she allowed us to play in their bedroom, *away from grown folks*. Ethel, Loretta, Vicki, and I were sitting on the bed arranging clothes on our paper dolls with the intensity of fashion stylists. I am not sure what set me off, but the moment Vicki and I reached for the scissors at the same time, I lost my freaking mind.

"Give me!" I demanded.

"I had them first!" Vicki yelled at me.

"So? They mine!" I proclaimed.

Somehow, we had made it to our feet in the middle of the bed and tussled back and forth. Ethel and Loretta tried to stop us, but we ignored them.

"This is My house, My scissors, and My paper dolls," I announced proudly. Knowing these things, I felt like I had a right to do what I damn well pleased.

"Give them to me," I demanded again.

"No!" Vicki stood her ground. Back and forth we went, pulling on the scissors.

"This is my house!" I laid down the law.

"But I got them first," Vicki contended.

"So!?" I snapped back. Then, suddenly Vicki either lost steam or lost interest, and loosened her grip. The scissors came up to my chest hard and I grabbed them in both hands and did a victory dance in the middle of the bed. Gloating, I showed her who was the boss.

"Na-na-na-na-nan," I teased, jumping high on the bed.

"Look!" Ethel hollered in a panic, pointing to my legs. "You're bleeding!" she screamed. I stopped jumping and followed her finger to see blood streaming down my legs.

"Georgia!" Ethel hollered. "Rae's bleeding."

"Ma-m-a-a-a!" I screamed, scared out of my wits.

"Did-dy!" Ethel called Tobie, as they referred to him.

Mama came to the door of the bedroom,

"What y'all hollering about?" she asked, as her eyes followed Ethel's finger to my leg. I couldn't speak. I stood frozen in the middle of the bed, hyperventilating. Mama's eyes got big as saucers when she spotted the blood streaming down my legs.

"Tobie!" she hollered, making her way to the bed. She raised my dress to see the damage. Blood was gushing out of my chest. Tobie came to the bedroom to see what the commotion was. Without saying a word, he immediately swooped me up and carried me to the car. Mama, Tobie and I made it to Michael Reese Hospital in minutes. When Vicki let the scissors go, my pull was so forceful that they stabbed my chest right next to the heart. What I find remarkable is that I did not feel a thing. I guess my adrenaline was so high from the fight and my ultimate victory that I was numb to the pain.

After we arrived at the hospital, my memory went blank. I don't know if they gave me some medicine to calm me down or what because the next thing I remembered, I was waking up at home in my bed bandaged up and in pain. I had three stitches on my left breast. Mama told me the doctor said if the scissors had gone deeper or they had waited to get me to the hospital, my condition would have been critical. I was afraid I would get in trouble but instead I only got a couple days out of school. Boy, was I relieved! After this incident, I still resented having to share everything, but I didn't express it out loud. Only time would replace the resentment I had with an appreciation for my siblings.

While I was still suffering from only-child syndrome, it didn't take me long to align myself with my new siblings around Mama's shenanigans. From the beginning of our families merging, Tobie gave Mama nearly complete authority over his children, and she ruled them worse than the wicked stepmother in *Cinderella*. Mama was cruel and it was hurtful not only to me but also my new siblings. While she did not curse and fuss all the time, she still found ways to wield her power over us. She distributed discipline between the younger siblings, including me, equally. As always, it took little to nothing to set off Mama. I didn't wish her wrath on anyone, but God knows I grabbed onto the rose any way that I could. She was so busy trying to manage the other seven I sometimes got lost in the middle.

The day she discovered a partially opened can of peas in the pantry, I surely thought Mama was crazy. She stood in the middle on the kitchen floor with the can of peas in her hand. "Rae, Pat, Ethel," she called. We toddled into the kitchen one by one.

"Who opened the peas and put them back in the pantry?" she asked. We stood frozen with blank stares. Mama had a can of peas in one hand, with the other hand on her hip.

"I said, who opened the peas?" We looked at each other, shrugged our shoulders and shook our heads. None of us knew how to cook and had no reason whatsoever to open the can. The truth is, we didn't know who opened the peas. Looking back, I wonder if Mama had opened them and forgotten because she was the only cook in the house. Whoever was the culprit, it was Ethel, Pat and I who paid dearly for that crime.

"Who opened the fucking peas?" she asked again.

"I don't know, Mama," I said. I knew trouble had landed in our lap and silence would make matters worse.

"Me neither, Georgia," Pat whispered.

Ethel was the stubborn one. She stood her ground and did not open her mouth. Mama started rambling off this stuff about wasting food. No one moved or dared to breathe a sound during her tirade.

"I'mo show y'all about wasting my food. Sit y'all asses down at this table," she screamed. She went to the sink and finished opening the can of peas, poured the liquid from the can into the sink, and divided the rotten peas among us. The stench from the peas was foul. We looked at our plate of peas and then at each other. Tears welled up in my eyes.

"You better eat every last drop!" she demanded as she left the kitchen.

We looked at each other and then at the peas. Mama really intended for us to eat spoiled peas. We did not touch them. We just sat there looking dumbfounded.

"You can sit there all day," she hollered back at us. "Just don't eat them and wait till Tobie comes home."

My tears fell. I was such a crybaby.

I whispered, "You gon' eat them, Ethel?"

"We ain't got no choice," she whispered back. We started eating the peas one at a time. I cried as I popped the peas into my mouth. Ethel whispered, "You better stop crying before Georgia whops you." I knew she was right, but I just could not stop. What in the world was wrong with Mama? She could figure out the most horrific ways to punish, but this was a new one to me. I started to feel sick, but I was too afraid to say anything. From time to time, she came into the kitchen to check on us.

"I mean, eat every last drop!" she yelled. Nobody dared speak. We continued to shovel peas into our mouths. She looked at me and hollered, "Don't nobody give a fuck about your tears. You better eat. Every. Last. One!"

We finished eating and rushed to the bathroom and took turns rinsing the taste out of our mouths. Ethel and I went back to our room until Mama called us to dinner. I was not hungry, and simply looking at the creamed corn and fried pork chops sitting in front of me made me nauseous. Mama walked into the kitchen and looked at my untouched plate.

"You better eat every last drop! I bet you won't waste my food no more."

"But Mama, I didn't open them."

"I don't give a fuck!" She hollered back, "EAT!"

I knew that was my cue to shut up and eat. After a while, I could feel my stomach bubbling and my food started coming up out of my mouth. I ran to the bathroom, holding my hand over my mouth. As soon as I made it, vomit exploded all over the toilet and floor. I dropped to my knees in the middle of all that foulness that came out of my mouth. When my body stopped jerking, I sat on the bathroom floor crying and cleaning up my mess with toilet paper. Mama came to the doorway and stood looking over me with one hand on her hip and a cigarette hanging from her mouth.

"I bet you won't waste my food no more," she smirked.

"But Mama, it wasn't me." She walked off in a huff, "Clean that shit up and get ready for bed." That punishment jacked me up and I never ate a green pea again. Even today at fifty-nine years of age, I pick peas out of potpies, Chinese-fried rice and any other dish containing them. While I can ensure that I never ate a pea again in my life, nothing has taken away the hurt and shame I felt toward Mama that day.

When Ethel and I went to bed that night, I whispered, "Was it you?"

"It wasn't me," she whispered back.

"Why Georgia so mean?"

I turned my back and went to sleep. I had no defense for Mama.

Six

NEITHER BLACK NOR WHITE

My old man's a white old man
And my old mother's black.
If ever I cursed my white old man
I take my curses back.

If ever I cursed my black old mother
And wished she were in hell,
I'm sorry for that evil wish
And now I wish her well.

My old man died in a fine big house.
My ma died in a shack.
I wonder where I'm gonna die,
Being neither white nor black?

—Langston Hughes

We outgrew my grandfather's house the day we became a blended family but made the space shortage work for almost two years. Before I finished third grade, we moved into a new house on the 6200 block of South Hermitage Street in Chicago's West Englewood community. Englewood had just begun to shift from white to Black residents west of Ashland Avenue. In 1971, we were one of the first families to integrate our block. As white families fled the city for the western suburbs, working-class Black families became first-time homeowners in Englewood. The white families that didn't move resisted integration and Western Avenue replaced Ashland Avenue as the new forbidden border for us. If Blacks breached this unspoken boundary, they were often met with white aggression—even violence. Children were forced out of public swimming pools and playgrounds, mostly at the hands of white teenagers, but white adults intimidated children in the area, too. If a person was caught on the other side of Western at night, that person ran the risk of being beaten or violently chased out of the area. On Hermitage Street, however, there were still white families, but not for long. I didn't understand white flight back then, but I was certainly a witness to the phenomenon. It seemed that every day a white family moved out and a Black family moved in. Our immediate area had no racial tension that I can recall. Other than neighborly acknowledgement and small talk, white people and Black people stayed to themselves.

Living near white people was new for me. My grandfather's Swann Street house was about five blocks east of the 47th Street epicenter, a thriving business area for Blacks in the sixties and seventies. The only white people I was exposed to were faculty at Beethoven Elementary School.

Prior to moving, I hadn't thought about race and skin color one way or the other. Of course, I've always known that I was half-white and half-Black, but I didn't really know what that meant. The white side left me dumbfounded because it was the thing that I could not physically see. I never questioned the Black side of me because I looked Black, at least to me. By this time, I was accustomed to Mama calling me out of my name, but after we moved the combination of living among white people and the fact that I was getting older and more inquisitive made race and skin color a complex maze for me.

I started to notice the difference between what Mama said to me about my skin color versus what she didn't say to the rest of the family. Whenever she called me bitch, she used an additional adjective to demean the color of my skin: *red* bitch, *yellow* bitch, *white* bitch. It was common for her to say to me, "Go sit your yellow ass down somewhere." However, she never used skin color to demean anyone else in the house. Dorothy, Tobie and Juan were also lighter in complexion and even when she was mad at Tobie, she never said to him, *you yellow motherfucker.* My other siblings were all a beautiful shade of coffee brown with a teaspoon or two of cream, and Mama never used their skin color against them. I know it may sound like apples and oranges, but when you are nine and ten years old, these words are hurtful and confusing. I thought a lot about Dorothy's skin color and what made her so much more special to Mama than me. The only defining difference that I could see was that my mother was white, and my siblings' mother was Black. Not knowing either side of my family other than my paternal great aunt Lula Mae exacerbated my confusion. She told me bits and pieces, but in the scheme of it all, she never had a kind word to say about my mother or grandmother. If I calculated into the equation Aunt Lula Mae, whose complexion was lighter than mine, and her dislike of the white side of my family, then the problem to me had to be the white side of me. My mother being white made me think I was defective.

If that wasn't enough, my peers on Hermitage Street only made it worse by asking me if my mother was white. Mostly, neighborhood children who hadn't met Mama or my siblings. It felt like a type of judgement was being placed on the question and me, and I, for one, didn't need any more judgements. I would just say, *none of your business*, all sassy-like, and keep it moving. My attitude didn't stop the bullying. They showed no mercy as they spewed spiteful one-liners at me about my light skin and sandy-brown-colored hair. No one on Swann Street had ever picked on me—other than Mama—because of my skin color. But on Hermitage, whenever there was the slightest misunderstanding among us the first thing they said was, "You think you white!" Well, I was half white, and I didn't know what it had to do with whatever they perceived I was doing that they didn't like. I didn't know which side of me was good or bad, which side to celebrate or hate.

What became even more difficult to address were adults inquiring about my racial make-up; both white, and Black. It was awkward when someone said to me, "You are so pretty. Is your mother white?" I knew Mama wasn't my biological mother, but they didn't know anything about me. That question was unsettling because it seemed to cancel or undervalue my blackness. I questioned what being pretty had to do with being half white. I wondered, *why couldn't I be pretty and half black?* Even at a young age I felt a certain kind of way about my Blackness being subtracted. I might not have understood what being half white and half black meant or if being half white made me damaged, but each time I looked in a mirror, I saw a Black girl and never doubted it. As I aged, I understood clearly that light skin and European features were celebrated over and beyond darker skin and African features, and I resented it with every breath in my body because it canceled my father and the entire Black side of my family. Even in dating, if a man was enamored with my skin color, I squashed any idea of us getting together. As a child, it was just confusing. Looking back, how ironic, and sad it was living in Englewood, on the border of white hatred and unrest, that it was the projection of self-hatred from my Black peers, and unwitting questions from Black adults that hurt me and made me doubt myself the most.

While I fought for my Blackness, I was scrambling to understand the problem with my white side. I had so many questions about my mother and grandmother, and no one to ask. I didn't dare ask Mama because she was way too territorial. While I didn't understand her jealousy, I had seen it with both Aunt Pam and Grandmamma Julia. I could imagine her saying *that bitch didn't even want your ass*. I figured Mama would find a way to use it against me. She was the master at taking a little bit of information and holding it over your head until the cows walked from Los Angeles to Chicago—like she did each time I received a Christmas card or birthday card from my grandmother.

"How much money did she send you?" It was never more than twenty-five or thirty dollars, so she wouldn't hesitate to say, "That's all you worth to that bitch?"

I focused on the good my grandmother did for me rather than the other three hundred and sixty-three days of the year that she was absent. I reasoned that the cards and Christmas call from her were indications that she wanted a relationship with me, contrary to what Mama and Aunt Lula Mae thought. With a smile on my face and a growing hole in my heart, I took the scraps from my grandmother's table and made it a meal. I looked forward to that five-minute Christmas call every freaking single year, like Santa was sitting in my bedroom with all the toys in the world just for me. The calls were short and awkward, but they still meant everything to me. I relished in the simple fact that my grandmother had called to talk to me.

I was perfectly fine being half white and half black until everyone created so much drama about my skin color. I hated being placed in this position, but all the contradictions and meanness had opened a door of no return for me. So, being my inquisitive self, I took the small gestures from my grandmother and my desperation to understand my whiteness and fixated on an elderly white woman who was friendly toward the children on our block. She always waved to the children and even placed a basket of apples from her apple tree on her front porch for us to take from time to time. Each time I laid eyes on her I wondered if my grandmother looked anything like her. I was too young to understand how to place someone's age. I concluded that since this lady was old and white, she must look like my grandmother. With that thought, she became my muse. I thought that in the long run if I studied this old lady, it would help me in some abstract way to experience my grandmother beyond the limited contact I had with her. I also reasoned that the more I learned about white people the more information I would have to fix myself, and maybe Mama would love me.

The little old white lady became my hope. I studied her every chance I got. Every time I saw her sitting on her porch swing, I would walk past just to get a glimpse of her. I always spoke as an attempt to engage a conversation, but her accent was too heavy to follow. I settled for waving at her, and she waved back. Occasionally, when no one was around, I walked up the six long steps of her big Victorian style house and looked inside the large front window to see what living white was like. If I got caught, I would get into trouble, but it was a risk I was willing to take. In my simplest calculation, I believed that if I knew more about my neighbor's life it would give me a glimpse into my grandmother's life. I reasoned that if I understood more about my grandmother's life, I would understand more about my own whiteness. But it didn't matter how long I studied that old white lady; the answers that I was seeking about myself were not there. But, I would learn that kindness bears no skin color; it just is.

Seven

❧ ✦ ☙

BROTHERS AND SISTERS

"Come celebrate with me that everyday something has tried to kill me and has failed."
—Lucille Clifton

Our new house was a castle compared to my grandfather's house. Most importantly, the larger size afforded me places to breathe like I had done before we became a blended family. I enjoyed my siblings, but I also enjoyed time with myself. This still holds true today. Being with myself requires nothing of me. It is a simple way of life, with no competing factors. It is a space where I am one with myself and God. Being alone was also another way to cope with Mama, and on Hermitage Street, I could escape for hours. Sometimes, I sequestered myself in my spacious closet and played with my collection of dolls, mostly Barbies, and those miniature Troll Dolls with the funny faces and wonderful hair in shades of purple, yellow, green, turquoise, and even red. When it was warm enough, I sat in our big backyard and made mud pies, picked dandelions, and pretended to cook.

The new house knitted us together but did not diminish who we were individually. The space alone created more boundaries and privacy than I had on Swann Street. When you walked into our front door, you landed in a spacious hallway. To the right of it was the downstairs living room. To the left was a long stairway that ended at a door that opened into the upstairs living room. The first floor had two bedrooms, one bathroom and a large kitchen. Mama and Tobie slept in the back bedroom off the kitchen. Ethel and I were given the front bedroom across from the bathroom on the first floor, but we mostly played together in the spacious unfinished kitchen upstairs. The second floor was the exact same layout, except that it had a small room in the very back that Junior eventually made his room. As the oldest, Kathy got the first bedroom, across from the bathroom. I think Dorothy and Pat got the middle room with bunk beds. The boys had bunk beds in the kitchen and there was still room to play.

All my elementary-aged siblings transferred to Earle, but Mama didn't move me until the next school year. It was the first time since we became a family that I felt like an outsider. Mama didn't explain her decision to leave me at Beethoven, and I knew not to ask. After school I went to Ms. Rachel's place until Dorothy picked me up. I liked having the time to play with Loretta before going home. However, I was downright jealous when Ethel told stories about her classroom inside a trailer at Earle Elementary. The school's main building sat between 62nd and 63rd on Hermitage Street, a three-minute walk from our house. The extension trailers, about a five-minute walk from the house, relieved the overcrowded classrooms and were located in the park between Hermitage and Paulina streets. Each trailer contained a single classroom. The idea of having a trailer as a classroom seemed so cool to me, and I wanted in. I might not have asked Mama why she kept me at Beethoven, but I did ask when she would transfer me to Earle. Her response was, "When I'm good and goddamn ready." I dropped the topic. My feelings were still hurt, but by then I had learned to compartmentalize every bad thing that came my way, and this was no different.

Englewood didn't have the tight boundary constraints that isolated the neighborhood like Swann Street had. We had corner stores on each end of Hermitage that sold penny candy and twenty-five-cent Hostess Suzy Q's snack cakes. I loved the double stack of cream between the two layers of chocolate sponge cake, and the two for a penny caramels that melted in your mouth. The neighborhood camaraderie, however, was just as it had been on Swann Street. Our house was an epicenter of the block, and so was Ms. Williams' house. Like us, she had a big family of eight, maybe, nine children—some, adult-aged. Her daughter, Teresa was closest to my age, and we became playmates. Theirs was the only house I recall spending time visiting because, for the most part, we were forbidden to go into other people's houses without permission. Mama allowed me free rein at the Williamses probably because she and Ms. Williams became friends and drinking buddies soon after they moved to our block. Tobie wasn't having it in our house, so Mama went down to Ms. Williams' place, and I would follow behind. While the grown folks socialized playing music and drinking, Teresa and I played with our dolls in her bedroom.

Summers on Hermitage Street were wonderful. Evenings lingered as people sat on their front porches. After dinner, even Mama would pull a chair from the kitchen and watch. Up and down Hermitage, children could be seen playing games. The girls from the block played Jump Rope and Hopscotch. I wasn't so coordinated for the girly games and much preferred to run off my energy. The real fun for me was when the boys joined in and we played Red Light, The Devil and the Pee Pot, and It. Mama would laugh at us arguing about who got caught and had to sit out. We had so much fun.

In fewer than four years, we had become a family. We looked and behaved like any other Black family on the block. On the surface, we had a good life. We had a two-family income, and I was amazed to see Tobie lay hundred-dollar bills on the kitchen table for Mama to get groceries. We always had a refrigerator full of food and even a full-size freezer that never went low. During the week, Dorothy and Kathy took turns cooking. Pat, Ethel, and I took turns washing the dishes because Mama said all of us girls had to learn. All the boys had to do was take out the freaking garbage. On Saturday mornings, we had breakfasts of grits with lots of butter and sugar, warm buttered biscuits and gobs of Log Cabin syrup, and those Parker House link sausages that Mama had delivered weekly. Sometimes, she even let us bring our plates upstairs to watch cartoons. On Sundays, Mama cooked big meals with fresh collard greens from her garden in our backyard along with macaroni and cheese, chicken, and pot roast. I am certain Mama believed she was a good mother, and in some ways she was. She put a sofa and television upstairs and it became the hangout for us kids. Often, we watched cartoons before and after school. There were even some memorable times that felt like love. On Easter, we dyed eggs with Mama and had Easter egg hunts. There were new outfits for all, and fresh hairdos for the girls and haircuts for the boys. On Christmas, we received lots of gifts and even more new clothes. Tobie's mother sent us crates of oranges, grapefruits, and fresh pecans from Florida. She even visited periodically. We had everything we wanted, even pets. We had the most beautiful German shepherd dog named Poncho. He woke Junior up for his paper route every morning and tagged along. Then we got Queenie, a beautiful Doberman/German Shepherd mix. She had a sleek black body and ears with a touch of brown. Eventually, Mama gave Queenie to Grandmamma Julia because one dog and eight children were enough in one house. Our house was like a revolving farm. Mama got us bunny rabbits and Guinea pigs; and we even had a bird. I think a cat was the only animal we didn't have. Affection from Mama took the form of bags of clothes and plenty of food. In the scheme of her life, I think she simply did not know how to give us what she herself had never received.

As good as Mama was with providing material things, she neglected to provide for us emotionally. Tobie wasn't the I-love-you, mushy type, either, but he didn't make life unnecessarily hard like Mama. In his eyes, children had a role and boundaries, and he expected us to keep them. By the same token, he took his responsibility as our father with the same respect he expected of us as children. Occasionally, he'd let a few of us ride with him on Saturdays to one of his worksites where men were cleaning and stacking bricks. It was amazing to watch them take rubble from a freshly demolished building and prepare them for their next construction. Even Allen and Junior worked the sites occasionally. While I didn't understand what it meant to work for yourself back then, I took pride each time he pulled a wad of money out of his pocket to pay his men at the end of the workday.

On Sunday evenings, he would smoke a cigar and have a beer or two. He'd call one of us girls to come down to the living room to clip his toenails. We all hated it but just like washing dishes, as we aged, we all got our chance. For me, I thought it was disgustingly funny sitting there on the floor giggling and clipping his toenails while some of my other siblings gathered around on the wall-to-wall red carpet watching television and listened to Diddy talk. Mama would look on, smoking her Winston cigarettes and slipping in the back pantry from time to time to get a sip of whatever was on her tap. By then she had moved on to Smirnoff vodka, the one with the red label.

When I put my relationship with Tobie into perspective, he made me feel as if I were one of his. I can honestly say he did what Mama never was able to do: he did not use who I was against me at any time in my life—not my mixed race or the fact that I did not share his DNA. Likewise, I give credit to his children because not one of them ever called me their stepsister. From the moment we became a family, they treated me like I was their blood sister.

While we were a solid core in our home, the division played out in annoying little ways. Sometimes, I went with them to their maternal grandparents' home, and I was acutely aware that I was not one of them. Nothing was ever said directly nor was I ever treated poorly. However, I could feel that the connection to their daughters' children was different from their connection with me. Likewise, Grandmamma Julia never asked for Ethel or any others to spend the weekend and go to church with her. Nor did Aunt Lula Mae invite them to her apartment. Our biological families belonged to us—just like the tragedies that brought us together. Growing up, I never considered that our family was birthed out of tragedy. At the intersection of our lives was a gigantic hole caused by the death of my grandfather and their mother. Their mother's death must have been a terrible blow to them, just as my grandfather's death was to me. Nevertheless, we were all mourning and thrown into a new living arrangement without missing a beat. We tucked in our sadness and kept it moving even through the chaos Mama created.

No one really talked about Mama's cruelty; it just was. I think each of us found our own way to cope. For me, in part, family time with my siblings helped me to hold onto something larger than Mama. I cannot imagine the sum total of the damage she would have done to me if we hadn't become a family. I don't know how my siblings felt about Mama when we were growing up, so I won't speculate. The fact is, they are the only ones who can truly articulate the impact living as a blended family had on them. I will mention, though, that none of them ever referred to Mama as anything other than Georgia, but I naturally referred to Tobie as Diddy, like the rest of his children. This would remain true until the day he left this earth. The other truth is that Tobie's laid-back personality made it easy for me to call him Diddy. While I did not know it then, I later understood that other than Granddaddy, Tobie was the only father figure I had in my lifetime.

Having all of them in my life added a rich texture to my world. My relationship with each of them was different in so many respects. I kept a little sister distance with Kathy, but I was curious about her, especially because of her silence. In the scheme of family dynamics, Kathy did what was expected of her. Her tone of authority was no nonsense to us younger ones, and we obeyed. In her free time, she mostly kept to herself. I think she did what I did and tried to stay the heck out of Mama's way. Especially since Mama was always nitpicking and trying to find fault in every single thing she ever did. I would catch myself staring at Kathy, wanting more, even though I couldn't tell you what that would have looked like. The *me* who I am today understands that the *me* who I was then wanted her love and approval. I also think parts of me wanted Kathy to engage me like Dorothy, but she never did.

Dorothy was exciting and fun to be with. A wild card both day and night, she was our family's bona fide bad girl. I tagged along with her every chance that I got as she roamed Chicago, doing what teenagers do. She took care of my personal needs like combing my hair, and Kathy took care of Ethel's. Spending time with Dorothy was my attempt to redeem who I was. Allowing me to tag along made me feel good about myself. I hoped if I was good enough for Dorothy, it would rub off on Mama. It never did. In the end, I would get to know Kathy as a young adult far more than I ever would Dorothy. I was even a bridesmaid in Kathy's second marriage. This is also true for Patricia, who I bonded with in my teen years after we were no longer one family. Patricia remained quiet and withdrawn during the years we lived as a family. She was most often curled up in a corner with a book in one hand and a thumb in her mouth with the other. Mama, of course, tried to break Patricia's habit by putting hot sauce on her thumb every time she caught her with it in her mouth, but it never worked. She was the middle child but came across as very mature. She was never about the foolishness. I stayed clear of her; when I didn't, all she had to do was give me a certain look and I knew to get out of her face.

By the time we moved to Hermitage Street, Junior had become the epitome of the African American teenager of the '70s. He wore bell-bottom slacks with turtleneck sweaters paired with stacked shoes, just like Richard Roundtree in the movie Shaft. His Afro was always perfect, with not a strand out of place. I looked up to him and he made me feel special. I cherished those days when Junior asked me to hook up his 'do. I had learned how to braid by watching the big girls on our block. He would sport the braids for the weekend, and come Monday, his perfectly shaped Afro was back in place, and I would share in his pride. Our relationship was everything to me—that is—until it turned dark. Juan and Allen were just boys. I saw them as my little brothers with whom I had nothing in common. In truth, I was a couple years older than Juan, but only eight months older than Allen. Nonetheless, they were quintessential boys through and through, which for me meant they were nuisances all the time and I treated them as such. The most interactions I had with them was when we all gathered to watch television. Beyond that, I couldn't be bothered with their foolishness.

Ethel's presence had a certain sass that soothed my spirit. She was the bedrock in our relationship, and I followed her every lead. Mama would buy us the same clothes but in different colors. Whenever I got a bag, she got a bag. We had our own friends, but we also played together. Sometimes she didn't want to be bothered. I sulked about it, but in the end, she made it easy for me to forget and forgive her independence and soon enough we were together playing with our dolls again. She was laid-back and easygoing. She didn't talk a lot, but she noticed everything. And she was fiercely loyal—you were either in or out; there was never an in-between with Ethel.

What I loved the most was that she refused to let Mama break her. God, did I admire that quality about her. One incident in our childhood speaks volumes about Ethel. We were taking a bath together and getting ready for bed; we started splashing our bath water on each other. Just giggling and having a ball. Mama opened the bathroom door, and the moment I saw her body moving into the bathroom I knew we were in trouble. In the smallness of the bathroom, the tub faced the door. Before we could say anything, she swung the brown extension cord, double-folded, across our backs. We both instinctively raised both arms over our heads to catch the blows.

"I told y'all about playing in this fucking tub," she hollered, still beating us. The first swing across my back hurt so much it could have been an axe coming down on wood and splitting it in half. Ethel and I pleaded as Mama lashed us indiscriminately. Then, as quickly as she'd come in, she left, screaming, "Get ready for bed!" And she walked out of the bathroom and slammed the door. Ethel and I looked at each other with hurt-filled eyes. Tears were streaming down my face, but Ethel held back and said nothing. She seemed to position herself inside with a determined attitude that reflected, *Whatever! Not tonight! I won't cry because of Georgia.* She was determined to keep her dignity and not allow Mama's madness to break her. Defiance was written in her body language and how she carried herself. She was one stubborn girl, and I admired her ability to take the hurt and hold all of it inside. I, on the other hand, would tear up if Mama even looked at me too long or too hard. We got out of the tub, dried off and went to bed. Mama was Mama, and that's is how it was growing up for me with brothers and sisters.

Eight

AUNT LULA MAE

" Though she be but little, she is fierce.**"**
—Shakespeare

My great-aunt was an amazing woman. She was feisty and proud, without a pretentious bone in her body. She might have been small in stature, but she was big on words. William Shakespeare's description of Hermia in *A Midsummer Night's Dream* best describes my Aunt Lula Mae: "*Though she be but little, she is fierce.*" Like Hermia, Aunt Lula Mae didn't take shit from anybody—not even Mama. I cannot tell you exactly when I met my paternal great-aunt, but when we moved back to Swann Street after my grandfather's death, she picked me up periodically for overnight visits. She started talking the moment our feet hit the pavement. She was animated when she talked, and that made everything she said seem to have an urgency about it. She is the only person I ever knew who could outtalk me, and that's saying a *whole* lot. After we moved to Hermitage Street, Aunt Lula Mae increased her visits with me, providing a welcome addition to my routine and a boost to my self-esteem. I felt proud when I was by her side.

She was petite with large hips and stood about five-foot-one; however, she walked with an air about her as if she were six feet tall. She was an educated woman and a retired nurse. She was one hell of a dresser who wore colorful silk blouses and well-fitted tailored suits. At home, she changed into pretty, quilted Stella Fagin-style floral maxi robes that were popular in the sixties. The ones she wore were made of satin, with a mandarin-style collar and bell sleeves that zipped down the front. Aunt Lula Mae had big beautiful light brown eyes. She kept her eyebrows thin and penciled in, like Joan Crawford's but with a light brown liner to match her eyes. She was always impeccably made up, even in the morning when she fixed my breakfast, and I wondered how she did that. Her signature look was a blonde or red curly wig, and typically, she wore beautiful shades of red lipstick that I absolutely loved! I would watch her with fascination as she pulled out her fancy gold compact, popped out her red lipstick encased in a gold-toned tube and shaped her lips perfectly like a 1930s movie star. Once I began wearing red lipstick, I reached into my memory and used her style to develop my lip glam. I loved everything about her.

My great-aunt believed that I should have been living with my biological family. Mama on the other hand, painted a picture of her altruism—that is, she had done me a favor because no one else wanted me. Then she'd turn around and contradict herself, by saying my grandmother told her she could take me, and she wore it like a badge of honor. I can't make this shit up. I was so confused until aunt Lula Mae cleared it all up. Every visit, she declared to me, "Your grandmother should not have given Georgia permission to keep you." Apparently, after my grandfather's death, Aunt Lula Mae reached out to my maternal grandmother, because someone from the family wanted to raise me. My maternal grandmother confirmed this in the letter she sent Mama about who should raise me. She didn't know my father's side of the family and didn't much care for Aunt Lula Mae. Apparently, Aunt Lula Mae had choice words about my mother that my maternal grandmother didn't appreciate. I can picture Aunt Lula Mae *reading* my grandmother about my mother and drugs. It couldn't have been pretty. I was in junior high school when I discovered the letter my grandmother had sent Mama, tossed around in a junk dresser drawer. It left no doubt that my grandmother did not want me. She thought since Mama had been married to my grandfather who, "took excellent care" of me, according to my mother, it made sense that I should live with my grandfather's wife. In the end, they acquiesced to my maternal grandmother's authority to have the last say because they believed, being the closest living relative at the time, that she inherently had the right to give me away.

Mama's worldview differed slightly, as it hinged on the racist social construct that "white is right," which disempowered African American authority. The roots go back to Black Southerners who dared not question white authority, mostly out of fear of retribution but also from some internalized belief that white opinions were superior to those of Black people. Mama said, "That white woman put a stop to that...." [referring to my paternal grandmother's family taking me]; and it was her epithet until the day she died. While she was bragging to me and her friends, she never said anything to Aunt Lula Mae about my maternal grandmother's authority nor did she display her badass persona toward her. It seemed to me that she was a little intimidated by Aunt Lula Mae because she worked hard at being dignified in her presence: no cursing or talking loud. As I got older, her failed attempts to speak "proper" around Aunt Lula Mae made me embarrassed for her. I would hear Mama trying to defend herself from Aunt Lula Mae's accusations that she was keeping me away from my family. Aunt Lula Mae didn't mince words or back down when she spoke to Mama. You could even see and feel her contempt about the situation. Many times, she said, "I'm taking RaeClara because she needs to be with her people." And she always placed emphasis on the words "her people" as she exited the house, wearing one of her tailored day suits and holding my hand. Mama never opened her mouth. She just stood in the living room in her house robe, smoking a cigarette and looking lost.

Looking back, I am in awe of Aunt Lula Mae's determination to know me. She was sixty-three years old when she began to pick me up from Hermitage Street. The trip from her apartment to my house would have been at least an hour on any bus route each way, and that speaks volumes about the woman she was. She picked me up every other month or so on Saturday mornings and brought me back on Sundays. Her apartment was small, and as usual, I was a little bit cramped and fidgety. If it bothered her in any way, she never said so. I was always free to be me.

Our ritual was pretty much the same. I changed into my play clothes and settled in for the visit in one of her vinyl retro chairs that stuck to my butt, with my legs dangling under the table. Sometimes she would put the Yellow Pages on the chair to raise my height to meet with the table. She would pour me a glass of milk, put two cookies on a saucer and pour herself a cup of coffee; and sitting next to me at the table in her kitchenette, the family lesson would begin. On each visit, Aunt Lula Mae cleared up more and more of Mama's contradictory information about family. She was a wonderful storyteller and I listened intently. First thing out of her mouth every visit was, "We are your people," and shaking her head in disgust, she'd say, "You should be with us." She never changed her opinion. Nevertheless, she didn't rock the boat, either. I think she let well enough alone because she believed Mama took good care of me and, for all intents and purposes, she did. I had a roof over my head, plenty of food to eat, and clothes for days. Suffice it to say, I did a great job hiding my misery. I thought about telling her about Mama's cruelty the beatings and name-calling on many occasions. But Mama scared the daylights out of me every Saturday morning while I waited on Aunt Lula Mae to pick me up. "I wish you would go over there and tell my business," she'd say, standing in the doorway by my bedroom with a cigarette hanging out the side of her mouth. "I'll beat the living shit out of you." Then she'd walk back to her bedroom. I knew she meant what she said.

Our visits together consistently provided me with a more intimate portrait of who I was. If not for Aunt Lula Mae, I would not have had a foundation on which to begin tracing my family roots. She anchored herself into my life like a tree planted by the water. It was through Aunt Lula Mae that I learned I was named after my parental grandmother, Jane Clara. Just the thought that my father kept the memory of his mother alive through me added another notch to my self-worth. And she paid homage to her sister every time she said my name, by pronouncing it as one word, RaeClara.

One visit she pulled out a photo album and pointed to a picture of me and my father. "RaeClara, that's your father holding you," she said proudly. It was the first time I had ever seen my father, but I thought she must have been mistaken. I did not want to refute her declaration, but the man she was pointing at was extremely dark. The baby he was holding looked nothing like me, either. Her hair looked black and mine was sandy brown. To me, the baby looked white. I just stared at the picture.

"Is this really my father?" I asked, looking up at Aunt Lula Mae.

"Yes, baby. That's your father." She took the photo out of the album and handed it to me. My name and birthday were written across the front of the picture. I turned it over and it read, *"Received Sept. 6, 1962, at birth, 3 lbs. 11 oz. May 22, 1962. Lula Mae Gibson's Great Niece."* I could not refute it.

"I was so little," I mumbled as I rubbed my hand over my face on the picture. This was the first time that I had ever seen a picture of myself as a baby, and it was overwhelming. If my grandfather had any photos, I never saw them. In many ways, I feel as if Mama just walked away from anything connected to my life before my grandfather's death. Holding the picture of my father and me on that day, I kept looking and tracing my father's face with my hand. That picture made him real, and not some imaginative construct. It also made my Blackness real, and after that day, I never allowed anyone to reduce me again.

My father's picture also created emotions in me that I never had. Until then, my grandfather was the only man I connected to emotionally. I could feel the pull on my heart both celebrating and mourning my father. Aunt Lula Mae was quiet for a long time as I soaked him in. It felt good to be able to put a face on him. He became alive in my spirit. He was more than a drug addict. He was my father, and his blood was running through my veins.

"You should have that picture," Aunt Lula Mae said, breaking my trance.

"Really?!" I asked.

"Keep it, baby," she said as she looked down on me grinning from ear to ear. We continued to look through the album at other pictures of my father in his youth. In one photo, he wore a sharp-ass, double-breasted suit and boxing gloves, kidding around. In the other picture, he was holding his saxophone. I am guessing he was somewhere between fourteen and sixteen.

"My daddy played that?" I asked, looking up at Aunt Lula Mae.

"Yes, he was a fine saxophone player." My birth certificate confirms his profession as a musician. Aunt Lula Mae took the other two pictures out of the photo album and handed them to me. I lit up like a Disco Ball.

Aunt Lula Mae told me that my father was deeply affected by losing his mother; however, without any details, I just didn't know what to think. Most times when she talked about my father and grandmother, she became melancholy and quickly deflected by saying, "We were all affected, RaeClara. Your grandmother was a wonderful woman." At other times she would say about my father, "Your daddy just got messed up with your mother." It was clear that she blamed my mother for my father's drug use getting out of control. Aunt Lula Mae gave me a place to start, but she left out more than she told me. Even though I was an inquisitive little girl, I didn't know how to frame the questions that needed to be asked. As I moved into my preteen and teen years, it never occurred to me to ask because I was too busy being a teenager.

Age and time have a way of knocking you over the head. Writing this book made me see the holes in my family history, and I felt the holes in my heart for the lack of knowing. I believe Little Rae is still searching for a family and the historian in big Rae cannot let it die. For me, the history of one's life gives you a specific place in the universe as well as in time and space. Alex Haley, the author of *Roots* put it this way; and his assessment resonates deep within my soul:

> In all of us there is a hunger, marrow-deep, to know our heritage – to know who we are and where we have come from. Without this enriching knowledge, there is a hollow yearning. No matter what our attainments in life, there is still a vacuum, an emptiness, and the most disquieting loneliness.

To seal this hollow yearning in my soul, I began exploring my family lineage on an ancestry website and researching vital statistics in the cities of record. I know now that my paternal grandmother, Jane Clara, was born in 1915. She had nine siblings. Her mother, Florence Shelton [Graham-Jones] was married twice with a set of children from each husband. I've also learned some of my paternal grandmother's siblings were still alive when my grandfather died, but I never met any of them other than Aunt Lula Mae. When I was a freshman in high school, Aunt Lula Mae scooped me up and took me to Aunt Geraldine's funeral. She was seventy-five when she passed and was in her mid-sixties when my grandfather died. I'm sure she saw herself too old to raise a child. Aunt Lula Mae did a herculean job trying to connect me to my family. On some Saturday visits, she took me to the church my second cousin, Ann Simington, attended. Ann was a Seventh Day Adventist, and had three girls—Lenora, Linda, and Lauretta—whom I would get to know. I would meet Ann's sister, Eleanor Jones, and her son, Kenneth, at Aunt Geraldine's funeral.

As a child, it never occurred to me that Aunt Lula Mae never mentioned my grandfather or his relationship with my grandmother. Back then, I didn't even think about it because I was so intrigued learning about my father and grandmother. Through my own research, I learned that my grandmother married Granddaddy at the age of eighteen in 1933. He was one year older. They had my father, Alfred Jr. two years later. What I find interesting is the lineage of the entire Black side of the family began in the small agricultural community of Charleston, Missouri near the Mississippi River. Aunt Lula Mae never ever mentioned Charleston. I have so many questions and they will get answered. I might not have finished my PhD in church history, but you better believe, I will get that PhD in my family history. While my grandfather was born in Charleston, my paternal grandmother, Jane Clara, was born in Chicago, and that's where they married. I had always assumed that my grandparents were married until her death. All Aunt Lula Mae would say was that she died young and had a hard life. After two years of research, I learned that I had been gravely mistaken, and Aunt Lula Mae hadn't even told me a fraction of the story.

My father was nine when Granddaddy remarried, but what in the world happened to Jane Clara? Standing in the courthouse clerk's office, on a fluke, I asked if you could obtain divorce records. I was sent to the archives of county records. With just the names of my grandfather's first two wives and the dates of their marriages, we found divorce records. According to the records, my grandfather's divorce from his second wife Earleen was amicable. After fourteen years of marriage, they had a quick divorce. They didn't even claim their children, Michael and Sharon.

It took a couple more weeks for them to bring my grandmother's divorce file up from the archives. It turned out that she and Granddaddy had been married for six years and separated for two prior to the divorce; my father was three years old. My grandmother filed for the divorce on the grounds of "extreme and repeated cruelty." I started hyperventilating. *WHAT IN GOD'S NAME?* I couldn't even continue reading. I called my good friend Luke Burke and asked him to stay on the phone with me as I read the file. On May 10, 1936, in my grandmother Jane Clara's words, "He [my grandfather; her husband] blackened my eye and cut me with his fist." On April 15, 1937, she stated, "He hit me and cut me again." Aunt Lula Mae had testified, and that jacked me up. She said that my grandfather treated my grandmother "very cruelly." On that day, May 10th, she saw my grandmother and she was "beaten up and her eye and lip were swollen." To top it off, my grandmother's mother, also testified that my grandfather was "cruel [to my grandmother] and always wanted to fight."

Whew! The man whom I cherished as my protector had been a wife-beater. This knowledge knocked me clear off my feet. I still don't know how to process this fact. It confirmed that I really did see my grandfather pushing Mama down the street one day. It also lends credence to the assertion that they were fighting, and Mama hit him over the head with a radio. Mama might have been many things, but the Georgia Lee that I know would never take a man hitting her sitting down. The fact that my grandmother walked away from a marriage at twenty-five years old with a toddler son is remarkable. In 1939, a woman filing for a divorce was a BADASS move—as it would be for any woman—with no income and a child. My grandmother makes me proud, and I'm honored to bear her name. What I've not been able to reconcile is that Aunt Lula Mae never mumbled a negative word about my grandfather. The way families keep secrets is mind-boggling. In the end, it does far more damage than good.

My father was a train wreck waiting to happen. I can see from residency records that he was the one driving the train—going from pillow to post most of his adult life. What I understand for sure is that trauma begets trauma. Drugs are never about the drugs, they simply numb the pain. I will never know the full extent of my father's wounds that are buried with him. Hopefully, the more I learned about my grandmother Jane Clara's life, which has been difficult—It's like she had disappeared into thin air—the more I will understand my father's life·

A unt Lula Mae took these secrets to her grave, and in the end, I believed she did what she thought was best for me. What I know for sure is that unpacking Mama's half-truths and misinformation placed me in a better position to protect myself emotionally. I can't even begin to explain the depth of power I was given with information from Aunt Lula Mae, which I used in the simple act of reframing my life—even if in a small way. Mama used information to tear me down and I used Aunt Lula Mae's information to lift me and shield my soul. It was one thing when Mama told me something hurtful and I saw her as an undeniable source, but with Aunt Lula Mae as a reliable source of the same information retold, I could begin to draw my own conclusions, even if they were flawed.

Each visit gave me a new piece of my life that Mama could never take away from me. They were the glue that helped to repair what Mama had ripped apart when it came to my family. Information is power, and I took the power Aunt Lula Mae gave me to fight back. Even the pictures of my father that I never showed to anyone became another tool to help me regain myself. I created a world in my head that was different from the one that I lived. Sometimes when I hid in my bedroom closet, I would have conversations with my dolls such as:

Aunt Lula Mae said she does, too, want me.

Aunt Lula Mae said it was my grandmother's fault that I'm stuck with Mama.

I imagined my dolls and me packing our clothes and heading to the family that loved us most. Even in a room full of people, I would withdraw into myself when Mama gave me a tongue-lashing. I would slip away inside my head and reunite with my maternal grandmother, who decided that she had made an awful mistake leaving me with Mama. Aunt Lula Mae was the North Star I needed to help me reshape my narrative. Those moments spent with her instilled a determination that helped me maneuver through the darkness. I thank God for my Aunt Lula Mae.

Nine

❧ ✦ ☙

BULLIES

❝Out of suffering have emerged the strongest souls;
the most massive characters are seared with scars.❞
—Khalil Gibran

Mama was the only one who hadn't settled in. Just like on Swann Street, she was a persistent source of tension for us. Every night I could hear her yapping to Tobie about one thing or another. When she got a cockamamie idea in her head that didn't sit well with her, she wasn't satisfied until she had rectified whatever that thing was. She sat on the side of the bed with a cigarette in her hand, making animated movements while Tobie watched television—and, Lord, you better pray your name wasn't mentioned because his punishment was a whooping with a red water hose that he kept by his bed. The one thing I can say about Tobie is that he rarely initiated a whopping unless you had committed some clear infraction. For sure, the most horrible punishments from him occurred when one person got in trouble. When we were all in trouble, we could lick our wounds together. But when Tobie beat one child, it was reminiscent of a slave being beaten for stealing from his master. Most of our beatings however came because Mama had accused us of something. And God help us all if Mama could not identify the culprit; she insisted that Tobie figure it out. If no one came clean, we all got our butts beat.

One time, someone ate nearly all the popsicles in like a day of Mama bringing them home—and she was pissed. As soon as Tobie walked through the door, he called all the younger kids to the kitchen. We stood in a line looking at each other. I was sure Allen did it, but snitching was not in my makeup, and certainly not over a hunch. You talk about painful to watch your siblings get their asses beat while you wait your turn? Those were some emotional calisthenics. I always hoped that Tobie would get tired by the time he reached me, but that never happened.

A beating with an extension cord is one-of-a-kind pain; it cuts and burns, and left scars on my body. Contrastingly, the rubber hose left no marks. But the force of the rubber meeting my body felt like the wrath of God crashing down on me. Tobie had one hell of a swing. Honestly, I'm not sure which was worse: getting a beating with his water hose or watching my siblings pleading futilely to him for mercy.

"Please, Diddy," we begged. "It wasn't me, Diddy." He didn't respond to our pleas. Instead, he beat that hose against our bodies reminiscent of Denzel Washington's character in the movie, *Glory*, being whipped across his back methodically and with precision. Tobie never moved from his spot during the beatings. Ever. We knew not to run or move around too much, or he would beat that person longer. You never wanted him to say, "Bring your ass back over here." While these beatings were physically painful, emotionally knowing that Mama had caused the beating was like Grandmamma forcing me to take castor oil for any old health issue that popped up—that is, having to taste every spoonful of that unnecessary bitterness. What was difficult for me to wrap my head around was that Tobie was sensible, and I never understood why he got caught in Mama's web.

Tobie gave us room to be children, but he was no doubt an unrelenting disciplinarian who believed in order. I know corporal punishment is acceptable in many Black families, and particularly so during the time when I grew up. It is rationalized as something for the good of the child in the long run. It guaranteed control, and control helped maintain respectability of the family. Just like Grandmamma Julia, Tobie adhered to the philosophy that you control your children at home, so they grow up to be in control of their own lives and not in jail or dead. Even in 2015, the American Psychological Association confirmed that African American parents are twice as likely to use corporal punishment than white or Latino parents. I know people my age who claim whippings made them better people. Maybe that is what one makes himself or herself believe to reconcile the conflict between the parents they love and depend on as the same parents who take a belt, an extension cord, or a water hose and beat the fuck out of them. There is not one freaking thing that I can muster up to make myself believe this type of degradation and depravation at the hands of a parent was good for me.

Interestingly, I didn't judge Tobie as harshly as I did Mama. My best guess is because he didn't curse or talk to us crazily like Mama did. Emotional and verbal abuse leaves a different kind of scar, and it just wasn't in Tobie's make-up. When I look over the sum total of my time under his parental supervision, hands down he was the lesser of two evils.

I clung to the good parts of Tobie as a child because the alternative would have been devastating for my young self. I needed to believe that at least one of my parents cared about me. Mama was relentless, and Tobie saved me many a day. Each time he intervened, I placed another check in the plus column for him. But at the end of the day, he is still the person who beat the crap out of us over some popsicles. If I am to be really honest about it, there were many times that Tobie could have stood up for us but didn't.

Mama was a bully and, most days, I was the target of her aggression. Yet, wasn't a wrong invented in Mama's eyes that could get Dorothy in trouble. Kathy said to me years later, "Dorothy got away with murder," and she was correct. Allen seemed to be another favorite. Once Mama realized that she couldn't break Ethel, she mostly left her alone. No one totally escaped her web but some, like Kathy and me, got it more than others. I remember Kathy saying to me in that same conversation, "It was as if Georgia had it out for me," and she was not lying.

Mama waited for Kathy to make any small infraction to report to Tobie, like a tattletale on the playground. One time, Kathy burned a pot of beans and Mama wouldn't let her throw them away. Before Tobie even got in the door good, Mama tricked.

"You ain't paying one bill in this house," he told Kathy. "Money don't grow on trees." He then ordered her to eat the pot of burnt beans. Mama stood in the doorway of their bedroom just off the kitchen with her cigarette dangling from her lips, watching every word out of Tobie's mouth like he was a carnival freak show. There was no logical reason for Tobie to render such a harsh punishment, and it remained one of those contradictions about him. Like I shared earlier, Kathy married her high school sweetheart and got the hell out of the house as soon as she could. Mama swore Kathy's motivation for getting married was that she was pregnant, which she wasn't. In the end, everyone in the house was a victim of Mama's madness at one time or the other. Mama's tight grip and bullying kept me on edge. It's a wonder I ever had normal cortisol levels as a child. I'm sure I had what Dr. Perry calls, "anticipatory anxiety"—meaning, anxiety over what will happen next. I was either trying to prevent the next assault, prepare myself emotionally for the next assault, or deal with the physical and emotional aftermath of an assault. Then, as if things couldn't get any worse, shortly after I started Earle Elementary School, one of my classmates started bullying me.

A girl named Clara, of all names, was the namesake from hell. I had Mama at home working against me and I had Clara at school. To make life even more unbearable, I absolutely hated attending Earle. I remember right after Ethel transferred, I desperately wanted to be with her. I thought it was so cool having school in a trailer. Now that I was in it, not even walking to school with Ethel could make me like being cramped in one room all day. There was nothing to stimulate my senses, no brightly colored walls and no art displayed on the doors, like at Beethoven. Staying in my seat all day in one room with windows too high to see out of was killing me slowly. We even ate lunch at our desks. The days of hot lunches with those wonderful butter cookies at Beethoven were over. We had cold lunch-meat sandwiches with a wad of butter on white bread accompanied with an apple and a carton of milk. I couldn't stand it, and I watched the big clock on the wall for 3:30 to arrive as if my life depended on it; eventually, it did.

The first time Clara bumped into me; we were getting supplies. I thought maybe I had bumped into her by accident; I am rather clumsy. But after she stuck her leg out and caused me to fall forward when I walked by her desk, barely catching myself, I knew she was picking on me. After that near-miss she passed me a note that said, "I'm gonna kick your butt." I stuffed it in my folder and took a deep breath. Aggression outside my home was new to me.

She stepped up her game. When I was getting supplies the next day, she bumped my back. It was so crowded I dismissed it. I was so gullible. When I turned to go to my seat, she was standing right there in my face, crowding my space. "I'm gonna get you after school," she snared, just above a whisper for only me to hear. I looked at her dumbfounded. My mind did jumping jacks as I wondered, *What the hell was this girl playing at?* I had done absolutely nothing to cause her hostility toward me. My feelings were decimated, to say the least. I had that *I-want-everyone-to-like-me* syndrome, and I had it bad! Let me clarify; wanting people to like me did not mean I wanted everyone to be my friend. Frankly, in my opinion, friendships were special, and everyone didn't qualify. I already had Loretta, Vicki, and Teresa. However, I didn't want people to find fault in me, either. I got enough of that at home. I couldn't take any more negative critics. That day, I just stood looking back at Clara. I didn't want to make matters worse. Our classmates were clearing out and returning to their seats. I think she didn't want to get in trouble because she turned and went to her seat. Likewise, I went to my seat, walking the two aisles over to avoid passing her desk.

As soon as the bell rang at 3:30, I shot my ass out of that classroom door and ran as if my life depended on it, straight to Ethel's trailer. She wasn't scared of anybody and, as soon she walked out of the trailer, I recounted the whole ordeal. Up to then, I hadn't told anyone about Clara—not even my teacher. I didn't want her to call Mama for any reason because she could flip the script with incredible ease. I knew that I could depend on Ethel. She listened attentively and when I had finished, she just shrugged and kept walking out of the school park. That caught me off guard. I walked in sync with her. This was important. Someone wanted to beat me up, and she was completely nonchalant. "But Clara," I started—and before I could get the rest of it out of my mouth, Ethel blurted her action plan loud enough so anyone in ear shot could hear, including Clara.

"I wish she would bring her butt over here and mess with you," she said, with confidence. "I'll beat her butt!" Ethel's declaration brought closure to my anxiety, and I walked home with her confidence by my side.

At first, I wasn't going to tell Mama. I knew I could count on Ethel to keep my secret. I also knew if Mama heard about it through the grapevine, I was a guaranteed at best a tongue-lashing and, at worst, an ass-beating. There was no way for me to come out ahead. I gathered my nerve that evening while she was sitting in the living room watching television and smoking a cigarette. I stood in the living-room entrance, close to my bedroom.

"Mama." She looked up at me, pulling the cigarette out of her mouth.

"Girl, what you want?"

"Mama, this girl at school is trying to fight me," I explained.

"If someone hit you, you better hit them the fuck back! You hear me?" she asked.

Lord knows I didn't want to fight anyone for any reason. I didn't respond to Mama at first. I simply stood there with my tummy doing flip-flops, wringing my hands.

"Do you hear me?" she asked again. I finally shook my head up and down.

"If I ever hear that you let someone hit you and you didn't fight back, I'ma beat your ass when you get home." I heard her loud and clear. Gloom fell over me like a London fog.

"Okay, Mama." I went to my bedroom and sulked. I was between a rock and a hard place. I understood that Mama wanted me to protect myself. To me, however, hitting of any kind was hurtful. It represented an ugliness of which I did not want to be a part. I had been hit so much that I didn't want anyone else to feel my pain. I could not imagine how hitting someone would protect me after the fact. It was just tit for tat. I realize that some may see it as a deterrent; however, to me, the hurt outweighs any justification. I don't want to control any being by the fear, humiliation and intimidation achieved by a beating. To this day, I have owned four toy poodles: Imani, Nambi, Sophie and Chloe, and I have never spanked them, nor do I allowed others to do so (although I will admit that Chloe works my nerves). I understood even then that Mama's threats were based on her desire to control my behavior. In so doing, she taught me through experience how hurtful hitting a person was; and I did not, for one moment, want that part of her to become a part of me.

My philosophy about hitting didn't change the fact that I was still afraid of Clara. Every day after school, I ran to Ethel's classroom to avoid my fate and she never told. One day for some reason that I cannot recall, Ethel and I were not together. As I was walking home, I felt a push against my back and caught myself so I wouldn't fall to the ground. "I told you I was gonna get you," I heard Clara say before I could regain my balance. When I turned, she was in my face with her hands on her hips; one of her older sisters was standing directly behind her. "Your sister ain't with you now," Clara's sister said, egging her on.

"Kick her butt, Clara!" People started gathering around us. I was scared shitless. I didn't open my mouth. I turned around and people started moving out of my way and before anyone realized what I was doing, I was running down Hermitage Street like Forrest Gump. I was not going to get beat up that day, and then turn around and get another beatdown from Mama because I got beat up.

Lord knows I dreaded telling her what happened, but I knew that I had to come clean, before someone else told her. After Mama changed her clothes that evening and sat in the living room to relax, I took a deep breath and stood in the doorway to explain the day's event. The shame I felt was eating me alive. I didn't want to go back to school the next day and face Clara and my schoolmates for running away, and I absolutely didn't want Mama to think that I was a chicken and beat my ass because of that fact. To my surprise, Mama listened without saying a word. When I finished telling her the story of how Clara and her sister double-teamed me minus the fact that I ran she called Dorothy into the living room. "I'll fix them bitches," Mama mumbled, to no one in particular. Something had stirred inside of Mama because the fight had been two against one and she wasn't going to let anyone double-team me.

"I want you to pick Rae up after school," she instructed Dorothy. "I don't know who these bitches think they fuckin' with."

The next day Dorothy was there right when the bell rang. She and I walked to Ethel's trailer, and we all walked home together. Dorothy continued to pick us up after school and Clara continued to taunt me. One day at recess she asked, twirling her hand in my face, "You think your big sister gonna stop me from beating your butt?"

"My big sister will beat her butt, too." I hadn't said anything to Clara, but that day, I got up enough nerve to ask her why she wanted to fight me.

"Because you think you cute," she responded. I could not begin to fathom what she was talking about. I looked at her like she was crazy. I didn't understand her reasoning. In my mind, I looked like her; she was my complexion and about my build. The only difference was our hair. My hair was about shoulder-length and Dorothy would put these little ponytails all over my head with different-colored rubber bands. Clara, on the other hand, had nappy little beads sitting on the top of her head. I didn't know what to say to her. All the girls in my house had shoulder-length hair and, most importantly, we were well cared for. I couldn't imagine that she wanted to fight me over something I had and that she didn't. It was like Mama fussing at me for doing something she had told me to do. Clara stood there with her hands on her hips. I turned away and walked to our trailer and stayed there until recess was over. Clara bumped into me every chance she got, and I continued to avoid her as best as I could. Then one day after school Dorothy, Ethel, and I were walking home and we heard someone say, "Get her!" We looked back and Clara and one of her big sisters (who seemed older than the one before) were closing in behind us. I guess Clara's big sister was the nerve she needed to fight me with my sisters by my side. What they didn't count on was Dorothy. She was a badass, for real. We stopped. Dorothy didn't move and didn't say a word. She just waited for them to get closer.

"I wish you would touch my sister, bitch," Dorothy told Clara's sister. My eyes got big, and my stomach dropped to my feet with anxiety. I looked at Dorothy and then at Ethel. They were both in fight mode.

"I will beat your ass!" Dorothy promised.

Clara's sister jumped in Dorothy's face.

"Bitch, I don't know who the fuck you think you talking to!"

Dorothy didn't flinch with the girl in her face. She matter-of-factly told her, "I'm talking to you, hoe!" My stomach dropped again. I hated being so scared. The Lord be my witness, I sure was thankful that day for my sisters.

"I will drag your ass up and down this street!" Dorothy declared, not moving one inch as the girl stood in her face. Clara's sister's disposition changed, and she slumped a little. You could see her calculating her probability for success or failure against my Dorothy, who had the confidence of David against Goliath. Dorothy stood there like, *Your move, bitch*. I was breathless, looking back and forth.

"Whatever," Clara's sister spoke, finally, as she grabbed her little sister's hand.

"I thought so!" Dorothy said as she declared her victory in earshot of Clara and her sister. And like that, we continued our way home as Clara and her sisters went on their way.

That evening, I was outside playing when I spotted a group of people walking down the street. As they got closer, I could see it was Clara and her sisters. I knew she had a large family, but I didn't know who was who. It looked like a family reunion when they finally made it to the front of our house. I ran into the house and told Dorothy they were outside.

"I wish they would," Dorothy said like a badass as she made her way to the porch.

"I see you had to bring your whole family, BITCH!" Dorothy hollered, looking right at Clara's big sister who we had the altercation with earlier that day. Dorothy was holding court, arguing with Clara's mama and sisters about who started what first. We all had made it to the porch and stood behind Dorothy in solidarity. They were going at it and our neighbors came out on their front porches to see what was happening. Tobie wasn't home yet, but Mama was. All of a sudden, she stepped out on the porch with Granddaddy's rifle in her hand. She cocked it up like she was going to shoot.

"I WILL BLOW Y'ALL'S MUTHA-FUCKIN' HEADS OFF." The argument froze.

"Who the fuck y'all think you are coming to my fucking house?"

Clara's mother finally reclaimed her backbone and stepped forward, big and bad.

"Your big-ass daughter was trying to fight my little girl," she hollered at Mama.

"That's a boldface lie!" Mama snapped back. I asked Dorothy to pick Rae up after school because y'all was picking on her." She relaxed the rifle as she attempted to explain the situation as she knew it, mother to mother. When Clara and her sister started talking over Mama, trying to drown out what she was saying, Dorothy went, "Hell to the no!" and started yelling back at them. Then Clara's mother stepped up, trying to be big and bad, like she was running something.

"Ain't nobody gonna fuck with my kids!" she declared.

Mama raised the rifle to show that she meant what she said and said what she meant. Everyone got quiet again. "Let kids be kids," Mama said to Clara's mother. "Ain't no reason all y'all want to fight my one child," she reasoned. Clara's mother was feeling herself trying to show her family that she was not afraid of Mama holding the gun. She kept right on yelling and cursing. And I could hear our neighbors instigating.

"Shoot that bitch, Georgia!"

"Get from in front of my fuckin' house!" Mama warned.

"Ain't nobody scared of you, BITCH!" Clara's mother sparred back.

"I'm sick of this shit," Mama mumbled to herself.

"Ain't nobody gonna touch my child! I'll kill all you muthafuckas!"

By this time, it seemed like everyone on the block was watching. You could hear them taunting and shouting all kinds of shit.

"Shoot they ass, Georgia!"

"They ain't got no business coming to your house!"

It was pure madness. There were so many people surrounding our house I couldn't tell where Clara's family ended, and our neighbors began. Everyone was chiming in. My head was darting from side to side, watching and taking it all in like I was at some rodeo and not the center of the debate.

PO-OW!!!.... The rifle fired; the shell casing fell clanging on the porch.

People ducked and scattered like cockroaches. I looked up at Mama in amazement. "WOW!"

Mama cocked the gun again. "I will kill all you motherfuckers!"

"Get from in front of my fucking house!" she warned, again.

The neighbors scattered to their porches but continued watching. Clara's family had stepped back.

"Just keep your daughter away from my daughter," Clara's mother said in defeat. Dorothy yelled, "Well, tell your little bald-headed daughter to stop starting shit!"

Clara's mother looked down at Clara, and said, "Just stay away from that girl."

"Why you want to fight her, anyway?" she asked. Clara shrugged.

"Come on here," she told her family, and they slowly walked away, trying not to look like they had lost a wager.

"Crazy bitch," she said, loud enough so Mama could hear it.

"That's right," Mama hollered back, "And I will blow your motherfucking head off!"

Mama continued to stand on the porch and hold the rifle in her hand, looking like a Black Annie Oakley, until Clara's family turned the corner off our block. Some of our neighbors came over to boost Mama's ego, laugh and talk shit. When it was all over, Mama called me into the living room.

"If that girl hits you again, I want you to beat the fuck out of her."

"Okay, Mama," I mumbled.

"Do you hear me?!" she screamed. I just shook my head up and down and went back to my room. Dorothy kept picking me up after school as a precaution, but the inevitable soon came to a head. One day we were walking out for recess and Clara pushed me hard. I fell on the wooden platform built around the trailer. It took me a moment to gather myself. My knee was hurt but my pride hurt worse. I was so over it all—Clara threatening me, Mama threatening me and the fear that loomed over me with so much power. I could hear Mama's voice that day: *Beat her ass or I'm going to beat yours when you get home.* I knew what I had to do, I got up swinging, catching Clara off guard. I hit her as hard as I could in the face. Her first reflex sent her hand up to the red spot I had just made on the side of her face instead of hitting me. Bullies never expect you to fight back. I swung again and again. "I hate you!" I declared. I kept swinging like a wild child. Our classmates gathered around, yelling, "It's a fight!"

Clara's pride shook her out of her daze, and we started fighting like two wildcats. We were tangled up when the principal tried to break it up. She had my hair, and I had her coat. "Break it up!" the principal demanded.

"You let go first," she said.

"Let my hair go and I'll let you go," I demanded. I had never wanted to fight her, but there was no turning back. It was sink or swim. I took my other hand and swung at her again. The principal was steaming. "I said break it up, now!" I felt someone pulling me back and I tried to jerk away but their hold was too strong. A teacher was pulling me as the principal pulled Clara. They took us to the administration trailer and the principal suspended us for fighting. I didn't care. I told my principal just that when he asked me why I was fighting.

"Clara hit me first," I declared, "and my mother told me I better fight her back." I crossed my hands over my chest and glared at Clara, who was sitting red-faced across from me.

"We will see about that," he said to me. I gave him a *"whatever"* shrug and continued to glare at Clara as she glared back at me. Of course, I knew that in ordinary times a suspension meant trouble. Neither Mama nor Tobie played with us on that issue. This was the one and only time that I was not worried. I had done what my mother told me to do. My fight was sanctioned. I expected Mama to be proud of me for not only fighting Clara back but getting the best of her. This I believed would be especially true after that showdown in front of our house. While I didn't like fighting, after that day, I was never afraid to fight again.

I was upstairs watching television when Mama called me down that evening. Dorothy stopped me in the hallway before I entered the living room. "Georgia just talked to your principal," she warned. I got a little nervous, but I immediately dismissed it. I had to have a clear head when I explained to Mama what happened. I stepped into the living room with confidence. Mama was standing in the doorway of the living room that led to the back. When my eyes reached her face, I knew I was in trouble. My eyes got large as I noticed the extension cord in her hand. I knew that time was of the essence, and I started rattling off the day's events as fast as I could.

"Clara pushed me on the ground and hurt my knee and I got up and I beat her butt." Mama didn't respond to what I had told her.

"Take off your clothes," she demanded.

"But Mama," I pleaded. "I did what you said."

Dorothy interjected, "Georgia, Rae was defending herself against that girl." She ignored us both.

"Take off your clothes, bitch!"

I was scared out of my freaking wits. The only other time she had beaten me without clothes was that time she caught Ethel and I playing in the bathtub. That beating was spontaneous and, while painful, it was quick. When you were called to a beating, you knew that only God could save you from Mama's wrath.

"Take them off or I'll beat them off!"

Tears streamed down my face. My stomach was in knots. Mama was embarrassed that my principal had called home. It was the ultimate sin. My mind was racing trying to figure a way out. Yes, I knew that I was supposed to act a certain way in public, especially with official kinds of people who mostly turned out to be white like my principal. *I didn't fight the principal*, I reasoned to myself; I had fought the person that Mama had instructed me to fight. Maybe if the fight had been off school grounds there would have been a different reaction, but it hadn't. I knew I was defeated. I was caught in Mama's web yet again and I knew there was nothing I could do to change that fact. This beating was going to happen. I didn't want to make matters worse, so I slowly complied. I took off my pants.

"Take them all off," she instructed. I pulled my shirt over my head, and I dropped it on top of my pants. I was humiliated, with tears and snot all over my red face. My heart was pounding, and my head was throbbing.

"Bitch, didn't I tell you to take them all off?"

"But Mama—"

"I don't want to hear that shit," she interrupted. "I'm going to show you about showing your ass at school." I pulled my T-shirt over my head; before it hit the floor, I felt the extension cord across my face.

"MA-MAAA!" I was screaming like a wounded animal.

"I'm gonna show you better than I can tell you!" A hot painful sensation ran down my spine. My body was on fire.

"Please, Mama!" I cried.

"You white bitch," she yelled as the extension cord landed on me in no particular place.

"You think you grown, bitch?!" The extension cord lashed into my flesh like a bird on the windshield of a moving car, hard and bloody. No sooner than she raised her arm the extension cord would land on my frail body with a quickness over and over. Her beating was chaotic and determined. Her words were methodical and calculated and they hit as hard against my spirit as the extension cord did against my body. BITCH! WHITE BITCH! YELLOW BITCH! RED BITCH! I was the bitch of the rainbow coalition— that is, everything but black. I could feel her anger as the extension cord tormented my body. It seemed like Mama was trying to beat something out of me. I believed it was my whiteness because she seemed to hate that the most. My tears became dry and all you could hear was the rhythm of me heaving. I could hear everyone pleading with Mama, but my vision was blurred by my swollen eyes. I could barely muster, "but Mama," out of my mouth. She continued to swing that extension cord into my flesh. I kept turning, trying to minimize my pain, but nothing could counter the hate I felt against my body.

"Georgia, that's enough." I heard Tobie's voice, but I didn't see him. He wasn't home when Mama started beating me. "Georgia, I said that's enough." He grabbed her hand and in that moment of stillness I could focus. He was standing behind her.

"This is my daughter," she hollered at him, trying to break away from the hold he had on her hand. I stood there in my panties; battered and broken.

"I'll kill her ass dead! Dead as she's got to die!"

"Georgia that's enough." Tobie repeated himself and wrestled the extension cord out of her hand. "Rae, go get cleaned up," he said to me. I went into my bedroom, but I had to squeeze past Mama because she was still standing in the doorway. I could feel her anger as our bodies touched and I got a hard cold chill down my spine as she looked at me with disgust.

I stood in front of the dresser looking at myself in the beautiful ornate mirror that I loved so much. What a contradiction my battered body was to the intricate craftsmanship and details that outlined the mirror. I felt unworthy of such beauty. How could this be? Life had presented me with so many contradictions at such a young age. Seeing the ugliness that had taken over my body that day, I began to weep. A deep sorrowful cry came out of my mouth, and it scared me into silence. I traced the two bloody welts covering the left side of my jaw over and over as close as I could get my fingers without touching the wounds. I had been branded like a cow. I was red, bruised, and bleeding. There was no part of me that had not been touched by Mama's violence that day.

I began to sink into despair. For sure, this had been the worst of beatings Mama had ever given to me. She threatened me with death many times, but now, I truly believed that one day she would kill me. Honestly, I don't know what would have happened if Tobie had not stopped her when he did. I truly believe that the ancestors were watching over me. Tobie was the first angel that descended in Mama's path. So, yes, maybe he got a pass for giving me whippings because his humanity showed through at some of the most important times in my life. My saving grace came together slowly in the aftermath of this beating. Something came over me, as if I had been given a jolt of strength to go on. I wanted to regain my dignity and clean my body. Yet, I didn't want to face Mama again and I certainly didn't want to see the helplessness in the eyes of my siblings. Within seconds of those thoughts, Dorothy eased into my room with a damp towel and a pale of warm water.

"You know how Georgia is," she said, "You'll be okay." And I believed her. Dorothy started to clean me up. Her touch was distinct and the opposite of what I had experienced from Mama. Her touch was attentive and careful, gentle, and loving, and I gave in to the moment. She was my Balm in Gilead, a soothing salve to my spirit. Each dab of that towel's softness was a reminder that there was something good in the world, even if it didn't seem to be in Mama. Dorothy finished dressing my wounds and I drifted off to sleep in my bottom bunk bed with my father's picture under my pillow to remind me that someone had loved me.

The next day Ethel went into the living room, like a gangster.

"Georgia, Rae was only defending herself," she said to Mama.

"She should've told me," Mama responded with a chuckle.

"She did," Ethel said. "We all did." She turned and came back into our room, leaving Mama sitting on the sofa smoking a cigarette. I had a one-day suspension and too many scars to go back to school the rest of the week. If you looked closely at my face, you could see those two round circles branded into my jaw well into my teen years. For sure, they were reminders of what Mama had done to me that day. Yet, for me, they became a symbol of what I survived that day and a source of strength of what I could survive in the years to come.

Ten

TAKE ME TO THE WATER

"Just give me a cool drink of water 'fore I diiie."
– Maya Angelou

My spirit was broken, and I was dying inside. That day Tobie stopped Mama's beating and branding, she told him that she had every right to "kill her [as] dead, as she got to die," and it felt as if she was doing exactly that in one way or the other. She was twisted in the head, and it was evident she believed she had every right to do what she wanted to me. She was ruled by the need to control me, and that made me her property rather than her daughter.

I have no idea what Tobie said to her after the beating, but she eased up on the physical abuse. On the flipside, she became manic with the verbal abuse. I tried to fight against the ugliness that came my way, but words are powerful, and spiteful ones linger like the smell of rotten meat. Mama began singling me out more and more. She was relentless. This was especially true as tensions mounted between her and Tobie. In retrospect, I believe her anger was more about her relationship with Tobie slipping away than it was about me. In my struggle to unpack those years, I realize that I was the only thing Mama could control and, at the same time, I was also the only thing she could show Tobie that she had control over. Experts believe the singling out of one child is often a source of displaced anger. In either case, some days I believed she hated me, honest to God. Her words hit harder than twenty beatings combined. Every night I tried to erase her words from my mind. I would float away to my make-believe world, where my father was alive and taking care of me until my real mother could get herself together and we could become a family. Withdrawing into my imaginative world soothed me for incremental moments. However, no amount of disassociation could match the power of Mama's words or the strength of their deliverance.

As God is my witness, I needed someone or something to save me from dying. And to tell you just how God works, She sent a soldier in Her army to plead my case. One Saturday, from the upstairs window, I saw Grandpapa Clayton's shiny silver Cadillac pull up to our house. I knew something was about to happen because Grandmamma Julia rarely visited. I immediately ran outside to greet them, with no coat, hat, or gloves. After I spoke to Grandpapa standing by the car, I eased into the house after Grandmamma. I sat next to her on the sofa as she got comfortable.

"Go get your Mama," she told me. I ran to the back and peeked in Mama's bedroom, saying, "Mama, Grandmamma and Grandpapa are here." Mama put out the old cigarette and lit a new one and sashayed to the front in slow motion, like she was royalty. She stood in the doorway to the living room, looking at Grandmamma. "What kind of shit you on Julia; over here so early on a Saturday morning?" she chuckled.

"Sit down, Georgia Lee. I want to talk to you about that child." My eyes got big. She never called Mama by her full name unless it was serious. Mama sat on the sofa, looked at Grandmamma, rolled her eyes and kept smoking her cigarette. She blew smoke into the air as if to say, *bring it on*. Meanwhile, I slid into Mama's spot at the doorway.

Grandmamma Julia sat very straight, looking regal with her hands folded resting on her pocketbook in her lap. She was wearing a royal blue walking suit with a matching tam adorned by a beautiful gold hat pin with a flower of pearls. Mama wore a faded housecoat, and her eyes were glassy from her morning drinks. She looked worn and weary. The air was thick with contempt—Grandmamma of her daughter's lifestyle and Mama of the mother who wrote her off long before she had a lifestyle that could be held in contempt.

"Georgia," Grandmamma started the conversation slowly. "That child needs to be in church." I sighed, knowing it was going to be the same old topic about Mama going to hell and that I didn't have to follow. I had heard it so many times that I knew it by heart. I left out the back and went upstairs to resume watching the Saturday cartoons. From the upstairs living room every now and then I could hear Mama raising her voice. "I don't give a fuck what you smell!" I heard Mama say, and I knew that Grandmamma had told her she could smell liquor on her breath. It was still morning, which was too early to be drinking, in Grandmamma's opinion.

"You don't run my life—just your mouth!" Mama spat. She was steaming, but I couldn't hear what Grandmamma said. She didn't raise her voice, not once. It got quiet for a moment, and I went to the top of the stairs to try to hear. I couldn't make out a single word. All I know is that Mama stopped hollering and cursing, which meant she was listening to Grandmamma for once in her life. I resolved that whatever they were saying to each other was reconciled between mother and daughter. After about an hour, Mama called to me. I answered and walked down the staircase and stood in the front doorway. She looked deflated and defeated standing in the middle of the living-room floor.

"Go pack your clothes for church," she ordered. For a moment, I was paralyzed by shock. Grandmamma Julia had won. I never saw it coming in a thousand years. I don't know why Mama gave in, but I am certainly glad she did. I generally understood that Grandmamma wanted me to go to church to save me from living my life like Mama had lived hers. What I didn't understand that day—and wouldn't until decades later—was that Grandmamma Julia was my cool drink of water.

"Go on and pack your clothes. You're going with Julia for the weekend."

"Okay, Mama," I said, and ran to my room. I thought about Ethel for a quick second, but I didn't want to rock the boat. I quickly threw whatever I could into a large brown paper bag and stood in the doorway ready to go. I so desperately needed this break from Mama.

I climbed into Grandpapa's Cadillac like Cinderella climbing into her magical carriage. We went straight to the fancy Goldblatt's department store and Grandmamma bought me a church wardrobe, right down to my panties. Goldblatt's had some of the prettiest dresses I had ever seen in my life. Unpacking my clothes at Grandmamma's, I knew that God had sent me a fairy godmother in the least expected person. Grandmamma was more at ease. She didn't fuss at me the way she used to. I'm sure this shift in our relationship was also due to age. I was growing up and developing interests that captured my attention. I played with my paper dolls for hours without jumping out of my seat. As long as I had something to occupy me, I was great. Sometimes, Grandpapa would pick me up on Saturday morning; other times, I would walk. They had purchased a house within just one block of Ashland on 57th about a ten-to-fifteen-minute walk from our house on Hermitage Street.

On those Saturdays, Grandmamma and I sometimes did house chores. She always gave me the responsibility of cleaning the bathroom. Grandpapa would occasionally drop us off at the laundromat and I was Grandmamma's little helper. Other times, Grandmamma baked a cake for church and would let me watch. Cake was the one dessert Mama didn't know how to make from scratch, and Grandmamma allowing me to watch was a treat. She started by beating the sugar and butter together by hand, no less until it was fluffy and light. Then she sifted the flour into a silkiness onto wax paper. Sometimes she allowed me to sift the flour while she watched and patiently gave instructions. Now I wish I had written those recipes down because she was the best cake-maker ever—especially with layered coconut cake. One Christmas, Carmen, Pam's youngest sister, and I ate almost the whole coconut cake. Grandmamma and Grandpapa laughed about it for years. Some of those hands-on instructions have stayed with me and my cake-baking skills are attributed to Grandmamma Julia and Ms. Shartiag, my home economics teacher at Chute Middle School. My pound cake is as good as Grandmamma's, but I'm scared to even try to make a coconut cake. Once the cake was in the oven, Grandmamma would let me lick the bowl and gave me the task of placing the large glass mixing bowl in the sink. These were some of the little things that boosted my confidence.

After chores and lunch, Grandmamma and I studied the Word of God, as she often referred to the Bible. She started teaching me the twenty-third book of Psalms, just as she had taught me the Lord's Prayer. She would say a line and I would repeat the line and we continued this method until I could recite it from memory. After working on the Psalm, we pulled out our Bibles and Sunday school lesson books. She sat in her chair by the entrance of her bedroom door, and we studied our lessons for Sunday together. This was such a contrast from three years earlier, when I sat in the middle of her living room dying on the inside while she read the Bible silently. On Saturday evenings, we did one of two things. We watched The Rock of Ages live gospel-music television show hosted by a Chicago icon, Ms. Isabell Joseph Johnson; then she'd make me a bed on the sofa, and I'd turn in for the night. Or Grandmamma dressed me up and Grandpapa took us to the live studio recording because Grandmamma was a featured artist for the night on Rock of Ages. I was proud sitting in the studio watching Grandmamma Julia sing her tail off. She could have easily been a recording artist.

I don't remember Grandmamma Julia ever saying, "I love you" and she wasn't much of a hugger, but God knows she nurtured me more than her daughter ever did. This time around she certainly rose to the occasion. I know she believed her mission was to save my soul, which, according to the Christian faith, prepares you for eternal life in the hereafter. What she didn't understand, however, was that God used her also to help save my living soul on earth in the here and now. This would also be true for Aunt Lula Mae and Ms. Rachel. The three of them were in my life at a critical time in my development. First and foremost, they provided time away from Mama, which provided me with emotional, physical, and spiritual protection from Mama's wrath. During the times I spent with each of them, I was able to regroup. That alone was like coming up from a body of water to get a breath of fresh air. God knows, I cannot begin to measure what it did for my self-esteem to be physically in a place where I wasn't cursed out all the time. What made the difference was their investment of time and love in me. An open and welcoming house was one thing but providing the food to feed a hungry soul was another. They encouraged me, educated me, and planted seeds that would grow in me. While it may also be true that I was extraordinary in that I just refused to give up, I believe throughout my life, God placed the right people in my path at the right times. What I find remarkable today is the research on childhood trauma runs parallel to my journey. Experts argue that children who live in toxic stress need a safe, predictable space at least part of the time." They call these people, buffers. I call them God's Angels.

When I look back over my life, I know God was watching over me. There is no other explanation for the glimmers of light that shone so brightly within the darkness of my childhood. Trauma can leave you hopeless. But every time I thought I was lost something from deep within would help me find my way. When I was knocked down, I got back up and looked for my North Star to freedom. Over the course of my life's journey my North

Star would show up through so many different people and in so many different ways.

Sunday mornings at Grandmamma's were everything to me. I would wake up to her angelic voice singing the songs of Zion, and the smell of bacon. I ate breakfast and got dressed as quickly so I could watch Grandmamma get dressed. Just like I watched Mama make magic in the kitchen, I watched Grandmamma Julia transform herself from a Campbell Soup factory worker into a stylish gospel singer. I would stand in her doorway as she did her thing. It was wondrous to watch how she carefully put on her stockings. My eyes were glued as she removed the stockings, one at a time, from the beautiful box and placed her hands at the bottom of the stocking, and gently pulled it on her foot and lengthened it smoothly over her shapely leg. Then, methodically, she would connect the stocking to the four hooks that hung from the lace garter belt around her waist. After that one was connected, she repeated the process, removing the remaining stocking from the package and, with the same precision, carefully brought it up her leg to the four opposite dangling hooks and connecting each one. There was something beautiful and sensual in the way she held the stocking and moved it up her leg, as if the stocking and her leg were being joined in matrimony.

Grandmamma's stocking ritual had such an impact on me that I started wearing stockings with a garter at the age of twenty. It became a ritual that represented Grandmamma Julia's gift of her fight for my Christian salvation, which became my life's salvation. The beautiful stockings and garters were financial splurges for me, and well worth it. Each time I laced my legs with those expensive silk stockings it made me feel beautiful and connected to my inner self. Yet, no matter how it made me feel in the moment, it wasn't enough to protect my self-worth and, eventually, my sacred ritual would become a sensual play on my part to capture love. But the intimacy of that beautiful space in time between Grandmamma Julia and me would never be blemished.

On those Sunday mornings, I soaked up every second of Grandmamma. After her stockings were on, she applied her makeup with perfection. I had only seen Mama put on lipstick; therefore, Grandmamma's makeup ritual was fascinating to me. She'd start with this cream foundation that made her skin look smooth and even. Her face powder was amazing — the pretty smell, the beautiful pink puff for applying the powder, and the bright orange and white box that held the Coty Airspun powder. After her face was done, she stepped into her dress and asked me to zip her up. I beamed with happiness! I cherished that responsibility and Grandmamma didn't mind when I popped off my shoes and hopped on the bed to complete the task. Once she reached for her reddish-blonde wig, I knew she was ready. Grandpapa dropped us off at the Old Ship of Zion Missionary Baptist Church, 4727 South Wabash Avenue around the corner from their old apartment. As Grandmamma reached for the door, he said, "Pray for me, nigga woman." Grandmamma slammed the car door, mumbling, "That old heathen! Ain't nothin' but the devil trying to mess with me."

I smiled and shook my head thinking; *the more things change the more they stay the same.* And that adage seemed to hold true for them for many years. In the seconds it took us to walk from the car to the door, she regained her composure and walked through the double doors into the church as the respected Sister Roberts, through and through. I headed to the children Sunday school class, and Grandmamma to the adult class. Sometimes after Sunday school, Grandmamma would let me go with the other children to the candy store around the corner on 47th Street. Next to chocolate and caramels, red chewy candy was my favorite. I would get those five cent boxes of Red Hots and Hot Tamales and by the time church started, my tongue was red.

Everything about church was amazing, the energy, the people, the music. Believe me when I tell you, I took it all in. Grandmamma's popularity automatically made me popular; everyone wanted to know Julia Roberts's "grandbaby." It was fun being popular but the person who had the greatest impact on me was the senior pastor, Reverend Otis Anderson, Jr. No matter what he was doing, as soon as he saw me, he opened his arms wide—just like my grandfather use to do—and I'd run and fall into them, and he hugged me into himself. I felt safe in his arms. After he released me, he never failed to ask me, "How you doing today, Rae Rae?" Then I smiled and twirled around in one of my pretty chiffon dresses.

Reverend Anderson was one charismatic man. He was a young pastor of thirty-eight. He was short in stature but larger than life to me. He was my complexion, with a thick, black, sexy mustache. At that time, I had no idea what he was saying—only that he sure sounded good saying it. I loved to watch him preach and, Lord, that man could sing. The command of his voice was magical, cycling up and down and then down again and repeating the cycle to effectively make his point. He talked a lot about salvation and the love of Christ. It sure sounded good to my young ears. The congregation would stand up and egg him on with a resounding, "Preach, PREACHER!" And I joined the crowd. Grandmamma never gave me that *"you're in trouble"* look for standing, so I went with the flow. People were shouting and hollering, and I watched in awe. I heard the other children laughing about adults getting the Holy Ghost and I was curious enough one day to ask Grandmamma what the Holy Ghost was. She said, "It is God's spirit moving inside of you." That sounded wonderful to me and tried to figure out why they were laughing but I didn't ask her about that because I was no trick; I didn't tell on my friends. I heard Reverend Anderson also refer to the Holy Spirit as the Comforter. Even at ten, the Holy Ghost sounded good to me—that is, the possibility that I, too, could feel God moving inside of me and providing me with comfort, and what that could mean for my life. I studied my Sunday school lesson each week because I hoped it would help the Holy Ghost hurry up and come to me.

After each sermon, Reverend Anderson walked out of the pulpit with the mic in his hand. As the music played softly, he proposed, "Won't you come?" The choir would sing softly, *"Come to Jesus – Come to Jesus – Come to Jesus just now."* Reverend Anderson extended his hands in front of him. "The doors of the church are open. Is there one?" I heard the congregation joining in with the choir's refrain: *"Come to Jesus – Come to Jesus – Come to Jesus just now. He will save you – He will save you – He will save you just now."*

One day he looked my way and that big, beautiful smile pulled me out of my seat. I could see Grandmamma as she got out of her seat in the choir stand. I started to walk down the aisle.

"That's my baby!" I heard Grandmamma cry out.

I got a little nervous and slowed my pace and almost stopped, but Reverend Anderson beckoned me to him. I made it to the front, and he opened his arms wide, and I landed in his embrace. I heard Grandmamma's strong voice cry out again, "Thank You, Jesus! Thank You, Jesus!" Reverend Anderson asked the deacons of the church to accept me as a candidate for baptism. I held my breath waiting and about to pee my pants if they said no. One of them spoke up and made a motion to accept me, another deacon seconded the motion and the church voted *yes* collectively, saying, "Amen!" At the end of church, Grandmamma gave me a hug, smothering me into herself.

When I got home that evening, I told Mama that I joined church and asked if she would come to see me get baptized. "We'll see," she said. I pretty much knew what that meant, and I just went to bed. I had to wait until the first Sunday of the following month for my baptism and I continued to ask Mama if she would come. It was an evening program and I hoped that she would come because she wouldn't have to get up early that morning. She continued to say maybe, and I continued to ask on those days I deemed her to be in a good mood. That Saturday morning before my baptism I reminded Mama before I left to go to Grandmamma's. She looked at me and I knew to keep it moving.

When I arrived at Grandmamma's, she had the prettiest yellow chiffon dress I had ever seen laid out for me on her bed. She pressed and curled my hair into a Shirley Temple ponytail. I felt so special.

It was a long day—two worship services with food in between. When it was time for evening worship service, the mothers of the church took me back into the choir room and changed me out of my dress into a long white robe, with a white swimming cap. Grandmamma stood and watched as they took care of my baptism needs. There were others being baptized that day and we all walked to the front of the church up by the choir stand to the pool.

As we made our way, I started looking for Mama. The music started playing and the congregation sang softly, "*Take me to the water – Take me to the water – Take me to the water, to be baptized.*" There was a girl before me, and my eyes grew big as Reverend Anderson dunked her into the pool and brought her back up with a quickness. I got butterflies in my stomach as the deacon picked me up and stood me in the pool in front of Reverend Anderson. He looked down at me and smiled.

"It's okay, Rae Rae," he whispered as he turned me to face the congregation.

I told the butterflies in my stomach to be still, and I took a deep breath to calm down.

"Sister Roberts and the rest of the family, please stand," Reverend Anderson requested. Grandmamma stood, and so did Grandpapa Clayton. I just grinned when I recognized him in the audience standing so proudly. Mama still had not arrived. Reverend Anderson prayed and then raised his hand over my head. Looking back on that moment, the power and authority in his voice could not be mistaken for anything other than the power of God working through him, and I felt a chill go up my spine. Nothing could take away the joy I felt in that pool—not even the absence of Mama. Pastor Anderson spoke slowly and with an exaggeration that he had not done with the girl prior to me.

"In obedience to the great head of the church," he said, and raised his hand over my head.

"And upon the profession of your faith, my child." He paused.

"I baptize you, my daughter." Another pause.

"In the name of the Father…" Then, he raised his voice.

"In the Name …. of the Son …. and in the name of the Holy Ghost!"

Just as quickly as he finished the words "Holy Ghost," I had been dunked into the pool and was already standing with water dripping down my face, smiling from ear to ear with unexplained tears running down my cheeks.

"You okay, Rae Rae?" I shook my head up and down as the deacon picked me up out of the pool and handed me off to one of the mothers of the church.

Grandmamma was crying and praising God, "*Thank You, Jesus! Thank You, Jesus!*" In the backdrop, you could hear the congregation singing "*None but the righteous, none but the righteous, none but the righteous shall see God.*"

By the second verse, someone had handed Grandmamma the mic and I felt like all the angels in heaven were singing to me as I made my way to change out of the wet clothes. I changed into my pretty yellow dress, but my hair had gotten a little wet and my Shirley Temple spirally ponytail had converted into a puff ball. I didn't care. I was all smiles.

The baptism service ended with communion. In the months that I had been coming to church with Grandmamma, I was never permitted to partake in communion because the Baptist doctrine believes communion is only for the converted and baptized Christians. Those Sundays when they served Communion, I protested as the trays were passed around me. Grandmamma would respond, "After you get baptized, baby."

That evening I stood in front of the congregation, my smile still beaming. This was my day. I was a full member of the Christian family. I now belonged to a family that wanted me. I cried tears of happiness as Reverend Anderson narrated, "This is the body that was broken for you: take and eat." I placed the small white cracker in my mouth. It was dry and chalky.

"This is the blood that was shed for you: take and drink." I drank the tiny cup of grape juice. It was sweet and I licked my lips.

I was too young to fully understand what it meant to become a Christian. The congregation was singing and clapping hands: "*I know it was the blood - I know it was the blood - I know it was the blood, for me. One day when I was lost, He died upon the cross - And I know it was the blood that saved me!*"

If I had not found the church when I did, I don't know how I would have made it through the war zone that I called Mama. Church became my bomb shelter, providing me temporary relief for the rest of my time living with Mama. It was the water that quenched my thirst and revived my spirit. What I know for sure today is that God heard my cry, literally, and created a path for me that shined a light to help me maneuver through the darkness in my life.

Eleven

BEING FAST

"We teach girls shame; close your legs, cover yourself,
we make them feel as though by being born female
they're already guilty of something."
—Chimamanda Ngozi Adichie

If I could freeze one moment of happiness with my siblings, it would be watching television in the upstairs living room cuddled under blankets on a cold winter night. Mama never came upstairs—and that meant our space was not polluted with the air of fear. We would laugh and cut-up without judgment of who we were, what we did or how we did it. We were one for all and all for one. It didn't matter what we were watching on the television; we had fun. Everyone loved watching the *Svengoolie* monster movies. I was a scaredy-cat. The monsters seemed real with the lights off and I would bury my face into the blankets when it seemed like the monster was going to jump out of the television and get us.

On movie night, everyone was always jockeying for the best spot in the living room. Sitting next to Junior, I felt like I had won a prize and I wore that badge of honor with a big smile across my face. I always felt special sitting next to him on the sofa, sharing a blanket. The third from the oldest, he was the cool big brother who could do no wrong in my eyes. He never made me feel like I was a nuisance, and that alone endeared him to me. I cannot recall him ever giving me that older-sibling attitude that said, "Girl, get out of my face," like I did with Allen and Juan. In my defense, my two little brothers got on my last freaking nerve. This was especially true of Allen. It never failed after he had spent his allowance, he would catch you walking out of the candy store and, before you could even get your bearings straight, he would yell "cobs" on your candy. If you weren't careful, he would snatch your shit and haul ass. He was a pain in the butt. I, on the other hand, had no flaws in my own eyes, although everyone else seemed to think that I talked too much and was a Little Miss Know-It-All. Junior, unlike my other siblings, never said I talked too much, which made me love him even more. I don't recall him ever telling me I was his favorite sister, but I certainly felt like I was.

On one of those Friday nights, Junior rested his hand on my thigh under the blanket. I didn't give it a second thought. We had been in close proximity before. Often when I braided his hair, as with everyone else, he rested his arms on my thighs while sitting on the floor between my legs. So, when he began stroking my thigh over my clothes, I didn't protest because it felt good. It had a calming effect and my normal fidgeting ceased with the magic I believed to be in his fingers. He would touch me in intervals, scattered throughout the movie. He stroked up, down, and around my thighs. The second someone moved for any reason, he snatched his hand away.

That blanket thrown over us was a symbol of concealment. It hid our bodies; it hid the ugly desecration that Junior thrust on me; and it hid the fear and shame that enveloped me as he groomed me for his pleasure. I can't tell you exactly when I became the object of Junior's pleasure, but I know his abuse began sometime in my second school year at Earle Elementary. I was ten years old and in the fifth grade. I don't remember Junior's age, only that he was in high school. Even that is a little fuzzy because I just didn't remember my siblings' grades as they matriculated. My calculation puts him somewhere between his sophomore and junior year. I've given what Junior did to me a lot of thought over the years. My gut tells me that the molestation began as an easy opportunity—not as a premeditated act. It would, however, become a calculated act based on access. The more successful his access to me; the more deliberate the molestation became. In the end, how it started does not take away any of the damage it did to me or the fact that it was a boundary that should have never been crossed.

Junior eventually made his way to the innermost part of my body. I could feel the pressure of his hand through my pants as he weighed down and around my clitoris. I didn't know what to think. Nor did I understand what he was trying to do. It didn't feel as good as his fingers did stroking up and down my thigh. I didn't dare open my mouth. I didn't want him to be mad at me. Each time we sat on that sofa; he pushed the limits to see what he could get away with. With time and precision, he became confident—and, with confidence, he became brazen, bold, and dominant.

The first time he slipped his hand down my pants, I tried to push it away. I knew that this was *being fast,* and I didn't want to get in trouble. He pushed my hand back and it scared me, and I stopped my protest. I don't know how many days or how long he stroked my clitoris through my panties, but in time I started to relax; once I relaxed, there was no turning back. When he moved my panties to the side with his hand under my pants, I protested yet again.

"Junior," I whispered, grabbing his hand. He looked down at me and shook his head, like, *You know better.* The friction of his fingers on my dry clitoris felt weird and uncomfortable, but he massaged me until my body said yes. Whew! I felt a sensation that jilted the pleasure senses of my brain, and my protest entirely vanished. My ten-year-old self was reeling in ecstasy, but my fear of *being fast* never left me.

The sensations I felt were remotely familiar to me and my mind worked overtime trying to figure out where and how I knew that tingly feeling that ran through my body. It was reminiscent of how I felt under the porch with the little boy on Swann Street. That incident seemed so distant, like an eternity ago, and the most vivid memory was not the feeling or the little boy, but rather the beating from hell I got from Mama. Remembering the beating gave me a cause to pause, but I didn't voice it to Junior. I didn't know what to say or do, so I dismissed the little boy and the beating—at least, in the moment—and concentrated on how Junior's hand between my legs made me feel. The feeling, however, was so intense that I couldn't dismiss my curiosity about what Junior was doing and how this was *being fast.* The only other times I had felt this good was when Aunt Lula Mae had given me Fannie Mae chocolates when I visited her. No joke: I equated Junior stroking my clitoris with how I felt the times I savored a piece of chocolate in my mouth to get the fullness of the flavor. Pleasure is pleasure—period. When I put it all together, there was no misery in the memory of chocolate like there was when I got caught with the little boy under the porch. My skill at diverting from the bad stuff served me well in my current situation, and I clung only to the good stuff because it made me feel good.

What I didn't understand was that my body had failed me. What I was feeling was a natural response to Junior fondling me. The body does not ask for permission; it simply responds. In this way, Junior had failed me, too. He awakened a part of me that should never have been activated at such a young age. I didn't understand sex and how the body worked, but I understood clearly that Junior's hand between my legs slowly zapped every second of peace that being upstairs had once brought me.

The first time Junior told me to meet him upstairs, I looked at him like he had two heads. I didn't want to get caught and get in trouble. I didn't want to *be fast;* I just wanted my big brother's love and affection.

"You trust me, don't you?" he asked.

"Yes…." I said, slowly, trying to buy myself some time. I knew what he wanted to do, but I thought going upstairs would be the death of me. This had nothing to do with trust; in fact, I had long stopped trusting him. Junior always got his way, and I didn't have any power to say no. It was a horrible position for him to impose on me; nevertheless, that's exactly what he did. He worked out a scheme to get me alone like he was sneaking a girlfriend—and not his little sister—in the house.

When we were on the sofa, I thought of clever ways to stop him—not because I didn't like it, but because I didn't want to *be fast.* I didn't want to get in trouble. I just wanted it all to stop. I wiggled and slid my legs close, grabbing his hand with my bony thighs and squeezing them into myself as tightly as I could. He leaned in and whispered, "It is okay." I stayed closed and rigid.

"I'm going to get in trouble," I muttered. And as if I hadn't said a word, he persisted, prying my thighs open with his other hand.

"It's okay," he repeated, but his reassurance did nothing to relax me. Meeting Junior upstairs became a thing and so did my fear of being caught. With each passing day, it became so overwhelming that I wanted to disappear—but there was no place to go. Mama had allowed the husband of a deceased friend to live with us. When Mr. Tom moved into the house, he took Ethel and my bedroom and displaced us to the upstairs sleeping quarters. Since Mr. Tom had my bedroom and we were not allowed in the downstairs living room unless Mama and Tobie were there watching television, I had no place to hide. The best that I could I think to do was to protest. I decided that the next time Junior told me to meet him upstairs, I was not going to do it. I tried to stick to my decision, but all he had to do was give me that look that told me, "Girl, stop playing," and my people-pleasing self would comply.

He continued to push the limits. On one of those days upstairs in the TV room, I was wearing one of my play dresses. Junior slid my dress up and pulled my panties down to my knees. It scared the daylights out of me. I also knew it was as wrong as two left feet. He really was trying to get my ass beat to hell and back.

"Uh-unnn." I uttered my only known objection and reached for his hand on my vagina. He pushed it away and I stopped protesting. I thought if I protested too much, he wouldn't love me anymore. This time what he was doing now seemed different. I felt a little discomfort. I couldn't explain it back then if my life depended on it, but now that I understand sex, he had moved from the top of my clitoris to the opening of my vagina. He continued to massage me, and after a while I started to feel the moisture like I had previous times as I settled into the mixture of pleasure and fear. Suddenly, pleasure turned into pain.

"That hurts," I cried. He had pushed his finger inside of me. Through reflex, I pulled my vagina back with the thrust of my hips. He pulled his finger out of my vagina as quickly as he had put it in, got up, and left the house. After that day, I stepped up my measures to protect myself. Pushing his hand away and squeezing my legs closed were futile. I stopped watching television in the upstairs living room alone. I spent as much time as I could at Teresa's house after school if everyone was not yet home. Once I guessed a good time when the house should be full, I left Teresa's and went home feeling somewhat safe. My efforts were never enough. When I least expected it, Junior would show up. I had to finally face the truth: there was no stopping Junior. He made me his mission and would magically appear whenever I was alone. I didn't understand how the two things I enjoyed the most Junior's attention, and the upstairs living room could have gone so terribly wrong. They were both stolen from me within the blink of an eye. Every chance Junior got; he took me for his pleasure.

One time while he stroked me, he reached over and placed my hand on his penis through his pants. It felt like a *freaking* brick, and I snatched my hand back. He gently reached for my hand and placed it back on his penis, pleading, "Rub it for me, please?" So, I did. Periodically, he took his other hand and squeezed it on top of mine and told me to rub harder. With my hand on his penis a war raged inside of me. I was frightened of both what I understood and what I didn't. What I had come to know by this time was that touching like this was *being fast*. I just couldn't name sex or its connection to it, and I absolutely couldn't name this particular kind of sex for what it was—sexual molestation.

I also understood that *being fast* would get me a beating straight to hell and back, but I still hadn't figured out why. Holding Junior's penis was like holding dynamite and there would not be a moment of peace until he was done. After he was satisfied, he dropped the enviable bombshell: "You know if you tell, we will both get in trouble." I shook my head up and down, even though I didn't completely agree with him. I had no reference to indicate the chances that Junior would get in trouble. I only knew for sure—at least, with Mama—that if she found out I was *being fast*, I would get my ass beat. I surmised that Junior wouldn't get in trouble because I had never heard anyone refer to a boy as *fast*. I tried and I couldn't figure out why or how he would get in trouble. Frankly, if there were even a tiny possibility that he would, he didn't have to worry about me because I was deathly afraid of what Mama would do if she found out. Just thinking about the beating I got for fighting in school made me want to crawl under a rock. And, God forbid, if Tobie beat me with the red water hose at Mama's behest.

One day Junior said, "You don't tell, and I won't tell." At the time I don't think he said it as a threat, but to reassure me. But his resolution hit me like tons of bricks. It was the first time I realized he held the power of a secret—his secret—over me. Locking me into his secret was the greatest power he had over me, and I held onto it like my life depended on it. Once I had that revelation, there was nothing that he could ask me to do to which I would say no.

My fifth-grade year was shot to hell. I cannot recall one thing about that year in school. Junior dominated my life, from my body to my thoughts. And if that wasn't enough, Mama gave me the responsibility to help take care of Mr. Tom. I knew Mr. Tom and his wife before Mama met Tobie, they would keep me when Mama was running the streets.

I have no idea how old he was, but if I had to guess I would say Mr. Tom was somewhere between sixty-five and seventy. He had difficulty walking on his own and held on to something as he moved. Although frail, his frame stood about six-foot-three-inches tall. He had curly hair and light brown skin. He was probably handsome in the days before alcohol ravaged his body. I never knew why Tobie permitted him to come to live with us. I only know that Mr. Tom signed his Social Security check over to Mama every month. Tobie was not money-hungry like Mama, so maybe he felt sorry for him. Who knows? But his move into the house was disruptive for me. Ethel moved her clothes upstairs, so she did not have to be bothered. On the other hand, I had to go in to get my clothes every day, with his eyes watching my every move. I hated going into Mr. Tom's room because it smelled like urine and cigarettes. It was a dreadful environment, like a one-room dive in a boarding house. In addition to the smell, it was always dark because he kept the window shade drawn. The TV provided the only light. Mama gave me the responsibility to feed Mr. Tom at lunch because Tobie told her his kids were not going to do it. I tried to get out of it; I whined and begged but there was no one else. I didn't want to overplay the hand Mama had dealt me, so I shut the hell up and did as I was told. The routine was easy because I had moved from the trailer classroom to the main building and school was less than a block from my house. However, I resented sacrificing my lunchtime. While my classmates were eating and shooting the breeze, I had to come home and make Mr. Tom's lunch. I made his sandwich as quickly as I could, then sat on the downstairs sofa waiting until he finished so I could collect his plate and run back to school.

One afternoon while waiting on Mr. Tom to finish eating, Junior walked in. I was shocked. He never mentioned to me that he was coming, but as soon as I started to say something he motioned his head to the stairway. I followed him upstairs and watched as he unzipped his pants and pulled his hard penis through the sleeve of his boxer shorts and sat on the sofa. I was unable to move. My eyes were frozen on his wee-wee. He gave me that look, and I knew to sit my ass down next to him. Immediately, he grabbed my hand and placed it on his penis and told me to rub. It felt harder than when I rubbed it with his pants on. I was curious because it looked nothing like the little boy's wee-wee when we were under the porch. Juniors was big and warm and hard and soft all at the same time. It felt somewhat like one of my dolls whose body was hard, and head was soft. I rubbed around his penis, and he placed his hand over mine. He guided my hand up and down. "Like this," he instructed.

After I got the swing of it, he laid his head back to enjoy being pleasured. After a while, I looked up at the wall clock and panicked; I was going to be late. I heard Mama's previous warning in my mind clear as day: "You had bet' not mess around getting back to school from lunch." I let his penis go and jumped up in a flash.

"I gotta get back to school!" I ran out the door and down the stairs, leaving him in the same position. There was no protest from him that day. He just showed up the next day, and the next, and the next after that. I tried pleading with Mama to let someone else feed Mr. Tom for a while, but she wouldn't budge. The pattern was set, and I had no way out. The only good thing was that Junior stopped showing up around the house when I least expected. That switch not only reduced some of my anxiety about being caught, but it also gave me back some of my personal space. It felt like a victory—even if it was a small one. With this new arrangement, however, Junior had the freedom to do as he pleased with me. With Mama and Tobie at work, he didn't have a reason to be cautious; as a result, he became self-assured, bordering on arrogant. He took full advantage of having the house to himself. Mr. Tom apparently wasn't an issue for Junior because he only left his room to go to the bathroom across the hall.

I wondered how he was able to come home from school at my lunchtime, but I never asked. These thoughts seem relevant now, but then, the situation was what it was. While I was uncomfortable with Junior coming home to meet me, I never thought about not showing up to feed Mr. Tom. If Mr. Tom told Mama I didn't come to make his lunch, there would be hell to pay with my ass.

After the first time, Junior instructed me to meet him upstairs immediately after I gave Mr. Tom lunch. As soon as my feet landed on the top stair, I saw him on the sofa waiting. He must have been pleasuring himself or anticipating me because he was already hard when I sat down. My body continued to fail me; the moment he touched my clitoris I became sexually aroused, but I had long passed the point where I enjoyed it. I just sat there wanting him to hurry up and finish. That first time he pulled his penis out and had me to pleasure him, had became a game-changer. I could never again relax as I had done before in those early days when he simply played around between my legs. His power over me rested in the fear of Mama's wrath, and it was greater than the magic in his fingers; but nothing eased the discomfort in my soul over what he was doing to me.

On one of those days when I ended at the top of the stairs, I didn't see Junior on the sofa. As soon as he heard my hard walking steps, he called out, "I'm in here." I followed his voice to the kitchen, and he was lying in the sofa bed under the covers. "Get in here with me," he said.

Déjà vu smacked me in the face. That's what I had asked the little boy to do under the porch. I got the beating from hell that day. I didn't move.

"Come here," he demanded. I walked slowly to the side of the sofa bed that was opposite where he lay.

"Get in here with me."

"I don't know, Junior," I mumbled, tears welling in my eyes.

"Girl, do what I told you."

Still, I didn't move.

"It's okay. I promise you," he coaxed, this time, in a softer tone.

"I don't know, Junior," I said again.

"You trust me, don't you?" He asked.

I didn't trust one word he was saying, but I knew he was getting mad. By then, his promises didn't mean jack shit to me. He had proven himself to be untrustworthy time and again. I knew this was trouble and my gut told me to run; however, his hold on me was overpowering. I didn't know how to do anything other than what he asked. I shook off my fears and sat on the bed.

"Take off your clothes," he ordered.

I undressed down to my panties and undershirt and got under the covers. As soon as I pulled the covers up, he reached over and pulled off my panties and threw them on the floor. I could feel the heat coming from his body and it felt good. I relaxed. The sensations from his nakedness and his touches between my legs were amazing. My young body was reacting in ways it never had before. I was besieged by the heat radiating from his body. All my fear and anxiety dissipated, and I was caught up as he manipulated my body with his hands. Suddenly, he knocked me out of my pleasure zone when he shifted his body on top of mine, consuming me into himself. He was heavy and I tried to push him up a little, but he didn't budge. He shifted only enough so that he could reach my vagina. He placed his upper body in a way that smothered my face and chest. I didn't want to complain but I finally managed to say, "I can't breathe."

He shifted his chest to the side, giving me some air. I could feel his thigh as he pushed my legs open. My mind started racing. I hadn't done any of this with the little boy. I had only laid on top of him and we moved around. I had no point of reference, so I took a deep breath to calm my little nerves. Junior reached down to my vagina, and I could feel him guiding his penis inside of me.

"It hurts," I pleaded, trying to grab his hand. But I could reach only as far as his arm. He pushed my hand back and continued to open my vagina with his penis. I felt like I was going to crack open. It hurt worse than any beating Mama had ever given me. He pushed the fullness of himself into me. Nothing could ease the pain I felt. I stiffened and grabbed his back, holding on to him for dear life as his rhythm picked up.

"Ohhhhhh," he moaned.

My mouth was dry. I couldn't speak and I couldn't move so I just held on, willing it to be over. He continued to push himself into me faster and faster.

"Ohhhhhh!" he cried out and crashed onto my body in the aftermath of his orgasm.

I didn't know why he had stopped, but I was glad he did. I tried to push him off me. He didn't move. Finally, he got up and his penis slid out of my vagina. As he pulled all the way out and started to get up, his penis dripped onto my stomach. He didn't say a mumbling word—just grabbed his pants and went to the bathroom. When I heard the door shut, I rolled out of the bed. I felt like I was on fire smack-dab between my legs. I shook off the pain. I didn't want to be late getting back to school. He was still in the bathroom when I walked down the stairs, grabbed my coat off the living room sofa and walked back to school.

At our bathroom break, blood and semen was dripping between my legs and thighs were sticky, like I had spread glue on them. I took some toilet paper, dipped it in the toilet, and wiped my raw vagina. The cold felt good and eased some of my pain. I did it again and again until it was time to go back into my classroom. That evening I wanted to tell, and I almost did. That is until Junior politely reminded me: "If you tell, we will both get in trouble." I didn't know what to make of him anymore. I just knew that once Junior penetrated me, that was a hurt that could never be taken back. My vagina was throbbing like a jackhammer from the pain he caused, and all he had for me was a threat on top of my pain.

I didn't even know the word *rape* but, in that moment, what Junior had done was to guarantee that his secret remained safe. That night, curled up in my bed, I knew that the special bond I thought I had with him had turned dark. I would come to understand it was never a bond in the first place. My sincere big brother-little sister relationship was one of grooming and manipulation for Junior's pleasure.

Junior continued to show up at lunchtime. Where he led, I followed. One day, he had not arrived by the time Mr. Tom finished his lunch. When I went to fetch Mr. Tom's plate, he was lying in bed holding his limp penis in the air.

"Get on top," Mr. Tom said.

I didn't think about it, I just did exactly what I believed I was supposed to do. Reminiscent of the day I removed my dress in the room with Mama and her date, I took off my pants and panties in one swoop and climbed on top of him. He was so tall that the top of my head could only reach the middle of his chest as he pulled me up until my bottom reached his penis. I became nauseated. He smelled bad, but even the strong smell of urine didn't make me stop. It was as if someone had hypnotized me. I felt his penis rise on my stomach. It was longer and larger than Junior's and that was scary, but I reminded myself this was what I was supposed to do. He couldn't find the opening of my vagina and started grinding and I followed suit. I felt his hardness and he wrapped his arms tightly around my body in a bear hug. After a while, I started to feel that tingly feeling I always felt with Junior and for some reason it made me feel weird about what was happening. I tried to get up, but he held me tighter and tighter, grinding harder and harder. I stop moving and laid there like a log. Finally, he released himself on my stomach and his body went limp. I crawled off, grabbed my bottoms, and went to the bathroom. I took some toilet paper and wiped him off my stomach, but I couldn't wipe the stench that had settled over my body and spirit. I went back to school smelling like sex and urine. After that, Mr. Tom popped his penis up periodically when I brought him lunch and sometimes even at dinner. I would drop his plate of food on the tray and pull the fuck up out of his room. I never climbed on top of him again.

The anxiety I felt each time Mr. Tom popped up his penis made me want to pee my pants and it was equal to how I felt about Mama learning that I had been *fast*. I'm not sure how I knew Mr. Tom should not be popping his penis up at me, but I knew. Maybe because of his age and our history, I believed that he should know better than to make me *be fast*. I wanted to tell Mama, but that thought was cautionary. Mama always found some way to flip the script. I had also witnessed her beat the heck out of Mr. Tom for shitting on himself. I didn't know how the wind would blow if I told. I figured I could tolerate his wee-wee pop-up every now and then rather than watch Mama beat this helpless man.

Without even fully understanding the hurt being done to me, I knew that both Junior and Mr. Tom had hurt me. There was something in my gut that said it was terribly wrong in a different way than *being fast*. I didn't know how to articulate what they had done or how to say it in a way to save me from Mama. Knowing that she already had such a negative opinion of *being fast*, I knew that without a doubt, if my hurt was interpreted by Mama as my fault, it would be the death of me.

As we got closer to the end of the school year, Junior slowly changed things. The molestation and rape were sporadic until he stopped altogether. I was relieved. He spent most of his time running the streets and I was able to breathe without the fear of him. All I had to do was keep his secret, and that is exactly what I did for nearly two decades. The damage had been done. With no point of reference to sex and rape, I was left to believe that something was wrong with me. It would be the most devastating part of the hurt: I now believed Mama's claim that I was *fast*.

I was glad when Mama told Ethel and I that we were going away on a summer vacation. Lord knows, I needed a break from Hermitage Street. I needed to go someplace where I didn't have to face the fact that I was this horrible little girl or face the two people who proved that fact to be true: Junior and Mr. Tom. Ultimately, I hoped that being away from them both would cure me of the defect of *being fast*.

Twelve

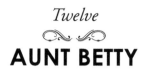

AUNT BETTY

"Abuse is never deserved, it is an exploitation of innocence and physical disadvantage, which is perceived as an opportunity by the abuser.**"**
—Lorraine Nilon

L ooking out the airplane window was transcendent. I couldn't believe Mama and Tobie had allowed Ethel and me to travel by ourselves. Honestly, I was even more surprised that Tobie allowed Ethel to go in the first place since we were visiting Mama's relatives in Red Bank, New Jersey. He was drawing the line more and more between Mama and his children lately. I was so glad that he had agreed. With Ethel by my side, I didn't have any doubts that I would be just fine. Her confidence continued to rub off on me, and her going into this new environment with me reduced the anxiety I was feeling.

That day the clouds were magical and, quite frankly, the plane could have dropped me off smack-dab in the middle. I could have stayed in the sky forever. Gazing out at the beautiful clouds, it seemed like the most peaceful place on Earth. I felt like I was at heaven's door, and I drifted into a daydream. My mind went to Pastor Anderson, who often talked about God sitting high and looking low, and we were definitely high above the clouds. If God's house was anything like this, then count me in. I could hear Pastor Anderson saying, "No more crying there." At that moment, all I could think about was no more Mama. No more *bitch* this and *bitch* that. Each Sunday, listening to Pastor Anderson gave me hope for a different life. He also said to *pray for those who hurt you,* and that's exactly what I did; but I ended up praying more for Mama to stop hurting me than I prayed for her goodwill. My prayers about Mama went unanswered, but I never gave up hope. Pastor Anderson made it clear that God's timing is not our timing, which meant that, one day, Mama would love me as I loved her—just not right now. That day in the clouds was reassuring. It was as if God whispered, *I got you, baby girl.*

I didn't know the Lawrences whom we were visiting and, honestly, Mama didn't know them either. Earlier that year, she had connected with her father, Robert Lawrence Sr., whom she hadn't seen since she was a little girl. Robert Sr. was retired from a career in the military. While stationed near Grandmamma Julia's hometown of Seal, Alabama, they hooked up and made Mama. One look at Robert Sr. and there was no doubt Mama was his daughter. They were twins. He had her smooth dark chocolate skin and those beautiful high cheekbones. He was short and stocky, with salt-and-pepper hair. His personality was laid-back, and he spent most of his time in his room off the kitchen where he slept. Like Mama, he was no stranger to hard liquor, but I liked him because he was kind and always had a smile on his face. His wife, Ms. Tina, was "grandmotherly" in both demeanor and actions.

Robert Sr. lived up to the Temptations song *Papa was a Rolling Stone.* With Ms. Tina, he had a son, Robert Jr., who was a taller version of himself. He had another adult daughter, Mary, who was closer to Mama's age, by a different woman. Mary lived nearby in Jersey City and was the short stocky version of Robert Sr., while Mama was the taller version. Then there was Betty. As the story goes, she was conceived during the Korean War. I don't know for sure how she landed in Red Bank without her mother, but I heard that Robert Sr. went back after the war and brought his daughter home for Ms. Tina to raise. I would say that Ms. Tina had to be a remarkable woman, raising another woman's daughter, birthed from infidelity, even if she seemed unremarkable day to day. Betty didn't look like anyone I had ever seen. Her complexion was light, with a yellow undertone. She was of medium build, about a size twelve. If you took the slight kink out of her hair and the Negro out of her nose, you could have taken her for a Korean woman right off the bat. She had just graduated from high school and often wore her school ribbon on her overalls.

With Ethel and me added to Robert Sr., Ms. Tina, Robert Jr., and Betty, their two-story home was full. While Ms. Tina's hospitality was genuine, there was something dark about the house, especially the first floor—literally and figuratively. The sun porch caught all the light, shielding it from inside so that the downstairs was eerie, and the darkness left me unsettled. Each time I walked in from outside, I had to adjust my eyes. The heavy dark wood furniture only added to the gloom that consumed the first floor. The formal dining room was cramped with a mahogany dinette set and a large sideboard. I loved the pretty wooden stairwell. It was carpeted all the way up to the second floor where the rest of the family slept, each in his or her own room: Ms. Tina, Robert Jr., and Betty.

Being in Red Bank was a new experience. On the surface, it was straight out of *Leave It to Beaver*. We had dinner together and often sat on the sun porch in the evening. The dinner table was alive with chatter and Robert Sr. engaging us with his charm. Red Bank was a lazy middle-class town that sat on the Navesink River. At the turn of the century, it became a thriving town, connecting the Atlantic Ocean to worldwide commerce; after World War II, it boomed. Neighborhoods were neat and uniform, like those that popped up all over the country after World War II. I liked the easiness in Red Bank and being with the Lawrences. It was a wonderful reprieve from Mama.

The most memorable moment of the trip was the day Robert Sr. took us crabbing for blue crabs. It was exciting each time he pulled the net from the water full of the pretty crabs with the bright blue tint on their claws. I had fallen in love with them, but I didn't translate them into food until we got home, and Ms. Tina plopped them into a gigantic pot of hot steaming water on the stove. I was horrified as the crabs tried to climb their way to freedom. I could relate to their misery—the tangle of helpless clambering for an escape, to no avail. After witnessing them be put to death, I had no desire to sample the "delicacies." Everyone was encouraging me to eat. In the meantime, Ethel was already enjoying them, as Ms. Tina gave instructions on how to dig the meat out of the crab. Ms. Tina turned to me. "Rae, it's only food," she reassured me.

"But I'm scared," I whined. Ms. Tina said, "Just try it one time for me and, if you don't like them, you don't have to eat any more." I picked at one on the paper she had spread out on the table. Robert Sr. said, "Girl, all that work we did catching these crabs—just give them one try."

I didn't want to explain that catching them was part of the problem, so I acquiesced. I picked the smallest piece and dipped it into the butter. I figured if I didn't like it, I wouldn't have to suffer much. It was a surprising delight, and I ate more. Still, the taste never changed how badly I felt about how they died, and I can count on one hand how many times I have eaten crab since. Crab cakes are the best I can do, and, to this day, I cannot pick a lobster out of a tank and have it cooked for my pleasure. Watching those crabs die was the beginning of my love for all of God's creatures. I believe this was the emergence of the Dr. Doolittle in me.

Ethel went home after the first week. I hated that she had to leave. Aunt Betty, stepped right in to fill the void. She reminded me of Aunt Pam in that she made me feel as if I mattered, but she didn't have any of the characteristics that I adored in Pam and wanted to emulate. Aunt Pam was glamorous and sophisticated. Her charm was endearing, and it made people stop and pay attention when she entered the room. Aunt Betty wore overalls, jeans, and gym shoes most of the time. I thought that she was a grown-up tomboy, and I liked the girly-girl look. In a couple of days, it seemed to matter less because she made up for it with the attention that she gave me. She let me tag along on errands, sometimes holding hands and swinging them back and forth. I loved the fact that she played with me upstairs a lot, especially when Ms. Tina ran errands. Betty and I would lay a blanket on the floor and situate my dolls, and she squatted down to my level as I combed their hair and changed their outfits. It was special to me that she came down to my level to play with me.

One day when Ms. Tina left for errands Betty said, "Let's play house." This became a defining moment for me at the Lawrences. My happy little Leave It to Beaver atmosphere had been ripped right from under me. Junior popped into my head, and it triggered my anxiety. I didn't understand why everyone believed that it was all right *being fast* with me when Mama thought it was the worst thing on the planet. I hadn't thought about *playing house* or *being fast* since I boarded that plane at Chicago O'Hare International Airport. This vacation was supposed to be a chance to cure me. Now, I was being pushed straight into the fire again. All of my fondness for Betty was canceled in a flash. I put my head down and tried to concentrate on combing my dolls' hair. I didn't want to meet Betty's eyes, as I continued to mull it over in my head—as if I had a choice. Yet again, I was faced with something I didn't want to do. I wondered what the consequences would be if we got caught. I knew how Mama felt about *being fast,* but what about the Lawrences? Would they beat me? Would they tell Mama?

I continued to focus on my dolls as she coaxed me to lie back on the blanket. I wanted to protest, but my need to be loved crept up on me like a thief in the night. The fear of rejection held its grip on me tighter than a vise. Pleasing people to get love was spreading inside me like a malignant and cancer.

Betty laid next to me and scooted close. My heart was beating so fast as she rubbed gently between my thighs, slipping her hand up the leg of my shorts. She pressed down on my clit for a while and then came back to my thigh. When she finished, she said, "You know if you tell anyone about this, we will get in trouble." I shook my head up and down. I thought maybe she would get into trouble—unlike Junior— because she was a girl, but then I didn't understand how two girls could *be fast* with each other. It was very confusing. I couldn't honestly fit everything I knew about *touching* and *being fast* into this same sex equation and that left me powerless in many ways beyond consent. For sure, I didn't have the power to say no, but I couldn't even figure out how much danger I was in or how much trouble I would be in if an adult found out about the abuse.

That day was Betty's testing ground and, like with most repeat offenders, success makes her cocky. She went from stroking me in my play shorts to eventually removing my panties and shorts when she fondled me.

One day, she shocked the mess out of me by undressing. I watched with unease as she shed her clothes. I had learned with Junior that less clothing meant more trouble. In a flash I tried to figure out how she could possibly hurt me, and again I had no point of reference or knowledge about same-sex relationships, much less same-sex abuse. She didn't have a "wee-wee" like Junior, so I wondered what could possibly go wrong. When she pulled off her panties my eyes got big as saucers. Wow! *She has an afro down there, just like the one on her head,* I thought. Seeing her naked created a thousand questions. I looked at her with curious awe. This was the first time that I had seen a naked woman.

Even living in a house with Mama and older sisters, we had always covered up.

She laid next to me on the blanket and stroked my clit. The moisture between my legs felt good. I relaxed. After a while, Betty reached over for my hand and rested it on her pubic hair. *What the heck?* It felt like the steel wool I used to scrub the pots and pans. I snatched my hand back. She shifted her body up so that I could have a better reach, placed my hand back between her legs and moved it around her clit. I remembered how I touched myself sometimes, which felt good, so I gave in. I fumbled around her clit much like I had done with my own, but it turned out to feel nothing like when I touched myself. It felt yucky in her wetness. It was all wrong and I could no longer concentrate on how I was feeling from her touches; I thought about what she had me doing to her.

When she penetrated my vagina with her finger, on reflex, I withdrew my hand and my body stiffened. Her fingers were unpredictable—in and out, and then around my vagina. It hurt, but I suffered through it in silence. She reached back over and placed my hand back between her legs.

"Don't stop," she whispered. I did as I was told. She moved even closer to my body, and I could feel her heat. Her invasion of my space was disconcerting. I could take everything she took from me, but her closeness was suffocating. In my eleven years on earth, space seemed to be the only thing I could claim as my own. It allowed me some control of my world on my own terms. My own space had been the safest place for me to be after my grandfather's death. It had been stripped from me—first, with seven new siblings. Then Junior took the living room—the one communal space I felt safe—and made it dangerous and dirty. Mr. Tom took my bedroom and my closet, which were the only two places I could think and reclaim myself. Now, Betty was breathing on me, sucking the air and the distance I needed as both literal and symbolic barriers between us.

Her clammy body was close to mine, and the smell of her sex made me want to magically disappear into those clouds I'd seen when I was high above the ground. I tried to go in my mind to the airplane, but like with Junior, Betty never got enough, and I was forced to stay alert. She rested her leg over mine and started grinding. *What the heck is she doing?* I kept asking myself. She pressed her hairy vagina hard onto my thigh, and it felt like little, tiny bugs crawling on me. She had my bony thigh in a gridlock, like a pit bull gripping its prey. The harder she grinded, the harder she jabbed her finger inside me.

O-h-h-h-h.

She moaned softly and pressed harder and harder.

Oh-h-h-h.

I laid there like a log, with my mind wandering through the universe and wondering when it was all going to stop.

O-h-h-h-h.

Her pleasure was my cross to bear.

O-h-h-h-h.

Her stifled moan let out a whimper and she finally went limp and pulled away, releasing my leg. I sprung up and went to the bathroom. I washed her off my body and sat on the toilet to regain myself. I felt like a lost puppy far away from home. Yet, at the same time, those eight-hundred-eleven miles between Hermitage Street and Red Bank were closing in on me. I couldn't get away from this demon of *being fast*. I tried avoiding Betty, but Ms. Tina would say, "You don't want to go with Betty? Are you okay?" I didn't want to cause any trouble for myself, so I pretended like all was well. Betty would grab my hand and say, "Girl, come on here." I was even more trapped than I was on Hermitage Street. In Red Bank, I had no playmates and no place where I could go to be on my own. Betty, on the other hand, went about her business like all was well in the world. She was emboldened and she held all the power.

One day, one of her girlfriends was over when Ms. Tina left to run errands. I had met her previously, but I didn't warm up to her. I can't explain why she made me uncomfortable, but she did. When she was around, I went downstairs with Ms. Tina, and I never wanted to tag along with them, even when they offered.

In part, some of my hesitation was that she acted more like a dude than any girl that I had ever met. She was short, stocky, and overweight, with an afro shaped like Junior and the other boys in the neighborhood. I never saw her wearing anything other than blue jean overalls, just like Betty. From the back, both she and Betty looked like dudes. In 1973, I had never heard the term "lesbian." I didn't understand what I didn't know to understand. Looking back, maybe it wasn't so much that she was lesbian, bisexual, or bi-curious or whatever she was; it was more about her unwanted closeness and stares. I'm sure I had picked up on sexual cues by now, and my intuition kicked in. She was dangerous. That day, I had stayed downstairs with Ms. Tina, but as soon as she walked out of the door, Betty coaxed me upstairs. When I think back to this time, Betty was as brazen as fuck. Robert Sr. was always in his room back off the kitchen and she didn't seem fazed at all.

There was no pretense whatsoever. Betty had me lie on the blanket and she got right to it. Her friend sat on the floor and watched as Betty jabbed her fingers in and out of my vagina. I felt exposed and on display; shame flooded my very existence. I just didn't understand why Betty would do this to me. Tears shimmered in my eyes, but I refused to let them see me cry.

After a while, Betty took her fingers out of my vagina and started kissing my body as she moved down to my vagina. She placed her face between my legs, spreading my thighs with her head. She hadn't done any of this before and I was at a loss. I felt her tongue and it tickled. I raised my head trying to see exactly what she was doing, but all I could see was her afro looking back at me. It started to feel good, and I relaxed. My mind slipped into pleasure and curiosity about what she was doing. I wondered if this was *being fast*, too. It felt like nothing I ever experienced before, and I surrendered to it.

Lost in the feeling I forgot her friend was watching. Betty lifted her face from my vagina, and I peered to see what was happening. Betty's friend was whispering to her; and Betty moved, and her friend eased into her spot.

"Aunt Betty!" I said in a panic.

She came up to the top of my body to reassure me.

"Un-unnn…. Aunt Betty," I begged. I felt old girl's mouth on me. I tried to lift my body up, but there was no moving her fat ass. Futilely, I laid back down, upset that Betty had allowed her to touch me. Tears fell and Betty wiped them.

"Make her stop," I muttered to Betty. But after she twirled her tongue around my clit a few times, I settled into the feeling. This shit—whatever she was doing—felt so good to me. Even better than how Aunt Betty had made me feel. I hated her for making me feel good and I hated myself for feeling good. Despite the alarm I felt, my body failed me again. Even in danger, there was no controlling sexual arousal. My body's reaction was like knocking over one domino causing the others to crash, each one on its own accord.

Then that heifer bit my clit! *Why the hell did she bite me?* I panicked and tried to get up again, but she pushed me back down. I tried to wiggle from her grip, but it was another exercise in futility. She kept on biting and licking. I eventually stopped fighting because I knew I could not win. She gnawed and bit and licked and consumed my clit with her mouth. Betty started kissing my stomach as her friend was working over my little stuff.

Tears ran down my face.

"Oh, God. Help me, please?" I prayed over and over again. Pastor Anderson said to ask, and God would answer but like with Mama, God didn't make them stop hurting me. They persisted, using me for their pleasure. The pain was more than I could bear. I ascended up to those beautiful clouds again and parked myself smack-dab in the middle. I was closer to God in that moment in time, and I stayed there until Betty's friend released me.

Those first few seconds when she finally let go of me, I couldn't move or think, and I could barely breathe. My vagina throbbed, radiating pain through the eight thousand nerve endings that compose my clitoris—pulsating up into my vagina like a jackhammer. Yet, something inside of me would not let me surrender into the darkness. My brain waves sent a signal of danger and panic gripped me. I had to get the fuck up out of there, but my body was still shut down. Moving slowly, I willed myself to get up. I had just raised my head and my upper back from the floor when, out of nowhere, Betty pulled me on top of her. She spread her legs and pushed me down between them. She pushed my face into her vagina, demanding, "Do me." I froze right between her legs looking down at the size of her clit that was pulsating at me like a beady-eyed monster. I didn't move. Betty started moving my head, pressing it down into her.

"Lick me," she told me.

The smell was awful. I licked and she moved her vagina into my face and fucked me hard. I had no more tears. When she was done, I tried to roll off her, but I could feel a grip on my arm. Within seconds, her girlfriend had pulled me on top of her body. She had stripped down. Like Betty, she pushed me down between her legs. I felt like I was going to suffocate with her heavy hand jabbing my head into her. I didn't have a prayer left and the clouds that held me had gone black. When she released my face, I ran to the bathroom and locked the door. I looked in the mirror to see what they had done to my face. It was red and wet, and it stank. The first thing I did was rinse my mouth out with water; I then took my facecloth, lathered it with soap and washed my face. I could still taste their vaginas in my mouth. I was determined to remove every ounce of their stench from my body. I thought about brushing my teeth, but I didn't know if their smell would transfer to my toothbrush, and I would be stuck with it. I settled on the soap as the best route. Lathering the towel again, I used it to wash my mouth. I scrubbed my tongue as well as the sides and roof of my mouth and rinsed until the soap no longer stung. Afterward, I washed my sore vagina—and then sat on the toilet and cried.

Thirteen

❦

TRANSITIONS

"Often when you think you're at the end of something,
you're at the beginning of something else."
—Mr. Rogers

When I came back from New Jersey, Mr. Tom was gone. I had prayed for him to leave after he started popping his penis up and God answered my prayer; he had moved out of town to live with his daughter. I stepped into my spotless room and the cleanness helped to erase the smell of his urine from my memory. *Thank You, Jesus*, I whispered. I stretched my hands out like I had seen the deacons do at Old Ship of Zion when they prayed, and I went to every corner of my room saying, "Thank you, Jesus!" I even stepped into the closet. "Thank you, Jesus!" I guess I called myself cleansing the ugly away; all I needed was a little olive oil. Ethel chose to stay upstairs and that was a blessing in disguise. My room became my sanctuary. I spent more time there than any place in the house.

Now that I was back home, I laid Junior and Betty side by side, and one rape intensified my feelings about the other one. I retreated to my room, and there, in solitude, I tried to make sense of what had happened to me that year. Every time I looked at Junior shame and fear gripped me. My heart raced and a combustion of anxiety initiated. I stayed as far away from him as I could. Surprisingly, it was easier than I had imagine because he was always running the streets.

I was relieved to be away from Betty. Good riddance was my sentiment. When Mama called to talk to her family, she always asked if I wanted to speak to Betty. I would shake my head no and Mama would carry on with her conversation. Ms. Tina had told Mama how I followed Betty around like a puppy dog, especially when we went to the submarine shop. Man, I absolutely loved those Jersey subs. Of course, that was before she used me for her pleasure. After that day she and her girlfriend didn't touch me anymore. She did not apologize. She did not try to explain it to me or justify it. She did not seem to miss a beat of her life while I was scared out of my freaking wits. Every time she looked at me, I wanted to crawl under a rock and just die. What made matters worse was that I didn't understand what they had done to me. I wracked my brain with the hope that answers would somehow relieve me of the emotions, hurt, and pain, but there was no understanding or relief. I pushed it all to the recesses of my mind and kept it there.

I started six grade at Earle that fall. There was nothing spectacular about school that year, at least nothing I can remember. Both my education and memory thereof were eclipsed by the chaos at home. Mama was all encompassing and kept me crazy and anxious. Should I talk? Should I be quiet? Should I sit? Should I stand? Am I looking at her the right way? (Even though I didn't understand the wrong way.) I was a mess. It's a wonder that I didn't lose my mind, but I didn't, instead I tried to be the perfect daughter. I was not a rule breaker. My behavior on my worst day as a good child was the behavior of a problem child on their best day. I mastered everything Mama asked of me, but nothing thwarted her wrath. Tobie continued to intervene with his magic words, "Georgia, that's enough," in a *don't-fuck-with-me-Georgia* tone. She'd snapped her neck at him with a look that meant *mind your fucking business*. As always, her comeback was, "This is my daughter and I do what the fuck I please!" She was no match for him as I was no match for her, but she typically acquiesced to him after having her say.

Then came an increase in the unrest between Tobie and Mama and that would cause the dissolution of our blended family. Sleeping downstairs, I could hear Mama and Tobie arguing all the time. Like always, I'd hear Tobie say, "Georgia, please stop it." She'd keep talking, and as usual he'd say, "Georgia, I don't want to hear that shit every single night." He had been saying the same thing to Mama since the day he moved in with us. *Georgia, you drink too much. Georgia, you keep too much shit going.* I knew it was bad, but I never expected it to crack the way that it did. I guess children never really understand the depth of a conflict until it explodes. The worst part of the fighting was when Mama used me against Tobie in a way that was similar to how Grandmamma Julia used me against Mama. And just like with Grandmamma Julia, I was the one to pay the price.

In the face of all the arguing she started bringing clothes home just for me, not even Ethel would get a bag. It was a horrible position for me to be in and I was riddled with guilt. I would stuff the clothes in the back of my closet to hide them because I didn't want Ethel to feel left out. If that wasn't enough, Mama made it uglier than it had to be. She would wait until Tobie came home and call me into their room to give me the bag of clothes. Tobie usually ignored it, but one night he told her, "Georgia, that ain't right to bring home something for one and not the other." It was the moment she had been waiting for. She put her hand on her hips and replied, "I ain't got nothing but one child." He just shook his head. I went to my room without acknowledging the bag in my hands.

After that night she kept baiting him, but Tobie didn't say anything else to her about bringing clothes home for me and none for his children. Then out of nowhere it all came tumbling down right on top of me – shattering me into a thousand little pieces. The week going into Christmas Tobie called all of his children into the living room and handed each of them Christmas spending money one by one. From the oldest to the youngest, he called each name and they stepped forward. Those crisp one-hundred-dollar bills popped like a firecracker between his thumb and forefinger as he separated the crisp bills. After he handed Ethel her money, I perked up expectantly, even though I had not been called downstairs. Ethel stepped back, and he called Allen. I looked around like *what about me*, but I knew in my heart that he was not going to give me any money. I stood there looking pitiful, twisting my hands trying not to cry. My eyes pleading, *don't make me ask*. After he had given Juan, who was the youngest, his money, I watched my siblings jump up and down with those one-hundred-dollar bills in hand. He sat there looking smug. I looked from him to Mama who was standing in the doorway to the living room with her hands on her hips. I couldn't take it any longer,

"Diddy, I don't get any?" I asked, in little more than a whisper. Tobie looked at Mama as if to say, *checkmate*, then turned his face to me, "Georgia is your mother, ask her." Tears fell on my twisting hands, but I was determined to not let my hurt show more. I looked at Mama. She looked at Tobie.

"You a dirty motherfucker," Mama said to him. I ran past Mama standing in the doorway as I went into my room. I fell onto my bed and wept. Tobie had never made me feel like I wasn't his daughter. That night he had hit the goldmine of getting even with Mama, and it hurt worse than all his water hose beatings combined, because the pain of Tobie's rejection cut deep into my heart. I felt betrayed. Mama opened the door and told me that she would have my Christmas money on payday, and that she did.

I don't remember exactly when, but sometime after Christmas, Tobie made the kitchen upstairs fully functional and moved up there with his children. It happened quickly. It never occurred to me in my wildest imagination that we would cease to be a family.

After the breakup, I became a true latchkey kid. I got home from school at 3:30 and Mama didn't arrive from work until after six in the evening. She had instructed me in no uncertain terms that upstairs was off limits, saying, "If I catch you up there, I'll beat the living shit out of you." And I never doubted her threats. I missed Ethel something awful and after I got Mama's routine down, I would occasionally sneak upstairs to play with her and our dolls after school.

It went downhill fast. Mama started drinking heavier than what she already did. I must admit, prior to this period I had never seen alcohol affect Mama's ability to function. Tobie walking away did something to her that I totally understand now, but back then, I was simply scared. Scared for her and scared of her. Each evening some of Mama's new friends from the neighborhood dropped by our house after dinner. They all seemed close to Mama's age, in their late thirties and early forties. The center of attraction was the man who Mama seemed to be friendly with. She was mourning Tobie, but already had a new man. They drank and listened to the music like they were in a juke joint. After a while, Mama would wander to the back and crash across the bed into a drunken sleep. I often peeked out of my bedroom to assess the state of things. I called myself watching the house since Mama couldn't. Once she was knocked out and her guy caught me looking out of my room, he would coax me out.

"Come on honey and listen to some music with us." It was exciting as all get-out. The beat of the music. The rhythm of their bodies as they grooved to the sounds of the seventies. I laughed, talked, and leaned in; completely engaged as Mama's boo taught me the words to the songs. As the night progressed and the visitors petered out, sometimes he and I would be the only ones left. Him cheering me on as I learned the lyrics of the song and Mama drunk in bed. Mama sometimes woke up and caught me in the living room with her company, and she'd pitch a fit.

"BITCH, if you don't get your *fast* ass out of these men's faces…." I went straight to my room, but I could hear any given one of her party buddies saying, "Aw, Georgia she was just listening to the music."

"I don't give a fuck what she was listening to. She ain't grown."

On Friday nights the house was especially full. It was scary that people we really didn't know had free range of our home as Mama was laid out drunk. On paydays I would go into her handbag and get her money and hide it even at the risk of getting in trouble. The first time it happened, after she woke up and I told her, she slurred, "Awwww, my baby is taking care of me." That became our routine for months. All I can say today is that God must have dispatched an angel to watch over me. No one tried to rape me. I can only recall a hug a little too long and a little too tight, and too sloppy of a kiss on the cheek.

Mama continued to spiral downward. Some nights after the drinking crew left and she'd had a good nap, she poured herself a drink, sat on the sofa, and listened to heartbreak songs. Her favorite was the Tyrone Davis hit, *If I Could Turn Back the Hands of Time.* With a drink in one hand and a cigarette in the other she sang the song with the sadness of a blues singer. The loss of Tobie played out in real time just like the 45 RPM on the record player. I could hear her in my bedroom singing loud as if to make sure Tobie could hear her:

> *Oh darling, I'm so lonely without you*
> *Can't sleep at night, always think about you*
> *But if I had the chance to start all over*
> *I would be wishing today on a four-leaf clover*
> *And leaving you would be the last thing on my mind*
> *If I could turn back the hands of time.*

Looking back, I get it. Lord knows I have sung a song to a man that walked into the arms of another woman, and I wondered if we could get a do-over. But back then, I just thought Mama was crazy. Each time Tyrone Davis got to the line, *start all over again,* she raised her voice and her glass to the ceiling as a plea to Tobie.

At first, I was mostly annoyed by the late-night music because I couldn't make myself go to sleep for the life of me with the music up so loud. If I thought it couldn't get worst, well, I was wrong. One night she rustled me out of bed. The music was blaring. She was drunk and wanted me to sit in the window and watch for Tobie. I looked at her trying to figure out if I heard her right. "Bitch, do what I say do!" I gathered myself trying to wake up to follow her command. "I said get up and tell me when Tobie get here with that bitch!"

I got my tail up before she beat me up. I dragged a chair from the kitchen to the living room and sat in the window on lookout duty. For sure, I thought she had lost her freaking mind. I was so tired most nights that my eyes hurt. It was sad and pathetic, and I was caught in the middle. Tobie had moved on with his life. After he moved upstairs with his children, I cannot recall him ever coming downstairs, nor any of his children. He didn't even use the front door that joined the two floors. Rather, he used the backdoor that was connected only by the outside stairs. To tell you the truth I don't even know how they paid the bills. It seemed to me that we were living totally separate lives. Tobie didn't seem to care what Mama did with her life. Not even once did he interfere with what was happening on the first floor.

Night after night I stayed up watching to see if Tobie had another woman with him. My eyelids felt as if lead was sitting on them. I honestly don't know how I made it through every night. If I even looked like I was dosing off Mama saw me and yelled, "Bitch, I'll beat your ass if you fall asleep." She had scared me shitless. In the meantime, she would go lay across her bed and take a cat nap. I couldn't believe it – the first night she took her ass in the back and didn't reappear. I got up to see if she was okay. I had assumed she was going to replenish her drink, but nooooo, she was laid across the bed, knocked the *fuck out.* I wanted to take something and throw it at her. It was the first time that I actually thought, *I hate you, Mama.* I got some Kool-Aid out the fridge and went back to my window-sitting. I knew if she caught me at her bedroom door there would be hell to pay. I decided which hell was the lesser evil for me to bear. After that night I started pushing the envelope just a little to give myself some relief by at least turning down the loud music. I'm still not sure why Tobie didn't come downstairs and make her turn it down. I guess when he was done, he was done.

Every now and then she sneaked up on me, "Bitch, didn't nobody tell you to turn down my fuckin' music!" And she headed straight to the record player and started Tyrone Davis all over again and went back to her room. It was an impossible situation. I was tired every day at school. I was so sleep deprived that I laid my head down at lunch time. When I got home from school, I took a nap. When Mama got home from work, she opened my bedroom door and asked me what I was doing asleep. She asked me that stupid-ass question like she really didn't know the answer. On Saturdays, when it was time for me to go over to Grandmamma Julia's for church on Sunday, Mama made me feel guilty.

"You gonna leave your Mama here all alone? You are all I got baby." She only called me baby when she wanted something. Some Saturdays I stayed to keep the peace. I would take my coat off and go to my room. When I had reached my limit, I called Grandmamma Julia and asked her could Grandpapa Clayton pick me up instead of me walking over to their house. I knew if Grandmamma Julia was involved Mama would back down, but she would always have the last word. As I walked out the door, she said, "You a lowdown dirty bitch." I didn't even look back.

At church I prayed for Mama to stop drinking. I prayed for all of it to stop. I prayed that God didn't let me fall to sleep. I even prayed that Tobie never brought a woman home. I was really afraid for him. Each night Mama pulled Granddaddy's hunting rifle out and laid it against the wall in the kitchen, mumbling, *I'm going to show that motherfucker.* My prayers couldn't match Mama's madness. She never failed. If Tobie's car was gone, I was on watch duty.

One night, Tobie pulled up about two in the morning with his new girlfriend Delores. I got up to inform Mama. I didn't want to, but I knew that Mama would beat my ass if I didn't let her know. She was sitting on the side of the bed smoking.

"Mama, Diddy home," I said it with such drudgery that she asked,

"What's wrong with you?" I shrugged.

"He got that bitch?" She asked. I shook my head up and down and stepped away from her bedroom door. She got up, grabbed Granddaddy's rifle, and was standing in the opened backdoor when he walked past.

"You dirty motherfucker!" She hollered. I'm gonna kill yo' ass!" She raised the gun. Delores' eyes got big.

"Mama!" I screamed, "Don't kill Diddy!"

"After all I've done for your kids," she hollered half hoarse and half out of breath. "You dirty motherfucker!"

Tobie stood in front of Delores, who was very pregnant. As Mama came closer, he knocked the rifle out of her hand. She fell backwards into the doorway. He placed Delores in front of him to go up the stairs, I presumed, in case Mama got back up. But she was defeated. He looked down on her and shook his head then followed Delores upstairs. Mama picked herself up and took her humiliation to sleep. I went to the front, turned the record player off, went to my room and thanked God that Mama hadn't killed Tobie. She never mentioned the incident, and nor did I.

Mama started a new job at the Evanston Inn, and I saw a change in her for the better. The Evanston Inn was about thirty miles north of Chicago's south side in Evanston, Illinois. It was a quasi-residential hotel made up of primarily wealthy white seniors. Some were permanent residents, and some were short-term. A woman, whose name I can't recall, moved in with us along with her toddler daughter. Allowing people whom she hardly knew to live with her became a *thing* Mama did that I eventually picked up, too. I have no idea where this woman came from, but one day she was there, just like Mr. Tom. She assumed Mama's duties of cooking and cleaning our house. She was in her early twenties, and it was great to have someone at home with me. Most days when I came home from school dinner was already done. Some semblance of peace even settled over our home. Come to find out, Mama had moved on with her life for real this time and had a new man. She came home one evening with this dude, Charles Turner. He was a resident at the Evanston Inn. To say the least, she was infatuated and showed him off like he was an Emmy Award. Charles was the polar opposite of Tobie, and I didn't know what to think. Tobie was a man's-man. Charles, on the other hand, came across as feminine. He crossed his legs like a woman and smoked long cigarettes. He picked up his glass of Johnny Walker Red Label Scotch Whiskey chased with milk as if he was the Queen of England. The days of beer and cigars were over for Mama.

Charles was brown skin; his nose was keen, and his lips were small. The word vain was his middle name. He kept his face clean shaven. He kept his hair cut short to mask the bald spot that was emerging in the very top, and he dyed his hair regularly. He was impeccably dressed, and his clothes fit his slim body as if they were tailor made. Looking back now, I would bet my best handbag that he was bisexual and living in the closet. Decades later I would hear a little chatter to that effect and from a reliable source. That wasn't the problem for me back then, I couldn't put my finger on it at first, but he scared me from day one.

The first time he looked at me with those piercing eyes something in my gut said that he was not to be trusted. It wasn't just one thing about him, but the sum total. He was eerily silent, more often than not, and it seemed to me that his eyes looked through me and everyone else in his view. Right before he spoke, he had a habit of turning his top lip upward like he had just smelled a whiff of shit. This way he had with his lips weirded me out. I kept my distance. When he stepped through the door of our Hermitage Street house I went to my bedroom. If it was still early enough, I could get away with going down to Ms. Williams's house to play with Teresa. I didn't want to be around him. Quite frankly, I didn't even want to be in the same house with him, but that wasn't usually in my control. My intuition told me that Charles Turner was dangerous, and it would be truer than true.

Fourteen

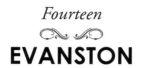

EVANSTON

"The Universe sends us exactly what we are ready for
at the exact time we need it in our lives."
—Kundalini Spirit

At the end of sixth grade, Mama packed up the first floor of our Hermitage Street house and moved us to Evanston. Evanston, for me, was a *Tale of Two Cities*. To borrow from Charles Dickens, "it was the best of times, it was the worst of times." When Mama told me we were moving to be closer to her job, I didn't know what to think—that is, until I got a glimpse of the town.

On Easter weekend, Mama took me to work with her because there was no school on Good Friday. I was in awe of the Evanston Inn and all its grandeur—at least, from the outside looking in, with its tall columns and grand entrance. Built in 1914, the five-story building was the first modern residential hotel in Evanston. On the inside, it had seen better days, but I was still in awe of the antiques that graced the lobby.

Twelve miles north of Chicago's downtown, Evanston was like a town I had seen in old movies that I watched on WGN-TV. The town was simply breathtaking, from the beautiful lawns to the Victorian-style homes and mansions. That day, Mama allowed me to walk over to the lake just a stone's throw from the hotel. I took in the view of the shoreline, with all the beautiful mansions with private access to Lake Michigan. I was in heaven—until Mama told me that she and Charles would be getting an apartment together. I was devastated. I didn't want to spend ten minutes with him in the same room, and now Mama was talking about living in the same apartment. This news had me tied in knots. Mama thought she had found a gold mine; I, on the other hand, believed I was walking on a land mine.

I spent most of that day helping Mama clean the rooms and trying not to think about Charles. For the most part, it worked. I loved going into the suites that the wealthier residents usually occupied. I had seen antiques on television, but I never imagined that people had furniture like this in real life. It was stunning: even a sofa with wear and tear had beautiful hand-carved legs. Whenever Mama left me alone to clean, I explored the built-in mahogany bookshelves with beautiful glass doors filled with all kinds of trinkets, porcelain eggs, crystal figurines and bowls, and fancy tea sets on the sideboards. It made an impression on me, and I could have spent hours looking at these exquisite items. I wasn't so much impressed with the standard unit—one room, with a bed and toilet. Those rooms made the Evanston Inn look like a run-down hotel. I would learn that day that being a maid was grueling work. I decided, right then and there, this was not the life I wanted for myself when I grew up.

When Charles came home from work, Mama sent me to his room to watch television until she was done for the day. I pleaded to stay with her, but she said I was in the way, and she needed to finish up. God knows I didn't want to go. I went from elevator to elevator, biding time until one of the other maids saw me. I didn't want to get into trouble, so I made my way to his room.

I knocked. When Charles opened the door, I said, "Mama told me to come here and watch television until she's done." He didn't say anything and just stepped back to let me in. I stood at the door entrance, assessing the room, and walked in. He lived in a one-room unit, furnished with a bed, dresser, and small desk. He had a hot plate on top of the dresser and there was a fancy small bar cart with a beautiful decanter and elegant shot glasses. It fit that hoity-toity image he portrayed. After he closed the door, he walked across the room to turn on the television, made himself a drink and sat on the bed. I decided the best place for me was on the floor in front of the television with my back to him. I couldn't stand his piercing eyes, and watching my back was all the shade I could think to give him at the time. I hopelessly tried to focus on the television program, but I was scared. If you had asked me why, I couldn't have explained for all the tea in China; I just was. Every now and then I would look up at the clock, praying that time would move fast. I wanted to look behind me to see what he was doing, but there was no way I was going to let him see my face until Mama walked into that room. I wished someone had told my bladder that I didn't want to move. I had to pee, and the more nervous I got the more the urge grew. I didn't want to walk near Charles. I looked at the clock again; it was getting closer to the time Mama got off. I prayed she would come before my pee came down, but no such luck. As life would have it, my body betrayed me again. I could feel a droplet in my panties. I jumped up and said, "I have to go to the bathroom." He pointed to the door and watched as I nearly ran across the room. The moment I entered the bathroom, I turned the lock and sat on the toilet.

When I came out of the bathroom, he grabbed me. I tried to push him back, but he pinned me up against the wall and smashed his face into mine, kissing me frantically— like he had been waiting his entire life for that moment. I smelled Johnny Walker and milk, and it nauseated me. I tried to hit him to make him stop and he pinned my hand against the wall above me. He was strong, but I kept fighting. He leaned part of his body into me sideways and grabbed my vagina hard and squeezed.

"STOP!" I demanded. He kept squeezing.

"Please STOP!" I begged, but he continued groping me.

"Oh, God," I called out. "Please help me."

He started to loosen his grip on me, and I kept fighting to get him off me. I swung and hit him hard on the face with my hand and arm.

"You little bitch," he snarled, and grabbed my nipple and pinched the shit out of me. The pain sizzled through my training bra like a hot comb on greased hair. I grabbed my breast, and he got an edge on me. With the weight and height of his body directly in front of me, he grabbed me between my legs again and held his hand there, squeezing. All of sudden he let me go. He stepped back and straightened himself up in a dignified manner. What the fuck was he playing at? This was some psycho shit. My heart was beating so fast I thought it was going to jump out of my body and run. For a moment, I didn't know what to do. When he walked toward the entertainment bar to make himself a fresh drink, I bolted toward the door. When my hand hit the knob, he called out to me. I turned around and saw him pouring milk into a glass. He turned up his lips and said, "Georgia told me about you." I looked at him. *What the hell was he talking about?*

"You know you wanted it, with your *fast* tail," he added. I didn't know which hurt the worst: that Charles had attacked me or that Mama had already characterized me to him as a whore, at eleven years old. I've often wondered, if she had given me half a chance, how my life could have been different with her. I turned around again and opened the door to leave.

"Rae," he called to me again. I stopped but did not turn around.

"If you tell Georgia, I will make sure you don't get any clothes for Easter."

Asshole! I thought. I shrugged and walked out the door. When I made it to the elevator, I took a moment to fix my top and recover before I faced Mama. Charles's threat didn't mean a damn thing to me. I couldn't have cared less about Mama buying me Easter clothes. What he didn't know was that Mama would beat my ass in the morning and bring home a bag of clothes the same night. Besides, I knew that Grandmamma Julia had a dress waiting for me to claim just like I knew my name was Rae. My problem had nothing to do with clothes, or Easter; it was Mama. She could not be trusted to protect me, and that is a fact she had proven to me over and over again. I weighed it out in my head while I was going from floor to floor trying to find her. All I could hear was, *You fast-ass bitch. What did you do to make him do it?* She had flipped the script on me so many times. I made the sage and safe decision to keep what had happened to myself. I found her and asked if I could go sit in the lobby until she finished. She was too flustered with work to give a hoot what I did. I sat in that lobby among the beautiful antique decor and wished my life was as pretty as the chair I was sitting in. The only thing I knew for certain was that I was afraid of both Charles and Mama.

I hated Charles worse than I hated collard greens with okra; he was like okra slime dripping down into the greens, spoiling a whole batch. But God, did I love living in Evanston! Fundamentally, I believe had we not moved to Evanston, I would have been lost to the world. The combination of the adverse changes that would occur in Englewood, my low self-esteem, my lack of stimulation at Earle, and the presence of Mama would have demolished me.

In 1974, Evanston had approximately eighty thousand residents, sixteen percent of whom were African Americans. Unlike most Black folks in Evanston, who lived primarily on the west side of town, we lived on the southeast side, about ten blocks from Lake Michigan. We moved into a red brick courtyard building on Seward Street. It extended around the corner, with three sections facing Sherman Street. Each section had three floors, with two apartments on each floor with facing doors. Our building was owned by an African American family. The patriarch, Leon Robinson, also owned the school bus service in Evanston. The large backyard connected the entire building and we each had a small back porch that could accommodate a couple of chairs.

We lived in a one-bedroom apartment on the third floor of one of two sections on the Seward side. Our apartment had shining hardwood floors, and dark wood doors with trim throughout. When you entered, you landed into the small foyer facing a closet that Charles used. The foyer opened into the living room that faced the front windows. You could see the entire living room from the foyer. Once you stepped into the living room, you faced a door to my bedroom and the large dining room to the left. To reach our kitchen, you had to walk through the dining room, which Mama and Charles made their bedroom. Off the dining room to the right, there was an opening the size of two doors that led to a hallway. Once you stepped in that hall, my second bedroom door was to the right, and the bathroom and Mama's closet to the left. With this layout, there was no place in the house where I could not be seen when I was not in the bathroom or my bedroom. Mama insisted that I have the private room, and it was the one and only thing she fought Charles for on my behalf. I heard her tell him that I was growing up and needed to have my own room.

Like on Hermitage, my bedroom was my refuge. In the five and a half years I lived there, I spent at least seventy-five percent of my time in that room. While my room didn't exactly protect me from the madness outside my doors, it gave me a place to call my own—a place to breathe. As usual, Mama indulged me the material things; my bedroom was laid. I had every amenity a girl could want. I had The Jackson Five and The Sylvers posters from *Right On!* magazines on my walls. I had a small white turntable and a black-and-white television. I even had a telephone in my room. I had twin beds in case I had company, but I didn't dare invite any of my friends into my reality show. I can count on one hand the friends who visited our apartment, apart from a surprise birthday party

Mama gave me. (That's a whole other story.) The truth of the matter is that I didn't want people to witness me getting a tongue-lashing or beatdown.

That first summer, during the day I was left to my own devices. I'd sleep late and kick it around the house until the afternoon and then I was off exploring Evanston. I discovered Ridgeville Park, a couple of blocks from our building, where all the young people hung out—unlike on Hermitage, where we mostly played on the block. This meant that no one who knew Mama around our apartment building had eyes on me, so I was free of neighborhood gossip. It was great not having the strict supervision.

I walked the neighborhood, getting my bearings. We didn't have corner stores like in Chicago, but we had a family-run neighborhood store, Gerard's that was one block up on Custer. I even walked up to Main Street, about five blocks from our apartment going north and ten blocks east of Mama's job. It was a thriving business area and I browsed around in the stores. This was new for me. I had never been in a store alone, other than the corner neighborhood store. Main Street was fascinating. It had a bakery that I had only seen on television, and there were craft stores and little boutiques. The Chicago-Main Newsstand on the corner of Chicago Avenue and Main Street was my first introduction to magazines. I could stay in there for hours, flipping though the magazines. Back then, it was a hole in the wall but, man, did it have magazines galore. I'd walk back home a different way to see more of my neighborhood. Our block was mostly apartment buildings, but we were surrounded by beautiful homes. The ones on Asbury, a street behind ours, and Ridge Street, which intersected with Seward, were beyond stunning. There was a beach a couple of blocks from Mama's job that I visited occasionally, but I wasn't so much of a get-my-hair-wet-and-have-sand-in-my-shoes kind of girl. Northwestern University, just a couple of miles away from my house, stood as a monument to classical education. It extended north on the shoreline with imposing architectural beauty. Once Mama got me my first ten-speed bike, I'd ride the lakefront. It was an easy way out of the house that Mama never questioned, and I never violated. I loved riding the lakeshore. Basically, I loved everything about Evanston, including the nineteenth-century-style streetlights. I paid attention to everything, and it was in the car with Mama that I found my new church home, Second Baptist, in downtown Evanston. She drove past it one Sunday and Black people were standing out front. I asked her if I could attend, and she said yes. The following Sunday, I backtracked to it on the train. It was only four stops and a quick ten-minute ride from our house. At first, I continued to go to church with Grandmamma Julia, but I hated that one-hour train ride to her house.

Second Baptist Church was the epitome of Black culture and education. The senior pastor was Reverend Dr. Hycel B. Taylor. At the time, he was also a professor of theology at Garrett Theological Seminary at Northwestern University. They had doctors, lawyers, educators and educated people galore. It was definitely the bourgeoisie church of Evanston. There were no drums or guitars like at Old Ship of Zion. Instead, the church had a pipe organ and a sanctuary choir. But I loved this new worship and cultural experience nonetheless.

It didn't take long for Mama to find her niche, either. Her new drinking buddy was Ms. Virginia Maddox, the matriarch of her family. Their large home sat on the Sherman Avenue side of our apartment building. They were a close knit, educated family, but were also heavy drinkers. Ms. Virginia was at least seventy, messy as ever, and Mama's biggest cheerleader. Out of the whole bunch I favored Ms. Virginia's daughter Barbara, who was maybe a little younger than Mama. She encouraged me and gave me beauty tips. Ms. Virginia's brother Humphrey, whom we called Humpie—asked me about school every time he saw me. He even suggested books for me to read and pushed me to think about my future, and that's exactly what I did. For sure, Evanston changed the lens through which I viewed life. I didn't understand the depth of how my world had changed or the importance of this change. However, I intuitively latched on, and didn't let go.

Fifteen

❧

CHUTE MIDDLE SCHOOL

❝The more healthy relationships a child has, the more likely he will be to recover
from trauma and thrive. Relationships are the most powerful therapy in human love.❞
—Dr. Bruce Perry

The day I first walked into Chute Middle School; I was entering the seventh grade,
but I was on a fifth grade reading level. On Hermitage Street, no one had seemed
smarter than me—which meant I had no idea what I didn't know. Whatever the
expectations were, I seem to have met them because each year I matriculated with my
classmates, thus normalizing my below-average performance.

Evanston presented a different set of standards than what I was accustomed to in
my Chicago environment. Between Chute and church, I began to understand that I was
missing a whole lot. Being behind was unsettling because I was such a Miss Know-It-All.
My peers at church seemed so much smarter than me. Between the Howlett clan and
Pastor Taylor's daughters, Chandra, and Audreanna (Audie), I wondered why I couldn't
be as smart. When our Sunday school teacher, Joyce Favors, asked people to read aloud,
I tried to make myself invisible. I was embarrassed when I stumbled over words. I wanted
to emulate the way the Taylor girls pronounced each word with precision. At the time, I
didn't consider the advantage they had with an educator mother, Ms. Ann, and a father
with a Ph.D. Thank God no one at church made fun of me. Most times they followed
along, helping me to pronounce the words. I started reviewing my Sunday school lesson
and reading the related Biblical scriptures twice before Sunday so I wouldn't stumble over
words; still, there were words I just didn't know how to pronounce.

Unlike at church, my classmates at Chute were not so kind. I will never forget how
they made fun of me because I said "liberry" instead of library. Thanks to Mama, I had
developed thick skin; I was never going to let anyone get the best of me. I practiced that
word like I was going to be in some kind of contest, until I got it right. In some ways,
peer pressure pushed me to perform. This was the first time that I had been personally
challenged and the Miss Know-It-All in me was not going to let anyone know something
I didn't know. I didn't envy anyone. Instead, I turned my shame into action and pushed
forward with purpose. I wanted to know more, do more and be more.

I look back on my Chicago education and can clearly see I had not been educated.
Instead, I went through the motions, obviously learning enough to get by—but not
to excel. Prior to entering Chute, I cannot recall ever reading a book— only my Sunday
School lesson and the passages in the Bible connected to the lesson.

I knew that a noun is a person, place, or thing because it was a catchy phrase. I
did not know the difference between a verb and an adjective, or how to use them in a
sentence. I learned the multiplication tables by memorizing them; however, within the
same school year, I forgot everything except the ones, twos, fives, and tens. I did not
learn the basics of phonics or even how to properly enunciate a word. I did not learn
the difference between a synonym and an antonym, which affected my ability to spell,

recognize words and comprehend what I read.

I've also tried to situate Beethoven into the equation, but I can't remember much other than I liked the spacious halls and colors on the walls—and those scrumptious butter cookies. I was probably already behind when I arrived at Earle. Educators argue that third grade is the most important year because that's when a child should be reading to learn; it's when a child should be able to focus on reading for information and comprehension. Whatever my condition was when I arrived at Earle, fourth through sixth grades were the most traumatic of my childhood that I can recall. I was going through the motions, and that's putting it mildly. When you combine the verbal and physical abuses with the sexual abuse, again, I had to have had a deregulated stress response system, which can mimic symptoms of ADHD, like short attention spans, hyperactivity, impulsiveness and even disrupted sleep. On top of what happened at home, I had to contend with the overcrowding at Earle and concentrating was difficult for me. Being locked away in the trailer sent me over the edge every freaking day. Plus, we had a predominantly white faculty who were given a task they never thought they would have to do: educate African American children. I don't know whose heart was in it. If there was a teacher who gave her all, that person didn't come across my path. I mostly remember having a difficult time staying focused at Earle. I would push myself to do the work I was assigned because a grade lower than C on my report card would result in a whopping from Mama. Furthermore, I had no help at home. My siblings and I went our separate ways when it came to education. No one asked for help, and no one volunteered it. We each learned on our own and in our own way. Patricia was the only sibling I can recall ever reading a book at home, and I never thought to ask her about any of them. Nonetheless, on Hermitage everyone had been expected to get a higher grade than C, and Tobie gave money to all of us for A's and B's.

Mama began making little snide comments here and there when I brought home an assignment with an A or when I said something she didn't understand. "You think you something" and "you just want to be white" were two of her favorite ways of trying to knock me down. It hadn't occurred to me prior to this time that Mama could barely read and write. Although she had told me she was taken out of school in second grade to work in the fields, I didn't fully understand how that translated into her day-to-day life. In Evanston, it was normal for me to sign my own absence notices and field-trip forms. By the time I became a first-year student in high school, Mama even asked me to read and explain her important business papers. I would be in my early twenties before I fully understood how well Mama hid her illiteracy. What was clear to me was Mama's jealousy, and it became another thing I had to be guarded about.

Picture this: I came to Evanston talking like a country bumpkin, splitting my verbs, and committing a multitude of other grammatical sins. This South Side Chicago accent that I still have only seemed to magnify my deficiencies, but any attempt to speak better was viewed by Mama as trying to be better than her. By high school, I had to shrink myself in front of her so she wouldn't squash me. Anything that came out of my mouth that she didn't understand or have knowledge of was, in some small way, a declaration that she was less than me. For instance, one day I was watering the plants and Mama was sitting on the sofa. I noticed the air conditioner wasn't in the window correctly. I turned to her and said, "Mama, I don't think the air conditioner is secure in the window."

"What the fuck you mean?" she asked. Dread came over me. I thought, *Oh, God. Here we go.* But that day I was thinking quickly, and it helped to minimize her sting. Something in my gut told me to repeat what I had said in a different way. "Mama, I was just saying that I think that the air conditioner is gonna fall."

"Oh. Why the fuck didn't you say so?" she asked. I didn't respond because it would have added fuel to the fire. I deflected and asked her if she wanted me to try and fix it. And to acknowledge her authority, I said, "I may need your help to hold it up so I can get it in right." Just like that, she became a different woman and got up to see if she could help secure the air conditioner in the window.

I could not celebrate my accomplishments in front of her because she turned them against me. Sometimes, she made me doubt myself. She even found a way to sour the joy of my eighth-grade graduation. A couple of weeks before graduation, she told me she would not be attending. When Charles dropped me at school that day, I left her sitting on the side of the bed in her housecoat, smoking a cigarette. Earlier that week she had taken me to Montgomery Ward's Department store to buy my outfit. (We didn't wear caps and gowns for the eighth-grade graduation.) After I got dressed, I asked her one more time if she would go. She responded, "If you ask me one more time, I'm going to make you take that goddamn dress off and you won't be going."

When the ceremony was over, she and Charles were standing by the car in the parking lot. She was just cheesing: "You thought I wasn't coming." I didn't even know what to say. It was just like that Christmas stunt right after my grandfather's death all over again. I didn't find it amusing. During the entire ceremony, all I could think about was that Mama hadn't come to the most important day of my life so far. The auditorium was too big for me to spot them. Mama kept me off balance. She certainly wasn't my cheerleader when it came to my education, and the more I improved myself, the more she punished me for my intellectual growth, despite the fact that she needed my intellect to help her maneuver through her own personal affairs.

I know I've said, "it was crazy" a lot, but I just don't have any other words to describe my life with Georgia Lee other than to say it was chaotic. The daily contradictions in her parenting methods were mind-boggling. She needed me to explain her important documents, fill out her job applications and complete paperwork. Yet I couldn't display my educational progress in my own right. The importance of my education only held value when it benefited her. Thank God for outside reinforcement from a village of caring adults.

Chute Middle School opened its doors in 1968—the same year my grandfather passed away. The school was named after Dr. Oscar Moody Chute, the superintendent who spearheaded the desegregation of Evanston's elementary schools beginning in 1956. By the time I arrived, Chute was fully integrated. Some African American children were bused from the west side of Evanston. Others, like me, landed there because we lived within walking distance of the school.

Wilbur George Quam designed the school structure to help facilitate interdisciplinary team teaching. We had multipurpose rooms on each wing of the third floor, with soundproof doors that separated the rooms into sections. The primary subjects were taught on the third floor, while the first floor was designed mainly for creative classes that worked the other side of our brain. Art, on the second floor with the lockers and language arts classes, was the exception.

I started the day with Mr. Jerry Murphy, my seventh-grade homeroom teacher. At first, I was a little leery of him because the only other male teacher I remembered was Mr. Frazier, my first-grade teacher at Beethoven, who slapped me. I had asked to go to the bathroom, and he said no. I was so close to peeing my pants that I got out of my seat, went to his desk, and pleaded my case. He stood up from his desk, looked down at me, "I said, no." He spoke through clenched teeth.

"But I gotta go bad," I whined.

"Go back to your seat," he demanded, and before I could get another word out of my mouth, he slapped me in the face. I grabbed my face and ran out of the classroom— leaving my coat and all my belongings—down the stairs and out the door. I didn't stop running until I reached my house on Swann Street. I have no idea why Mama was home, but she was. She looked at me, tears running down my face,

"Girl, what you doing here?" she asked.

"Mr. Frazier," I said, breathless, "hit,"—snot and tears all lumped together on my face— "hit me." I was still holding my face to dramatize what had happened. Mama got up from the sofa and examined my face that still bore my teacher's handprint. Mama had me go clean up and use the bathroom and marched me right back to school. She didn't even stop in the office. She went straight to my classroom and cursed Mr. Frazier the heck out. I stood behind her as she read him the riot act.

"If you put your hands on my child again, I will come back up here and beat the living shit out of you," she said. My eyes popped. Mr. Frazier turned cherry-apple red. He tried to explain but before he could even get it out, Mama hollered, "I DON'T GIVE A FUCK WHAT SHE DID!" She was boiling mad.

"Don't nobody but me have a right to put their hands on my child," she added. "You BET' NOT EV-ER do it again," she said. She looked down at me. "Girl, you can go to the washroom anytime you want." Then she looked back at Mr. Frazier, "And you BET' NOT say a MOTHER-FUCKING-THING!"

"Go on back and sit down," she ordered me, then turned on her heels and went back home. This didn't erase the memory or the fear that set in toward white male teachers. I always avoided them in the halls.

Mr. Murphy helped ease that fear. He wasn't uptight, like Mr. Frazier had been in his suit coat and tie. Instead, he was a laid-back and easygoing man in his mid-twenties. He often wore khakis paired with Oxford button-down shirts. His tawny eyes blended with his pale white skin. He had curly dark brown hair that almost looked like an afro. He called it his Jewish afro because of the wiry texture common among people with Jewish ancestry. From day one, he took me under his wing, so to speak—or so it felt like it to me. Often, he would ask me to run classroom errands for him. I felt appreciated and valued. The homeroom teachers at Chute were primarily responsible for language arts and social studies. However, Mr. Murphy's seventh-grade homeroom was the only class at Chute that had two teachers and an aide. We had a ninety-minute class period. Mr. Murphy taught social studies and Ms. Randi Ehrenberg taught language arts. Additionally, Kathy Manchester, a Master of Arts in Teaching candidate from Northwestern University, worked with them in a coordinated curriculum.

I tracked Mr. Murphy down to chat with him about teaching at Chute when I first began to write this book. We met at Starbucks on Main Street, just a few blocks from where the Evanston Inn used to sit. I shared my hopes for my memoir; he shared his teaching philosophy, and how he addressed my educational and emotional challenges when I landed in his seventh-grade homeroom. He said his starting point was "to recognize a student's strengths and weaknesses." He used a child's strengths to help build his or her confidence and to simultaneously correct that child's weaknesses. For example, my reading comprehension was below average, but he explained that I was a vocal girl who quickly understood concepts. Rather than have me to read aloud, he had me participate in small group discussions where I could shine. He had Kathy tutor me in reading and comprehension three days a week outside of the class to help correct my weaknesses. I remember sitting with her like it was yesterday. Some days we just pulled two desks out in the hall. She was patient with me, and I was eager and hungry to learn. The individualized help made a world of difference for me. Being able to read and actually liking it opened a whole new world for me.

Mr. Murphy hit the nail on the head. The better I could read and comprehend, the more my self-esteem was boosted; and the more confidence I had, the better I performed. By the time I left Chute, I was able to analyze written concepts—not just topics from our discussions and the films we watched, but also from the larger topics discussed in class. My ability to unpack topics from reading, research and observation has remained one of my greatest strengths. Even though I still struggle with spelling and sentence syntax, I am an endless vault of research, ideas, and concepts. The fact is Mr. Murphy didn't try to kill my quick thinking and verbal skills the very thing I had been admonished for the most at home but helped to build my self-esteem. During our conversation that day he also described his teaching model as "child-centered and relationship-based," and explained that the overall environment at Chute during this period helped to facilitate his approach to teaching. He credits our principal, Mr. Edward Pate, for his openness to innovation in the classroom.

Mr. Pate, who is African American was recruited to Evanston in the early sixties to help integrate the pool of teachers in the elementary schools. His wife, Clara, was the first African American principal of Oakton Elementary School, just up the street from Chute. They would both retire from Evanston School District 65 as legends. Mr. Pate began as the assistant principal the day Chute opened. By the time I arrived, he was in charge. He called us Pate's Kids. He explained before his death that he "sought to have the best teachers he could to ensure his students had the best education." No doubt, he provided a nourishing environment for children to grow.

I've mentioned that trauma experts believe children can overcome when they have an alternative environment—a "buffer" that nurtures the soul. I had always credited Chute with getting me on track academically, but it wasn't until I watched the 60 Minutes special, *Treating Childhood Trauma* in 2019, when Oprah Winfrey interviewed Dr. Perry, did the light bulb in my head go off. Oprah, who also lived in toxic stress as a child, credited her fourth-grade teacher, Mrs. Duncan, as her buffer. Overall, she credited school for giving her a "sense of value and connection." This resonated with me wholeheartedly. Mr. Jerry Murphy and Dr. Lorraine Morton were to me what Mrs. Duncan was to Oprah. They helped me to believe in myself, and that was the one tool I didn't have in previous years. It became the catalyst that catapulted my growth and development.

Interdisciplinary teaching was a godsend for me. Moving to different classrooms for different subjects, combined with different teachers with varied personalities and passions, helped to provide an outlet for my short attention span. My mind is always racing, and I quickly lose interest. Exposure to new disciplines kept me stimulated and expanded my thinking in ways I didn't even know one could think.

In addition to the primary subjects, we had industrial arts. I had never heard of such a class. We had state-of-the-art machines for a woodworking shop that included plastic molding and silkscreen. In art class we had painting and pottery, which I could never get a handle on, although I did make a lopsided bowl. Home economics was my absolute favorite. Our teacher, Lois Shartiag, was a petite woman with a lot of personality. She seemed like three people in one because she was always by your side when you needed extra help. Even today, she's on Facebook cheering us on. We had full-range stoves and sewing machines. I can still remember making Rice Krispies Treats and learning how to level off dry ingredients—something that has stayed with me to this day. Every time I bake a cake, I imagine Ms. Shartiag taking a butter knife to demonstrate how the success of a cake involved leveling the exact measurements from the recipe. I watched Grandmamma Julia bake cakes, but she didn't seem to measure off anything. But that was old-school Southern generational cooking. I credit them both for putting me on the path of being a great baker.

My weakest area was sewing. I wanted to learn, and Grandmamma Julia was an expert seamstress, but it was her craft and hers alone. She didn't make clothes for anyone other than herself. When she sewed, my curious eyes and questions left her irritated and me deflated. I eventually let it go because I didn't want to ruin my time away from Hermitage Street by making Grandmamma mad at me. I understood the concept of sewing but I was never able to follow the patterns well. It required me to use the other side of my brain, whereas I wanted to be creative. Years later, sewing with Mrs. Jacqueline Jackson was my cup of tea. Our starting point was always with a vision. Then we found the fabric and measured, cut, and sewed with not a single pattern in the equation.

Our gym was substantial, with doors that opened to a large outdoor field for use during the warm weather months. We even had a basketball court with bleachers. The athletic program had everything: basketball, baseball, calisthenics, and gymnastics, with equipment. My lack of coordination made gymnastics a challenge, and that's an understatement. Likewise, I couldn't play a lick of basketball, but I joined the girls basketball team so I could hang out with my friends Annie Schofield, Lena Hicks, Sadie Ruff and Rennée Jones. All except Annie were in my seventh-grade homeroom. None of them lived within walking distance to my house, so I only spent time with them at school. It was a great advantage that Mama had no access to them—and I didn't tell any of them about my home life. Annie and I talked a lot on the telephone. I also made friends with other girls on the team, Gail Stephens, Cameryl Hill, Pamela Andrews and Patsy Powell, who was the star of the team and eventually played semi-pro ball. Until I moved to Evanston, my friendship pool was meager. I can't remember any friendships I established at Earle other than Teresa, and that's because her mother and Mama were friends. When I combined the friends from Chute with those from church, many of whom attended Chute, I had more friends than I could have ever imaged. I truly believe this move was a blessing. Mama came to Evanston chasing a man, and it was the best decision she ever made for herself that had a positive outcome for me. Even living with Charles, Evanston represented the best (and worst) of times for me. It changed the trajectory of my life.

Ms. Kris, a former nun, was both the gym teacher and basketball coach. Everyone loved her and she, in turn, loved us. I could never figure out why she gave me playing time on the court, because I couldn't dribble a ball while standing in place. But those two minutes every now and then made me feel as if I was doing something. One sport that I absolutely loved was badminton. I became so skilled at Chute that, in my first year of high school, the teacher in charge of the team asked me to consider trying out. I was excited, but Mama said no. If I could have gotten away with it, I would have done it without permission, but high school sports required too much of a time commitment to do them behind her back.

While the extracurricular activity enriched my life, it also gave me a safe place to be after school and more time to hang out with friends. I didn't dare tell Mama. My gut told me if I asked for permission, she would say no. Instead, I counted on most of our activities taking place right after school. I could get away with activities that didn't require me to be home past the time Mama got home from work. I joined everything I could at Chute, including the chorus. My singing skills were even worse than my basketball skills. But I figured that if Belinda Hubbard, the minister of music at church, and Francine Markell, the chorus teacher at Chute didn't care, then why should I? I was in chorus both years. I gave up basketball after the first year.

Sadie, Rennée and Annie were in chorus with me in addition to the basketball team, and we ate lunch together and stuck close in most of the school activities. Annie had one of the strongest personalities in the group and was, more or less, the leader of the pack. During our eighth-grade year, she decided that we were going to form a girl group for the annual *Chute-O-Rama* all-school talent show. Annie was the lead singer, and Sadie, Rennée, Lena (I believe) and I were her backup singers. We rehearsed our behinds off after school and sometimes at lunch. We were so cute, singing Natalie Cole's "I Can't Say No If You Ask Me." You couldn't tell us jack; we just knew we nailed it. It was these times, events and friends at Chute that kept me going. It was, in part, how I made it through the first two years, which were the most difficult after Charles and Mama became an item.

My absolute favorite teacher at Chute was Dr. Ray Mena, who taught Spanish. He was larger than life in my eyes, and my first and only schoolgirl crush. He was from Cuba, and he was HOT! He had a sexy accent but spoke perfect English. The fact that we shared a first name meant everything to me. Every time his dark brown eyes made their way to me, I wanted to melt. He was our version of the singer Tony Orlando, with his dark shoulder-length hair. I loved the smell of his spicy cologne that announced him loud and clear. He was impeccably dressed every single day. He wore those silky dress shirts that were popular in the seventies, with slacks and a blazer. The first few buttons of his shirt were always unbuttoned and from his neck there hung a gold chain and medallion. He topped off his style with a thick gold ID bracelet. He was charismatic and magnetic, and sucked me all the way in as he taught.

I did my best to keep up, but I was still trying to get my verbs correct in English, making Spanish even harder for me. He never made me feel as if I couldn't learn, and that endeared him to me. I wanted to be in his presence every chance I got; therefore, I joined the Spanish Club and the Spanish chorus both years. I still couldn't sing and could barely pronounce the words in Spanish, but my ass was front and center whenever we performed. You couldn't tell me anything! I learn the words to "Feliz Navidad" and performed the first three repetitions very well. But enunciating that second line, "prospero año y felicidad," was like singing a song when you don't know all the words and you just make something up.

When I left Mr. Murphy's seventh-grade homeroom, I was ready for eighth grade and my new homeroom teacher, Dr. Lorraine H. Morton. By the time I arrived at Chute, Dr. Morton was the matriarch of the school and already a legend in Evanston. She was the first African American to teach in an Evanston public school outside of the predominantly Black Foster Elementary School. In 1957, Oscar Moody Chute recruited her; and together they spearheaded the desegregation of Evanston's elementary schools. The year after my graduation from Chute, she would leave to become the principal of Haven Middle School, taking Mr. Murphy with her to serve as the assistant principal. I cannot say it enough: I genuinely believe God placed the right people in my path at the right stages in my life.

Mama Morton—as the Chute students called Dr. Morton—would have certainly been classified as one of DuBois's Talented Tenth. Born in a prominent African American family in Winston-Salem, North Carolina, she completed her master's degree in curriculum education from Northwestern University in 1942. By the time I started speaking, she was long since retired from education and had entered politics. She was a member of the Evanston City Council during 1982-1991, and in 1993, she became the first African American and Democratic mayor of Evanston. She was also the longest-serving mayor of Evanston, serving four consecutive terms totaling sixteen years. She passed away in 2018 at the age of ninety-nine. Mama Morton was tough, and some students dreaded being assigned to her class. As for me, I watched her with deference. She dressed like she was a corporate executive every day. She stood about five-foot-two in stature but when she looked at me from under her tiny wireframe lenses, I knew to sit my tail down and shut the heck up.

I discovered that social studies was my favorite subject from Mr. Murphy's classes, but it was in Dr. Morton's class that a whole new genre Black history opened up to me. Black history was taught right alongside American history and the U.S. Constitution, which we were required to learn in order to graduate. I got my first real understanding of slavery and the civil rights movement in her class. Once Dr. Morton unleashed us in the library and I discovered the section containing books by and about African Americans, there was no turning back for me. I developed a love for books and reading became a new way of life for me. I went to the library after school, sat on the floor and perused the small section on Black history. It would be in high school that the world of Black literature really opened for me, but I have never forgotten my introduction to both came by way of Dr. Morton's class. She made me want to learn, and I consumed it all. She often said to us, "You can be anything you set your mind to." I believed every word that came out of her mouth. I was walking that glorious labyrinth and I savored each and every moment at Chute Middle School. Mama and Charles made it complicated and dangerous, but I reasoned that if I could hold onto the joy I felt at Chute every time I walked back into that apartment on the third floor of 802 Seward Street, I would be all right in the end.

Open house was a big event at Chute. Everyone was involved. It was wonderful, and students were the focus. Chute faculty worked hard at making our talents shine. Dr. Mena always had food and music. He placed the students in charge of explaining Cuban cuisine to parents as they savored the variety of dishes. It was so much fun!

Dr. Morton decided we would re-enact historical events. She gave us a stack of speeches and events, and everyone had to pick something. We could do it with a fellow classmate or by ourselves. I was going through the pile when a speech by Sojourner Truth caught my eye. Born into slavery, Sojourner Truth was an abolitionist, a women's-rights activist, and a spy in the Civil War for the North. She delivered the now-famous speech at the Women's Convention in Akron, Ohio, in 1851. Reading it, I was captivated. I was already drawn to the liberation of Black people, but this was the first time I had been exposed to the plight— specifically, of a Black woman in and of herself. Truth's demands seen through a lens of her own humanity has never left me.

I asked Dr. Morton if I could do it in open house and she said, "Certainly." I took that speech home and I rehearsed it until I could repeat it in my sleep. I asked Mama if she would come; I wanted her to see me shine. Silly girl—my heart was still holding out for her to see me, value me and support me. "We'll see," she said, like always.

On that night of the open house, Dr. Morton had prepared a nineteenth-century costume for me. She had a skirt and blouse for me and tied my head in a wrap. I watched the door until it was my turn. I brilliantly transformed into Sojourner Truth from the first to the last word in her speech, "Ain't I a Woman?"

Hearing me—and now old Sojourner ain't got nothing more to say."

When I was done, the teachers and parents gave me a standing ovation. Dr. Morton hugged me with tears shimmering in her eyes. That night I no longer had any doubts that I could do anything and be anything that I set my mind to.

Sixteen

CHARLES

"I have been in Sorrow's kitchen and licked out all the pots. Then I have stood on the peaky mountain wrapped in rainbows, with a harp and a sword in my hands."
—Zora Neale Hurston

"Rae, bring your ass here!" I heard Mama calling me out of my sleep. The tone of her voice said I was in trouble.

"You hear me?" she hollered.

I wiped my eyes, tumbled out of bed, and grabbed my robe.

"Don't let me call you again."

"I'm coming, Mama." I looked at the clock, and it was 11:45 p.m. I wondered, *What in God's name is this about?* My heart was pounding. *Oh, God,* I thought. I immediately recapped everything I had done in between the time Mama finished cooking dinner and fell asleep, tired from a day of cleaning other people's toilets and buzzed from *Christian Brothers* to relieve the humdrum of her life. I completed my homework. Check. I washed the dishes. Check. Put them up. Check. Cleaned the top of the stove. Check. Cleaned the kitchen table. Check. Swept the kitchen floor. Check. I couldn't think of another thing that would get me in trouble. I hadn't even been on the telephone, which I had free range to, sometimes.

Since moving to Evanston, most nights Mama was knocked out just as soon as she had finished making dinner. Sometimes she would take a nap and then get back up and watch television; other times, she would sleep until the middle of the night. Either way, I would eat my dinner, clean the kitchen and head straight to my bedroom to be as far away from Charles as I could. I hated when I had to be in his proximity, and dinner was one of those times. Mama wouldn't let me eat in my bedroom, so the kitchen was it. Charles never stopped watching me—and every minute of it was creepy. Sometimes, while Mama slept, he would make himself a cup of coffee and sit across from me as I ate. He was a living, breathing nightmare sitting there in his pajamas drinking coffee, all grand.

He hadn't attacked me since that day at the Evanston Inn and I still couldn't make sense of it. I knew what he had done was wrong. I knew that his actions were sexual in nature. I knew he should not have been grabbing his woman's daughter. What I didn't understand was the cruelty that had come with it. What kind of pervert was he to grab my breast and grip it like a vise, making me hurt so bad? While he hadn't touched me again, he still made my life a living hell. Every time he looked at me with his eerie smile, I got squeamish. I couldn't eat my food and clean the kitchen quickly enough to get away from him. I tried my best not to look at him looking at me, but it was hard. If I took a quick glance, he pursed his lips as if to say, *I'm watching you.* That particular night, as I ate, he sat on the side of their bed in his pajamas with his legs crossed, smoking a cigarette.

I stood in the hallway between my bathroom and the bedroom. "Yes, Mama?" I asked, half-asleep. She looked up from her side of the bed. Charles was sitting on his side with his back turned from both me and Mama.

"I thought I told you to clean that fucking kitchen?" she asked.

"Mama, I did," I said in a panic as I made my way to the kitchen to point at my proof. My eyes landed on the sink. *WHAT THE HELL?* I thought. It felt like I had been punched in the gut when I saw dishes in the sink, and I instinctively grabbed my stomach. To calm my nerves, I took a deep breath before I turned back to them. Charles was within inches of me, and I wanted to ram those lips pointing at me into his mouth. I moved to the center of the room. I didn't want to be within arm's-length of Mama; if I was going to get a beating, she would have to get up from that bed and make the effort.

"Mama, I don't know what happened, but I cleaned that kitchen," I said. Our eyes met briefly, and then she rested her head in her hand. That was always a sign that she was frustrated.

"So how did those dishes get in the fucking sink?" she asked, looking at me from the corner of her eye.

"I don't know, Mama." My eyes sank to the floor.

"Look at me, bitch, when I'm talking to you!" I raised my head, and I started praying, *Please, God: don't let me get a whopping. Please, God.* I kept repeating that prayer in my head.

"I'm gon' ask you again," she said, taking a drag on her cigarette.

"How did those dishes get in the sink?"

"Mama, I cleaned the kitchen," I repeated. I took a deep breath I knew I had to say it. There was no way out. But I also knew that I couldn't flat-out accuse Charles of making the mess after I had gone to my room.

"Maybe Charles had something else to eat?" I suggested, as meekly as I could.

"Charles told me those dishes were in the sink when he went to sleep." She looked straight at me. I knew this was bad.

"But Mama, I'm not telling a story," I cried. Mama turned around to Charles for reinforcement. He had shifted his body so that he could watch the show, but he never met her eyes, or responded to her question. "So, he's lying on you, huh?" she asked. I didn't dare open my mouth again.

"So, he's lying, huh?" she repeated.

My eyes darted at Charles with defiance. He had trapped me. I knew it was my word against his. If I said no, I would be admitting to not cleaning the kitchen and lying about it. If I said yes, I would commit one of the biggest taboos ever in Mama's eyes: calling an adult a liar. I continued to pray. When Mama looked back at me, I knew I had to say something. "Mama, I'm sorry. I thought I had." It was the only way out: take the blame and pray that she would have mercy on me. And I waited, mentally preparing myself for the blows however they came. The thirty seconds it took Mama to determine her next move were excruciating. She was resting her head in one hand again and holding the cigarette in the other one. Of course, she knew by now he was lying, but what's a woman to do? It was her daughter or her man. She found the middle ground. No beating.

"Get your ass in that kitchen and clean it up."

"Thank you, Jesus," I whispered under my breath.

"And I bet' not have to tell you ever again."

"Okay Mama." I hurried to the kitchen to clean the dirty dishes Charles had deliberately left in the sink after I had gone to bed. Why would an adult even bother to behave this way? This was some psycho shit. I had to give it to him: he won that round, but at least I didn't cry. After I finished cleaning, I was much too mad to go back to sleep. It was clear that Charles was far more calculating than I could ever have imagined. That night I learned a valuable lesson: I couldn't ever let my guard down.

Charles was a puzzle to me, and so was their relationship. Mama and I knew very little about him. He was secretive. Dude even put a lock on his closet door. I was like, *Dang! There are only three people living in this darn apartment.* I was in the living room cleaning one Saturday when I heard Mama ask him why he was putting a lock on his closet. He told her, "Because I want to." I looked back at him like, *you dirty dog,* and shook my head. Mama dropped it just like every other time they got into a disagreement. She never raised her voice at him the way she had at Tobie. I have no idea what happened to her backbone. Charles had her wrapped around his finger. Later, she had someone come and put a lock on her closet. It was all so pathetic.

I never saw him lay money on the table for food like Tobie did. Even when she asked him to pick up KFC for dinner, she went into her purse. I know they split the rent, but all the utilities were in her name because she would sometimes send me to the currency exchange to pay the bills. He didn't allow her to drive his car, either. That bronze-and-black soft top Buick Caprice Brougham was like his God and he kept it spanking clean. I had to hand it to Mama, though: she showed him. Before the end of that summer, she bought her own car. I wasn't *even* mad.

Charles came home from work (smelling like oil from his factory job), bathed, put on a fancy pair of pajamas, and poured himself one of his whiskey-and-milk concoctions. When I went with them to visit two of Mama's friends on the South Side—sisters, Gertrude and Mary he drank more. Their home was a frequent hangout for Mama and Charles. They owned a two-flat home, one sister and her family lived on the first floor and the other sister and her family on the second. And those times, the more he drank the quieter he got, but those damn eyes of his took in everybody and everything.

When I heard her tell him that my father was white, I thought maybe he had put some voodoo on Mama, for real. He wanted to know why I was so much lighter than Mama and she lied to maintain her legitimacy as my mother. She forbade me to tell him otherwise. Since she was claiming to be my biological mother, at least she stopped saying, "No one wanted your ass but me." Of course, once her relatives from Grandmamma Julia's side of the family started visiting from Alabama, that cat slowly crawled out of the bag. It took some real self-hatred to lie about your child to impress a man. It was also another contradictory thing about my skin color and mixed race that she kept up until I was out of her house. It was BATSHIT CRAZY!

Charles was divorced, with two adult sons. We met them sometime between my eighth- and ninth-grade years. His eldest son looked to be in his early to mid-thirties. He was a choreographer in the entertainment industry. At the time, he was traveling with the R&B group The Whispers and gave us complimentary tickets to the performance. Before he left town, he stopped by our apartment. He was quite engaging and spent most of the time talking to me, mostly about his career. I thought he was so cool, especially when he pulled out a photo album filled with pictures of him and entertainers of the day. I stopped cold when I saw a picture of Michael Jackson—yes, *the* Michael Jackson, with his big afro and wearing a blue turtleneck, standing at a pool table leaning on a cue stick. "Woo-o— is this really Michael?" I asked. He took it out and handed it to me, saying, "Sure is." He told me that I could keep it; and I have—all these years. I met the other son, who seemed to be in his early twenties, when we had dinner with him on our only family vacation, to Detroit. I didn't like him. He was aloof and sarcastic when Mama mentioned anything about her and Charles's relationship. He had Charles's brown complexion, unlike his brother, who was my complexion and way taller than both of them. Beyond meeting his two sons, Charles never talked about his life.

The evil stunt Charles pulled with the dirty dishes was only one of many. He played on Mama's weaknesses like a master violinist. The combination of her need to please him and the animosity she felt for me made the conditions prime for him to play her against me. He worked on Mama, planting disparaging seeds about my character that were not true. I could hear him talking to her about me sometimes after I had gone to my room. He would straight-up lie on me. I'd have my ear pressed to the door, thinking, *WHAT THE FUCK?!*

"Georgia, I saw Rae in Humpie's face," referring to Ms. Virginia's brother. That was his favorite topic *me being fast*. It was just stupid. I was in seventh grade, for crying out loud! My idea of a dream man was a teenage boy who looked like Michael Jackson—not a fifty-plus bald man who worked for the railroad. Nonetheless, I watched myself when I was around Humpie in Mama's presence. While I was careful, I kept right on talking to Humpie. I couldn't allow them to take everything from me. Humpie always had my back; I liked that about him. Whenever he witnessed Mama's verbal abuse, he would pull me to the side and tell me to hang in there. Occasionally, he would caution his sister, Virginia, when Mama was slut-shaming on their porch. I heard him tell her, "Don't encourage Georgia in her foolishness."

Those nights when Charles reduced me to a whore, Mama listened, not saying much.

"You need to stop her before she gets out of control," he'd say. Every now and then, she would interject.

"She been that way her whole life. Just too *fast* for her own good," Mama said, like I was a hopeless case. Those late-night conversations between them made me feel lower than low. Boy, did I miss Tobie. Charles made me remember the gem I had in Tobie, flaws and all.

Children should never be made to feel less than human by a parent, but he was relentless: "Georgia, did you see that Rae wasn't wearing a bra?" Mind you, I was a skinny girl straight up and down. I had no hips, no butt and, certainly, no breasts. I had nubs until I started taking birth control when I was sixteen. After I got my period, I moved from a training bra to a 32A, and I didn't even fill that out. You would have thought I was slinging breasts like Cardi B. How he knew all of this was beyond me. Once he was home from work, he rarely went out. Every blue moon, he sat on Ms. Virginia's porch—and I mean, every blue moon. When the weather was nice, I spent little to no time on my block, purposely staying out of sight. Nonetheless, after I heard their conversations, I'd rack my brain trying to figure out if I had done what he said I had done. I knew he was lying from the get-go, but I still questioned myself. That's just how messed up Charles had me. It was debilitating having to be on alert all the freaking time.

Just months after we settled, my worst nightmare became true. Charles asked Mama to marry him. Mama was tickled pink. I didn't realize then how much older he was than Mama, which I should have figured out because he had adult sons. While researching for this book, I found their marriage license. He was fifty-seven and Mama was forty. She was close to his oldest son's age. I will admit, he wore his age well, but I was young then, and I didn't have a concept of age.

They were married on November 30, 1974, at Evanston City Hall. She wore this beautiful royal blue two-piece skirt suit with a white corsage of orchids Charles had given her. I was dabbling a little in make-up and I hooked her up. She looked great, with no signs of being up late cooking for the guests. They went to City Hall to tie the knot, and I stayed home to finish cleaning the house and preparing for our guests.

Mama was in her element; the food was plentiful, and the music was blaring. We had a full house. Our friends from Swann Street Ms. Rachel, her daughters, and children; and Mama's friends, sisters Gertrude and Mary and their families came over. Her friends from Evanston piled into our apartment, too. It was going great that night. Mama was happy, and I was glad she was happy. I knew to stay out of her way as she entertained. I was not going to get into trouble, so I found a seat in the living room and sat my ass down. I listened to the music, bopping my head, and talking to Loretta. Mama had asked me to play the music, so occasionally, I set up a new round of hits on the Atomic 45 rpm turntable, then took my tail right back to my seat. It was a fun night of people drinking and talking; every now and then, someone would even get up and bop in the middle of the living room.

Everything was great until I looked up and saw Mama coming at me with a quickness in her step with one of those big ass old fashioned Polaroid cameras that was popular in the seventies. I raised my hands attempting to catch the blow but not soon enough. I heard the camera crack against the bones of my back as it landed with each blow. I was hunched over on the sofa wailing, "What did I do, Mama?"

"You little whore," she hollered.

"Please, Mama. Please, Mama," I cried.

"I'mo show you better than I can tell you." Each time the camera landed on my back I sunk deeper into my lap with my hands covering my head, and tears falling. I could hear people's voices above my pleas telling Mama to stop. *Georgia, stop! Georgia, stop!*

"This don't make no sense, Georgia," I heard Ms. Rachel holler to Mama.

"Why you beating that child like that?"

Mama didn't respond to anyone. She just kept beating me with the camera. Finally, someone tussled the camera out of her hand. I ran into the bedroom and hid on the side of my twin bed closest to the wall. I scrunched down as low as I could to protect myself. *Please, God,* I frantically prayed in my mind until my tears dried. My heart was beating so fast I thought it was going to explode. I couldn't make myself calm down. I was so ashamed of Mama. I wanted to crawl under my bed and stay there for the rest of my life. People were still pleading, *No, Georgia, no. Gimme that. Come on, Georgia.*

"Oh God," I moaned. I knew she was coming for me again, and I stayed curled between the bed and the wall with my arms wrapped around my head for protection. *Please, God—help me, please.* I could feel the bristles of the broom as they met my arms over my head. She was swinging the broom across the bed. Thank God, someone had blocked me into the corner so she couldn't get to me directly.

"What did I do, Mama?" I moaned.

"You fucking bitch!" She was out of breath and could barely talk but she continued swinging the broom over the bed, yelling, and gasping for breath.

"You ain't nothing but a whore; you better stop this shit! I'm gonna kill you dead. Dead, as you got to die."

Terror consumed me to the point I couldn't even beg for her mercy anymore. I simply accepted that she was in a zone and was going to beat me until she had enough. She didn't even care about all those people witnessing her madness. I could hear everyone pleading futilely with her to stop hitting me. Someone finally stood in front of her to stop the blows and then they pulled her away from the bed.

"Come on in here, Georgia," I heard Ms. Rachel continuing, "This don't make no sense." I raised my head as they were taking her out of my bedroom. I heard Ms. Rachel asking questions to try to get to the bottom of the madness. Everyone chimed in, including an unfamiliar voice that asked, "Georgia, what the fuck is wrong with you?"

When Ms. Rachel finally got Mama to calm down, she explained that Charles had seen me in the hall foyer kissing Poochie's boyfriend. I was still hunched on the floor on the side of my twin bed. I shot up and came to my door that led into the living room. I didn't get too close to Mama, but I was not going to let that lie hang in the air.

"Un-unn, Mama." I said with all the strength I could muster. She turned to me, hand on one hip.

"So, Charles is lying, huh." Her look threatened, *Bitch you bet' not challenge me.* I backed off and turned quickly to Ms. Rachel, saying, "Madea, I didn't do that," I said, with my eyes pleading.

"I know, baby," she said to me so Mama could hear her.

Helen and Ms. Rachel called Poochie into the house at the same time. She and her boyfriend, Jesse, must have stepped out on the back porch to get away from the madness. She and Jesse walked past Mama standing in the doorway between the living room and dining room, glaring. Ms. Rachel repeated to them what Mama said.

"Hell-fucking-no!" Jesse shouted. "What the fuck do I want with a little girl?" Jesse was headed for his twentieth birthday in a month. I was twelve. He and Poochie were later married and had a child together.

"That's just not true," Poochie stated, matter-of-factly. "He's been by my side all night."

"So, Charles lying on all y'all?" Mama asked.

"Hell, yeah!" her boyfriend said adamantly.

"Georgia we all been in this living room all night. Where I'm sitting, I can see straight into the hall," Ms. Rachel said, and "ain't nobody seen what Charles said he saw."

Charles sat on the side of their bed with his legs crossed, a drink in his hand, looking all grand, as usual. She called to him to seek his confirmation.

"I saw what I saw, Georgia," he said, never moving to the front, but sounding irritated in a certain way, and Mama knew to stop talking to him.

"Well, if you saw me, you're a MOTHERFUCKING LIE!" Poochie's boyfriend shouted toward the back where Charles was still sitting.

"Georgia, this is not true. Charles is trying to pull the wool over your head," Ms. Rachel said to her. No matter how hard they tried to convince her otherwise, Mama stood by Charles's accusations with her hands on her hips, trying to look defiant but, instead, looking pathetic. Charles had made a fool of her in front of a house full of people—and on their wedding day, no less.

"You know better, Georgia." Ms. Rachel added. Everyone seconded.

"Get y'all coats and get ready to go," Ms. Rachel said. Other people already had their coats on listening to Mama trying to defend that psycho she had just married. Once everyone spoke up, I left well enough alone, went back to my bedroom, and sat on the floor between my twin beds. I couldn't process what had just happened. I took deep soothing breaths to regroup myself.

After the last guest left, Mama hollered into my room for me to clean up. I went into the living room and picked up the scattered glasses and plates. When I entered their room to go to the kitchen, they were both sitting on their respective sides of the bed. Mama was smoking a cigarette with her head down. Charles had a glass of Jack Daniel's-and-milk chaser, sipping it with a smile on his face—as if he had just had the best orgasm of his life. Back and forth to the kitchen, no one said anything. When I started to clean the kitchen, Mama told me to just put the food up and wash the dishes in the morning. She never mentioned the incident again. I wanted to feel sorry for her, but I couldn't get past getting the fuck beaten out of me with a Polaroid camera.

Seventeen

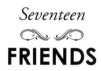

FRIENDS

"One loyal friend is worth ten thousand relatives."
—Euripides

Second to school, fostering friendships contributed to my survival and intellectual growth in Evanston. Looking back, it was as if Evanston were living labyrinth—a place for me to journey and find myself. Each turn I made was one step closer to learning who God created me to be, rather than what Mama made me believe. The friendships I developed while walking this labyrinth helped me to see my worth. Chute and church both served as vehicles for me to meet other young people my age and foster friendships. However, the first friends I made outside of school would have the greatest impact on my first two years in Evanston.

I believe with my whole heart they were all a part of my destiny, like the ancient Chinese belief that an invisible thread connects those who are destined to meet, regardless of time, place, or circumstance. Holly Campbell being my first friend in Evanston was not an accident but was something God appointed. I don't remember how we started hanging out at Ridgeville Park; we just did.

Holly was the cutest little girl. In my eyes, she was the Black version of Shirley Temple, whom I loved. On Saturday mornings, locked away in my bedroom, I devoured every Shirley Temple movie I could. I lived vicariously through her movies, in which she was often pitted against a villainous caregiver; however, in the end, she was rescued by some nice person or long-lost relative. It was my hope that one day my "real" family would take me away from my life with Mama, just like with Shirley Temple. After I met Holly, it was like God had sent me my very own Shirley Temple in place of my relatives. She had cute dimples and naturally curly hair with tight ringlets, just like my child hero—except Holly's hair was the color of Nutella, with perfectly matched eyes. She was short, with a beautiful smile. She was a year younger than me, and her sister Ginger, a year older. We all shared the same complexion, and I wished we were sisters. Her family moved to Evanston about a year prior to mine and lived in an apartment building on Elmwood, about four blocks north of our building. Her mother, Jean Hayes, was divorced and, through my lens, she was the quintessential mom. She was the coolest and hippest modern woman I had ever laid eyes on, except for Aunt Pam; but she wasn't a mom. It was at Holly's where I first witnessed a mother-daughter relationship that resembled something I had seen on television. It was a revelation. In my life, I had no examples of a mother who held a conversation with her child that had nothing to do with giving some kind of order. Jean actually laughed, hugged, and talked to her girls as if what happened in their lives was important to her she talked to them as if they mattered. Mama had never held an uplifting conversation with me and certainly never showed me any affection, ever. We just co-existed. Witnessing a different way to interact with your mother was revolutionary.

That summer when I wasn't exploring Evanston, I was in and out of their house while Mama was at work. Even on Saturdays after I completed my chores, I would go over Holly's and hang out all afternoon. Surprisingly, Mama was cool with it as long as she had a telephone where she could reach me. In a small way, I guess she was allowing me to grow up. I don't know; I just took it and ran with it. I loved everything about Holly's life, and I wanted as much of it as I could get. Those Saturday's Jean made us lunch and we all chatted away. She made me feel like I mattered, in a way similar to what Aunt Lula Mae did. I had my very first grilled cheese and omelet at Holly's. Mama made scrambled eggs with cheese, which I loved, but omelets were a new culinary delight. Every time Jean made one, I watched. I called myself trying to replicate Jean's omelet at home one Saturday morning. Mama asked, "What you putting all that lunch meat in that egg for?" I just shrugged. I didn't dare explain what I had learned from another woman.

Sharmayne Williams was another friend I met that summer, but at church. She also attended Chute, like Holly. Interestingly, I spent almost no time with either of them at school. Holly was in sixth grade and had a different schedule than me. Sharmayne and I were the same age and grade but in different homerooms, although, we did have gym together. She was a gifted gymnast who did double flips on a balance beam in the blink of an eye. She tried to teach me, but the most I learned to do was walk straight on the beam and pray I didn't slip and fall. While Holly and Sharmayne were overlapping friends from the neighborhood who also attended Chute, my friendship with them were separate from each other, and from my other friendships at Chute.

After school, I met Holly at the lockers, and we'd walk home together if we had no extracurricular activities. I was always looking for a place to be other than my house after school so that I didn't have to be home alone with Charles in that two-hour timeframe before Mama got home from work. Unbeknownst to Holly, her house was my safe place almost that entire school year.

Sharmayne and I started hanging out after her mother, Marilyn Barnes gave me a ride home from choir rehearsal. One evening, it was extremely cold; I was walking out of church at the same time as Sharmayne, and she asked me how I was getting home. I told her I was taking the train, and she offered me a ride. That's how Sharmayne and I discovered that we lived only a few blocks from each other. In the beginning I didn't tell Mama because I was forbidden to get in other people's cars. I could have asked Mama to pick me up, but she was just going to ask Charles because she wasn't going anywhere after she had gotten comfortable. I much preferred to take the train, even in the cold, because I didn't want to be alone with him. I dreaded the times Mama instructed me to call home after rehearsal so Charles could pick me up. I hated getting in that car with a passion. As soon as I made it to the car, he would turn his skanky lips up, and I headed for the back seat. On some Sunday's I walked to Sharmayne's apartment and rode to church with them. After church, I'd go up to their apartment sometimes and hang out just long enough so that Mama wouldn't question my whereabouts. I was able to get away with this because Second Baptist worship service ended almost two hours earlier than Grandmamma Julia's church. Mama was accustomed to me coming home sometime between three and four o'clock. For the most part, she didn't know what I did after church. If she found out, there would have been hell to pay. But by then I was sure, as day turns into night, it was a price I would be willing to pay—not just to spend as much time as I could away from my house, but to soak up environments that added value to my life.

It was the following summer after I first met Sharmayne that she overheard Mama cursing me out on the telephone and asked me about it. We had gone bike-riding and it started to get late. I called to see if I could spend a little more time at her house and Mama went off the deep end. I was embarrassed. Mama had never met Sharmayne, but by then she knew of her as a friend from church. That day, I told Sharmayne, "Another time; another day...." and got my tail on that bike and headed home so I didn't get my ass beat. Sharmayne wouldn't let it go, and I finally gave in and told her about my crazy life.

Sharmayne was horrified when she learned that I was being abused and insisted that

I talk to her mother. Marilyn was concerned and decided to have me talk with a friend of hers to explain my circumstances. Officer Washington was a policeman assigned to Evanston Township High School. One Saturday she had him come over to their house to meet me. I had just begun my first year at Evanston Township that fall of 1976. Marilyn thought maybe he could help, particularly because Mama was not my biological mother. He was incredibly sympathetic but because I hadn't come by way of the state, he didn't see a way out. He watched out for me, and I continued to give him updates from time to time. In the meantime, Sharmayne's mother made sure I was included in their after-church activities, and that I knew her door was always open to me.

Just like Holly and her mom, Sharmayne and her mother had a great relationship. Neither Marilyn nor Jean cursed or hollered at their girls that I ever saw. There mothers seem to have reasonable expectations of them. Equally important, they were active in their children's lives. To say the least, it was an eye-opener being exposed to a world that didn't look like the one in which I lived. My only other friends prior to this move were Teresa, on Hermitage Street, and Loretta, on Swann Street. Even though their mothers treated them way better than Mama treated me, I saw slight nuances with these Evanston parents that were different than what I had known.

When I look back, my first thought was that maybe Sharmayne and Holly's mother's positive interaction with their children had something to do with their socioeconomic and education levels; however, upon deeper examination that assumption didn't hold. In actuality, the education and socioeconomic status of my friends' parents varied, and I couldn't blame those as the root causes of Mama's maltreatment of me. My friend Melanie Hall for example, was in both of my homerooms at Chute and lived in the neighborhood. Her mom, Joan Hall, was another parent who was nice to me. When I think about it, Ms. Hall, Ms. Barnes, and Ms. Hayes were all divorced and single heads of household and had entirely different relationships with their girls than Mama had with me. I'm sure none of these families was perfect, but they were a whole hell of a lot better than what was waiting for me at my house.

Back then I never compared Mama's education or profession to my friends' parents; it was just about how they interacted with their children. The only positive similarities I perceived were that Mama provided me with a place to live, food to eat and as many clothes as I wanted. I understand now she was raising me out of her own experiences, and limitations and it defined her parenting.

Even at church the adults treated the young people as if they mattered. They chatted with us about school and the extracurricular activities we were pursuing. This also happened at the coffee hour after church, where we were not relegated to our seats like I was accustomed to. Seeing children in adults' faces was a big no-no from the world where I had lived prior to moving to Evanston. Without question, none of the adults at Second Baptist saw me and the other children as their peers or vice versa. Rather, it was an acknowledgment of my humanity and place in the world, even as a young person. They encouraged us to talk about our lives, celebrated our accomplishments and offered us advice. No one told me to sit my *fast* tail down, or that I talked too much.

I can honestly say that the adult-child relationships at Second Baptist that I witnessed were informed by the African proverb: "It takes a village to raise a child." It didn't matter that I was not their biological child; I still belonged to them. Our minister of music, Belinda Hubbard, hugged me just as she hugged her own daughter, Veela. Pastor Taylor and his wife, Ann, extended the same kind of warmth to me that they did to their own children: Chandra, Audreanna and Hycel III. The Howlett family clan did the same, treating me as they did with their children, nieces, and nephews. All of the parents were kind to me. I absolutely loved Ruth and Warren Howlett who were uber kind to me.

I remember after the *Essence* cover story Ms. Ann Taylor, our former first lady at

Second Baptist and her daughter Chandra, came to hear me speak in Nashville. That gesture was more than enough but the next morning they came to the airport to see me off. Ms. Taylor sat next to me at the boarding gate. She held my hand and asked if she had failed me because they never knew the conditions under which I lived at home. Of course, she hadn't failed me. But it meant the world to me that she cared enough about me to ask. Second Baptist saved me in a different way; in that the role it played in my life was a testament to the environment of love and nurturing it created, like at Chute.

I was learning what positive interpersonal relationships and emotional support looked like. Something in my gut told me that as long as Mama was the primary influence in my life, I was not going to win. All I can say is that God had my back. I paid heed to my intuition, and the universe continued to show me the way. I never looked back. I made a deliberate paradigm shift. I took the face value of those positive influences I encountered and transformed them for my benefit. I sat my tail right smack-dab in the middle of that village of friends and took in everything I needed—not only to survive, but to thrive.

I didn't just have friends; I had friends and their lives. I couldn't get what I needed from Mama, so I lived the lives of my friends by default. I took every chance that I could get to spend time with my friends and their mothers. This was the truest with Holly, Sharmayne and, then later, with Coré and her mother, Reverend Dr. Jeanne Cotton. As sure as my name is Rae, this saved me from total self-destruction. These parallel worlds I crafted for myself were the key to my survival. I think it was nothing short of extraordinary how I maneuvered them. The trickiest part of living in both worlds was keeping them separate from each other.

In spite of all the wonderful friends I made my first year, not everyone liked me. Go figure. At Chute Wendy Williams began bullying me right away. She said she didn't like me because I thought that I was "bad," being that I came from the South Side of Chicago and all. I was scared of Wendy. She looked rough. She was bigger than me, and fully developed, like she was already in high school. I didn't want to chance a fight because I might get beat up and, Lord, then I'd have to answer to Mama. Honest to God, I would leave from the side door at school rather than the front door to avoid Wendy. At some point, it somehow resolved itself. Lo and behold, her father and his wife moved into my building, right across the hall from us. The first time I walked out of our apartment and bumped into her making it up the stairs to her father's apartment, I froze. She looked at me, rolled her eyes and jerked passed me into her father's door. After that, thank God, she started speaking when she saw me at the building and stop taunting me at school.

Then this Filipino girl—Marilou Ynot, who was in my homeroom—hated me for reasons I never figured out. But it seemed like everyone in my class got involved, going back and forth between us. Our classmates informed me that Marilou was some kind of martial arts expert, and she was. I had absolutely nothing to trump a black belt, and I bided my time. I was relieved when that phase went as quickly as it came. In fact, Marilou lived across the street from Chute, and I started meeting her at home before school and we walked across the street together. Rosalind Shorter came to Chute for a year, and she didn't like me, either. I thought I was going to have to fight her. Then one day, just like that, we became friends. We share the same birthday and remain friends to this very day.

The problem that wouldn't resolve with time was Kathy Williams. She hated me and expressed it on many occasions throughout the school year. Like with Marilou, she never told me why she didn't like me; she just didn't. I always hated those blanket and unfounded declarations, and I still do. People make shit up in their heads and believe it. At least Wendy declared her reasons, even if she had made herself believe she was supposed to fight me because I was from the city.

I never understood bullying. If I had a problem with someone, you'd best believe I could name it. I also understood that it was my problem, not theirs, and I didn't have to expose myself to whatever it was I didn't like. I was friendly with everyone, but like when I attended Earle, I didn't want to be everyone's friend. I knew when to stick around and when to keep it moving. Nor did I think everyone had to be my friend. By the time I got to Chute, I had spent too much of my life trying to prove my worth to Mama, and I wasn't going to do it with my peers. I used to say, "Like me or lump me." I didn't give two hoots.

Kathy was a tall skinny white girl with long reddish-brown curly hair and freckles to match. After she declared that I was on her shit list; our classmates, being who they were at twelve and thirteen, egged her on. I tried to avoid her in some cases and ignore her in others. I really wasn't trying to put myself in a position to get in trouble over some stupid shit. I had no beef with her. One day as we were crossing the outside corridor, which is the quickest way to reach the other side of the building, I felt something hard against my butt pushing me forward. *WHAT THE FUCK!?* I thought, trying to maintain my balance so that I didn't fall face-forward. When I got myself together, I turned to see who had so violently pushed me forward. Kathy Williams was standing in my face.

"Yeah, I kicked you. So what?" she asked matter-of-factly.

This bitch must be feeling her oats. I thought and swung at the same time. I kept hitting her as hard as I could. She hadn't expected this response and, by the time she started swinging back like a wild cat, I had the best of her. I could hear Mama in my head: *If you don't fight back, I'm going to beat your ass when you get home.* Some teacher pulled us apart. As I was sitting in Mr. Pate's office waiting on my punishment, I heard Mama's voice again: *I told you about showing your ass and embarrassing me.* It was that situation with Clara all over again. Gloom took all of the glory out of my kicking Kathy's ass.

After school, I went to Holly's house instead of going home. At least I could delay Mama's wrath by the time it took me to get from Holly's house. Right about the time Mama was supposed to be home from work, she called Holly's to see if I was there. Charles had informed Mama that I wasn't always home when he arrived, and she asked me about it. Once I explained, she was okay as long as she knew where I was. But typically, I made it home before she did. That day, I was in no rush. As soon as I got on the phone she said, "Bring your ass home!" The dial tone was the next thing I heard. Before I could place the telephone back on the receiver, I was crying. Holly and her mother tried to reassure me that Mama would understand that I was defending myself. I had been there before, and I knew the truth. Whatever it was they said to me that day didn't stick. All I can remember is, *but you don't know my Mama,* repeating over and over in my head. I just couldn't say it aloud. As of yet, I had not told one living, breathing soul in Evanston about my home life. I was too embarrassed, and I was afraid of Mama. The misery she and Charles thrust on me was my cross to bear, and mine alone. I dried my tears, hugged Holly and her mother, and made my way home. I walked at a snail's pace; yet at the same time, it seemed to be the fastest walk ever. I couldn't figure out how to approach Mama. When I reached our apartment, I went straight to my bedroom. Before I could put down my book bag, I heard Mama's voice.

"Come here, young lady," she said. I took a deep breath and prayed, "Please God, don't let me get a whopping." I went back out my door leading to the living room the farthest away from Mama. As usual, she and Charles were sitting on their sides of the bed. Charles stood up when I entered the room.

"What happened at school today, Rae?" Mama asked.

"Mama, this white girl named Kath-." I stopped mid-sentence because my eyes had focused in on the bed. The covers looked like there was a hump in the bed; something was there under the covers, and I knew that Mama always made her bed before leaving for work. As I focused in on the bed, I could see what looked like a thick piece of wood sticking out a tad from the side of the covers.

"I'm talking to you," she said, demanding that I continue my story. But I was frozen. It was as if a force greater than me had closed my mouth and fixed my eyes on the bed. Charles noticed me straining to see and he took a quick anxious look at the bed. It all seemed to come together in slow motion, like on television when two people are running toward each other, but it really happens in a flash. The realization hit us both at the same time. Charles grabbed a belt from beside the bed. I turned and high-tailed my ass out of the house leaving the door open. I pounced down those stairs in a flash. I ran my ass off around the corner, then hit the alley, and ran past Ridgeville Park. I didn't stop until I reached Holly's house. Thank God Mama didn't know where she lived. Holly's mom calmed me down. At first, she thought I was exaggerating.

"Rae, I'm sure you didn't see a thick piece of wood sticking out of the cover." My head was shaking up and down, trying to get it out. Crying, wiping snot, and trying to explain at the same time. Jean looked doubtful. Tears streamed down my face. *You don't know my Mama* was on replay in my head. She was struggling, trying to believe me. I knew she wanted to, but it seemed completely far-fetched that a mother would actually beat a child with a thick piece of wood. But my fear was undeniable. Jean said, "Let's start from the top." I knew it was time for me to explain.

I started with the fact that Mama was not my biological mother. When I finished, Jean gave me a tight hug. I had never experienced this kind of compassion. The weight hovering over us was so heavy you could cut it with a knife. Jean was outraged. I was relieved. For months, I had been living in these parallel worlds hiding my secret one from the other. I felt as if I had an ally. Jean talked to me like I was her daughter. She consoled me and tried to think through solutions to help me. She suggested the idea of going to talk to Mama, but she saw the fear in my eyes and let it go. It was the first time that someone had named what was happening to me as abuse.

With the exception of a few, when Mama's friends witnessed my degradation, they dismissed it, saying, "You know how Georgia is." It was the era when people didn't interfere with how a parent raised a child, especially when the degradation is accepted as discipline rather than abuse and neglect. How she disciplined me was her business, and hers alone. When I think back on those days, I would give anything for more of her peers to have said, "Georgia, you are wrong." Tobie was gone and Charles seemed to get pleasure from my misery. When I think about it, Tobie was the only adult and family member who ever told Mama she was wrong. For as much as Grandmamma Julia and Mama were at odds, she only seemed to be concerned with my soul for the hereafter, not my living soul slowly dying from the cancer called Mama.

Jean was determined to help me. When the police arrived, she explained that I was an abused child. We filled the police in on the day's events and they took me home. Lord knows I didn't want to go. Tears formed in my eyes, and Jean and Holly tried to reassure me everything would be all right.

I was scared to death.

Please, God. Please, God. Please, God, let it be okay played in my head. I had broken one of her cardinal rules: discussing her business outside the house. Sitting in the back seat of that police car, I tried to work out every possible scenario. When Mama answered the door, she was shocked to see the police. She listened and looked at me as they addressed the situation. The police seemed to be on my side in their approach to Mama, explaining that the fight at school was not of my own making. While fighting was never condoned, it was self-defense, they explained to her. At one point she looked at me.

"Why didn't you tell me that, girl?" she asked.

"I tried Mama, but you was going to whop me," I said, pathetically. Mama shot me that look, and I knew to shut the fuck up. As the police filled her in, it was clear that Charles had not told her what really happened. He was the one who had spoken with Mr. Pate and relayed the message that I had a one-day suspension, but Mama didn't appear to know that it was because of a fight. She was embarrassed, and it was written all over her body. She slumped a little and her glassy eyes lost all the fight. Charles had made a fool out of her yet again, at my expense. I never found out what he actually told her, other than I had been suspended. When she shut the door, I went to my room and exhaled. Thanks to quick thinking and Jean, I was spared the rod.

After a while Mama called me into their room. I went to the entrance of their bedroom from the living room, again keeping my distance. They sat in their usual spots like nothing had happened. She lit a cigarette, and he was drinking a cup of coffee like all was well with the world.

"Yes, Mama," I answered, with bated breath. Charles shot his eyes at me and pushed his lips out, his Adam's apple bopping up and down from the gestures with his lips. He was so freaking creepy. Mama took a deep drag on her cigarette and blew the smoke in the air.

"Rae, I don't want you over that bitch's house anymore," she said, defeated.

"Who, Mama?" I asked, trying to play dumb.

"Whoever that bitch is that called the police on me," she said. I stilled myself and held my breath. I knew one wrong word or move, and I would get the shit beaten out of me, police and all notwithstanding.

"If I catch you, or even hear of you going over there…" she paused and looked me straight in the eye: "I'm going to beat your motherfucking ass."

I didn't know if I should respond so I stayed still.

"You hear me, bitch?"

"Yes, Mama," I said, meekly, trying to hold back tears.

"Where do they live anyway?" she asked.

"On Elm Street," I said, pleading with my eyes.

"Where on Elm Street?"

"Over there by the hospital," I said, trying to keep it vague, and hoping she didn't ask for the specific address. That seemed to satisfy her.

"Get out of my face," she demanded.

Charles didn't say anything, he just watched me intensely while drinking his coffee. Mama never looked his way. Often, she would turn her body toward him for reinforcement, but her back stayed toward him and her eyes were focused on me.

The next day, my friends told me that Mama and Charles were walking up and down the street looking for me after I fled the house.

"Your mother is a crazy bitch," one of them said.

"They asked us if we had seen you."

"We just shook our heads," someone else explained.

They all laughed and joked, explaining that Mama had a two-by-four in one hand. "It looked like she had been at a construction site," someone laughed. They explained that she had an extension cord in the other hand and Charles had a belt in both hands.

"That shit was fucked up," another voice chimed in. Shame slid into my gut like vomit.

They all chimed in when someone said, "Damn, girl—you are living like that?"

All I could do was shake my head up and down and try not to cry.

"Well, girl, we got you," someone else said.

"Crazy-ass motherfuckers," another person mumbled.

Gratitude immediately replaced my shame. They had all seen me running toward Holly's house and they didn't tell Mama. They had protected me that day. I was thankful to God for my friends.

Eighteen

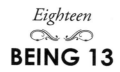

BEING 13

dark phrases of womanhood
of never havin been a girl
half-notes scattered
without rhythm/no tune
distraught laughter fallin
over a black girl's shoulder
it's funny/it's hysterical
the melody-less-ness of her dance
don't tell nobody don't tell a soul
she's dancin on beer cans & shingles
—Ntozake Shange

I was maturing. My Barbie dolls and stuffed animals were neglected and finally placed on my unused twin bed as a monument to Little Rae. My flat chest grew buds, and I went from an over-the-head training bra to a grown-up bra that clasped in the back, which made me incredibly happy. I had been envious of my new neighborhood girlfriends Teresa's and Anita's beautifully rounded breasts. I was a wonderful mystery unfolding before my eyes and I had lots of questions—and nowhere to turn for answers. I was NEVER, EVER in this lifetime going to ask Mama anything that had something to do with my body. I had already experienced so much shaming at her hands that I figured I should leave well enough alone. Instead, I navigated the terrain on my own, picking up how to take care of my body here and there.

Mama, on the other hand, didn't need me to tell her anything about my maturation; she had eyes, and she laid down her laws of antiquated wives' tales about the female body. When hair started to grow under my arms and on my legs, she forbade me to shave, saying it would "ruin my nature"—whatever the hell that meant. I never figured it out. My girlfriend Sharmayne shaved, and I didn't see what the problem was. By the end of my freshman year at Evanston Township High School, I would defy that rule. For one, I hated the odor of my underarm hair, and I detested the dark brown hair that grew on my legs that made them look dirty. I learned how to shave by trial and error. There were many a day when I shaved off a layer of my skin right along with the hair on my legs. The underarms were easy breezy, except that it itched like crazy once it started growing back. I tried Nair—a hair-removal cream—in high school after seeing my girlfriend Stevie use it. I probably burned off a layer of my skin using it.

The most intriguing was pubic hair. Watching it emerge into a little afro was nothing short of amazing to me. I wondered how God did that. Then my amazement turned into disgust when I started my period. I didn't like the fact that my pubic hair held an odor or that the blood created clunks of matted hair around the vulva edge. I wanted to cut it off, but I was too afraid that I would cut my stuff right along with my hair. The point is that I muddled through maturation with no help from my mother and with a fear that, if she found out what I had done to my body contrary to her demands there would certainly be hell to pay.

I watched Mama uneasily observe the physiological changes that took me from childhood on the path to womanhood. Whatever insecurities she had about herself as a woman showed up in her discomfort about my growing up. Public shaming became even more prevalent, as if she could demean this process. I remember it like yesterday. Sitting on Ms. Virginia's porch, Mama would tell her, "She think she grown now that she got some titties." I mean, where did that come from? I'd twist my face up, making Ms. Virginia laugh. If Barbara were there, she'd say, "Now come on here, Georgia." Sometimes, I'd pretend not to hear or get up and go to the park, leaving them laughing at me. The worst was when a breeze hit my breasts and caused my nipples to harden. One time I walked across the street to tell Mama I was going to the park. Before I could get anything out of my mouth she told me, "Get Your Hot Ass In The House," emphasizing every word, "And Change Your Goddamn Shirt!" Of course, everyone sitting on the porch looked at my breasts. All I could do was shake my head and go back to the house to change.

Some days Mama made me feel so low I wished I were a boy, in spite of the fact that I loved being a girl. On other days, she'd give me everything I wanted. We were in Montgomery Ward's department store one day and I saw a sign for the Wendy Ward Charm School. "Mama, can I go?" I asked, pointing to the sign.

"What's that, girl?" she responded. I explained and she asked me how much it cost. She allowed me to go upstairs to the school to get the information. After her next pay period, I had my first Wendy Ward class. These bizarre dichotomies she created for me to live by were the most difficult to live with. She kept me off balance. Honestly, most days I really didn't know if I was going or coming. I just did my best and adjusted to the contradictions as if they were always part of the plan.

When I started Wendy Ward, Mama was already an Avon representative, but I did all the work. I went door to door and pitched the product. I wrote the orders, counted the money, and delivered the items. Makeup samples came, and Mama let me fix my face as practice. I was learning to apply makeup at Wendy Ward and having the Avon samples made it all the more fun for me. Wendy Ward polished me and made me shine. I thought I was all that and a bag of chips.

On our summer vacation to Detroit, where we met Charles' youngest son, I was feeling my "13" oats. Mama had purchased me all these new clothes and I had two outfits for each day, just in case. Lawd! It was really exciting. We had a day trip to Canada and to the famous amusement park, Boblo Island. Well, the morning we were going to the park, we were rushing from the hotel to have breakfast before we got to the Boblo boat. I hadn't quite finished pulling my "look" together and when we arrived at the restaurant, I went into the bathroom to glam up. I pulled my Avon samples out and got to work. I rationalized that if I could sample the makeup at home and at Wendy Ward, then I could certainly use my skills on a day that I should be looking fabulous. As soon as I sat at the table, Charles nudged Mama and waved his head my way. Mama looked up and the expression on her face said, *HELL TO THE NAW!* I knew I should have gotten up right then, but my hormones told me, *Gurrl, you look-ing fly!* I was *snatched*—from head to toe—in my white slacks, powder-blue top and white stacked-heel sandals, and a beat face to match.

"BITCH!" Mama spewed. "Who the fuck do you think you are?" It seemed to me like everyone in the restaurant looked our way.

"Get yo' ass in there and take that shit off your face!" By the time she said, "You ain't GROWN!" I was already out of my seat. Oh, my God—I was so embarrassed. When I came back with a clean face, she darted an eye at me, but she didn't say anything else about the makeup.

Looking back, that was the most authentic mother-daughter interaction I had with her during this period in my life. Makeup was still one of those age-appropriate topics that floated among mothers in the mid-seventies. Here my ass was, sitting down all big and bad, with a full face. In hindsight, I probably could have gotten away with the soft pink blush and lip gloss, but I was doing way-y-y too much with that blue eye shadow. To this day, I don't think I've worn blue eye shadow ever again.

By now, I had been living with the secret of Charles's attack for two years. I had made the sage decision to keep it to myself. At the time, I had no way to predict that Charles would become a fixture in our lives. My hope was that she would get him out of her system quickly, but that didn't happen. Once I learned how demented Charles was and the power he held over Mama, I knew she could never know this truth.

Then Claudette came into our life. She was a new maid at the Evanston Inn. She and Mama quickly became friends. Their friendship would continue a few decades until Claudette died from cirrhosis of the liver. Of all Mama's friends, I really liked Claudette. She was younger and hipper than Mama. She was undoubtedly my biggest ally among Mama's Evanston friends. She was never afraid to tell Mama what she thought, and she always held her ground. She intervened on my behalf quite a few times and I was grateful for her. I can hear her saying, "Georgia, you are so full of shit. Let the girl be a damn teenager."

One day Claudette pulled me to the side and asked why I rode in the back seat of the car when I was alone with Charles. I looked down at my feet, avoiding her eyes. I could hear Mama in my head: *You bet' not tell my business!* In the aftermath of the incident with the police and Jean, I had been wary to talk about my home life. I shrugged my shoulders. "I don't know," I said.

"Yes, you do," Claudette insisted. For a moment, our eyes locked and mine said what my mouth couldn't *You already know. Don't make me tell you.*

"You can trust me," she said. I thought about it for a minute, and I felt that I could trust her in the same way that I could trust Jean. Claudette had proven herself to be on my side. The problem was weighing the benefits of telling. I knew that once I told, there could be no turning back. She seemed like a worthy opponent because she won Mama over on other things. I thought maybe she could win her over on this, too. Obviously, she was concerned about my well-being because she had approached me with her observation. On the other hand, I wasn't too sure I wanted to break this rule of talking about Mama's business again. This was one of the hardest decisions I ever had to make, but that day I let go of the secret because the burden of holding it felt like Charles was still holding me against that wall. Standing in the corner huddled with Claudette—and contrary to everything I knew about Mama—I made myself believe that telling would somehow benefit me in the end.

"I'm scared of Charles," I whispered, as if saying it any louder would be the death of me. She leaned back to get a better look at me.

"What do you mean you're scared of Charles?" she asked.

"I'm just scared," I said, shrugging my shoulders and looking back down at my feet.

"Why?" she asked. Claudette grabbed my hand and led me out of the corner of the hotel and outdoors away from where Mama could've seen us.

"Talk to me, girl," she said, in a serious manner.

"Charles tried to rape me," I said, and my entire body exhaled. I knew then, no matter how it played out, I had made the right decision. Claudette embraced me and let my tears fall onto her shoulders. I told her about the day in his room before we moved to Evanston. How he had pushed me up against the wall, groped me then threatened to get me in trouble if I told Mama. How I was afraid to be alone with him because I believed that one day, he would actually rape me. At least if I rode in the back seat and he tried to attack me, the barrier would give me time to get out of the car. After I had recounted all the details and we were headed back into the hotel, all of my bravado went straight out of me, and I started to panic.

"Please, don't tell Mama," I begged.

"You just let me handle Georgia," she said, and she hugged me again.

That Saturday after Charles left the house, Mama called me into their bedroom. I stood at the doorway closest to the bathroom. She was sitting on the side of the bed, cigarette in hand.

"Claudette told me that you scared of Charles," she said. The fact that her starting point was about me being afraid of Charles rather than what Charles had done to me made me nervous.

"I am, Mama," I mumbled.

"What kind of shit you trying to pull?" My nerves were a mess. I braced myself, already hating that I hadn't entered her room from the living room closest to the front door.

"Nothing, Mama," I said, barely audible. "I'm just scared of Charles."

"So why you scared of Charles?" she asked all too calmly. I had seen that kind of calmness before and once ignited, it caught on like wildfire. Anxiety took over. I wanted to jump out of my skin and leave my body to contend with the firestorm I felt coming my way.

"Because he grabbed me that time Mama," I pleaded with my voice. She wasn't giving an inch. She just sat on the side of the bed watching me squirm. As I recalled the story of that day in the hotel with Charles, I found my voice. The cat was out of the bag and there was absolutely no point in backing off my truth. I told her about every single detail with absolute clarity. She listened, taking deep draws on her Winston. After I had said all that had been done, I shut up. Those seconds it took for her to speak felt like hours.

"So why you just saying something now?"

"I was scared to tell you, Mama." I twisted my hands and prayed to God I didn't get the shit beaten out of me.

"But you weren't too scared to tell Claudette." Mama had just checked me for telling Claudette. I backed up an inch closer to the hall toward my bedroom.

"But she asked why I rode in the back seat. You never did." I tried to explain and got tongue-tied. I was all jumbled up. I continued to explain why I had told Claudette. She watched me fumbling over my words and, for a moment, I didn't know if she was listening to me or just watching me fall apart. Finally, she spoke.

"Bitch, take yo' ass somewhere with these lies!"

"But Mama, he did. I'm not telling a story!" I said, without hesitance. (And without thinking.)

"Who the fuck you raising your voice to?" she asked.

"I was just trying to explain, Mama. I'm not telling a story, Mama," I pleaded.

"Charles ain't done shit to you!" she insisted. At that point I knew there was nothing else to be said on my part. Once Mama made her decision, it was final. She had chosen Charles, as I predicted the day it happened. Now, all that had to be done—which was typical since Charles came into our life—was for her to justify her decision.

Mama had never known me to be a liar. I just didn't have it in me, and I still don't. I may not have told her everything I was doing but, in the end, if she had ever asked, I told the truth. In spite of what she said to me that day and all the days that followed, I didn't believe she thought for one moment I was lying. I knew in my heart that Mama knew I was telling the truth, as was the case in many other incidents that had occurred between us since Charles. Surprisingly, I didn't shed a tear. I just listened to her diatribe as she crafted her defense.

"You ain't nothing but a fucking whore! I'm not going to let you fuck up my shit!

Charles don't want yo' ass! Get the fuck out of my face!" Those were her last words. I hurried from the hall into the bathroom and locked the door. I figured if she was going to beat me, she would have to break the door down. I sat on the toilet, trying to make the hurt go away. It was no use. When I heard Mama on the telephone I went to my room and changed clothes to get the heck out of the house. I stopped at the doorway to her room. She looked up at me.

"Excuse me," I said. "Can I go outside?"

"I don't give a fuck what you do," she said, and went back to her telephone conversation.

One day the following week, Mama had Charles drive me someplace I can't recall. Before he pulled off, he shifted the front view mirror to get a good view of me.

"Georgia said that you are afraid of me," he said. I took a deep breath, thinking, *What- The-FUCK?* I couldn't believe Mama had set me up in this way, leaving me so exposed. Rather than protecting me by facing Charles and pushing back—as I had seen her do countless times with Tobie— she threw me under the bus. I couldn't even fathom what he was going to say. I braced myself for his madness, thinking, *Here the psycho goes again.* "If I want your little ass, I'll get you in the front seat or the back," he said then pulled off, but kept the mirror so he could look at me when he stopped at red lights. He never mentioned it again, but I carried that fear of him until their relationship ended.

Not too long afterward, Mama continued to shape her narrative and spread that lie. She knew that Claudette knew the truth and she had to make sure that if it got back to anyone, she had covered her behind. "Yeah, that bitch out here trying to say Charles want her ass," I heard Mama say on the telephone to one of her friends. I didn't know who she was talking to, but I understood that this was the beginning of the BIG LIE, just like Donald Trump and the 2020 Presidential election. Mama could shape a lie and keep it going, like, forever. I wondered if her friends believed everything that she told them. My God, she was good at it. She'd sit on the sofa—always closest to my bedroom door for my benefit—smoke cigarettes in her housecoat and tell her version of the story with the ease of a telephone salesperson. She was relentless with her propaganda, casting me as some wild child. It never failed; just when I thought some topic was out of her system, we were back at the same old story. Like the time I almost got a beating for fighting and Jean called the police to protect me from her. Mama must have told every friend she had, to put it in her words, "…what that bitch did," speaking of Jean. "I should have beat her motherfucking ass after the police left," speaking of me. The fact that I had told her business to a stranger and that Jean had called the police was the whole story.

Mama's narrative never had anything to do with the fact that Charles duped her, or her fundamental treatment of me. It was always about me being "out of control," in her words. You would have thought I was running with the wolves. The fact is, at this stage in my life, I was still a virgin on my own account. I was home every evening on time until the day I no longer lived with her. I was too afraid to do otherwise. If not, she knew where I was. I never smoked a cigarette or a joint. In fact, I've never used any illegal drugs in my entire life. While I have had an alcoholic beverage, you could gather all the drinks I've had over the fifty-nine years of my life, and you would maybe have a gallon of booze. I've never had a beer or a glass of wine—just mixed drinks with more mix than alcohol. I simply never acquired a taste for alcohol. Yes, I was precocious. Yes, to some adults, I came across as "acting grown." Yes, I talked a lot, masking all my pain. If I kept talking, I didn't have to think about what was waiting for me when I returned home each day. If I belonged at school, or at church, or my friends' houses, I didn't have to dwell on the fact that I didn't belong in my own home. It was a very difficult time for me. I was trying to find my place in the world as best as I could. It was bad enough that Mama used everything against me. When her friends played into the lies it was even more painful.

One day spinning her narrative I heard her say, "I put them together and she denied it." I jumped out of my bed and stood with my ear to my bedroom door. *You have got to be kidding me!* I thought. She was telling someone she had confronted Charles in front of me and I denied it. Of all the stories Mama had ever told about me, hearing this lie caused something to die inside of me. It never happened, but she kept that lie going until the very end. That day, my mouth flung open in disbelief. "Little whore," she spun. "I'm not gonna let her fuck up my shit." Whoever it was must have given her an amen. "Yeah," she said, "Charles been too good to me." I rolled my eyes. "I'm not gonna let that bitch run my man away," she continued.

It was unfathomable she would go this far. I didn't know what to think about her. She never failed to surprise me with her depraved treatment toward me but, in this case, she totally threw me for a loop. Years later, I concluded that she threw me under the bus because she understood that by staying with Charles, a man who had sexually assaulted her pre-teen daughter, she had broken the basic bonds of a mother-daughter trust. Mama might not have had a formal education, but she was far from stupid. She told Claudette that same lie, of course. Claudette circled back and told me, "I don't believe an ounce of what Georgia said." She continued to encourage me and push me to think about my future. One day she told me, "Georgia is not the end-all-be-all, Rae. Just stay in school and make a way for yourself."

Mama advanced slut-shaming to a whole other level after she learned about Charles's attack on me. Without one doubt in my mind, she used my coming of age as a weapon against everything wholesome and natural about growing up female. Attacking me was how she addressed the war raging inside of her. While I had speculated prior to this period that Mama resented me and it manifested in our daily relationship, at thirteen I was able to pinpoint this new escalation. I believed that, in her mind, I became her competition. In the scheme of things, it was a combination of conditions the start of my maturation, the advancement in my education, a shift in me because of my newfound information in Evanston. And above all of these there was the same narrative she had been touting since I was six: that I was *fast*. She told herself this one thing: that Charles wouldn't want to fuck me if I wasn't *fast*. She told herself this lie so often I think, at some point in her life, she started to believe it. What neither of us understood then—and Mama never would— was that Charles never wanted to *fuck* me; he wanted to control both of us. Divide and conquer was the method he chose, and it worked. Mama never would understand this because to let go of the BIG LIE would make her less of a mother.

When I couldn't be out of the house, I retreated to my room and my music. On Hermitage Street, music was Mama's thing. But coming of age in the seventies was a time that R&B was thriving, and without a doubt I absorbed the messages in the music, and it carried me. Music was cathartic. It soothed my soul and gave me hope. I'd sit on the floor in front of my little turntable and little album collection, and the music helped me through a mood, a moment and Mama. I had 45 RPMs, too, because I couldn't always afford the whole album. The theme song from the movie Mahogany, starring Diana Ross and Billy Dee Williams made me think about my future. I teared up every time I heard Diana's angelic voice asking,

> *Do you know where you're going to?*
> *Do you like the things that life is showing you?*
> *Where are you going to? Do you know?*

I didn't have a clue what would become of me. Mama never asked about my dreams and aspirations, and I had none—other than to grow up and get the heck out of her house. This song made me think, *What happens next?* I had been working so hard since moving to Evanston to just get ahead. Now music was pushing me to think beyond leaving Mama's house. Day in and day out, I'd sing to those songs that inspired me, pushing Mama and Charles out of my head. On happier days, I played the music of the young recording artists I had fallen in love with, like every other thirteen-year-old girl. First came the Jackson Five and then came the Sylvers—another popular R&B family musical group similar to the Jackson Five. To make it official, I added a poster of the Sylvers to the wall in my bedroom, right next to the Jackson Five. I put on the Sylvers' 45 RPM, Boogie Fever and danced it out in the middle of my room. I loved to dance, even if I still couldn't get the beat down like Mama. I daydreamed and created scenarios about meeting and marrying one of them. It didn't matter which one, because they were all gorgeous. The only person who could dethrone any one of them was Michael Jackson. He was already my king. I knew all the words to all the songs, especially that one about being under the apple tree. Sometimes I would dance with that photo of Michael that Charles's son had given to me. It was a hoot.

Earth, Wind & Fire was the male musical group who made songs that touched my heart and soul. Named for the mighty elements of the universe and founded by Maurice White, the band's sound was a mixture of R&B, soul, pop, and funk. *That's the Way of the World* was the first album I ever purchased. Every song on that album was a hit, but my favorite was "Shining Star," which rose to the Billboard Hot 100 and Hot Singles charts. Shining Star became my battle cry. I played it repeatedly until I learned the words. I wrote the lyrics down in my notebook and sat on my floor and sung along. Once I knew it by heart, I'd stand in the mirror, with a hairbrush for my microphone, and sing that song as a mantra to what I could be. The chorus is a powerful two-liner,

You're a shining star
No matter who you are
Shining bright to see
What you could truly be (What you could truly be)

I even wrote it down on all of my school folders as a reminder of how special I was and could be. Whenever I started to feel unworthy, I'd read it again. To survive, I did whatever I could to rebuke everything Mama ever told me I was and everything she declared I was never going to be. As many times as I can tell you that Mama was never my cheerleader is about as many times that she said to me, "You ain't never gonna be shit." Music did what she was not willing to do: it validated me.

I loved gospel music more than any music in the whole wide world. Grandmamma Julia had done her job well. On top of going to church with her and to the Isabel Joseph Johnson Show, I tagged along on Sunday afternoons when she was the guest soloist at 3:30 for musicals, anniversaries, and special occasions typical in the African American religious tradition.

We went to large churches like Pilgrim Baptist where famed gospel composer Thomas Dorsey got his start. Other times it would be Progressive Baptist. I was awestruck by how large some of the churches were and by all the fancy clothes people wore. Grandmamma was always dressed to the nines, and I wore one of my pretty dresses. Then the magic happened. Grandmamma would look at me and say, "Stay seated." The music would start, and she would rise and start singing as she made her way down the aisle to the front. There was so much fanfare in her performance that the audience went wild. "Sa-ang, Julia!" people shouted.

Even back then, gospel music seemed to tell my story of suffering, and I leaned all the way in. Just like R&B was on the rise in the 70's, so was contemporary gospel. Reverend Walter Hawkins and his family dominated the genre. I had their first *Love Alive* album and played it religiously. One song, God Is Standing By, felt like it was written just for me. It reassured me that God had my back:

Everywhere you go, there is trouble
And everywhere you go, there is strife.

111

Everywhere you go, there is something that worries you,
But remember, my God is standing by.

It also illuminated a scripture I had latched onto in John 16:33: "In the world ye shall have tribulation: but be of good cheer; I have overcome the world." The scripture informed me with an understanding of my suffering and survival. This verse said to me that no matter what I faced, in the end, God would make it all right. I appropriated those songs to my life in the same way slaves took scripture and created spirituals to get them through the degradation of slavery. When our minister of music, Belinda Hubbard taught us that song, I took it as confirmation that God understood my life and would see me through the hell that I was living in. This is when I first fell in love with Tramaine Hawkins. I listened to her single, Changed, over and over and continued to pray for a change to come over me.

It was heartbreaking that, at my age, I had to latch onto songs about suffering. My thirteen-year-old self was robbed of the simple pleasure of singing for the Lord. When my choir members where rejoicing in the songs, I was weeping loudly and unapologetically. I had so much bottled up inside of me and, Sunday after Sunday, church was the place where I released my anguish. Many of those songs we sung were my invitations to let go of the pain, if only for the time I was at church. I arrived at church for Sunday school and stayed until Second Baptist literally locked the doors. If I didn't have somewhere in particular to go, like with one of my friends and their mother, I went over to Marshall Field's and perused the fine China department and I loved looking at crystal and porcelain figurines, like I did when Mama worked at the Evanston Inn. When I thought it was time to show my face. I'd go to the candy department to get me a few Frango mint chocolates and head home, ate dinner, and played me some more gospel music for the rest of the night. Sundays belonged to God.

I played my gospel albums as if playing them would change my situation. But most days, it only numbed my pain, like taking an opioid. It provided a euphoria that made me feel as if I was no longer hurting, even though I was. When I think about the role of gospel music and religion in this way, I partially agree with German philosopher Karl Marx's analysis about religion. He argues, "Religion is a sigh of the oppressed creature, the heart of a heartless world and the soul of soulless conditions. It is the opium of the people." Here, he is talking about the state using religion as a stronghold over the people's unwillingness to challenge their conditions and their suffering. While this bears truth, on a micro-level, I can see how this is exactly what gospel music did in my life. I was so powerless in Mama's house that the best I could do was to numb the pain with church and church music. Even though I can attest to how Marx's theory manifested in my life, I also understand that religion and its tools are not one-dimensional for me and most people. Listening to Tramaine sing, Goin' Up Yonder—about a better life in the hereafter—may have numbed my pain, but it also soothed my soul, which was living in a soulless situation. It's like this: When you get a reprieve from pain—any kind of pain, whether physical, emotional, or mental—you can think a little more clearly. There's nothing like popping a Tylenol to tackle a headache to bring you back to your senses. That's what gospel music was for me. It gave me a reprieve from my pain, and, in that moment, I could center myself. I took these songs as literal, and they helped to sustain me. I apportioned my suffering and, by doing so, I found the strength to carry on.

I got my period at Ms. Rachel's while visiting Loretta. I was surprised that Mama even allowed me to visit Ms. Rachel's house after she challenged Charles's accusation about me and Poochie's boyfriend kissing. I was glad my period had come at Madea's rather than at home because I didn't have to deal with Mama right off the bat. When I saw the blood, I called Loretta to the bathroom, "What you want, girl?" she asked, peeping through the crack in the bathroom door.

"I think I came on my period."

"How you know?" she asked. "Let me see," she added, stepping into the bathroom. I showed her the bloody toilet paper I had just used to wipe.

"I think so, too," she said, cheesing. She already had her cycle, and I was a little jealous. She stepped out and brought a box of sanitary napkins and told me to put one inside my panties and then she went and told Madea. I didn't want to tell Mama, but Madea said not to worry. She said she'd call her.

"Every girl gets her period," Madea said, "I don't see how Georgia can find fault in that." She was trying to reassure me. Still, I breathed a nervous sigh. Nothing was normal with Mama. She could find fault in a hard turd. Medea called Mama and I heard her trying her best to explain to Mama that getting my period did not mean I was having sex. *Here we go again*, I thought. Loretta and I looked at each other. Madea explained that it wasn't too early, adding that Loretta already had her menstruation and that our ages were so close together that it was probably my time. When they got off the phone, Madea said, "Georgia just a fool," shaking her head.

Loretta asked, "Do she have to go back home?" We all knew the answer to that one. Decades later, Loretta told me that every time I came over to visit, she asked Madea if they had to send me back to that hellhole. She said, "Georgia treated you so bad, and I felt so sorry for you." In the end, it didn't matter where it happened or who talked to Mama on my behalf; my period was Mama's proof that I was a whore. The next day after I came home, my period went away. I thought Mama must have scared it away. It didn't come back until several months later. This was normal, although I didn't know it at the time. Some girls going through the *menarche* phase would have one period, and it would stop then come back later. Looking back, if we consider all the stress I was living under, it's a wonder my period wasn't delayed altogether.

From the moment I walked back into the house from Ms. Rachel's until my period came back permanently, Mama ran a marathon campaign of humiliation. "Bitch, I know you fucking," she declared. "I'm going to take you to the doctor," she threatened, but never did. She did, however, tell every one of her friends about my period and her theory. It didn't matter when or where. She repeated the story to the point where she started lying. She told some people that she had taken me to the doctor, and he told her that she needed to watch me, implying that the doctor was trying to tell her I was already having sex. She was preoccupied with my vagina in the worst way possible. Instead of guiding me through the beginning phases of menstruation, she denigrated me in every way possible. "I knew she was fucking," she told her friends. "She always been too *fast* for her own good," she would add, recalling the time she beat my ass for *fucking*—her word to describe me doing whatever it was I was doing with the little boy under the porch at six years of age. I would sit in my bedroom and listen to her phone conversations and wonder how she kept it all straight. One day she was the one who caught me under the porch and other times it was my grandfather who caught me. She told her friends, "Al," speaking of my grandfather, "caught her *fast* ass under the porch and beat her ass." As crazy as it might sound, I considered those phone conversations a blessing compared to the public shaming. Sitting on Ms. Virginia's front porch one day, she said, "Her *fast* ass say she got her period." I wanted to hide inside my skin.

"Don't nobody get a period for one day," she stated, taking a sip of her drink.

"Naw, Georgia, I ain't never heard of anything like that." Ms. Virginia egged her on. I swear Mama talked about my period to anyone who would listen. I had heard about the beginning of my whoredom, according to Mama, since right at the time I believe molestation entered into my life. You would think, by then, I would have been used to years of name-calling and labeling that projected me as a Jezebel. But this time, it felt different than when I was younger. I think my bourgeoning awareness of my own sexuality and my ability to name sex and understand these terms jilted my sensibilities. It felt like the ultimate betrayal that she had thrown away my virtue before I even understood the term, and it settled over me like the aftermath of a nuclear bomb. When my period came back a few months later, Mama handed me a blue box of Kotex sanitary napkins and said, "You think you grown now." And that was the entire conversation.

If I thought that starting my period was enough humiliation, well then, developing a bladder infection was the *crème de la crème* for Mama to use against me. I began having pain when I used the bathroom. It scared the daylights out of me. I didn't know what the hell was going on and, Lord knows, I did not want to tell Mama. I went to the school nurse a lot that week, leading her to believe that the pain I was feeling in my lower belly was because I was getting ready to come on my period. This at least gave me a chance to nap during the day, and I took Midol for what I believed to be pre-cramps when I got home.

After that first week, the pain got so severe I couldn't keep it a secret anymore. The worst of it was the pain when I used the bathroom. Every time the urine stopped and started it felt like a sharp object had shot through my bladder. Mama took me to see a doctor and they did a urinalysis as the first level of testing. She asked the doctor to give me a pregnancy test. I wanted to disappear under the examination table.

"Mama, I'm not having sex," I said, defending myself in front of the white doctor. I wasn't having sex. I hadn't even kissed a boy. I was so embarrassed I couldn't even look at the doctor.

"I don't know what your hot ass been doing," she replied. The doctor gave me a look of sympathy, cleared his throat, and tried to explain that based on the symptoms I probably had a bladder infection.

"She got it from fucking," Mama said, shaking her head as if she were agreeing with the doctor but explaining that it was because I was having sex. She was comfortable in her ignorance.

"I want her checked out," she demanded. This was her chance to receive validation. The doctor looked at her like what she acted like: an uneducated, ignorant-ass Black woman. He cleared his throat and again tried to explain that there was no need for a pregnancy test. She insisted, and the test came back negative. The urine test for the bladder infection came back inconclusive. They wanted to hospitalize me and run more tests. Rather than showing concern, she kept beating a dead-ass horse. Her narrative never changed. I was fucking and that's why I was sick. She was just like President Trump. No matter what the experts claimed, it was fake news to her. She never strayed from her worldview. She did not have Twitter to spin her narrative like Trump, but God, she had that damn telephone. Some days I just wanted to snatch the cord from the damn wall. Without a doubt in my mind, this was the lowest point in my life since moving to Evanston. My body was changing, I was sick and scared, and Mama had no compassion whatsoever.

I was hospitalized for what I now know was a procedure called a cystoscopy. The doctors didn't fully explain what they were doing except I remember him saying that it would hurt a little. They gave me a shot of a mild sedative in my arm. It made me drowsy, but it didn't take away the pain when they inserted the tube into my bladder before they took me upstairs for the procedure and knocked me out. The pain was beyond anything I could articulate at thirteen. But the shame I felt with all those white men looking at my private parts was unparalleled to any experience that I'd had up until then—even Mama's public shaming. I felt exposed. I didn't understand female anatomy, including the difference between the little hole for pee from the hole for my vagina. It was all the same to me.

When I woke up after the procedure, Charles, of all people, was sitting there looking at me with those piercing eyes. Mama hadn't made it from work. Pain was radiating from below and I wanted to tell the nurse, but with Charles looking at me I just slid down in the bed and turned away, wishing I could pull the covers over my head. After almost a week in the hospital, it turned out to be an aggressive bladder infection. When the infection wouldn't go away, I had to have a second course of treatment. I was also told to drink lots of water and stop holding my pee when I needed to use the bathroom. I couldn't even deny it. I was good for holding on to my pee until I had no choice but to get up and go. Most nights I tried to wait until Charles was asleep because I didn't want him looking at me in the short distance from my room to the bathroom. ``

Mama's failure to support me when I was sick hurt me to the core. One day, walking home from school, I thought about the dismal reality I had to face each time I put my key into that door at 802 Seward Street. I couldn't read enough books, stay in my room long enough, listen to enough gospel music or go to church enough to rid myself of the pain I felt in that apartment. I was determined to find a way. I arrived home from school one day and went straight to the bottle of pills I was taking to treat my bladder infection. I got a glass of water and sat on the side of my bed. I thought about how many times Mama had threatened to kill me in the seven years since my grandfather's death. I thought about the vengeance and hatred that embodied her declaration, and how easily it rolled off her tongue, like a nursery-school rhyme. I thought about how many times she had proven herself capable of killing me with any number of the beatings I had received. I put one pill in my mouth and drank some water.

I thought, *I should save her the trouble*. I put another pill in my mouth and took a sip of water. At least I would have control of my own destiny. Another pill. Another sip.

What was the point of being a girl if the very nature of me was foul? Another pill. Another sip.

If God could not come to me, I would go to God. Another pill, and then another, and another.

I laid down and waited. The philosopher Fredrich Nietzsche wrote, "If you gaze long enough into an abyss, the abyss will gaze back into you." I had entered into the bottomless pit that I had gazed into every day of my life since my grandfather's death.

On top of my sheets fully clothed, shoes and all I waited for death to do what it does, but it didn't. My overactive mind took over and the moment I started to feel really sick I jumped up off my bed, grabbed my coat and ran to Holly's. A flutter of thoughts flooded my head. I didn't really want to die. I wanted to stop the pain. My life was racing through my head and my feet were racing for my life. I wanted to prove Mama wrong, and it would never be achieved if I died. I picked up speed. Looking back, I have no idea how I made it to Holly's as sick as I was. When I entered their apartment I shouted, "I took some pills." By then, I was sure I didn't want to die.

Holly's mother, Jean, took me to the emergency room at St. Frances Hospital adjacent to their apartment building. I was ushered into the back and given this nasty concoction and told to drink it down as quickly as I could. For a moment I balked at the taste and the nurse told me if I didn't get it down right away, they would have to pump my stomach. That scared the daylights out of me. Vomit came pouring out of my mouth and tears poured out of my eyes.

The police arrived and I tried to explain the unexplainable. When Mama arrived, I was thankful that the police were still there. Jean had left after the police arrived. The first thing out of Mama's mouth to the police was, "Aww, ain't nothing wrong with that bitch. She just wants some attention." The police took her to the side and had a private conversation with her, neutralizing her antics while the doctor continued to take care of me. We were referred to a child psychiatrist who specialized in family issues, but it should have been reported to child-welfare services. Mama and I never talked about the suicide attempt.

The following week, we went to see the psychiatrist in a big fancy office. I will never forget Mama sitting on the sofa next to me, all smug. When the doctor asked me to talk about what was going on with me. Mama jumped in before I could even open my mouth, "Ain't nothing wrong with her; she just *fast*." She dominated the hour, and that white man didn't have a clue how to regain control of the session.

After the dust settled, Jean had a long talk with me. I had never stopped spending time with them, and she supported me in my defiance. Her house was a safe haven for me, and I was not going to relinquish that safety net. I figured if Mama were going to kill me, at least it would be over something of my choosing. Jean asked me how I felt about her going to talk with Mama. She told me I could come and live with them if Mama gave her permission. Under any other circumstances, I would not have supported her talking to Mama. This time, though, I thought that maybe it would be in my favor because a part of me honestly believed Mama didn't want me, and another part of me wanted a new life—the one I had witnessed in Holly's home over and over again.

That evening, when Jean walked through our door, I knew it was a mistake the moment Mama saw her. She rolled her eyes and stepped back to let Jean into the house. I knew in that moment that the color of Jean's skin and the way that she was dressed were two strikes against her. But Lord, when she opened her mouth and sounded all proper, she had reached the third strike and the conversation hadn't even started. I'm not sure why Mama took her back to the kitchen and sat her at the table. Jean sat on one end and Mama sat facing her, with contempt written all over her face and body. The more Jean explained, the tighter Mama became. She listened politely to what Jean had to say. Jean explained that given the two incidents she had been involved in with me, it appeared as if Mama had her hands full. I have to admit: Jean was bold and not one of Mama's mean looks shut her up. She flat-out said to Mama, "If you don't want Rae, I will gladly raise her with my girls." I could hear Mama trying her best to talk proper.

"Ain't nothing wrong with that gal. She just too *fast* for her own good. Rae don't want to live by my rules, and I done told her ain't nobody gonna run over me." Jean continued to explain her position as she saw it. Even if I were out of control, it was clear that I needed help. As Jean saw it, there was a problem and Mama's methods were not "appropriate."

Finally, the Georgia Lee came out in Mama: "Ain't nobody gonna take my baby away from me." Then she said something to the effect that she would kill me before she let me or anyone else run over her. Jean tried to explain that she wasn't trying to supersede Mama's authority but was seeking it. Mama said something like, *I don't give a fuck what you gotta say.* That ended the conversation. I looked up from my seat on the sofa and Mama was walking toward the living room, escorting Jean to the door. No words were spoken, and Jean left. Mama walked back to the kitchen, and I went to my bedroom. After Mama got her a sip of liquor from her stash in the pantry, she called me into the bedroom. I stood in the doorway nearest the living room entrance. She lit a cigarette, took a deep draw, and exhaled the smoke into the air.

"If you ever bring somebody to my house again, about my business, I will kill you," she said as slowly and clearly as I had ever heard her talk.

"I will kill you dead, [as] you got to die," she said. Then she let out the full amount of the anger and humiliation she must have been feeling at that table with Jean. She started talking to no one in particular—saying what I think she had wanted to say to Jean: "Who the fuck does that white bitch think she is coming up here? I'm a grown-ass woman. This is my muthafuckin' house," and on and on. Then she turned back to me.

"What goes on in my house stays in my house!" she said. "I'll kill you before I let someone take you from me!"

I was sweating all between my legs and under my bra. I was too afraid to say anything and too afraid to move. She continued to wail at me.

"I mean it, bitch! Do you hear me? "Don't let me have to tell you again!"

"Now get the fuck out of my face before I beat your ass," she added before picking up the phone to call her girlfriend Mary. "Thank you, Jesus," I mumbled under my breath as I made my way to my bedroom thinking, *Whew! She didn't beat me.* There was never another intervention, but this suicide attempt taught me a valuable lesson: there is life beyond that one moment of gazing into the abyss. I reminded myself of this fact daily.

Nineteen

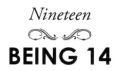

BEING 14

" An abnormal reaction to an abnormal situation is normal behavior.**"**
—Viktor Frankl

I liked boys. I *really* liked boys and, even better, they liked me. My attraction for boys started in the seventh grade with LaTodd Johnson, who was an eighth grader. He pursued me that entire school year, but he didn't get far. I liked him, but Mama's rule said boys were forbidden. I figured if I was going to rock the boat it should be with a boy I really liked. He was David Miller from my seventh-grade homeroom. David was such a nerd that I could never get his attention. As adults, he, and his wife Donna Miller, who is also a friend, laugh about the fact he didn't have a clue I had a crush on him. By eighth grade, Mama had made it clear I was not old enough to have a boyfriend. *(As if I needed to be reminded.)* Like with most things during this time, she didn't say it directly to me. I heard her tell her phone buddies, "I wish she would come up here talking about a boyfriend." I heeded her warning at first. I didn't want to give her anything else to shame me. Then my teen hormones took over, and it was a wrap. I was still afraid of Mama, but the forces of nature were so powerful I didn't know how to stop myself.

Before eighth-grade graduation, I gave in to my curiosity and all the attention I was receiving from Darwin Brown. We started as enemies. One day between classes he grabbed my breast—well, what there was of it. Its small size notwithstanding, the pain sizzled, and I held my little breast hoping for relief. Then I kicked his ass right in the nuts. Dr. Morton caught the end of it and stopped dead in her tracks.

"Young lady!" she said, looking at me. "What in God's name do you think you're doing?" she asked, watching Darwin keel over like he was dying.

"He grabbed my breast," I said defiantly. I folded my hands across my chest, mad as hell. Dr. Morton went on about how I could have hurt him for life. Darwin was still holding his dick while she scolded me good before she sent me to the principal. No one, not even Dr. Morton, could tell me that an injustice had not been inflicted on me. After she stopped talking, I asked her, "What about Darwin?" She looked down at me through her glasses, "Rae, that was not lady-like and what you did to Darwin—it was dangerous."

I stormed off mumbling to myself all the way to the principal's office. "His Black ass should have kept his hands to himself. Who the fuck does he think he is?" Shit, my nipple is still hurting. I only wore a 32A, but Lord knows that handful of breasts had no volume, and it hurt!

I got the same spiel from Mr. Pate as from Dr. Morton, but he couldn't make me budge, either. Like Dr. Morton he implied that Darwin's body was more important than mine. Darwin was not punished for grabbing my breast. If I had an ounce of sympathy, it began to fade. I resolved that he deserved that kick. Mr. Pate wanted a parent to come to school the next day to stress to me how dangerous it was that I kicked Darwin in the crotch. I shrugged him off and went home prepared for my punishment. To my surprise, Mama had my back, but she wasn't taking a day off for, in her words, "this bullshit." She added, "You should have kicked him in the dick."

Mama sent one of her girlfriends to school, and Mr. Pate gave her the same story about the damage I could have done. Every time she tried to ask about Darwin grabbing my breast, he deflected back to the fragility of the penis. She stared at him like he was crazy. I got suspended for a day. What a crock. When she made her way to the door, she asked if Darwin was also going to be suspended for grabbing my breast. It was Mr. Pate's turn to look crazy. I'm sure this was my introduction to misogyny. None of it set well with me and, looking back, I'm proud of myself for standing my ground. I never apologized to his ass. But then I turned around and kissed him. I couldn't make this life up even if I tried. Apparently, Darwin was trying to get my attention. After he soothed his hurt feelings—and his penis—his pursuit of me was relentless, even endearing. Eventually, he wore me down. He became the first boy to have the privilege of giving me a sloppy-ass tongue kiss, and he even got in a grind or two.

The summer after graduation, I was feeling myself. Maybe smelling it too, as the grown folks used to say back in the day. I turned fourteen right before my eighth-grade graduation. It was official: boys became living, breathing things. My interest in boys skyrocketed, and it frightened me. Outside of the fact that my outright defiance of Mama could lead to disaster, I thought maybe I really was *fast*. I just couldn't stop thinking about boys. I didn't understand that sexual maturation is a natural part of every teenager's growth and development, even if our parents try to will it away. Sex hormones not only affect your physical growth, but your mind, behavior, thoughts, moods and impulses, or lack thereof.

I couldn't explain the changes in my body, but after I started hanging out with Theresa it was comforting to know that I wasn't the only girl who felt this way about boys. Theresa became my neighborhood sidekick by default. I knew her from hanging out at Ridgeville Park, but we hadn't spent any real time together. Now that school was out, my Chute friends were on the other side of town. Annie tried to talk me into coming to her house while Mama was at work, but I wasn't brave enough. Sharmayne was in gymnastics camp most of the summer and, with my fear of being caught going to Holly's, Theresa became my new best friend. Right off the bat, she and I bonded over the topic of boys—that is, who we liked and who we didn't, who we would let kiss us, and even who we might do it with—although I had not done it yet. Boys clung to Theresa like bees to honey, and I clung to her like we were conjoined twins. I was already at a place of no return, and it was nice to have a friend who was on the same page. Besides, Theresa had way more freedom than I did. She was always in the know. I marveled at her independence. She seemed to run her own life, unlike me.

Mama met Theresa by default on one of those summer days, she was sitting on Ms. Virginia's porch and we happened to be walking down the street. Mama asked her if she was white. Theresa's father was African American and her mother was Caucasian and a stay-at-home mom. Theresa gave an uncomfortable laugh, and I said no and let it be. She was much lighter than me and could have passed for a white girl. She had light-colored eyes with brown and green hues, and light-brown, bone-straight hair. Later, when I got home the first thing out of her mouth was, "That girl got titties like a woman. I know she fucking." I went straight to my room. After that, I made sure Theresa never visited me at home.

I never thought about Theresa's age because she was much more physically developed than I was. She stood about five-foot-seven and was fully developed in all the right places. Physical appearance aside, she was two years young than me. We were the blind leading the blind. We both had teenage guys macking us more than boys closer to our age. I don't know what they saw in my tail; physically, I didn't have a fraction of Theresa's body. It could have been as simple as a teenage boy didn't much care who he was able to get it on with—just as long as he could.

Theresa and I spotted these fine-ass brothers and cousins around the same time. All of them were drop-dead gorgeous and could have given The Sylvers and The Jackson 5 brothers a run for their money. We spent a lot of time trying to figure out who was who. You could tell they were related because they had similar features in skin tone and all-around fineness. They became our favorite topic; however, they looked a little too old. Then, one day I spotted James coming out of their apartment building. I had never seen him in the park, and he looked younger than the others.

After that day, I started hanging out on my block instead of at the park so I could meet him. Determined, I walked by their building every so often hoping to draw him out of it and into my arms. Then, one day I heard this voice say, "Come on over here and talk to me little mama." I looked up and he was standing right in front of me. I thought I was going to melt right then and there. We exchanged numbers. James was nineteen and had just graduated from high school. I didn't have a relatable concept of an age-appropriate relationship because Mama had the same reaction about the male species, from 13 to 113, which was, "Get out of his face!" I figured any guy who was a teenager was fair game. If he had "teen" in his age, he was still a "teenager," even if he was five to six years older than me. At fourteen, I was going into high school and thought it was a perfect match. Or maybe my hormones told me that stupid shit. What I didn't know at fourteen was that dating someone who was five years older than me was on an entirely different level than kissing my eighth-grade classmate in some corner of the school.

James' family was from Arkansas, and he was visiting his older brothers for the summer. He had beautiful skin with the color and smoothness of a hazelnut. His afro was perfectly stacked at least six inches, and he had the nerve to have all this baby hair around the edges. He was tall and lanky, and his jeans fit his slim waist like they were tailor-made. We talked on the telephone a couple of times before he invited me over. I'd go out my back door, walk through the alley and approach their building from the side so nosey-ass Ms. Virginia didn't have eyes on me. She was always sitting in her picture window that provided a panoramic view of Seward Street.

We pretended to watch television—but actually, we'd be making out. His tongue swirling in my mouth was nothing like those sloppy kisses from Darwin. They were slow and methodical and made all of me say, *Give me more and more.* Looking back, we really had nothing in common and absolutely nothing to talk about. Yeah, he was macking—telling me how pretty I was and all that jive. Beyond that, you couldn't close the miles of space between us if you tried. I thought I had died and gone to heaven, and you couldn't have told me otherwise. That night, I retired every single *Right On!* poster that hung on my wall. I didn't need the posters when the guy was living three buildings away from my front door.

We had made it from the sofa to the bedroom after a few visits and all in one week. The first time in his bedroom, I was nervous and unsure what to do. I looked at him and then at the bed. But I needn't have worried because he was as smooth as ice. He pulled his T-shirt over his head and came so close to me that I could feel his breath when he bent down to kiss me. He was in no rush, and I could nearly feel his heartbeat as we scooted to the center of the bed. He removed my shirt and bra and gathered my little breasts into his mouth. I was swept up. He slipped his finger up my inner thigh through the side of my shorts right to the center of me. I surrendered to the touch of his hand, and when he finally slipped my shorts and panties off in one fell swoop, I could feel my wetness. He stood to remove his jeans, and butterflies tumbled nervously in my stomach as I admired how good he looked. Damn! He was fine! Even his penis was fine. He laid down and pushed his finger deep inside to make sure I was ready for him. I felt his penis throbbing against my leg and my nervousness turned into desire. It was all-encompassing as he slipped on top of me and guided his penis into me with ease, but the pain caused me to stiffen.

"You alright, baby?" he asked.

"Yes," I muttered after a deep breath. It hurt, but I was alright. I wanted him, and I wanted this. I never told him that I was a virgin, but I suspected he knew. My age and lack of experience was obvious. The deeper he went, the more his concern showed, asking again if I was okay. After he was all the way inside me, he rested there before he started moving. He pulled back a little and then pushed himself back inside me, back and forth. My body intuitively responded, meeting his back-and-forth, deeper and again. As we moved in sync, I felt pain and pleasure. His penis grew inside of me as he went deeper, and he pulled back and went deeper again, and faster. I matched each move until he exploded. I hadn't fully grasped the concept of an orgasm, but I understood clearly that we had just finished having sex. He collapsed on top of me and moved beside me and pulled me closer.

Now that it was over, I became anxious thinking about the fact that I had just had sex. It was disconcerting. I had broken all the rules. I thought about what could happen if Mama found out. The agony in my head and the pain between my legs told me to go home. I nudged him gently and said I had to go. When I got back home, I ran a bath and undressed. I could still feel semen mixed with my blood and the wetness of my vagina between my legs. I immersed myself in the warm water. Lying in the tub, I started to feel melancholic and began to cry. I had lost my virginity. I had given up a part of myself that I could never regain. I had moved into the *fast* lane, both literally and figuratively. I couldn't put my finger on it, but I knew that having sex was a game-changer for me.

Since that first time I gave myself to James, I have viewed it as the actual moment I lost my virginity. In my mind, it was the day *I decided* to have sex for the first time. My belief that I lost my virginity at fourteen, of course, contradicts the fact that I had already had sex through rape and molestation. In those prior years, it had not been my decision. Consent is the cornerstone of any sexual relationship. In those instances when I was violated, there was no consent nor could there have been. I subconsciously tucked away the abuses and gave them no power over the day *I* chose to have sex. It would be the way that I held on to as much agency as I could at my age.

After my first time with James, I visited him as often as I could. I loved everything we did up until the point of penetration: that took more time for me to adjust. Learning enough about sex to be pleasured wouldn't happen until the following summer. However, I loved spending time with James and started to view him as my boyfriend even though he never asked me to be his girlfriend, which was customary back then. I decided that sex was somehow a commitment to each other in and of itself.

One day Theresa came over to James's with me. She and I were sitting in the living room with him and one of his cousins. We were talking and laughing, and Theresa kept giggling. That shit got on my last nerve. Here I was trying to act mature, and she was acting like a child. James told her, "You keep on giggling. I'm going to take you in the back and give you something to giggle about." I looked at him like he lost his fucking mind!

"Stop playing like that," I demanded.

"Ain't nobody playing. I'm for real. Let her keep it up," he said, kind of jokingly. I started laughing too, having decided that he had to be joking. It all seemed to die down, but then James began instigating and manipulating Theresa. He would look her way, and then quickly turn his head as if he wasn't looking at her. Every time he did that motion, Theresa started giggling all over again.

"Didn't I tell you what I was going to do?" James asked after a while, as he got up from his chair, walked over to Theresa and held out his hand.

"What did I tell you, girl?" he asked. She just laughed. Then she reached up and grabbed his hand, and they started walking toward the back.

"Boy, you crazy," his cousin said.

I laughed it off, still thinking, *He has to be joking.* Sometimes a situation is so awkward, embarrassing, and unbelievable all you can manage is a distorted laugh. Then there was silence. James and Theresa didn't come back. It became so uncomfortable for me that I didn't know what to think or what to do.

His cousin spoke up. "You gonna let him get away with that?"

"What?" I asked, defensively.

"You know what they're back there doing," he said. "Don't play dumb."

He was right. I did know, but I didn't want to face it.

"You should teach him a lesson," he said. He stood up and reached for my hand. It took a second for me to compute. He nodded his head toward the back as if to say, "Let's do it." I was appalled that he would even think that I would have sex with him. Being in a relationship with James wasn't a game for me. I cared about him as much as any fourteen-year-old could. Back then, I genuinely believed that giving your body to someone meant something. My feelings were hurt, and I was confused.

Then came my moment of clarity. I had no control over Theresa and James, but I did have some control over me in that moment. I got up and walked past his cousin and straight out of the apartment. I was more ashamed than heartbroken. I felt as if James had made a complete fool out of me. Later, Theresa rang my doorbell, and I came out to talk with her. She said she didn't know what else to do but go along with it. I believed her because I hadn't known what to do, either. While I didn't fault her *per se*, I still felt betrayed, and I would slowly drift away from her. I never went over to James's again. I decided he did not deserve me.

Regardless of how it played out back then, today I understand we were two young girls who were way out of our league and caught in a powerless situation. I was fourteen, and Theresa was twelve. Neither one of us was in a place of consent, even if I thought we were. That day, I wanted to take back every single thing James and I had done. Instead, I learned the hard way that once you surrender your body to someone, you cannot take it back. Honestly, I'm thankful that I was not raped or that leaving Theresa alone didn't cause more damage for her. It could have turned out differently, resulting in a lot more pain for both of us. It also taught me to respect my friends' relationships, past and present. I hated how I felt about James and Theresa, and it has stayed with me. I decided then and there that the guys my girlfriends dated were off-limits to me; I don't care if she fucked him a thousand years ago.

I spotted James a couple of times after that on the street, and he was always trying to holla. One day as I walked past his building, he seemed to think I was going to stop. He was all smiles. I walked straight on by like he wasn't even standing there.

"Why you trippin' girl?" he hollered after me.

"Fuck you, nigga," I hollered back and kept on walking. Fool me once, shame on you; fool me twice, well then, I'm the fool, for real. I wasn't trying to hear it. I missed hanging out with him. But every time I thought about going over there, I would think about the silence that consumed their apartment when he and Theresa didn't return to the living room. My stomach would drop in despair all over again.

Rather than hanging out at Ridgeville Park, I started to focus my attention elsewhere. I joined the youth branch of the NAACP. Joyce Favors, our choir director of the Young Gifted and Black Youth Choir at Second Baptist, was also the youth branch advisor. As a result, many of us in the choir joined. The NAACP was my first official introduction to politics and community advocacy. At the time, the NAACP was running a nationwide grassroots campaign, canvassing fundraisers for the Legal Defense and Educational Fund (LDF). We were given collection cans at a chapter meeting, and I hit the streets to canvass. I went door to door in my neighborhood using my Avon route, hitting up some of my customers first. I had my little script down and everyone gave. You couldn't tell me one thing. I was in those streets for the cause, and it felt better than being in the streets chasing boys.

Soon after I call myself quitting James, I got my first official job and my own money. I thought I had it going on. Tommy Gerard—who helped his father manage the neighborhood grocery store, Gerard's—asked me if I would like to be a cashier, and Mama gave me her approval. I had my first official job, at fourteen. Mama also took me to the bank to open my first savings account. It only took one time for her to withdraw some of my money for me to switch up the game. After that, I asked Mr. Gerard to cash my check, and then I only put some of it in the account and hid the rest in the back of my closet. I didn't want Mama to know what I was making, anyway. Money was some kind of thing for her that I never understood. She was always scheming on how to get more money—even money that wasn't hers to have. So, I decided it was best to manage my own. Every time I asked Mama for something, and she said no, I marched to whatever store it was and purchased the item for myself. I must say, I had one hell of a work ethic. I was never late, and I worked as many hours as I could. Money blew through my pocket like the Chicago wind, and I didn't learn a damn thing about saving. Nonetheless, I was pleased with how my life was transforming because of work, church, and activism.

I developed a new friendship after I took the job at Gerard's. Anita's family owned a house on Custer Street across from the store. We were in the same eighth-grade homeroom at Chute and were friendly. Every time she came into the store, we would chat it up. One day she invited me over to her house after work, and as the saying goes, the rest is history. Anita came from a middle-class family, and both her parents worked. She had a sister, Crystal, who was a couple of years younger than us. Both of her parents were really nice to me, and I was in and out of her house often after work. Mama said the same thing about Anita she had said about Theresa: "That girl got titties like a woman. I know she's fucking." They also met by default, like with Theresa. Mama saw us walking down the street while sitting on Ms. Virginia's porch. Mama liked Anita for some reason and gave me more leeway with her than with others. Still, we didn't spend time at my house because I never wanted to be there. Mama saw us outside together, and she never had anything negative to say about Anita once she got the breast observation out of her system.

Anita was the opposite of Theresa and me for that matter. She was laidback and low-key; there wasn't a hyper bone in her body. She wore the latest styles and seemed to live in bell bottoms. She had beautiful brown skin a mixture of oolong and black tea steeped exactly two minutes. I was always envious of her perfectly shaped afro. In seventh grade, I begged Mama to let me have an afro and dye it red which was the trend back then until she gave in. Loretta's mother, Helen, did the coloring but I could never get my afro to do right and gave up on it by the middle of eighth grade. Anita seemed mature for her age; maybe because she had put away all the trappings of a pre-teen. She was my first friend you could have called a *bad girl*. She smoked cigarettes openly well, at least away from home. I was still a scaredy-cat when it came to risk-taking of this kind. I was so afraid I didn't want to walk beside Anita for fear that I would go home smelling like cigarette smoke and get the shit beaten out of me. Besides, Mama smoked enough for everybody, me included. Anita never tried to get me to smoke, and I liked that about her. In fact, over the years, my friends who dabbled in vices didn't try to force me to join in. It was an unspoken mutual understanding to respect our differences and embrace our commonalities. Loyalty and trust were my two barometers for friendship, and it only took one infraction for me to walk. Anita was fun. She always had something for us to do outside our neighborhood. One Saturday, she wanted me to go with her to meet some dude and his friends at the Burger King on the Chicago side of Howard Street. I asked Mama if I could go with Anita to get a burger, which was only a little lie. Anita and I ate, sat around, and talked shit and laughed with these guys. Time passed and I looked up and the sky was drifting into the darkness. I was on shaky ground. I knew I had to be home by the time the streetlights came on. We walked fast and thought of excuses why it took so long for us to get our hamburgers. We settled on the story that Burger King had been very crowded. Anita came upstairs with me to help explain. Mama took one look at us and shook her head.

"I don't want to hear y'all's bullshit," she said. "It don't take that long to get no hamburger," she chuckled. Her light-hearted response was a sign that she was okay with me being late. I exhaled a sigh of relief.

"Y'all full of shit," she added. We looked at each other and cracked up. I was glad that Mama was comfortable with Anita. With all the tension around Holly and her mother, at least she wasn't looking over my shoulder, so to speak, like she had done after Jean came over to have that failed woman-to-woman talk about me.

One day, Mama and Charles were planning to go to visit her friends Mary and Gertrude. I didn't particularly care so much about going because neither of them had children my age. They were either younger or older; however, staying home by myself was never an option. I asked Anita if she wanted to come because there would be nothing for me to do but sit on the porch while the grown-ups sat around drinking and visiting with each other. If she came, I would have someone to talk to. She agreed.

That day, Gertrude's son Danny was there. Before I knew it, he and Anita struck up a conversation. Danny was a handsome guy and somewhere in his early to mid-twenties. He was a bad-boy-gangster type who was in and out of jail all the time. He carried a gun; I saw it nestled boldly in his waistband one day. He had a limp gossip claimed was due to a gunshot wound. His swagger could not be denied. He was well-dressed in slacks, silk socks, killer gator shoes and a brim on top of his head. I can see why Anita was attracted to Danny, but I had never thought about him that way, maybe because I had known him since I was much younger and never viewed him as my peer.

Danny was chatting up Anita and she was all the way in. His friend Mickey tried to talk to me, but I wasn't interested. He was a little scary. He looked to be even older and more gangster than Danny. He had a big-ass head, and he was thick, not fat. He was broad-chested and something about him made him appear to be seasoned like a real grown-ass man. Honestly, I didn't know what to say to him. If I thought James and I had nothing to talk about, then Mickey and I had even less than that. I couldn't imagine what Danny was saying to Anita, but they were in a groove. I gave in because I didn't want Danny to change his mind about Anita, like we were a package deal or something. If I believed they were too old for us, then they were. My experience with James had taught me a hard lesson and I was at least trying to be more thoughtful about men. Mama came out on the porch where we were sitting, and I was surprised she was so nonchalant about it all. I kept waiting for her to tell me to get out of Mickey's face, but she never did. The irony blew my mind. On the one hand, she was always on my ass about being *fast*. Yet, she had nothing negative to say about Anita and Danny, or Mickey's interest in me—and neither did Charles. It was another one of those contradictions I had to live with.

Anita and Danny exchanged numbers. When I looked up that following Saturday, he and Mickey were at my front door. I don't remember if they previously arranged this date—just that Danny asked me to call Anita and let her know he was at my house. Anita came over and we were all sitting in the living room. Mama looked in and said, "Alright, now, I don't want no shit out of ya'll." She left to go to the store, leaving us alone. Charles wasn't due home until later. Mama's approval of the entire situation was baffling. After she left, Anita and Danny took a walk and Mickey suggested we go into my bedroom. I don't even know how I got sucked in but here I was in this precarious— if not outright dangerous—situation. I gathered he probably wanted to make out, and I didn't want to.

I was only trying to keep him company while Danny and Anita were hanging out. I also knew if Mama caught us in my room, I would be in trouble. On that point, I was not confused.

"Come on, baby. It ain't gonna hurt nothing," he said.

"If Mama catches us, I will be in serious trouble," I insisted. He kept begging, and the pressure was getting to be too much on me. Finally, Mickey said, "We can leave the bedroom doors open." Then, I agreed. He pulled a chair close by the window. I sat on the edge of my bed close to where he was sitting. Eventually, he nudged me his way until I was sitting in his lap. He removed his gun from his waist to get more comfortable and laid it on the floor next to the window. I wasn't surprised he had a gun, just nervous as shit with it sitting on my bedroom floor. He started feeling between my legs, and my anxiety shot up.

"Un-unn," I said," trying to push his hand away. If Mama catches us, Mickey" I said.

"Shhhh," he whispered and kept right ahead.

I didn't reciprocate. I didn't want to do this. My mind was thinking one thing and my body was doing its own thing: I started to get wet. After a while, I could feel Mickey moving around. Before I knew it, he lifted me up a tad, pushed my shorts to the side, and penetrated.

WHAT THE HELL!? I felt like he had just shoved a bat inside me. He was big; I mean, really big. And it hurt; really hurt.

"Mickey, un-unn!" I said.

"Shhhh, it's okay," he insisted.

I thought he was going to bust me wide open between the small gap he used to penetrate and his big-ass penis, hard as a brick. I couldn't breathe; I couldn't think.

"Move a little," he whispered.

"Mickey I-" was all I could get out of my mouth.

I tried to say it hurt too much to move, but nothing else came out. When Mickey realized that I wasn't going to move, he tilted back in the chair so that he could get a better angle into my vagina. He went deeper and harder, pushing my hips forward until he exploded. After his orgasm, I could feel the tension leave his body, and he raised me off him. I looked down as he stuffed his softening penis back into his pants; even then, it was still huge. I went to the bathroom and locked the door.

"WHAT THE HELL JUST HAPPENED?" I screamed over and over in my head. I knew we had just had sex or, should I say, he had sex with me. Today, of course I would name it rape. Back then, I just couldn't wrap my brain around it. I couldn't believe he just did it like it wasn't a big deal. I was throbbing and aching; I wanted to wet my towel and put it between my legs to soothe me, but I was too paranoid. My mind was racing. *God forbid if Mama spotted my wet towel and asked me what was up.* As an alternative I dipped some toilet paper into the toilet and wiped away the blood and semen. I was mad at myself for letting this happen. I knew I shouldn't have allowed him to come into my bedroom. I heard Mama's voice and pulled my shit together in a hurry.

"Nigga, what you doing in there?" she asked Mickey about being in my room.

"Aw, Georgia, just sitting here looking out the window," he said.

"Nigga, get your slick ass into that living room," she demanded.

I stood in the hall between the bathroom and my bedroom, listening.

"Aww, Georgia, the doors are open. Ain't nothing happening."

"You ain't got no business in her bedroom. I let you come to see her. I don't want no bullshit from you."

When I heard him rustling to go into the living room. I came into the front from the opposite way as if I had never been in the bedroom when Mama looked up and saw me.

Keep that nigga out of your bedroom," she said. She didn't have to worry because I was never going to see him again. I told Anita again that I didn't like Mickey. I'm not sure how much longer she continued to see Danny, but I had had it with Mickey, James, sex, and the male species in general the whole fucking shebang.

Anita and I continued to be friends, but I decided to chill all the way out.

Twenty

EVANSTON TOWNSHIP

" I have the nerve to walk my own way, however hard, in my search for reality, rather than climb upon the rattling wagon of wishful illusions."

—Zora Neale Hurston

Evanston Township High School was a maze, and so was my freshman year of high school. You could have put Chute inside ETHS three times and still have room. It is a sixty-five-acre campus with 1.2 million square feet inside, making it the largest high school facility under one roof in the United States. I was like a mouse in that maze, circling around trying to find my *freshie* way, literally and figuratively. I was still getting lost in that maze of a building by my senior year, and the maze of my life had me running around in circles and hitting brick walls until the day I got my diploma.

Back then, the school was divided into four halls based on the main directions: East, West, North and South. Students were assigned to a specific hall, and that was the administration we reported to and the cafeteria where we ate lunch. I was assigned to West Hall. My dean of students was Arthur Williams, and our principal was Dr. McKinney Nash—both African American. Dean Williams got to know me pretty well and became an ally. I told him bits and pieces about my home life, and he was always encouraging. I remember the first time I was invited to speak at ETHS by Denise Martin, who started as a history teacher at ETHS when I was a student there. Eventually, she rose to the positions of dean of students and assistant principal before she retired in 2006. My counselor Mr. Horn attended. Afterward, he came over to me and apologized for not being aware and knowing the chaos in which I lived. It was an awkward moment. I appreciated it, but I didn't know how to respond, he had never been my cheerleader, especially when I needed him the most.

ETHS had a curriculum about as large and wide as the building. Even the required course selections within specified categories were large, and the electives were endless. The volume of choices had my head spinning. The best description I have for my academic performance at ETHS is that I muddled through. Chute had done the best it could in preparing me for high school; however, it took a huge adjustment. The workload was far more substantial than in junior high and it required different study habits. I had no academic cheerleaders like Mr. Murphy and Dr. Morton. I did my best with what I had to work with. I wanted to excel, but staying focused was a challenge, to put it mildly. I was anxious all of the time either because of what had recently happened to me at home or from trying to stay out of Mama's target zone to prevent something from happening. When there was any drama with Mama, what little academic discipline I managed to develop crumbled right before my eyes. I never knew when or how the drama was coming, and after it came, I had to adjust and keep on with the rest of what was required of me despite what I felt emotionally. I no longer had the luxury of disappearing into my head or hiding in my room, like I did when I was a little girl. I had a life that required me to be physically, emotionally, and intellectually present at school and at home. I put on a good face, but it was more than a notion to keep it all together. Some aspects of my life suffered and in part, my education was one of them.

One Friday morning during my freshman year, Mama called me out of bed at 5:30 a.m. When I appeared in the doorway, she asked me about her hairbrush and accused me of misplacing it. I hadn't seen her brush, but I immediately started looking.

"Bitch, find my brush!" she demanded, and walked off to the kitchen. I'm looking and praying. *Lord, please don't let me get a whopping this morning.* I'm all over the dresser, pulling everything back, checking and double-checking. Mama came back to her dresser with a glass of water. I didn't dare meet her eyes. She must have gone to the pantry to get a sip of Christian Brothers because I could smell it as she approached. By now, I'm all inside the dresser drawers. My heart is pounding so fast I think it is going to explode. I'm still praying, *Lord please don't let me get a whopping this morning. Please, God.* I'm trying not to cry, and Mama is still hollering. "I know you had it! Bitch you better find it or I'm gonna beat yo' ass!"

Please, Lord, help me find this brush. Please, Lord. Please, Lord. Please, Lord.

"FIND IT, BITCH!!" She hovered over me. At times like these, I tried my best to stay at least an arm's length away from her so she couldn't hit me as quickly. That morning, I was cornered. After fumbling in one drawer as long as I thought I could get away with it, I turned toward her to get to the other drawer. Suddenly, I felt ice-cold water running down my face and my neck, dripping into my robe. In an instant, she had doused me with her glass of water. I didn't wipe my face. I just kept looking and praying. *Please, God, help me find this brush. Please, God, don't let me get a whopping.* So much adrenaline was rushing through my body, it's a wonder it didn't jump out of my skin. I knew something had to give—either me or the brush—because Mama was never going to give. With my hands deep in that drawer fumbling around and buying time, I stopped moving. I took in a deep breath. *Oh, God,* was my plea. I exhaled. Before I knew it, I was asking Mama if her brush could be in her purse. "Hell, no. It ain't in my purse!" But my gut—my shining star, the universe, the ancestors, God, Mary, Joseph, and Baby Jesus—intervened. I shifted my body toward her purse sitting on the dresser and pulled her brush out, in full view.

"Oh, I thought you had it," she smirked. I handed her the brush and she began brushing her wig. I went back to my room, mumbling, "Thank you, Jesus." When I heard the door slam, I knew she'd left for work, and I let the tears flow. I held myself and cried until all the misery seemed to have dried up. Then I bounced back like a ball against a wall. I had to get ready for school. Once I entered that door at 1600 Dodge Street, I had to pretend to be a normal girl, even though I was living in an abnormal and abusive home. Like I said, I was bouncing off the walls every freaking day.

The night after the early morning brush incident, I walked the block home from work and braced myself for whatever was ahead of me—good, bad, or indifferent. Mama had made dinner, and, like most paydays, she had something for me. This time, it was a leather maxi coat that I had begged her to get me. I was already developing expensive tastes, and maxi coats were the latest fashion craze. I never thought about it then, but it had to have cost a good chunk of her paycheck. My coat was fly. It was a beautiful color not quite burgundy and not quite wine. It reached to my ankles and was belted at the waist, with big buttons going down the front. It had a wide hood that was cute and did nothing against the Chicago cold. But I sure looked good. For a moment, I was that little girl again, sitting in the middle of all those toys and not thinking about the agony Mama had caused me that morning. I couldn't stop the pain, but I could cover it up with things.

The cruelty and unpredictability in my life made it hard to stay focused. On top of that, right after school—when I should have been studying—I was working, and I did so through most of high school. Mama didn't make me work. But a punishment could consist of a tongue-lashing; a hit upside my head with whatever was at hand; the telephone being locked up before she went to work so I couldn't use it when she was not home; or no money for the bus or lunch. That made working a necessity. Eventually, I signed her name to my paperwork for free breakfast and lunch, but I still had to deal with bus fare. After school, I went straight to work. At the beginning of that school year, I switched jobs. Ms. Ann, the owner of the dry cleaners just a couple of doors down from Gerard's Grocery Store, wooed me away from Gerard's with ease. I thought it was so cool to work for a Black woman. I loved to see a Black woman in a leadership role running things because it made me hopeful for my own future. I had a lot of responsibility and it made me feel good to be trusted. I was the only employee working from right after school until closing at seven o'clock. After she closed the cleaners on Custard, I worked at her other location on Howard Street a couple of days each week after school. I had study time and was glad I didn't have to cram after work. But then I lost my house keys in the dead of winter and, for one month, Mama made me stay out in the cold until they got home.

"Keep your ass out in the cold," she said. "That will teach you about losing my keys." The front of our building had two outside doors. One let you into the foyer, which is where I would stand to get out of the cold; the other door leading to the stairs was locked. When someone went in or out, I skillfully slipped inside the door, sat on the stairs, and half-studied and half-kept watch for Mama and Charles from the window. If I saw one of their cars pull up out front to park, I hauled ass back outside. One day I got engrossed in reading a book, and Mama caught me sitting in the hall. "If I catch you in this hall again, I'm going to beat your ass," she said.

My inability to focus made freshman algebra especially difficult. Try as I might, I could not make a lick of sense of a string of letters that represented unknown numbers that had to be figured out according to mathematical rules. I barely made that C. Working after school prevented me from getting a tutor. As a result, I never learned math well enough to successfully make it through sophomore geometry, where I would earn another C. Those were the only math requirements; after those courses, I didn't take another math class because I hadn't learned enough to move forward. My lackluster performance in math would follow me for the rest of my life. It was most reflective in my ACT and GRE scores.

My love for social studies and anything to do with history grew as did my love for literature. Many of our English classes centered around literature, and I became one reading Black girl. Our library had far more books to explore than at Chute and I went to the Black authors section on my free periods to peruse the titles. Scouring the library was how I was introduced to authors from the Harlem Renaissance. However, it was during Black History Month at Second Baptist that Chandra, one of Pastor Taylor's daughters recited a poem by Langston Hughes, which put him on my radar. Then at ETHS I found Hughes' books and, as the saying goes, the rest is history. While I loved to read, I continued to struggle with grammar, and my spelling was horrible. This made writing assignments more of a challenge. I could get away with it in some classes because my reading comprehension was so good that my teachers would dismiss a misspelled word for great answers to questions.

Making friends my freshman year was difficult in such a large building. I was still friendly with my closest friends from Chute, but being assigned to different schedules and halls made it challenging to get together. On top of that, Mama forbade me to participate in extracurricular activities, which was the natural place to meet friends. As I've mentioned, Mama had already said no to me joining the badminton team, so I joined the newly formed Black theater company, Thunder, without her permission. That took some moxie, but I really wanted to be part of it. We'd had programs at church during Black History Month that highlighted poetry and dance, and I was always intrigued. This would be my chance to be directly involved in something similar. Chandra, and

Pastor Taylor's other daughter, Audreanna, and other classmates from Second Baptist had joined. I hoped that when the time came to tell Mama, she would give in because I was already participating.

There was no running with the wolves in Georgia Lee's house; it hadn't been the case in junior high, and it apparently wouldn't be the case in high school, either. I've heard people say they had to be home by the time the streetlights came on. Well, that was my truth, for real, with few exceptions. Those winter months when the time changed were dreadful. If I wasn't working, my tail was sitting in my bedroom by 4:00 p.m. I wasn't going to risk getting home after the lights came on. I did get to attend the track meets that occurred right after school and went to the Saturday football games held during the day. Basketball games were out because they were held in the evening. I simply waited with bated breath for the time change to come around again. I wanted in Thunder so badly that I held out some hope that she could say yes. I gave her the permission slip to sign, and I'd be lying if I said I was surprised when she said, "You need to bring your *fast* ass on home after school." Still, I felt utterly deflated.

"But Mama," I whined, "I already joined." She looked up at me from watching television and said, "Well, you can unjoin." And she went back to watching her program. I realized that I could have signed the permission slip; however, there'd be no way to explain why I was coming home late. My classmates wanted to know why I stopped coming, and I just shrugged it off. I was too embarrassed to tell them that my mother was tripping. This kind of isolation was an adjustment from what I had been accustomed to at Chute. Church and anything to do with it was the exception to Mama's rule. Whatever Grandmamma Julia told her that day on Hermitage Street must have stuck like Super Glue. Therefore, the majority of my socialization took place at church and at NAACP meetings. I was elected vice president of our chapter and participated in the statewide convention that was held in Evanston that year. All the young people were socially and politically conscious, and I fit right in. I met a host of new friends, mostly from other parts of Illinois, and we became pen pals. I met a guy named Anthony who lived on the South Side, and we started a telephone romance. Our friendship would span another five years before we lost contact.

The combination of Second Baptist, the NAACP, and the abundance of Black literature I read complemented and piggybacked one another. I would sequester myself in my room on cold winter days and devour book after book. The suffering of Black people resonated with me in ways I didn't quite understand at first. Maybe it was my own suffering that grew my compassion and left me hungry to learn more. Don't get me wrong: I'm not comparing getting my butt beat by Mama to Jim Crow, but there were tiny nuances that connected me on a deeper level than just learning for the sake of learning.

At school, I was mostly drawn to upperclassmen. I became friends with Stevie Harrell. She was a super-cool junior and was very popular. I felt privileged to be her "little sister." We sometimes hung out on my free periods and sat together at lunch. She was friends with a lot of the football players. That's why I started going to the Saturday games. She and her mother lived a ten-minute walk from my house, and their home became another place for me to be other than at home. Stevie was my lifeline on all things female, and she caused a revolution of self-realization in me. She was a free spirit who was comfortable in her skin. She unabashedly wore oversized T-shirts with no pants in the house like it was no big deal. I couldn't do that at home. Her comfort level with her body made me pay attention. I had been taught to hate my body. I started developing Stevie's unadulterated liberation of the female form. I became carefree in the gym locker room. Once I was out of Mama's house, I didn't have to carry the shame of my body anymore. I mentioned earlier that it was after watching Stevie shave her legs that I got some backbone and shaved mine, cutting my skin down to the bone in the process.

Granted, my path to liberation was fraught with trial and error, but I was doing it my way.

My hair was another mess Stevie helped me work through. I really didn't know anything about taking care of my hair and Mama didn't either. After Tobie and his children moved upstairs, I was on my own. Mama took me to the hairdresser every once in a while. Grandmamma Julia hot-combed my hair for special occasions at church. I had done the best I could, but by the time we moved to Evanston, my hair was badly damaged. I'm sure dying it red and trying to have an afro didn't help.

Stevie's hair was always perfect. It was naturally curly, and she went from curly to straight styles with ease. I had never been able to do that. My hair was naturally curly, bearing the roots of both my white mother and Black father. When it was wet, I had natural waves, but once it was dry it was a fuzzy mess. I'd wash my hair, put it in braids and hot-comb it when it was dry. Then, I rolled it up section by section with those pink sponge rollers to get curls. I wanted to get that straight look like Stevie had, so I decided I was going to give myself a perm. I purchased a jar of relaxer and worked it through my hair until it was silky. I was quite please after I rinsed, washed, and conditioned it. Back then, Black girls weren't really blow-drying their hair. I slicked it back to let it air-dry and went about my day. A couple of hours later, my hair had become brittle. I called Stevie in a panic, saying, "My hair is hard. I need to talk to your mother." Stevie's mother, Linda, was an instructor at the now famous Pivot Point Beauty School. Stevie told me to calm down and tell her what I had done so that she could tell Linda.

"But it's falling out every time I touch it," I said, frantically. Of course, it was. I had purchased a single jar of Afro-Sheen perm rather than the whole kit because I thought I could have what was left over for another time. Little did I know the neutralizing shampoo in the kit was necessary to bring my *pH* level back to normal. Linda knew immediately what was wrong, and she had me come up to Pivot Point to save my hair. Most of it had to be cut. I didn't know how Mama was going to react. I had gotten permission to go, but then this was Mama. When I walked into the house she asked, "Girl what you done to your hair?" I told her and she said with a shrug, "That's your head. You can cut it all, for all I care." I continued to use Pivot Point when I had extra money, and I'd perm my hair four more decades. For a very short period, I even had a Jheri curl, yes, a Jheri curl. Just like with my red-dye and afro phases, my Jheri curl was in and, as always, it had to be fly.

I stayed away from guys when I first began the school year. After James and Mickey, I had had enough of being hurt. Therefore, when I first met Robert Young, I had no romantic inclinations toward him. I met him hanging out in the cafeteria during my free periods. Some days he would catch me in the cafeteria looking sad and ask what was wrong. His concern for my well-being was endearing. Eventually, he gained my trust. If I'd had a particularly harsh tongue-lashing from Mama, I confided in him. He was a junior and started calling me his "little sister," like Stevie. (I guess that must have been a thing back then.)

I cherished our talks, which evolved into taking walks together. We found areas away from the hall monitors and talked about my crazy life. Those talks didn't solve my problems, but I certainly felt the lifting of a weight from my shoulders. We sometimes continued our conversations on the phone at night. After a while, we started holding hands; then, one day, he kissed me. Things spiraled out of control after that and, before I knew it, we were doing the do. Yes, we were having sex in school, of all places. First off, space and freedom made it easy to do anything you thought you could get away with at school; plus, we had an open campus. Mama called herself having a tight leash on me; little did she know it would never stop me from having sex if I wanted to. It got so good, Robert and I started sexing like bunny rabbits. We didn't bother to undress fully; we only did the bare minimum to make it work. Often, I sat on his lap and that was all she wrote. Our encounters were all intense quickies and if we had time left, we resumed our walks. You talking about a boost of endorphins in the middle of the day? I would bounce my tail back to class, and then off to work I would go.

I had not stopped to consider the possible implications of my actions—that is, until my menstrual cycle was late. I panicked! For three days I could not sleep. I was consumed with the thought, *What if?* I avoided Robert like he was the plague because it was the only way I could say no to him. I sure as hell wasn't going to play with fire and have sex with him again. I knew as sure as my name is Rae that Mama would beat that baby out of me. I was headed straight to hell. I prayed every single night: *Lord, don't let me be pregnant. Lord, please don't let me be pregnant.* But after each prayer reality set in and I said to myself, *You should have thought about that before you lost your mind fucking in school.* When my period finally arrived, I thought I had been reborn and given a second chance. You'd better believe that I didn't run out to see Robert. However, I knew I couldn't hold him off forever. I finally told him the deal: I thought I was pregnant. I told him I didn't want to get pregnant, and that meant I couldn't have sex with him anymore. I was done. I cut him off. I thought he would understand because he knew Mama was crazy. I told him many times what it was like to live with her. We had spent hours talking about her. As it turned out, he was like most high school dudes. He wasn't trying to hear that I was cutting him off from sex. He wasn't even offering any solution, like condoms. He only wanted to keep going. But that pregnancy scare had changed everything for me. It knocked me back to my senses. We didn't have any business screwing in school anyhow, and I told him as much. I was cool being his friend, but he certainly couldn't have any more benefits.

About a week later, Robert came to my job to "talk some sense into" me. At the time, I was still working for Ms. Ann at the cleaners. I was pissed.

"Dude, what if my Mama or one of her friends sees you?" I asked. "That would be *my* ass *and my* job." I was giving him all kinds of attitude. Ms. Ann had told me not to have friends hanging around, and sometimes she came back before closing. His self-centered reaction made me think that sex was the only thing he wanted, and that turned me off for real. I was not trying to hear it. He had the nerve to tell me that if I cut him off, he would tell everyone at school what we had done.

"Everyone is gonna know you a hoe," he exclaimed.

I pleaded with him not to, but he was not trying to hear me. I put him out of the shop. In that moment I decided, *Fuck it. Do what you got to do but consider me and my pussy dead to you.* I was done. In hindsight, I think if he had given me a little time to get over the pregnancy scare, he probably could have gotten me back. But no-o-o; he wanted to punish me, and betrayal wasn't something I took lightly. The next day, a male friend pulled me aside and told me that Robert was spreading a rumor that I had sex with him at school.

"You really think I'm that stupid?" I asked. I hadn't thought about how I would defend myself if he followed through, but I was thinking fast. I flipped the script, and vehemently denied it. I couldn't deny that he and I spent time together. Everyone saw us, but then, that was perfect, too.

"He just mad 'cause I won't give him none," I said, thinking deflection would work. Guys did that all the time to ruin a girl's reputation. I hadn't told anyone that Robert and I were having sex, and it helped make my denial believable. Stevie had heard the rumor and I denied it again but confessed that I wasn't a virgin. She gave me some big-sisterly advice about guarding my reputation. She also told me about Planned Parenthood, where I could get birth-control pills without parental consent. I didn't hesitate. I figured even if I wasn't having sex, I would be prepared when it happened again.

After my mess with Robert, I told myself I was done with boys—like I had with James. It was just a lie, similar to how we promise God that if She delivers us from whatever the mess is, we won't do it again. The fact was that my hormones were on fire and my self-esteem was low. While this was only the beginning of many more mistakes and men, I did manage to avoid sex the rest of that school year.

The early part of the summer I was very active with the NAACP. In addition to being elected to serve as the vice president of our youth chapter, I was selected to represent the chapter at the national convention. Joyce Favors, our advisor came over to the house to ask Mama's permission to attend. Joyce was everything. Full stop. She wore many different hats: advisor, Sunday school teacher and choir director while she was a graduate student at Northwestern University. I don't know how she pulled it off. But when she agreed to come over and meet Mama to ask for permission, I knew she was the real deal. I hadn't confided in Joyce about my situation at home other than my mother was very strict and sometimes a little crazy. I told Joyce, "I don't know what might come out of her mouth," but from the moment she walked in, she had Mama eating out of her hands. With her congenial personality, that beautiful smile of hers and beautiful, dark round face to match, Mama said yes. With Joyce as my chaperone, I got to attend the NAACP National Convention in St. Louis, Missouri for almost an entire week

The convention was an amazing experience in many ways. I got to meet up with all my friends whom I met at the state convention that winter. Anthony and I met and got to spend a little time together. We made out, but I didn't violate Joyce's trust. I kept myself in check. Attending the youth workshops was fascinating. Each session provided information on how youth could be politically active. It would take me years to fully understand the significance or the privilege I had been afforded to hear Roy Wilkins' outgoing speech, and Benjamin Hooks' incoming address.

Twenty-One

SHAME

" Shame is the intensely painful feeling or experience of believing
that we are flawed and, therefore, unworthy of love and belonging."
—Brene Brown

I learned through my friends' lives that my life was not normal. It would be somewhere between the ages of 15 and 16 when I started to believe I wasn't normal—that something was wrong with me, but I couldn't put my finger on it. I'd stumble into situations, not thinking. I may even have stayed stuck for a time, but I had this uncanny ability to walk out of the fire and keep it moving, leaving the smoke to linger in my spirit long after it was all said and done. Like with Robert and sexing in the corners of ETHS. In all of my years of transparency, I had only shared that story with my therapist because I was too embarrassed. I share it now because I see it as the beginning of a pattern in a cycle that took root in me and would define my dating pattern for decades, ultimately, leading to me becoming infected with HIV.

From my teens and well into adulthood, I lived in parallel worlds that created, in me a deep sense of pride on the one hand, and abject shame on the other. Different from my earlier years, now, I not only had to contend with how Mama treated me; I had to deal with my own behavior and the misery it brought me. In the aftermath of each blunder, the self-loathing began. I was merciless on myself, asking poignant questions: *What the fuck is wrong with you, girl? Why can't you ever seem to measure up?* It would take decades for me to answer these questions. By then, the damage had taken root, requiring a massive effort to stop the cycle.

I had always believed I was damaged in one way or another. Mama had killed my self-esteem over the years. On top of her accusation of me *being fast*, my lack of self-worth was compounded by Junior, Betty, her friend, Mr. Tom, and Mickey. I wondered, *Why was I such an easy target? What is it about me that made them think it was okay to make me be fast?* The only answer was that something was wrong with me. After that horrendous year of abuse, I pushed it to the back of my mind so I could cope with the burdens of their abuse and the shame I had about *being fast*—until it all came back, forcing me to try to make sense of what had happened to me.

My memory was bound to be triggered at some point. In retrospect, I believe it began with Junior's death in August 1975, as I was entering eighth grade. One morning, Mama came to my room and told me Junior had been shot by the Chicago police. It was weird because I sensed that I already knew. That night, I'd had a dream that I was falling, and Junior attempted to save me, missed my hand and fell to his death. It was so real that I woke up startled; I tried to shake it off and go back to sleep, but I couldn't. When Mama entered my room, I sensed what she was going to tell me, but to hear her say Junior had been shot by a Chicago police officer left me speechless.

Just like in 2021, there are often two versions of a police officer killing a Black male; however, in 1975, there were no videos to disclose the truth. The police account of Junior's murder went like this: Two Chicago police officers, James Moylan and Daniel

Dixon, spotted six Black teenage boys attacking a white teenage boy. The patrol stopped and chased them away. The alleged victim also fled. Junior had somehow evaded the police, doubled back, got into the parked police car and allegedly tried to run down Officer Moylan, who then fired six shots at the moving car, killing Junior with a bullet to the chest. The version of area residents and people at the scene was recorded by several city newspapers, and it went like this: The fight was over by the time the police arrived. Junior, according to witnesses, was not a part of the group or the fight. He was however, intoxicated; he got into the police car and started to drive away. At the time, Junior was not in Officer Moylan's view; rather, he was chasing one of the young men in a gangway between two houses. Then, he noticed that the police vehicle was moving; he fired at the car, shooting Junior. When Officer Moylan reached the crashed vehicle, he discovered Junior was wounded, opened the door and dropped him in the street. By the time Junior arrived at Holy Cross Hospital, he was already dead. Junior was eighteen years old.

The police department's Office of Professional Standards investigated the shooting and considered reprimanding Moylan for leaving his keys in the car, but it never did. It was my understanding that Tobie sued the Chicago Police Department, receiving a settlement a few years later. This pattern—in which accountability is replaced by money from police departments across the country—has continued for decades.

Mama and I went to Junior's funeral; this was the first time I had seen or spoken to Tobie or any of his children in almost two years. After the funeral, to my surprise, Mama allowed me to rekindle my relationship with Ethel. We started out talking on the phone, and that led to an overnight visit. I was so excited for Ethel to sleep over. Her visit was ruined when Mama bolted into my bedroom at 2:00 a.m. and beat me out of bed to wash the dishes. Ethel and I had been having so much fun that the dishes slipped my mind. Ethel never spent another night and I never asked anyone else to sleep over.

After Junior's death, every detail of the abuse rushed into my head like a torrential flood. I spent a lot of time trying to make sense of what happened. I could now name sex and I asked myself poignant questions: *Did I really have sex with my brother?* I was horrified at the thought. *Was I really that "fast?"* I remembered that I didn't want to and how I had gone along so he wouldn't be mad at me. I also remembered that in the beginning it felt good with no understanding that my body failed me and I asked, *What does that say about me?* Junior's death and my subsequent trigger coincided with Mama's accusations around getting my menstrual cycle and the bladder infection. Trying to make sense of this memory in that climate was futile, so I pushed it out of my mind again. Ten months later I had sex with James and thought about Junior again, but quickly decided it was James who had taken my virginity because that gave me some agency over my body. Then when Mickey raped me a month after I stopped seeing James, I asked myself, *Weren't Mickey and Junior precisely the same because they had both penetrated me when I didn't want them to?* Within weeks of Mickey, I had another trigger. I came home from work one Saturday and my father's siblings, Uncle Michael and Aunt Sharon, were sitting in the living room talking to Mama. I recognized them immediately, although I have no memory of meeting Sharon prior to this day. I have no idea what brought them to our living room that day. Everyone looked up at me when I came through the door. I stood in our small foyer, trying to digest the situation.

"Girl, ain't you happy to see your people?" Mama asked, trying to propel me into a conversation. Aunt Sharon walked around the coffee table and gave me a big hug. Michael stood, and I knew my feet were supposed to move in his direction, but I was stuck. I could see that ruler coming down on my little hands. If I had never seen him again in life, it would have been too soon. "Girl, what's wrong with you?" Mama asked. I started moving in his direction, and he bent that skinny body down to hug me. I hesitated, but then I could feel all eyes on me, and I reached up to hug him back. I felt dirty—the same kind of dirty I felt after Mickey. I pulled away and moved to the other side of Aunt Sharon and sat down. Mama went into the back. Then everything went blank. It was like I had an out-of-body experience. Darkness settled over me like a cloud before the storm. I know the three of us talked because time passed, but I have no idea what was said other than "Goodbye" and "Keep in touch" when I walked them to the door.

I shut the door behind me and went straight to my room and sat on the floor between my twin beds. I was overwhelmed and anxious as thoughts roamed my head trying to conjure memories that would not come. However, I couldn't shake that feeling of dirtiness and sexual familiarity. *Had I had sex with my uncle? Why can I remember the alphabet lesson and ruler, and nothing else?* I was so weirded out by their visit that, after they left, I went into the bathroom, locked the door, tore up the paper with their telephone numbers and flushed it down the toilet. I didn't understand what was happening, but I didn't want any part of it, not even a piece.

Only months after I saw my aunt and uncle, Betty came walking back into my life. Robert Sr. was visiting his sister who lived in Chicago and Betty had come, too. Mama, Charles and I went over one Saturday to hang out. Betty walked into the kitchen, and every sordid detail of her and her friend came back. My stomach turned into painful knots. I had a crippling, helpless feeling, and I didn't know what to do. I stood frozen until shame overtook my pain, and I went into the bathroom. Just thinking about her girlfriend made me feel like I was going to throw up. I bent over the toilet waiting for it to come, but all that came was shame. At that moment, I viewed what happened to me with Betty and her friend as a sexual encounter gone awry. *How could you have had sex with that girl? With your own auntie?* I was horrified and ashamed. The fact that they were females confused me and compounded my shame. I stayed in the bathroom until someone needed to use it. When I came out, I made it a point to not be in the same room with Betty. She came upstairs; I went downstairs. She came into the kitchen; I went into the sitting room.

Seeing Betty brought on a catastrophic meltdown. I couldn't sleep and I had crying spells at school. Just imagine: All of this happened within a fifteen-month span—dealing with Junior's death, having sex with James, being raped by Mickey, seeing my uncle for the first time after he disappeared and seeing Aunt Betty after all those years. I was so confused I couldn't tell you up from down. I was learning about incest in health education. My situations with both Betty and Junior constituted incest, but then Betty's friend made it more complicated. I understood what she had done to me was sort of like rape, as I had believed with Mickey because I didn't want them to. However, even in 1977, rape was being taught to us as a violent act by a stranger, not by someone who you considered to be family or a friend. Even incest, as I understood it, was more about consensual sex rather than rape and molestation. I was creating a road map for my future self, and the lens through which I viewed sex had been so distorted that I couldn't determine consensual sex from molestation and rape, not with Betty and her friend, Mickey, Mr. Tom or Junior and only God knows what happened between my uncle and me. What is certain is that I couldn't shake the sexual familiarity I felt around him that day. The myriad of convergent thoughts was too much for me to take in at fourteen, and I wanted to stop the chaos circling in my head. The easiest answer was to assume all the blame by believing I really was *fast*. It was like Mama said when Claudette told her Charles attacked me: If I weren't *fast*, he wouldn't have wanted to have sex with me. I was the problem. Mama had been drilling it into me for so long that, now that I was sexually active, I could see myself from her point of view. Anything to the contrary would force me to confront the fact that I had been violated by those who should have protected me. I was still living in chaos, and it was more than enough trying to manage Mama's betrayal and Charles' cruelty. I was on toxic overload; to add more to my plethora of emotional scars would have been too much.

In the end, I protected myself by taking another hit to my self-esteem—by accepting that I was this girl Mama claim me to be. Being gravely wounded by those sexual violations would cause the abnormal way of life to influence the parts of me that were normal. As a result, my abnormal response to my abnormal situation became normal behavior for me.

After these triggers, I would have a couple of normal, age-appropriate relationships. One was with David "Dee" Russell, who I met when visiting Pat and Ethel right before my sophomore year; the other was with Mark Caselberry, during that school year.

Following Ethel's visit, Mama allowed me to stay at Tobie's every now and then. I returned home from the NAACP convention and Mama shocked me by allowing me to visit them for almost a month! I took it and ran. Tobie had an entirely different vibe than when he and Mama were together. He laughed and talked, and it felt like a family. In some ways it was as if we all picked right back up where we had left off, minus Mama. I wish life had been this easy when we were a blended family. During my visit, Tobie at least acknowledged that Mama had a drinking problem and kept mess going. It seemed he felt sorry for her. I didn't pry.

Patricia was the big sister in charge. She took her role seriously and we took her seriously. It was me, Ethel, Pat, Allen and Juan. Dorothy was on her own by now. Tobie's girlfriend, Delores—yes, the same one Mama pulled a gun on—and their son Buddy were around but didn't live with them. Delores seemed to bring out the best in Tobie, and she was fun. Even though Tobie had cheated on Mama, he at least kept it out of her face until the very end. I had never laid eyes on Delores until the night Mama pulled the rifle on them, and Tobie came home every night. He did, however, replace Mama with a younger woman, and that had to have hurt. Nonetheless, I liked Delores and she was kind to me. Being over there was the same neighborhood experience like on Hermitage: lazy days kicking it around on the front porch. It was priceless and gave me peace of mind.

That summer, Pat was the big sister I didn't know I needed. She taught me how to use tampons and freed me from those bulky-ass sanitary napkins. I came on my period and there wasn't a sanitary napkin to be found.

"I got tampons," Pat laughed.

"I don't know how to use a tampon," I complained. It had been almost three years since my cycle came on a regular basis and I was still struggling with taking care of myself during what seemed like the longest seven days in the world. I wanted to ask Stevie, but I thought it was a tad too personal.

"Well, you gonna learn—*today*," Pat emphasized.

"But Mama said I couldn't use them." With Mama, tampons and shaving were forbidden for the same reason: They would ruin my nature.

"Don't nobody care about what Georgia say," she said flatly.

I was still the scaredy cat, asking, "But what if she finds out?"

"How she gonna know?" Pat asked. "You planning to tell her?"

"Girl, come on here. Ain't nobody got all day," Pat demanded.

I will never forget Pat standing by the bathroom door with one hand on her hip and a tampon in the other. She handed me a tampon and instructed me through the crack of the door on how to insert it. It was funny as all get-out: me on the toilet and Pat trying to explain how to slant the tampon into my vagina so it wouldn't hurt.

"It hurts," I kept whining.

She was patient. Each time I put one in wrong she would have me take it out, and she'd hand me a new one, with slightly different instructions, until I got it right. By the end of that day, I felt brand new and I never turned back. At home, I hid my tampons in a shoebox because Charles searched my room occasionally. Now, that's a whole other story.

The summer was going great, and it got even better when I met David. He lived up the street from the Toblers, with his mother and sister. He was new to the neighborhood and girls were gunning for him. I came in with all my sass and assertiveness and swooped him right up. David was six-feet-two-inches tall, with this big, beautiful smile and his dapper style. He was entering into his senior year at Dunbar Vocational High School. He was ultra-cool and a ton of fun. He was genuinely a nice guy. He was dark chocolate and smooth as a Godiva truffle, both in and out of bed. The contrast when our bodies met was tantalizing.

I enjoyed spending time with David. We talked and laughed—and had sex. It wasn't like it had been with Robert; trying to find a corner to do it in; or James, for whom sex was the end game. David and I explored every inch of each other—touching, caressing, taking long baths and, after sex, having long talks about life. He was very philosophical. Come to think of it, David was the first guy to capture my mind; I liked that trait in him. It has stayed with me forever. If you're not a critical thinker with some enlightening conversations, then don't think about looking my way—period.

Pat and Ethel covered for me when I was over at David's. Our mornings turned into afternoons, and he made me feel as if I was on top of the world. I had my first orgasm with David, and he has always held a place in my heart. It was the best summer fling ever, and it created a decades-long friendship. After spending time with David, I knew I had been an absolute fool messing around with Robert in school. *That was so uncouth,* I thought, reading myself the riot act. *You better have some self-respect this school year.* The problem is, I didn't give myself or my hormones a chance. This is why I'm a big advocate of teaching young girls about sex and sexuality. Something has to give other than *keep your legs closed.'* That demand, in and of itself, made me feel like I was already a failure.

I started dating Mark Caselberry at the beginning of my sophomore school year. He was a senior and on the varsity football team. We never had sex but, lawd, did we make out! I'd bike over to his house and right before we could get our clothes off, his mother always came home. I guess it just wasn't meant to be. In fact, Robert would be the only guy I actually had sex with during my years at ETHS.

Mark and I shared lockers that school year, and I wore his varsity jacket. I would go to the football games and cheer him on. I still had a curfew, so I was never able to spend any time with him outside of school. It was my most normal relationship when I look back on the sum total of my dating experiences. I pledged to get through my sophomore school year with no bumps and, for the most part, I did. I didn't work that school year, which afforded me more study time. Academically, it was my best year at ETHS. I even got an A both semesters in English, which propelled me to Honors English the following year. My teacher thought I was wasting my time in regular English, but I guess Mr. Horn was looking at my overall performance and didn't think it was a good idea. A whole new world of literature opened up for me in Honors English. I read *Catcher and The Rye,* by J. D. Salinger; *Moby Dick,* by Herman Melville; and *Native Son* and *Black Boy,* by Richard Wright. I was in my element reading and analyzing books, and I shined.

Veronica Slater and I became more friendly; by the following year, we had become close. Our friendship has spanned decades. She was a popular girl with a lot of personality. Her brother Darryl was two years older, and he was the total opposite. He was completely laid-back cool. Veronica was a Willie Wild Cat our school mascot and she performed at games. I thought dressing up in the wildcat costume and being silly at the games would be so much fun. I asked Mama if I could try out and, as anticipated, she said no. I joined the Student Council instead, not asking Mama for permission. Our advisor, Ms. Robin Tucker, recruited me, she said, because of my outgoing personality. Council met at seven-thirty in the morning, and I could get away with it. I got up early and as soon as Mama walked out of that door, I made a mad dash for the bathroom to get ready for school. I saw Student Council as another way to continue my activism along with the NAACP. I thought I was *so* politically savvy. I also developed new friends in Student Council, including Nancy Williams, our president; Jill Adams; Rodney Williams; and Kim Buster. I looked up to Nancy. She was so darn smart; a senior, she was headed for the Ivy League. She took me under her wing that school year. Kim lived up the street from me and sometimes I would study with her after school before Mama came home. I loved being active in Student Council. I even participated in my first blood drive that school year. Being a voice for my classmates in West Hall made me feel as if I was doing something for the greater good—and took me out of my own misery.

My other closest friend, Coré Cotton, came into my life around this time by way of church. She and her mother, Reverend Dr. M. Jeanne Cotton, moved to Evanston from Little Rock, Arkansas during the summer of 1977. Dr. Cotton relocated to Evanston to attend Garrett Theological Seminary, at Northwestern University. Subsequently, she came to Second Baptist to do field study work for the M.Div. program. I was impressed with Dr. Cotton from the day Dr. Taylor introduced her to the congregation. She was statuesque and poised, with short curly hair and walnut-colored skin. Her diction was flawless. She had both sophistication and Southern charm. I described her style of dress as Neiman Marcus meets Queen Nefertiti. She wore a fragrance with a deep spicy smell and floral undertones that I loved. One day, I finally got the nerve to ask her the name of the scent. It was Royal Secret, by Germaine Monteil. How fitting that it had the word royal in the title. It was the first department-store perfume I ever purchased.

Coré was a couple years younger than me and in the eighth grade, but she seemed so much older. Like her mother, she was a licensed and ordained minister with an incredible voice. She joined the Young Gifted and Black Choir. Coré was aloof, but after we became friends, she told me she was homesick. Dr. Cotton encouraged me to befriend Coré. I'm not sure why she picked me, but I took her request seriously. I don't think other members of the choir knew what to make of her. A minister as young as Coré was new to us, and I think everyone saw her as a child prodigy in that she preached like a seasoned adult minister so they didn't push it, unlike me. I was determined to get Coré to say more than two words. I kept at it until she finally gave me her number. We quickly became close friends. She confided in me about missing Little Rock and I confided in her about my home life. Frankly, some of the things I went through at home were unbelievable, even to me. I think for every story I ever told Coré and Veronica, there were at least three more to match that I didn't tell. Who wants to recount such madness or disclose their life as a living hell, when on the other side, their friends' lives are sunny and bright? Mama liked the fact that Coré and her mother were ministers and allowed me to spend as much time with them as they would allow. The few times Coré visited my house, she had Mama eating out of her hands. Coré liked Mama and Mama liked Coré far more than she ever liked me. Mama laughed and joked with her in a way that she never did with me.

"Co-Co," she'd say, referring to Coré by her nickname, "You just full of shit, girl."

"Aww, Mama Georgia," Coré would say to Mama, and Mama would start grinning from ear to ear. I was happy that Mama gave me free rein when it came to the Cottons. By the time I met them, the void in my life had grown by leaps in bounds. I latched onto them and swore not to let go. When I think about it today, I felt in my heart there was something special about the entire family. Maybe it was the love I saw between them and the fact they'd done so well in life. I placed them on a pedestal, especially Coré. She was smart and talented, and she had been raised in a loving atmosphere that I would have given my life to have. It was something to watch them interact, particularly when they were singing. Coré was the baby of the family, with four sisters and a brother. When they came to visit, I never stopped being in awe. The oldest sister actually moved to live with them, and she didn't like me. I stayed out of her way as much as possible. Inevitably, the circle of life always comes back around. Nearly four decades later, her sister confirmed what I had always felt. I was at Coré's for Thanksgiving and that sister told me that back in the day she didn't want me to hang around Coré because she thought I was a bad influence, but that I had made good on my life. That day, I was that lost teenage girl all over again. I didn't dare show my hurt. Instead, I talked about my accomplishments more, still trying to prove my worth.

Being friends with Coré was like a two-for-one deal because I got to spend time with her and her mother. Dr. Cotton was often invited to sing and preach at church programs, and she allowed me to tag along. It was reminiscent of my days with Grandmamma Julia. In the evening, Coré and I would spend hours on the phone laughing. Mama never picked up the phone ordering me to "get the fuck off the phone," as she did with other friends. On Saturdays I walked over to Coré's a good ten to twelve blocks from my house, and we'd have Bible study. She was serious about her religious studies, and I became serious about mine. We read the Bible, looked up references, and checked and double-checked different scholarly interpretations about biblical texts. Her sister was worried about my influence, but I wonder if she ever considered Coré's influence on me. Prior to hanging out with Coré, I only read the Bible for Sunday school assignments. Our Saturday Bible studies opened a whole new spiritual world for me. We listened to gospel music together. Sometimes we listened to Reverend Donald Parson's sermons on the record player. Suffering began to take on a new meaning. I was able to appropriate scripture to my own life. Many of those prayers I had made over the years had gone unanswered, leaving me to wonder if God was up there looking down at my life of hell, twiddling Her thumbs. I came to understand that God might not have taken me out of the storms but helped me to weather them. I am still amazed that I wasn't devoured by the trauma or that I didn't totally self-destruct. I started studying the Bible on my own and grew spiritually by leaps and bounds. The church was no longer a place solely to numb my pain. It became a place to experience the presence of God. Hanging out with Coré was as if I had been reborn. I spent less and less time with Sharmayne and her mother so that I could be with the Cottons.

I made it through that school year without any major mishaps. Well, Mark and I didn't end so well and, when I look back, that was normal, too. I broke up with him. Don't even ask me why. I think I was embarrassed I couldn't spend any time with him outside of school. I couldn't even go to homecoming with him. Rather than keep making excuses, I walked away. His feelings were hurt. When I opened our locker the next morning, his ass had torn up my library books. I was livid. I confronted him in the cafeteria while he was hanging out with his boys.

"The rats ate them," he said, and everyone around burst out laughing. I was embarrassed, but my payback was to hold his varsity jacket hostage. Toward the end of the school year, he had his father call Mama, and she made me give it back. Mama called me in her room that night, asking, "What's this about some boy's jacket you got?"

"Mama, I kept his jacket because he tore up my library books." I guess she was too tired that night to fuss. She took a draw on her cigarette: "Give that boy back his jacket. You ain't got no business with it." She had me call him right away, and he and his father came over to get it. Then, Mama asked his father, "What about the books he tore up?" He said Mark would have to pay for them. That was the end of my dating life in high school. Other guys liked me, sure, but I wasn't budging. I flirted with them here or there. Some even got in a feel or two, but none of them got any further than that.

The biggest observation I can make about the next ten years of my life starting from the beginning of my sophomore year is that I was able to soar despite the chaos, when I was in a safe environment with no distractions and no one preying on me. However, the moment I stepped outside of that bubble and was left to make my own decisions, things went haywire for me. I'm not trying to absolve myself from my choices, but I am saying that my life had been so distorted all it took was one person or decision to make me ask myself, yet again, *What the heck is wrong with you girl?*

That's what happened in the summer of 1978. I started a new job at the McDonald's about a fifteen-minute walk from my house. I had just turned sixteen and could legally work. Most weeks, I clocked forty-five to sixty hours. By the time Mama came home from work, I was already at McDonald's. I often closed, which landed me at home each night after ten and, on weekends, after twelve. I liked working at McDonald's and became proficient at it. Like always, I wanted to learn how to do everything, even fry burgers—and I did.

When I started at McDonald's, boys were the last thing on my mind. I was doing well, and I was proud of myself. I hadn't had any toxic or dangerous relationships. I flirted and all that, but I had avoided real trouble. Most importantly, I had managed to stay out of the web of men who were too old for me after Mickey and James. Still, I thought I was all of that. I also perceived myself to be far more experienced with sex and men than I actually was. In the wake of the back-to-back triggers, I would view myself through the lens of *being fast* for nearly two more decades. *I've been having sex since I was a little girl. Of course, I'm good in bed* is what I told myself. The truth is I was green as a country collard and had no idea what the hell I was doing. But by the time I reached nineteen, I had made that misnomer my truth.

Upfront, I liked the chase. I was drawn to the banter between a man and a woman as well as the sexual tension leading up to the sex. The chase was more exciting sometimes than sex itself. That's what happen with L.D., one of my managers. He started macking me, and I got all caught up. The next thing I knew, we were headed to a hotel. On the ride there, I asked myself: *Do you real-l-ly want to have sex with him?* "No" was the answer. I just didn't know how to put on the brakes. After we finished having sex, I felt and looked like he had sucked the life out of me. I had hickey's all up and down my neck and even on my breasts. I looked at myself in the bathroom mirror with disgust for having sex with L.D. I was my own worst enemy. I didn't understand that having agency over my body through the ability to say yes or no didn't mean that I had control. I had walked into a powerless situation thinking I was a badass, but really L.D. was the wolf and I was Little Red Riding Hood. He was sixteen years older than me; he had the experience and, most importantly, he was my boss. It was a boundary that he shouldn't have crossed. No matter what I thought going into the situation with L.D., I had been taken advantage of in the end.

Trying to hide hickeys in the summer ain't cute, but somehow, I managed to keep them away from Mama. A few days after my rendezvous with L.D., another manager, Randy Hoskins asked to see me in the office at the end of my shift. Before I could sit down, he said, "Don't you EVER let a man do this to you again," waving his hand up and down beside my neck. Stunned and embarrassed, I put my head down. He lifted my chin and said, "You are not a damn animal," adding in a softer tone, "You are a young lady and should be treated as such." Randy and I talked for over an hour. I told him that L.D. had already tried to get me back between the sheets and I didn't want to. Randy said he was going to put a stop to it, and he did. I don't know what he said to L.D., but dude made a 180-degree turn and totally ended things.

That one day in the office with Randy turned into another day, and another, and then another. Randy was so easy to talk to. He was smoother than ice and wise beyond his twenty-six years. We didn't talk about sex; instead, he asked me about my future and what I wanted out of life. We talked about Mama and Charles. He told me if Charles ever touched me again, he would kill him and ditch his body, and I believed he would. I learned in the years that followed, he was more capable of making good on that statement than I could ever have imagined. He started scheduling me to work his shifts, especially for closing, so we could spend more time together. One night sitting in his cramped office, he said to me, "Girl, I'm going to marry you." He leaned in close, tracing my lips with his tongue. I blushed so hard. Randy didn't ask to take me to a hotel; rather, he asked me to be his woman, and I said yes. He didn't rush into having sex. Instead, he eased into the moment, never forcing me to do anything or assuming that he could do anything to me. Instead, he always asked permission every step of the way. One day he whispered into my ear, "Can I lick you?" I nodded my head and drifted away into ecstasy. Another hot summer day when he asked if I would lick him, I blurted out, "I don't think so! That's nasty." He never brought the subject up again. He just created magic with his tongue between my legs, and I came to a place where I wanted to give him the same pleasure that he was giving to me. The day I slid down and took him into my mouth, he reminded me of the way I often sucked his finger and told me to do it the same way. He had been teaching me how to pleasure him, but also how to be pleasured. Being with Randy was about a connection—one I had never had with a lover or any other living being.

"You belong to me," he declared one day. And I believed I belonged to him. By the time school started in the fall, I was so deep in love and happy I couldn't see the forest for the trees. Coré began her freshman year at ETHS, and we were locker partners. I was happy to finally be with her during school hours. We ate lunch together and now the tables of friendship had turned for me: My closest friend was a freshman and now I was a junior. Now, I was the big sister showing my little sister the ropes.

I was also trying to juggle my relationship with Randy between school and work. The first half-day we had at school, I didn't tell Mama. I went over to Randy's and spent the afternoon at his apartment. Time flew by; before I knew it, I was late for work. I called the manager on duty to tell him I would be about thirty minutes late. I walked into McDonald's with my backpack slung over my shoulder and went straight toward the counter, heading to the back. Before I even got to the other side of the counter, I heard Mama's voice.

"Let's go, young lady," she said. I almost jumped out of my skin. I turned in slow motion, and she was standing by a table in the small lobby. I walked out of the restaurant and straight to the car. That five-minute ride home in silence was hell on earth. It felt like judgment day. When we reached the apartment door, she asked me, "Where the fuck was you, bitch?"

"I was with Randy," I said, matter-of-factly. I thought I might as well tell the truth and get it over with. I knew I was going to get beat no matter what I said. She went into her room to get the extension cord. She came back in the living room with one hand on her hip and the extension cord in the other, firing questions at me. "Who the fuck is Randy?" she demanded.

"He's my boyfriend," I said. The questions kept coming, "Where did you meet him? Before I could get it out of my mouth, I felt the extension cord hot across my back. I cried and took the blows and accepted that I had brought this on myself. For the first time, I couldn't claim Mama to be in the wrong. The blows across my back matched the insults from her mouth.

"You fucking whore!

"You white bitch!"

"I'm sick of your *fast* ass!"

"I'll kill you!"

"You ain't shit!" She beat me until I was hunched over on the floor, and she was out of breath and almost hoarse. Then she called Charles and handed him the extension cord. His blows burned like a fire deep in my soul. My tears turned into anger. This was the first time she had allowed him to beat me. I was defiant. Lick after lick, I sat on the floor with my hands and arms over my head, and I showed no reaction. I just took the blows. I had made up in my mind the moment he stepped into the living room that there was nothing he could do to hurt me; he had already done it all. I think my lack of reaction caused his lack of interest, and he stopped soon after he started. I went to the bedroom, cleaned myself up and nursed my welts.

About an hour later, Mama made me call Randy. When he answered, I told him that Mama wanted to talk to him.

"I'm going to put your ass in jail!" she hollered. Randy was smooth, and whatever he was saying to Mama shut her down quick. Then I heard her say, "You can have the bitch if you want her." I figured he must have told her he wanted to marry me.

"I'll sign the papers!" she hollered. Mama turned to me and asked, "Do you want to marry him?" I didn't answer right away. My head and stomach were during flip-flops. It was a lot to think about in that moment of chaos, and I was a wreck trying to figure it out, with Mama mean-mugging me to hell and back. Sure, I loved Randy, and I believed he loved me, but I was afraid of the unknown. I didn't know what it took to be a wife. As crazy as it might sound, the scariest of all was leaving the security of my home. Mama was abusive, but I never had to worry about a meal. I wanted to be with him and hoped that one day after I finished school, we could get married. But on that day—at sixteen years old, standing there—I thought that maybe I should stay with the devil I knew.

"I don't know." I shrugged, looking stupid.

She instructed Randy to never see me again, or she would have him arrested. After she hung up the phone, she handed down her punishment. The orders rolled off her tongue quickly and with precision like she had rehearsed it.

"Quit that fucking job. I bet not find you near it. I bet not catch you with him again, or I will kill you. Don't use my telephone. Come home right after school. Don't ask me for any money."

I broke my silence and interrupted, "How am I supposed to get to school?"

"I don't give a fuck. Crawl!" Mama responded.

"Can I go to church?" I asked. She hesitated for a moment: "I don't know. Co-Co's Mama might not want a whore like you around her daughter." Shame gripped the whole of me. For a moment, I lost track of what Mama was saying.

"Call her!" she demanded and brought me back to my senses. My eyes watered. "Call her now, and let me ask her," she said. The first thing I thought about was that time Dr. Cotton's sister, Dr. Dee Bennet, got me straight in a hurry. One Sunday, she and another sister were in town visiting. We were all on our way to Springfield Baptist Church, up the street from Dr. Cotton's office. They were having a high-spirited conversation about who was going to sing, and I butted in. They were old-school in their belief that children did not jump into grown folks' conversations when not invited. I never did that again because I never wanted to give Dr. Cotton a reason to turn away from me, and now Mama was putting the worst of me dead in her face.

I dialed their number with Mama breathing down my neck. When Coré answered, I told her that Mama wanted to talk to her mother. When Dr. Cotton got on the phone, I handed it to Mama.

"I don't know what to do with this girl," she said to Dr. Cotton. "Her and these men." Mama listened to whatever it was Dr. Cotton was saying; I expected that because she rarely showed her behind when she wanted someone to think the best about her. Then I realized that she was hanging up the phone and I felt relieved that she hadn't asked about Coré. But then she turned to me and said, "Dr. Cotton is coming over. Let's see what your hot ass got to say now." Within an hour, Dr. Cotton was ringing our doorbell. The three of us sat in the living room. Charles went into the kitchen.

"Go on and tell her what your hot ass did," Mama said. She sat on the sofa, looking like she had caught the cat by the tail. This was worse than any beating she could ever have given me. Shame rose up in me violently, like vomit coming out of a drunk. I was ashamed—not so much because I had been with Randy that afternoon, but I knew our relationship was socially unacceptable. I believed that Dr. Cotton would not approve and,

Lord knows, I never wanted her to think the worst of me. The fact is that I hadn't ditched school; I just hadn't told Mama that I had a half-day. If I hadn't been late for work, she would never have known the difference. Nevertheless, here I was recanting the day's events and my relationship with Randy. It was excruciating to explain that I had been laid up with a man all afternoon a man ten years my senior. I cried tears of shame.

There were many counterproductive views about teenage sex. And truth be told, a ton of hang-ups in the Black community were about sex. Everybody was doing it, but nobody wanted to take ownership. Neither Dr. Cotton nor Dr. Taylor was the fire-and-brimstone type of preacher, like many other Black pastors I knew who tried to preach the hell out of its congregants over and over. Dr. Cotton was, however, a woman of high moral standards, and I knew I had failed miserably.

After I finished talking, I sat wringing my hands and thinking about what a failure I was. I also braved up for what I believed was coming next. Mama sat there, content in her smugness. The moment Dr. Cotton opened her mouth, everything changed. Instead of shaming me, as Mama had done, she showered me with God's grace and mercy and showed me what that looked like in the here and now. The wisdom she imparted to me was the most critical advice I had received in all my sixteen years, and I would carry it with me for the rest of my life. She expressed her disappointment, and even that was affirming and not judgmental. She said, "Rae, when Jesus walked up the hill to Calvary, he fell down—but he got back up."

She continued: "It's not that you fall, but that you get back up. It's not about how long you stay down, but that you don't wallow in the mess while you're down."

I could have jumped up and done a two-step! That was a sermon, and the church in me said, "Amen!"

"You can be better than this situation," she affirmed, then continued. "And when you do get back up, remember to be the best. No matter what it is, just be the best. Even if you are a garbage worker, be the best garbage worker you can be."

Mama didn't get the expected outcome she had hoped for. She said, "I know you don't want her *fast* ass around your daughter anymore."

Dr. Cotton didn't respond right away. I was on pins and needles. Lord knows that giving up Coré would be painful. When she spoke up, she addressed me, not Mama.

"I'm not going to forbid Coré from seeing you, Rae. That is her decision, and if it's fine with Coré, then it is fine with me." That was all she had to say. Mama didn't know what to do. Dr. Cotton asked to pray with us. Mama stood up from her chair slowly. Dr. Cotton asked us to hold hands, and I had to grab Mama's because she was not trying to catch hold of mine. Her little shaming scheme hadn't worked. In the end, what Mama would never understand was that it had worked on a whole other level.

The next day I learned from Randy what had unfolded the previous evening. The head manager on duty called my house after I called in late. When Mama told him that I was supposed to be at work, he said to her that she should check into my behavior. She came to McDonald's after their phone call.

"That muthafucka just mad that I got you, and he didn't." Randy said. In T.J.'s defense, he was the one male manager that didn't try to take me to bed. Mama's punishment was the undeniable truth. She unplugged the telephones when she went to work and locked them in her closet. She did not give me money for months.

Twenty-Two

❧

PERSONALITY, POETRY, AND PURPOSE

" Suffering breeds character. Character breeds faith. And in the end,
faith will not disappoint. Faith, hope, and dreams will prevail."
—Reverend Jesse Louis Jackson, Sr.

Randy made sure I had enough money for the bus to get to school and extra for spending until I finally found a job at Montgomery Ward, in the Old Orchard Shopping Center. Taking that bus out to Skokie in the dead of winter was murder on me. The buses ran on schedule and there was no jerking around after school. I had to make that bus to be at work on time. Most evenings, I didn't get home until after 9 p.m. and if I had to work until closing, I barely made that last bus. I tried to cram on my free periods, but I was perpetually tired. I went to school, worked, and came home. On Sundays, I wanted to stay in bed, but church was the only place Mama allowed me to go.

Every time I saw Dr. Cotton, shame crawled through my skin like ants marching in formation—up, down, and all around. She had extended God's grace to me, but I didn't feel as if I deserved it. There was a part of me that believed I didn't deserve Coré, either. She was wholesome, and here I was—a hot freaking *fast-ass* mess. I had accumulated five sexual partners of my own free will, and then there was that blurry area involving rape and sexual molestation that amounted to another five people. Yeah, I was everything Mama said I was, and I certainly saw more goodness in Coré than I ever did in myself. I was glad she hadn't turned me away.

I had started the school year off with a bang. I had my sidekick, and our first adventure together was to join the Thunder Theater Company. Mr. Sincere Thunder had left after that first year and another teacher, Ms. Philander Coleman, revived the company at the beginning of the school year. I told Coré that she and I should try out. She was not sure but came along, anyhow. Ms. Coleman gave me a poem to learn and perform on the spot. Coré and I went out in the hall, and she coached me until I was ready. I finished my audition and was accepted. Ms. Coleman asked if there was anyone else who wanted to try out. Coré was not speaking up, so I shouted, "My friend can sing!" Everyone turned and looked at us, and I turned to Coré and said, "Go on up there and show them what you can do." She was more than embarrassed but it didn't stop her from going up front to try out. And as I expected, she blew it out of the water. I was smiling from ear to ear. That evening, when Mama came home, I told her I had joined Thunder with Coré, and that was the key. She didn't say for me to unjoin, like she had done before. She was all things Co-Co which was always to my benefit. I guess Mama allowed me to continue to participate because she thought Coré was going to save me from the girl she had helped create. As usual, I just ran with it and didn't look back. Thunder's rehearsals, however, became mostly a thing of the past because I went straight to work after school. Ms. Coleman gave Coré my poems for the first show so I could practice on my own.

Thunder was everything to me. It gave me a sense of pride that connected me culturally to the Black experience. At the same time, it placed the arts within my reach. At one

145

point I even thought about majoring in Theater when I went to college. Veronica and I dabbled in theater after high school. She always had a new adventure going on and pulled me and some other girls together to rehearse Ntozake Shange's choreopoem *For Colored Girls Who Have Considered Suicide When the Rainbow is Enuf* to see if we could actually have our own production of it. Veronica was Lady in Red, and I was Lady in Yellow. Lady in Yellow's first line was everything: "It was graduation nite and I waz *[sic]* the only virgin in the crowd." I loved re-creating this natural flow of exploration of a girl going into womanhood. Too bad that wasn't my experience; Lady in Red was my real story.

Thunder was our launching pad and acting allowed me to be someone other than Rae, if only for a few minutes. I would move into politics because it felt like that's where I belonged. Veronica, however, had never given up on acting after Thunder. After retiring from the airline, she fulfilled her dream and got her first paid acting part at fifty years old. Now, on her third career, she is an actress with some movie and television credits to her name.

Veronica's mother, Sherry Slater, was a volunteer for Thunder; it was around this time she became a fixture in my life. Sherry was educated and polished like Dr. Cotton, but she was different than most traditional Black mothers. First, she insisted that we call her Sherry, and talked to us like we had common sense. She acknowledged and respected our free will. Sherry understood that young people were going to do what they wanted to do. Her goal was to make sure that we had the best information to make the most educated choices. Sherry was like the aunt every young girl needed. She was easy to talk to, you could ask her anything and she never judged you. But she did voice her opinion when you had done or was going to do something stupid. Whenever she said, "Well, Rae, first of all…." I knew it was coming and would brace myself for some real talk. As Veronica and I became closer, I also became closer to Sherry because I was always around. When I moved into my early twenties, she was the adult who provided me with the most thoughtful advice; that's why Sherry was the first adult I told that I was infected with HIV. Veronica was the first person I called the day I learned I was infected. I was sitting at my desk at SANE, where I worked at the time. Veronica didn't know what to say or do other than to tell me to call her mother. I didn't give the suggestion a second thought. I hung up from Veronica and called Sherry. The first thing she said was, "You are not dying, Rae. Get that out of your head right now." She was an early convert to the manifestation of positive thinking, and when she finished her lecture, I calmed my tail down and went back to work.

My participation in Thunder would become one of the most important places for me to grow, develop friendships and experience camaraderie around a shared goal. Those of us participating in Thunder that year became a close-knit group. There were many of us who participated: me; Coré; Leon Towns, my student council buddy; Ernie Bibbs; Eric Smith; Marcie Wilson; Barbie Howlett; Nikki Henry Jones; Ruth Taylor-Hamilton; Angela Henry; Sylvester Miles; Craig Thompson; David Weeks; David Hamilton; Darryl Clark; and Jacqueline Williams, who also has some acting credits behind her name. Those from the Sincere Thunder production and Ms. Coleman's group included Veronica Slater, Audreanna Taylor, Theresa Norris and Chandra Woodruff-Thomas. We rehearsed, hung out together in and out of school, and became a family. Our first production was a choreopoem written and directed by Ms. Coleman. Some of us were more talented than others, but Ms. Coleman made sure everyone had a role.

The production focused on the struggle and perseverance of Black people in America. Ms. Coleman drew from the works of Black authors like Langston Hughes, Claude McKay, James Weldon Johnson, and Gwendolyn Brooks. I don't recall the author, but I remember the poem I did, and I can still perform it like it was yesterday. This poem has stayed with me to the point that I sometimes say it, shaking my head, when I get bills in the mail.

Bills Bills Bills
All I pays is Bills
Ma Bell
Con Ed
I even owe the undertaker
And I ain't even dead.

We packed the house each night. It was a magnificent feeling to belong to something greater than myself. Mama told me flat-out that she would not be coming. I tried not to allow her to steal my thunder, but a sadness swooped over me watching my cast members' families congratulate and give them flowers. I kept my poker face on and my hurt inside.

That Christmas, Mama and Charles put up the Christmas tree, but she didn't get me anything for Christmas. I never saw that coming. This was her way of showing me she was disappointed in me, and I got it. I had proven her to be right about me, after all. Before it had all been supposition, but now Randy was proof. I think, more than anything, she was embarrassed I had proven Charles right. I could hear Mama and Charles talking after they learned about Randy.

"Now, do you believe me? I told you she was a whore," Charles said to Mama.

"She's been that way her whole life," Mama said, sounding defeated. "I just don't know what to do with her." Ironically, Mama had been the one to craft the narrative before my grandfather's grave even got cold. Charles was the match that lit the gasoline that Mama poured on me time and time again. In many ways, I was just being a teenager. Randy was my first love. Period. I fell hard because I believed I had found in him what I had dreamed of since my grandfather's death: someone to love me for me.

That January, Randy moved to St. Louis to help one of his brothers manage a McDonald's. Before he left, he asked me again to marry him. I was still afraid of the unknown, so I told him I couldn't. I found a way before he moved to spend one more day with him. We made love; then he held me, and we cried together. He moved and I tried to get on with my life. When the Christmas rush was over, Montgomery Ward let me go, and I was looking for a job yet again. Mama started to loosen up; by the spring, she gave me bus fare. I had switched over from English honors to regular English the second semester. It had been such a difficult four months at home that the volume of work was more than I had to give to one class. I just couldn't cut it.

I met a new guy, Rickey Daniels, when I was a tour guide for him and other students from his high school who visited our high school. He and I flirted the entire time. We exchanged numbers and I was all giddy again. He lived on the West Side of Chicago, and the distance placed limits on our relationship. Mama had given me back my telephone privileges that spring. Rickey and I talked every evening. That was cool because I loved talking to him. He was very bright—wiser than his seventeen years—and somewhat eccentric. Our conversation was lively and thought-provoking. He was also a musician—a drummer—in a rock band no less, and often shared stories about his escapades. I was getting my life back to normal and seemed to be mostly on track.

Thunder began rehearsal for its spring production right away. Ms. Coleman chose two plays written by African American playwrights that we performed back-to-back. The first play was *A Day of Absence*. It is a short satire written by Douglas Turner Ward in which all the Black people disappear in a Southern town, and white people are left to maintain their daily routines without the presence of Black people. After intermission, we performed *The Amen Corner*, written by James Baldwin. This is a three-act play that confronts religious idealism in the backdrop of real-life experiences. I had a small part in *The Amen Corner*, and Coré and Veronica had significant roles.

It was also in Thunder that Coré and I had our first falling out over a boy, of all things. On the last night of our spring performance, I entered the stage for my small part.

When I finished talking, I looked out into the audience and spotted Rickey sitting next to Dr. Cotton. *WHAT THE FUCK is he doing here?* I asked myself aloud. I was so mystified that, when I exited, I looked back at him and fell off the stage. At the end of the night, I found out that Coré had not only invited him, but she had also worked it out so she could pick him up from the train station and bring him to the play. I was hot! And I was hurt. I felt as if Coré had taken away my control. Truth be told, I had never forgotten that feeling of betrayal with Theresa and James and I wanted to know, *Why the hell was she talking to my boyfriend?* The fact we had had a three-way phone conversation once did not mean she could talk to him without me. It didn't feel right, and that loyalty thing was a trigger. Rickey tried to reassure me nothing was going on between Coré and him. Honestly, I didn't know what I thought was happening between them. I know only that my ego was crushed to hell and back. She said she was trying to surprise me. I don't remember what was said about who initiated the call and, honestly, I didn't care. At the end of the day, I felt that if Rickey made the call to Coré, then she should have flat-out told him, *You cannot call me without Rae's knowledge.* That's it and that's all. If I had wanted Rickey there, I would have found a way to make it happen. With all the issues around Mama and Randy, it was a surprise that could have backfired right in my face. On the way home that night I asked Coré, "Why were you talking to MY boyfriend without MY knowledge?"

"And who gave you the right to invite him?" It was intense. Coré said to me, "I don't want your boyfriend."

"I ain't even worried." I responded, "Why would he choose you over me?" The moment I said it, I regretted it—but you can't take words back. I knew this better than anyone. But insecurity will make you do and say hurtful things.

The next morning when I came to school, Coré had moved out of our locker. The damage had been done. Rickey and I remained friends, even to this day. I'm not sure what hurt Coré the most—that I implied she was talking to Rickey in the dating context behind my back, or that I implied I was better than her. Either way, looking back, it was my low self-esteem talking because it was the opposite of what I believed. Hands-down, I thought Coré was better than me, even as we aged well into our thirties. I saw myself as a needy fuck-up, especially after I was diagnosed with HIV. While I was living in shame with HIV, she had finished law school, passed the bar and was a practicing attorney on top of being a lead singer in a Grammy-winning musical group. I didn't believe I could ever accomplish enough to catch up with her. God, however, would prove to me that my gifts and talents have a place in the universe. Years of therapy I would learn to love myself as much as I love Coré. I don't know if I added any value to her life, as only she can answer that, but I acknowledge the value she and her family added to mine and I'm grateful for it.

Coré and I never had a heart-to-heart conversation about boundaries or the fact that we both could have handled it differently. Not back then or ever. I simply wanted back into her life. I dropped my feeling of betrayal, whether it was warranted or whether it was my imagination and insecurities running wild. It took a lot of pleading for me to get back into her good graces. By the time Project Advancement Gospel Ensemble (PAGE) choral activity came around later in the school year, Coré and I were friends again—but we never shared lockers again.

I knew back then that I had a complicated personality. I knew that I had a way about me that rubbed people the wrong way. I also knew that people said behind my back that I had no couth. I was seen as too assertive or too pushy. I was still that Miss Know-It-All and had no problem letting people know that they were wrong, and I was right. Even today, I will pull out my cellphone and Google in the middle of a conversation. That part of my personality is what it is. On the other side of me, I am a generous person, and fiercely loyal. But my in-your-face honesty doesn't sit well with people: It didn't back then and still doesn't now. The difference is, back then I wanted to belong, and, at the same time, I rejected conformity—the very thing that would have helped me fit in.

Dr. Karyn Purvis, founder of the Karyn Purvis Institute of Child Development, has said, "Behavior is the language of children who have lost their voice." That resonates with me. Outside of my house was the only place I had a voice and I'd be damned if I couldn't be free to say whatever the hell I pleased. The problem with my desire for freewill was my deregulated stress response system. I was very easily triggered and unable to reach the most efficient parts of the brain, like reasoning. It's a wonder what came out of my mouth.

When a stressful situation occurs these days, I intentionally calm myself, before responding. The goal is to step back from a situation so that I can work my way from the lowest part of the brain the brain stem up through the diencephalon to the limbic system, and finally up to the cortex, where we are able to reason, think critically and reflect. Back then however, I had no tools. I was always hypervigilant and had a heightened sensitivity about everything. Well into my forties, a simple question could lead to a defense rather than an answer. And when you stage a defense, people react. After I calmed down, I would tell myself, *Girl, you went a little too far.* But by then it was too late. I was fighting for myself the best way that I could. In part, some of my connection to Coré was one way I pushed myself. If I was her friend, then just maybe I wasn't as bad as I felt on the inside.

I was probably one of the least talented members of PAGE. We were an elite choir with some incredibly talented young people. Coré and I used to laugh about my singing. She insisted, "You are a strong alto when you get on key." When I was off key, thank God, she would sing in my ear to steer me back on key.

PAGE was organized by Herman Ruff, a hall monitor at ETHS. His sister Sadie was one of my close friends at Chute and was a member of PAGE, too. Our sponsor was James Ingram, and I still don't know what he did at ETHS. Herman recruited the gifted, but he didn't turn away the less talented, either. He was a talented musician and singer, and we flourished under his leadership. We were ahead of our time. Our choir was equal to some of the popular groups today. Nothing like PAGE has ever existed since then at ETHS or in Evanston. We were a hot commodity and were often invited to sing as special guests for church anniversaries and various events. We also had concerts. In my senior year, we even recorded an album. In the end, both PAGE and Thunder gave me something productive to do that kept me from totally self-destructing. My participation in PAGE also helped in my spiritual growth. Herman was serious about his faith, and many of my peers who belonged to PAGE shared this faith walk. God became a living and breathing thing moving inside of me. On Saturday mornings, I woke up to my chores and the *Reverend Milton Brunson Gospel Hour* on the radio and went straight into the *Father Hayes Gospel Hour.* By evening the house was spotless, and I would end my day by watching *What a Fellowship Hour,* a recorded television broadcast from the previous Sunday's worship service of the Fellowship Missionary Baptist Church that featured the Reverend Clay Evans. I opened my Bible each night and followed his sermons. Nine years later, I would become a member of the Fellowship Missionary Baptist Church; twelve years after that, Reverend Evans would become my father in ministry, licensing me to preach on August 20, 2000. You may not know why people and places are in your life at the time, but I'm here to tell you there are no coincidences. It is all by God's design.

My most significant life-changing event happened one Easter Sunday. I arrived at church at Second Baptist, and there was a buzz all over the building. The civil-rights leader Reverend Jesse Louis Jackson Sr. was the guest minister for our Easter Sunday service. Before that day, I knew who he was, but I had not given him a lot of thought because my political activism at the time was with the NAACP. When he sat on the pulpit with Dr. Taylor, my mouth flew open. *My God, this man is fine.* All the other girls in the choir were giggling and whispering and trying to act cool all at the same time. Honestly, it was hard to focus on the worship service; that is, until he opened his mouth. I was no longer thinking about how fine Reverend Jackson was, but about the depth and breadth of his words. Sure, he was charismatic, and that had its own appeal, but by now, I was the person to open my Bible and follow the sermon. Never had I heard an Easter interpretation of the life, death, and resurrection of Jesus like the one Reverend Jackson delivered that morning. Tears streamed down my face. He had reached the epicenter of my soul, and I received the most significant theological revelation of my young life. Jesus' suffering on the cross was not in vain: It was for the greater good of God's people. If Jesus could suffer for the greater good, then why not me? I took Reverend Jackson's sermon into my heart and spirit and kept it there. I latched on to the idea that everyone had a purpose that was bigger than themselves. One day, God would use my suffering for the greater good. Everything I had experienced - every tongue-lashing, every beating, the loss of my family and the rejection that had deeply wounded me was about something higher than me. I didn't have the language then, but it was clearly this idea of the suffering servant. I appropriated my suffering as a tool to help me better understand suffering in order to help those who were suffering. It wasn't that God allowed me to suffer for this purpose, but because I had suffered, it would be used for a greater good. I profoundly believed that God's plan and purpose for my life would be revealed one day. In the meantime, I saw everything I had experienced and would experience afterward as a training ground for what God had in store for me. No matter what Mama did or what came my way, all I needed to do was keep holding on. I was confident that God would see me through, not only for me, per se, but for the plan I could not see.

When the worship service was over that day, Belinda remained on the piano, and she and Dr. Cotton had a little gospel jam session. Coré joined in. Reverend Jackson loves music and singing, and that day was no different. He grinned from ear to ear while they sang. He invited Dr. Cotton to sing at the morning forum that was held at Operation PUSH every Saturday. The forum was composed of a live radio broadcast that was half church service and half political meeting. I tagged along, right by Coré's side. Every second of the Saturday PUSH experience was electrifying. I had never experienced anything like it.

The NAACP meetings I went to were nothing like this—not even the conventions. Don't get me wrong: At the NAACP meetings, we talked about the plight of Black people in America and the fight that was ahead of us. But Reverend Jackson made you want to walk straight out of the building and head to a picket line. There was nothing like that moment when he rose to the podium and led the call and response, "I am somebody!" The audience, me included, lit up with roars and cheers, repeating each phrase after him.

I am, (I am), somebody! (somebody)!

I am, (I am), somebody! (somebody)!

I may be poor, (I may be poor), but I am (but I am) somebody! (somebody)!

I may be Black! (I may be Black)! but I am (but I am) somebody! (somebody)!

I wanted to believe him, but it would take years for me to acknowledge and embrace my self-worth. Nonetheless, I believed that God could use me even in my brokenness, and days like these would carry me until I could love even the broken parts of myself.

Twenty-Three

TWO SIDES OF THE SAME COIN

"Life and death are two sides of the same coin called destiny."
—Muhammad Haider

"SUR-PRISE!!!" was the first thing I heard as I entered our apartment. My eyes focused and Coré was the first person I spotted, smiling ear to ear. I looked around the room; Veronica, Ethel and a bunch of my friends from Thunder and PAGE were sitting in my living room. I scanned over everyone until my eyes landed on Mama standing in the doorway between the living room and bedroom, grinning. It was unbelievable, but it was as real as real could get: Mama was throwing me a surprise birthday party! This was one of those contradictory moments I relished in while living with Mama, eleven years since my grandfather's death. It had been slow going between us after she found out about Randy. Some days, she just looked at me with disgust. I walked a tightrope for months. For real. I honestly didn't think she would ever come around. While she had loosened up some, she had totally stopped bringing home bags of clothes. I overheard her tell a friend (on the phone, of course), "I wish I would buy that ungrateful bitch a muthafuckin thing." This seventeenth birthday gift was like thirty bags of clothes in one swoop.

Mama had never celebrated my birthday. She gave me an occasional card, but never a cake, a gift or a party. I thought either the world was coming to an end, or something was changing within her. I took the birthday party as a sign of better days. Coré told me it was Mama's idea and that she just helped to make it happen. I wasn't so sure, but nonetheless, Mama had agreed and laid the spread of food out as only she could do. I basked in the joy of that day. We laughed, talked and ate. Coré sang "Happy Birthday," and Veronica and Ethel stayed until late in the evening. I didn't think I could ever be this happy in this apartment, but that one day would be my best day ever in the six years since we moved here. Mama seemed to have loosened up all around. At the end of the school year, she gave me my first official curfew: midnight.

The summer of 1979 was great. Before the end of the school year, I began working at a clothing resale store in Evanston called Crowded Closet, not far from my house. However, business wasn't so great and, after they reduced my hours, I begin working at the movie theater in Evanston. PAGE had singing engagements almost every weekend. Between gigs and rehearsals, I was keeping busy.

I can honestly say life felt really good to me for the first time, ever. Then all hell broke loose. On August 1, 1979, I came home from work earlier than usual. I could hear Charles moving around. When I walked past the entranceway from the living room to their bedroom, I saw boxes everywhere, and then I saw Charles. He looked up but didn't speak and went right back to packing. I went on to my bedroom, but my curiosity got the best of me. I went to the kitchen to get some Kool-Aid. It was the perfect excuse to be nosey. Sure enough, dude was packing. I mean, he was packing ev-er-y-thing he owned. I got my Kool-Aid, sat on the sofa and watched. I was dumbfounded as he made those trips through the living room to his closet and laid clothes on the bed to add to the boxes. I wondered what the heck was going on. When he finished packing, he sat in his usual

151

spot on the side of the bed and smoked cigarettes. I got up and looked into his closet; sure enough, every piece of clothing he owned was gone and his psycho ass had put the key into the lock, leaving it dangling. I went to my bedroom and picked up a book. I didn't want any part of whatever the hell was going on.

When Mama walked into the house, she didn't even make it past the living room before she asked him about the boxes in the middle of the floor. Charles informed her he was leaving.

"What do you mean, you leaving?" she asked, confused.

My eyes bucked! *Whoa, this was deep. Mama didn't even know. Heartless bastard.* After almost seven years and Mama paying almost all the bills, he was just walking away flat-out cold. My heart ached for Mama.

"Just what I said," I heard him tell her in that *don't ask me any more questions,* irritated tone he often gave Mama. She wanted answers this time, and she asked.

"Why?" I could hear the tears in her voice. Charles didn't respond. She finally asked, "What have I done to you, Charles?"

"I don't want to be around your bitch-ass daughter anymore," he said.

Aw, hell naw, he didn't! I was seething. Lord knows it took everything I had inside of me not to confront him, but with Mama, there was no way to predict her reaction. I don't know why I was surprised he had made me the fall guy. He had done it effortlessly from day one.

"When she's gone, I'll come back," I heard him say.

Ye-ah, right. (I almost shouted it from my bedroom.) After that, he started loading his car. Mama sat on the side of the bed, smoking a cigarette. She didn't look up or say another word as he made the trips up and down the stairs. He finished, shut the door behind him and left. Mama was shattered. I had no idea what to say to her, so I said nothing.

It should have come as no surprise that I was happy he was gone. He had made my life a living hell. "Good riddance" was my sentiment. During those first two years of Charles living with us, I was totally mixed up in the head. For Mama's sake, I actually tried to develop a relationship with him. I was always respectful when he spoke to me. I even asked him to help me with fatherly things. One day, on one of my attempts to "make nice," I asked him to help me with my camera. He asked to see it. I handed it to him and instead of taking the camera he grabbed my nipple and squeezed the life out of it. It happened so quick that by the time I reacted, he already had it and then, like before, let go. I laid the camera on the dresser and ran out the house; I stayed out until Mama came home from work. Later that night, I heard him tell her that he had helped me with my camera to pre-empt me from telling her my side of the story. This was after Mama learned about the attack at the Evanston Inn. Now ask me why I was still trying to get his approval. The only answer I can come up with was that I was trying to get Mama's approval. I stayed trying to get him to like me because I wanted her to be happy. Yes, they had me mixed up in the head. I even continued to buy him Christmas and birthday gifts with my little hard-earned money. By the time I was a freshman in high school, I learned my efforts were all for naught and I stopped trying. The tipping point for me was the Christmas he let his gift from me sit under the tree, unopened. After the tree was taken down, I put it on top of his dresser and it remained there unopened for another few months. I heard Mama ask him if he was ever going to open it. He told her he would when he was good and ready, and she dropped it. I was glad that he was gone, but Mama was in so much pain; it hurt me to see her so distressed.

It didn't take long for Mama to spin the narrative. I heard her talking (yes, on the telephone): "That Bitch ran my husband away." She wasn't going to take ownership for that, either. It hurt me right down to my bones. I'm not even sure why I expected her to handle this differently because I had always been the problem, according to Mama. I don't know: Maybe a part of me believed that with Charles gone Mama and I had a better chance, especially in the aftermath of the party. I had always believed this, even to the point that I had prayed for Charles' departure. It was a sick irony I had seen Charles as the problem after Mama had shown me time and time again that she was the root of the problem. Silly me, yet again. Mama didn't care about the emotional carnage she left behind. Within days she became cold and hostile.

Now Charles was gone, and our relationship became even worse. There was nothing I could do to please her. I decided to stay the heck out of her way. I took advantage of my new curfew. After work, I would hang out until my new boo, who was a freshman and star running back at Northwestern University, finished practice, and I would stay with him until 9:00 p.m. or so. I had met Jeff while I was riding my bike on the lakefront by Northwestern's campus.

When school started after Labor Day, I continued to stay out of Mama's way. I was not going to give her any reason to bring her wrath down on me. She continued to be hostile, but I tried not to take it personally because she was hurting. I was not going to give her a reason to fuss at me. Mama would sit by her side of the bed, smoking and looking lost. As much as I hated Charles, this was painful to watch.

I began a new job at Selig's, a men's boutique of fine clothing in downtown Evanston. It was a part of the vocational studies program at ETHS. The store was owned by the Rosenberg brothers and had a stellar reputation. I loved working in the land of tweed sport coats and slacks. I was out of school two days a week at noon so that I could go to work. Between work, school and PAGE, I stayed busy. I continue to see Jeff when time permitted and, on Saturdays, I would go to Northwestern's football games.

That October, I decided to attend Northwestern University's homecoming dance with my friend Jamie Foster, who was also a senior at ETHS. I don't even remember how we became friends, but we hadn't been hanging out for long. I was geeked, to say the least. I had never been to a party in my life because of my curfew. I was really there to see Jeff, but he kept disappearing on me. After a while, Jamie and I figured out he was juggling me with his real girlfriend. I was the side chick. I wanted to be mad but, honestly, I wasn't invested in him. Other dudes were asking me to dance all night, and I danced Jeff right out of my system. I had so much fun losing myself in the music that time slipped away from me. I don't know what made me look up at the clock but I did, and it was five minutes to twelve. It felt like my heart stopped beating. Mama was going to kill me! I went looking for Jamie and interrupted her dance.

"Girl, you got to take me home." She kept on dancing. "NOW!" I hollered over the music and started pulled her away from the dance floor. After I had her attention, I explained that I was past my curfew.

"My mama don't play," I told her.

It took a solid fifteen minutes for us to get out of Northwestern Student Center in Norris Hall into the car to drive to my house. I put my key in the door at 12:15 AM. I kept trying to turn the lock, but it wouldn't move. I finally realized that Mama had the double lock on the door. I knocked and knocked, but there was no answer. Jamie was outside in the car, waiting for my signal that I had gotten in the house safely. I came back out, scared. I remembered those first months after Tobie left her, and it was nothing nice. I had hoped that nothing was wrong and that she hadn't heard the door because she was knocked out drunk. I had Jamie drive me to a pay phone. When Mama answered on the first ring, I was relieved. I didn't think about the possibility that she could be—and apparently was—sitting by the phone waiting on my call. Likely, she was smoking a cigarette in the living room when I knocked on the door.

"Mama, the double lock is on the door," I said.

"I know, bitch! Go back where you just came from!" she exclaimed and hung up the freaking phone. I looked at the phone receiver like, *What the heck?!* I called back, but Mama didn't answer. Jamie took me to her house, and her mother let me spend the night. She told me to let my mother cool off a bit. I followed her advice and let it drop for the night. The next morning, I called Mama and I asked her apologetically,

"Mama, can I come home?"

"Come get your shit, bitch!" she demanded, and I could hear the dial tone buzzing in my ear again. I didn't believe it for one second. I told Jamie that I might as well go home and face the music. I would get this beating over and done with and move on. Jamie stayed in her car again, waiting for me to give her a sign that everything was all right. When I walked into the apartment, Mama was standing in the living room with a hand on her hip and a cigarette hanging out the side of her mouth.

"Go pack your shit," she demanded. "I want you out of my house." Her tone was freakishly calm as she stood there, never raising her voice—not once.

"You don't mean me no good," she said.

"You ran my husband away." I traipsed past her on the way to my room, expecting her to knock the mess out of me, but she didn't, to my surprise. I sat on the bed, thinking that I would let it all blow over.

"Bitch, get your shit and get out of my muthafuckin' house," she yelled.

"Mama, I'm sorry," I said with tears dropping out of my eyes.

"Don't nobody care about your tears," she spat. "I want you out of my house."

Not in my wildest imagination did I think Mama would put me out of the house. I got my suitcase and started packing. She watched, standing in my doorway with that cigarette still hanging out the side of her mouth. The first thing I thought about was that I might as well have gone with Randy, but it was too late now. Too afraid to speak, with my heart racing, I did as I was ordered. I had no idea what I was going to do. After I had gotten all the things from my dresser, I went to my closet, and she lost it.

"You bet not touch a muthafuckin' thing in there!"

"But Mama, what am I going to wear to school?"

"I don't give a fuck! Go naked."

"I bought that shit!" she said. "You's a ungrateful bitch!"

I got my bookbag and the suitcase she had allowed me to pack, and I left. Jamie's mother offered me their home until I could figure things out, but I knew I would soon have to find a permanent place to live. I called a couple of times to ask if I could come home, and Mama told me that she didn't give a fuck where I lived. She said I just couldn't live with her anymore.

Twenty-Four

GOD'S TIMING

"God may not come when you want him, but He's always on time."
—Pastor Otis Anderson Jr.

Mama had lost her freaking mind over a man. I often wondered if the reason she didn't let me come back was that she was holding out, hoping Charles would come back. Well, if that was it, I could have saved her the agony because I knew Charles was never going to look back—and he never did. She only knew where he was living because she heard the info through the grapevine.

The first few weeks after I was thrown out, I was really at a loss—and scared. I couldn't have had more than a hundred dollars to my name. Mama was still holding my clothes hostage and Jamie let me borrow hers from time to time, but I was basically living out of one suitcase. I continued to go to school and work, but it was all a blur. Most days, I just went through the motions. I remember being hungry a lot. When you're living in a stranger's house, you don't open the refrigerator whenever you want something to eat. It doesn't work like that in the real world. I went into survival mode. Instead of taking the bus, I walked to school most days from Jamie's and walked the fifteen blocks or so to work after school. I started getting up for school early enough to get my free breakfast despite the fact that I didn't have a class until second period. I also made sure I got lunch before I went to my minimum wage, two-days-a-week job. There was no point in asking for more hours. The store closed at six in the evening, and I was already working the store's late days. Occasionally, the owners purchased dinner for the late evenings on Tuesday and Thursday, and I ate until my stomach felt like it was going to burst. I kept calling Mama and she kept telling me, "You don't mean me no good" and "You can't live with me anymore." She'd hang up the phone, and that was that.

Pride and shame are monsters. When I added my low self-esteem on top of them, I couldn't think clearly for the life of me. I was stuck about how to move forward. I thought no adult on this planet, except maybe those who knew Mama personally, would have believed that I had been put out for being fifteen minutes late for my curfew. It was unfathomable even to me, but it only took a few days for me to figure out Mama had really thrown me out because Charles left. I had no doubt, in my mind, that explaining this to an adult would have left me looking crazy. As a result, I didn't broadcast my situation. Coré knew; however, I couldn't face her mother again, so I never talked to her about my situation. After I didn't get an offer for shelter from Coré, I decided to leave well enough alone. Veronica graduated a year early and was away at college. I didn't have a phone to call long distance, but I did go over to their apartment one evening and waited for Sherry to come home. It turned out her apartment wasn't an option, either. With both of her children – gone Darryl enlisted in the military – she had just taken in a roommate. I probably should have told Dr. Taylor about my situation, but I had left Second Baptist to join Dr. Cotton when she organized her church. I thought it would be tacky to seek help when I was no longer a member. It was immature and fatalistic thinking but that was all I had around this time. I was stuck in the shame of my entire situation.

I didn't move forward until it became clear that I had worn out my welcome at Jamie's. The only person I could think to call was Ethel. I knew Tobie wouldn't let me stay homeless. He would either talk some sense into Mama or give me a place to live. A part of me was still hoping Mama would take me back. It was scary not knowing where my next meal was going to come from. Mama was all I knew, and the thought of leaving her before I had finished school was unsettling. I had also gotten a taste of what it meant to be on your own, and I didn't like it very much.

To my surprise, Tobie was preparing to move out of state. He was taking the two youngest, Allen and Juan, with him, but Ethel didn't want to move. She was a senior, like me, and intended to finish her last year at Tilden. Patricia had just gotten married and had a baby. Her husband was in the military, so she and Ethel were getting ready to move into a two-bedroom apartment that was the upstairs of a two-flat owned by their grandparents. Their mother's brother and his family lived on the first floor. Pat and Ethel invited me to move in with them and share the expenses. Tobie thought it was a great idea and advised me to leave Mama in her misery.

The house was on 57th and Justine, a block down the street from Grandmamma Julia and Grandpapa Clayton. After I moved, I reached out to Grandmamma, but she was speaking Mama's madness about me needing to get my act together. I felt a deep sense of betrayal. She knew Mama better than anyone, and to place all the blame on me was just plain wrong. From time to time, I would go and speak to Grandpapa, but I left Grandmamma alone during those times. It was enough trying to keep myself together. If she wasn't offering to help, then I didn't want to hear it.

Each morning I was out of the house no later than 6:00 a.m. I took the bus to the train station. The commute on the train was from one end of the line, starting at 63rd Street and Ashland Avenue, straight through the city going north to the other end, Howard Street. It was an hour ride. After I got off the train, I had two options to get me to ETHS: I could take the Evanston train at Howard Street to downtown Evanston and take another bus, or I could take a Howard Street bus all the way. Neither was faster than the other and the total commute could take anywhere from an hour and a half to two hours.

After school, I went to work at Selig's. My wages were not even close to what I needed to pay for my share of the expenses. I couldn't quit because it was connected to my grade. The only other solution was to take a second job, and I returned to the same McDonald's where it all began. Most nights, I didn't start my trip back to Chicago's South Side until well after 8:00 at night, or after 11:00 p.m. if I closed. I studied during free periods at school and breaks at work; I tried to study on the train but didn't accomplish much. I was tired as shit when I woke up and tired as shit when I went to bed. Many mornings, I slept on the train. It was a struggle, but at least I wasn't living on the edge that is, Mama's edge.

Pat, Ethel, and I got along exceptionally well. As the oldest, we often deferred to Pat, but we lived as equals and helped take care of Tyrone Jr. This is what our sisterhood looked like. We wanted the best for ourselves and each other, and we moved forward as a team. It wasn't easy for us. The money from those minimum-wage jobs Ethel and I had didn't go very far. Pat wasn't working the first few months because of the baby and depended on support from her husband. Toward the end of the month, when money was getting low, we would pull our meager resources together and get a bag of white potatoes and chicken wings; that would hold us over until the first of the month. One day, I was talking to someone regarding my situation. They said that I should go to the Social Security office to see if I could be declared independent from Mama and start collecting my own check instead of her. I figured it couldn't hurt, and I'm glad I followed through.

Because I was seventeen and Mama had not adopted me, I was allowed to have my father's Social Security benefits diverted back to me. This was a great help when my work study ran out at Selig's, and I only had McDonald's.

Things were working out, and I hadn't seen a reason to inform the school I had been kicked out of the house. One day, I was called to the school office. When I walked into the conference room, I was shocked to see several people waiting for me. My eyes scrolled around the conference table. I saw Mr. Horn, my counselor; Officer Washington; Dean Williams; and then, my eyes landed on Mama. The scowl cemented across her face let me know this wasn't going to be pretty. I sat diagonally from Mama on the other side of the table. Dean Williams spoke first.

"Rae, I understand that you have run away from home."

"That's not true," I said defiantly. "I was put out."

"So, I'm lying, huh?" Mama interjected.

"Actually, you are lying, Mama," I said confidently. I had been out of Mama's house for two months now, and her power over me was gone. That moment was like the celebratory song in the *Wizard of Oz*: *"Ding-dong, the wicked witch is dead!"* I looked her in the face for a moment. All these years she had wielded her power over me in the worst ways possible. At this point, I had nothing to lose. *What else on this earth can she do to me?* I thought. I turned back to Dean Williams and recanted the story of the curfew and the events that followed.

"She's a muthafuckin' lie!" Mama hollered. Everyone looked at her. It was my turn to be smug and I thought, *Now you're seeing the real Mama.* She regained herself and explained the same old story about me being *fast*, out of control and not wanting to follow her rules. She was convincing, I had to hand it to her. She came across as a helpless mother raising a girl out of control. After she finished talking, Mr. Williams interjected that I was well-behaved at school. She had an answer for that, too I was slick. "She got y'all fooled." I gave Dean Williams a helpless look and he gave me a reassuring nod. I think my counselor, Mr. Horn, was scared of Mama because he wouldn't look her way. He cleared his throat and looked at me.

"Well, Rae, why haven't you said anything about this abuse before now?" he asked me.

"Because she told me that she would kill me for telling her business," I replied. Poor Mr. Horn's eyes bucked! It was true that I hadn't told him about what was going on at home. But I had told Dean Williams bits and pieces, but never enough for him to try to have an intervention. After Jean's failed rescue attempt in high school and then Officer Washington that day at Sharmayne's and her mother telling me that nothing could really be done, I didn't want to add insult to injury. Mama wasn't playing about telling her business. I might have been crazy, but I wasn't stupid. Now I was sitting here with scary old Mr. Horn who had put me on the spot, suggesting that I was lying. I mean-mugged his ass and turned back to Dean Williams. However, before I could say anything, Officer Washington—who had been quiet the entire meeting—spoke up.

"Actually, I believe Rae is telling the truth," he said. Mama's mouth dropped.

"I have known her for a long time, and aspects of her home life have been shared with me in years' past." Mama didn't know what to say. I exhaled and silently thanked Jesus. Officer Washington had full control of the room. He turned to Mama, continuing: "From what I understand, Rae is not your biological daughter, and you did not adopt her." Mr. Horn didn't even know that, and he looked completely confused. Dean Williams nodded in agreement; I had at least told him how I came to live with her.

"But I've been taking care of her ass since she was a baby," Mama interrupted. I rolled my eyes; there were just lies and more lies.

"That does not matter," Officer Washington quickly replied.

"Technically, she's a ward of the state, and without any history of being in trouble, at her age the state will declare her independent." My eyes bucked then!

"She does not have to go back home," he explained.

Mama was mad, saying, "I don't give a fuck what she does."

He looked at me and asked, "Do you want to go back?"

I looked at Mama's angry face, and I knew I could not go back. I had been too afraid to leave when I was given a chance with Randy but being on my own had given me courage. Everyone was looking at me, waiting for me to declare my independence.

"No, I don't want to go back," I said.

"You fucking bitch!" Mama lit into me. "You dirty bitch!"

She said something to the effect of, *You went down to that Social Security office and told them lies! And they stopped my check!*

It had taken a short forty-five minutes for the truth to rise to the top. Mama didn't give a fuck whether I came back home. She was concerned about that check.

"No, Mama," I responded. "They started giving *me my own check*."

As far as the school officials were concerned, the meeting was over. They all stood up. Mama stormed out of the room. Dean Williams said to me that as long as I wasn't truant, they would waive the residential requirement to attend ETHS because it was my last year and I was in good standing. I went back to class knowing, without a doubt, that God had my back. I recalled that day at Sharmayne's—explaining to her mom, Ms. Marilyn, and Officer Washington how horrible my life was I wanted to be rescued right then and there. Instead, disappointment settled inside of me when nothing came of it. But God had a plan I could not see. Pastor Anderson was right after all: "God may not come when you want Him but He's right on time." I couldn't wait to get home and tell Pat and Ethel what Mama tried to pull.

After that meeting, it was more than clear I would not be going back. I called my cousin Kenny Bowman. We had stayed in contact off and on after great aunt Geraldine's funeral. I hadn't called Aunt Lula Mae because I didn't want her to worry about me. She was close to eighty, and I knew that I couldn't live in her senior building, anyway. I thought Kenny should know what was going on. He told his mother, Eleanor, and she called Mama about the rest of my clothes. I don't know what she said to Mama but, before long, they were picking me up to go get my things. I was a nervous wreck. Mama stood at the door of my bedroom, mean-mugging me, but she didn't say a word. When I shut the door behind me at 802 Seward Street, I knew I had ended a chapter in my life.

Twenty-Five

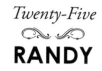

RANDY

And I cried.
For Myself.
For this woman talkin about love.
For all the women who have ever
stretched their bodies out anticipating
civilizations
And finding ruins.
—Sonia Sanchez

I had made it through my first semester of school with no hiccups. I was proud. The holidays were great. I spent Thanksgiving at Eleanor's, and Pat let me take Tyrone Jr. with me. I loved that little boy. Kenneth was home from boot camp, and all of us were glued at the hip. Eleanor's sister, Ann, and her adult daughters were over that day. Linda, the oldest of Ann's daughters, lived on the North Side of Chicago and offered her apartment those late nights after work when I didn't want to ride to the South Side. I took her up on the offer, and it made a world of difference in my commute. That Christmas, Pat, Ethel, and I cooked food ourselves. We didn't have a lot of money for tons of gifts, but I would have sacrificed a thousand bags of clothes from Mama for the kind of peace I had at this juncture in my life.

One evening right after the New Year, while working the cash register at McDonald's, I looked up and Randy Hoskins was flashing his gorgeous smile at me from across the lobby. My heart skipped a beat—maybe two. He was the same old Randy. You wouldn't call him fi-i-ine; he was more like average. But he had so much charm, it didn't matter. He was an average height, about five-foot-nine, with a brown complexion and beautiful brown eyes. Randy was shaped like a bulldog from head to toe. He was not someone to be taken lightly. He was a streetwise brother in a McDonald's uniform and tie, and he moved between the two worlds with ease. He had relocated back to Chicago, and that night we resumed our relationship as if we had never been apart. The year since he had been gone had felt like an eternity.

While I had the freedom to be with him, the circumstances weren't ideal. Randy was a manager at the new McDonald's in Evanston, and he was getting back on his feet with no place of his own. He bunked where he could lie his head; most nights, he was with one of his brothers. He told me as soon as he could, he would get us settled in our own apartment. Those first few months, we were inseparable. At first, my priorities were school, work and then Randy. Before he came back, I went on dates here and there, but there were no big distractions. I was singularly focused on graduation, and I kept my eyes on the prize. I don't even know when it changed, but it just evolved into Randy, work and then school. I went to school and when I got off from work, I'd hang out with him while he worked instead of going home. Some nights, we would crash at one of his brothers' places. Other nights, we would come back to my place. Ethel and I shared a room, and she would give up the bed and sleep on the sofa or go down the street to her boyfriend's place.

Randy encouraged me to finish school, but he did nothing to provide the necessary structure I needed to succeed. I don't think he even thought about the late hours we were keeping. When we slept at either of his brothers' place, we spent most of the night having sex. The next day, I was dragging and barely able to awake during my classes. Even on the nights I wasn't with him, I was so sleep-deprived that it was hard to focus on my assignments. I remember one night, I was trying to finish an important paper for my English class. I stayed up all night, and Pat typed as I wrote. It was grueling, but we got it done. I received a well-deserved F on the paper. I was on my way to flunking senior English.

Ethel and Pat had no idea what was going on with me. I always came across as if I knew what I was doing. They assumed I was doing what I was supposed to. I was always good at masking my reality. My cousin Linda, on the other hand, was older and wiser, and she peeped my card as soon as Randy came into my life. One night when I was waiting on Randy to pick me up, she asked if I knew what I was doing. She wasn't against the relationship; she was more concerned with the late hours I was keeping.

"It's late, Rae, and you do have to go to school in the morning," she said. In my mind, I was, like, *Girl, I'm grown*. I didn't want to seem ungrateful because I was appreciative of her allowing me to stay at her house. I got over myself quickly and reassured her that I had things under control. The fact that I was using her place to wait on Randy rather than for its original intent was a sign that I was already in trouble, and that F confirmed it. I started to spiral. I slept through classes, snuggled in Randy's arms. I would wake up knowing I needed to get my ass out of bed and to school, but I wouldn't even breathe loudly because I didn't want to wake him up. I knew I should have, but I didn't want to leave. Sometimes he would wake up a few hours after we had drifted off, and we'd have sex again and fall back to sleep. A part of me knew I was just fucking my life away— literally and figuratively—but I didn't know how to reel myself back without rocking the boat. I didn't want to do anything that would cause a breach between us. I thought I needed Randy like I needed to breathe.

One morning I was brushing my teeth, and I started to vomit. Randy came into the bathroom with a big grin on his face. "You're having my baby," he said.

"Get out of here. I'm not pregnant," I said, playfully shoving him out of the bathroom. All the time he used to say, *We just had some baby-making sex*. But I didn't pay any attention to his crazy talk. I knew I wasn't ready for a baby and had been taking birth control pills since after I dated Robert my freshman year. I was in denial until one morning on the train, when the smell of someone's perfume caused me to vomit all over myself. After school that day, I went to Planned Parenthood in Evanston, and the people there confirmed I was pregnant. Needless to say, I was none too happy with myself. *How the hell did I let this happen?* This time, the answer was easy: *Fucking like a goddamn rabbit and forgetting to take your birth control pills and doubling up when you remembered.*

Randy was a happy camper. We talked about it extensively. He argued that this baby was a part of him and a part of me; that it was the best of us together. My reluctance had nothing to do with our love for each other, but everything to do with my childhood. Call me old-fashioned, but I wanted the fairy tale, and Randy wasn't offering marriage like he had before he moved away. There was also the uncomfortable fact that he didn't have his own place. Nor was he bringing home baby booties. My childhood had been jacked-up, and I never wanted to bring a child into a less-than-ideal situation. I agreed to have the baby, not because he made an offer that I couldn't refuse but because I couldn't find my power. Within a month, it became harder. Some mornings I was so sick I didn't even make it to school. On top of that, I was still working at McDonald's and keeping late hours with him.

One day, I was having back pain to the point where I could barely walk. I could not find Randy anywhere. I called every McDonald's I could think of. I called both of his brothers; he was nowhere to be found. I will never forget taking the bus to Cook County Hospital, crying the entire way. I was even more overwhelmed when I walked into that jam-packed emergency room. The wait at Cook County Hospital is notoriously long, and there is nothing more painful than waiting by yourself all evening, through the night and well into the next morning to see a doctor. Every time I went to the pay phone to call Randy and I didn't reach him, my stomach churned. My fear of bringing a child into jacked-up circumstances help me gain my power. The doctor told me that the back pain was because of the pregnancy. He wanted to know my mother's history, which, of course, I did not have to give. That only added fuel to the fire. He speculated that with these symptoms so early on, I might have a difficult pregnancy. After he conducted the ultrasound, he told me that I was almost three months along. I was stunned. Neither Randy nor I had thought about how far along I was or about prenatal care. It had been two months since I found out I was pregnant, and this was the first time I had seen a doctor. When the doctor started asking me questions about my plans, reality hit me like a ton of bricks. I accepted, for the first time, that I was headed for a place of no return. I thought about my miserable-ass life, and I knew as sure as my name is Rae that I didn't want to bring a child into this world under these circumstances. Forget all that figuring-it-out-as-you-go crap; I wanted to know now. It felt like the weight of the world was on my shoulders as the doctor talked to me. From out of nowhere, I asked about a possible abortion. He asked, "Are you sure?" Frankly, I really didn't know. In any case, he wrote me a referral for counseling, and I was discharged from the ER. I took the referral next door to the Fantus Clinic and got a consult.

When Randy finally appeared with his bullshit excuse, I told him I had scheduled an abortion. He pleaded with me but, by then, I had come to terms with my reality as it related to having a child with him. I was exhausted with all the arguing and pleading, and I told him that my decision was final. He finally acquiesced. Afterward, we made love and I cried myself to sleep in his arms. I wanted him to be that man I had fallen in love with when I was sixteen, but he could not rise to the occasion. A week later, with a heavy heart and a clear mind, I had an abortion.

Easter weekend, Dorothy decided that Mama and I needed to make up. She called Mama and arranged a meeting. I, Dorothy, Ethel, and Allen—who had moved back to Chicago and was living with us all went over to Mama's.

Mama waltzed around with a cigarette in her hand like she was entertaining dinner party guests. She had cooked a delicious dinner for us. Dorothy made some kind of speech about Mama being my only mother, and that she and I needed to make peace. Mama said the same old thing about me being "too grown" and how I wasn't "gonna *run* her." *Same old shit, just a different day.* I failed to understand how Mama could just lie and lie and lie.

"She already ran my man away," Mama said. I just rolled my eyes. *I have been gone now for six months,* I wanted to say, *and Charles still ain't came back.* But that was a battle I was not going to win. She held on to that lie until the day she died. Nothing had changed.

"I want to know why she got rid of that baby."

My eyes bucked. *HOW THE HELL DID SHE KNOW?* Then it hit me. A friend of Mama's had seen me in downtown Evanston one day. I guess I must've *looked* pregnant because she asked me if I was. Of course, I denied it, but she had apparently told Mama her assumption.

"Ain't nobody pregnant, Mama," I said as calmly as I could.

"You was," she said, with certainty.

"No, I wasn't pregnant," I said trying to sound mad about it being a rumor. "I don't know who told you that, but I wasn't pregnant," I repeated.

"You could have given it to me," she said. "I would have raised it," I looked at her as if she was crazy for real. *Ain't no way on this planet I would let you, of all people, raise a child of mine,* I affirmed silently.

"Well, whoever told you that was wrong," I said. That was the last thing I said about it. I never was good at lying and was relieved when she eventually dropped the subject. That day nothing was resolved between us, but it did open the door for me to come back into her life. Sensing she was lonely, I started calling to check in on her, but I didn't make many trips out there to see her.

From the outside looking in, Patricia, Ethel and I seemed to be doing well. If Ethel had any problems along the way, she didn't voice them. She graduated with her class. Patricia had started secretarial school at Robert Morris College. I, on the other hand, flunked English, and gym. How does one flunk gym, you might ask? Well, let me tell you: by being pregnant; hiding your baby bump; and every time you try to jump up and down for any reason, feeling like you are going to throw up, so you ditch class. I didn't talk about how the pregnancy had affected me, so no one knew I had messed up royally until the very end. I knew I had messed up with school and I also knew that my relationship with Randy was part of the problem. Still, I couldn't bring myself to walk away. One day, Allen came home and told me that he thought Randy had another girlfriend. He was working at the McDonald's in Evanston with Randy, who had hired him at my request. You could not have paid me to believe that Randy was cheating on me after all we had been through. Even though I had certainly felt for months that something was not right, I shook it off. Thank God Allen didn't let it go. He came home from work one day and told me exactly who she was. She had moved here from St. Louis, and she and Randy were living together. He pulled out a piece of paper with their telephone number on it. "Call it if you think I'm lying," he said to me. My too-smart ass picked up the phone and got the shock of my life.

This woman confirmed everything Allen told me. In fact, she knew all about me. I just didn't know about her. She also told me she knew that Randy was still in love with me, and she assumed we were together. I didn't know what to think. Listening to her talk about her relationship with Randy, I felt like my heart had been cut out of my body. The betrayal I felt was unlike anything I had ever known. Randy was the first man I ever loved, and the first man who ever made me feel loved. The fact that I knew he still loved me made it even worse. I was devastated. I called Randy at work, and I couldn't even speak coherently. I mostly screamed and sobbed. I told him I never wanted to see him again. I was done.

How could I have been so stupid? When I thought about the many nights that he had fucked me from pillar to post—even while carrying his child—and that he was actually setting up house with another woman, it tore me apart. I sacrificed everything for him, and all he had done was take and then take some more. It didn't matter to me if I ever saw him again in life. Randy, however, was not accepting the end. He kept calling, asking if he could come over and talk. I said no, and I continued to say no. I wanted closure, but I didn't know how to express what I was feeling. It wasn't just about him cheating, but about my long history of rejection and betrayal. All those feelings came to the surface. The one and only person I had counted on the one who made me feel worthy of love—had now made me feel as if I wasn't enough.

One morning, he came unexpectedly to my house. It had to have been close to 5:00 because it was still dark outside. I hadn't seen him in a few weeks. I continued to say no every time he called. If Pat or Ethel answered his calls, they told him he couldn't talk to me. That morning when he knocked on our door, he was still wearing his work uniform. We sat on the stairs leading up to our apartment and talked, cried, and talked some more. He wanted me to give him some time to get the woman settled on her own. After going over it again and again I became weary. I couldn't think and, before I knew it, I had made a pallet on the floor in the living room for us to take a nap. We dozed off and, when we woke up, I could feel his nature rise. No one had stirred in the house but us. He shifted his body and kissed me as if his life depended on it. He moved his tongue down my body and gathered me up into his whole mouth. It fueled those empty places, and I gave myself over to the loving. He took his time as he pleasured me. Every time I tried to reciprocate, he wouldn't allow it; he just shifted his body and whispered, "Lay back, baby." I gave up and soaked him in. When Randy made his way back up, he asked if he could have me. I knew that meant more than my body, more than this act. I nodded my head, and he entered my innermost space. As quickly as he found his pace, he stopped.

"You've been with someone," he said, matter-of-factly. I couldn't lie to him, so I didn't. "Yes," I said, surprising myself.

Randy always told me if I fucked around on him, he would be able to tell. "I know your pussy like I know the back of my hand," he'd say to me. I'd laugh it off, saying, "You crazy." But sure enough, he knew. A few days earlier, I was feeling low and called David Russell. We remained friends and kept in contact over the years. He picked me up that particular night, and we ended up all sexed up, like back in the day. Randy didn't pull out of me; instead, he grabbed my side. His eyes grew large with anger, and his nails dug deeper and deeper as he broke it down for me through clenched teeth.

"This is my pussy. You belong to me."

"Randy," I cried.

"Don't you ever, I mean, not ever, let another man touch you. Do you hear me?" Tears fell from my eyes like a quiet storm.

"Randy, you're hurting me."

"Randy—stop, please," I begged. He dug deeper and deeper with his fingernails.

"Do you understand? Answer me!" he demanded.

"Yes. Yes. Yes." I pleaded, "Please, let me go."

He looked down at the blood that was covering his hand and dripping down my stomach, and he let me go. His eyes bucked.

"I'm sorry, baby. I'm sorry," he pleaded emphatically and jerked his hand away.

"Oh God," he said, jumping up.

"I'm sorry. I'm sorry," he kept saying as he dressed. I'm sorry. I never meant to hurt you," he added. He put his pants back on, rushed out of the door and down the stairs. I ran behind him, holding my side. When he hit the front porch, he looked back at me and said, "I love you, Rae. I'm never going to stop loving you."

When I came back upstairs, Pat had awoken from the commotion.

"He hurt you?" she asked as her eyes made it to my bloody side.

"I wish that nigga would come back over here." Allen wanted to go up to McDonald's and kick his ass, but we convinced him not to. Pat helped clean me up just like Dorothy had cleaned me up that day years before when Mama beat me senseless.

Later that day, I sat on the porch with Minnie Riperton's song, Lover and Friend, on repeat blasting it from our upstairs window. I repeatedly played our relationship in my head. And then I replayed what he told me that morning about the woman. He explained that he got into some trouble with the law in St. Louis and lost everything. She supported him through the mess. She bailed him out of jail. She stood by him, and he felt as if he owed her. He said if I had married him when he asked me, he would never have met her. He said that, at least, I owed him some time. But what did he owe me? I looked at our relationship with nothing but regret. I had lost everything because of him. Who the fuck was going to bail me out?

Twenty-Six

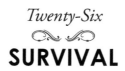

SURVIVAL

& they call us
"hard women."
As if survival could ever be delicate.
—Clementine von Radics

On May 22, 1980, I turned eighteen years old. It was a stark contrast from my seventeenth birthday, when I had been on top of the world. Instead, I was an emotional wreck. I asked myself often, *How could I have messed up my life in the short span of twelve freaking months?*

I was so deep in survival mode, I never considered that it all began with Mama. In my mind, she was somehow secondary to my entire situation. I viewed her throwing me out of the house because of Charles as just another item in the long list of things she had done to me in the twelve years since my grandfather's death. It goes without saying, but I will say it anyway: Mama sent me down this path. I wonder what my life would have been like had I not been thrown away like trash. Randy's betrayal even seemed secondary to what I considered my own self-inflicted wounds.

As usual, I did a good job masking my shame. I could take a licking and keep right on ticking. I got myself right together. Before the school year ended, I was all set to begin night school in the fall. To complete my high school diploma, I had to take two English classes and an elective of my choosing; they waived gym class. I remembered Dr. Cotton's advice the first time around with Randy: "It's not that you fall, but that you get back up." That's exactly what I was doing. I was getting on with my life. I started working at the McDonald's on Dempster Street in Skokie, a suburb north of Evanston. The manager, Jim Jackowski, asked me to come work at his store. *What the hell.* Maybe I needed a change of scenery from the Evanston store and everything it represented. Veronica was home from school for the summer and arranging our social calendar. Hanging out and meeting guys was a perfect way to get Randy out of my system. One Sunday, she and I went to a summer boat party at Jackson Park Harbor. We were sitting out on the grass when I saw a man walking across the lawn, heading for the boats. He was carrying two McDonald's pickle barrels. I could see that he was wearing a white polo shirt with white tennis shorts and boat shoes. He had a pair of gorgeous legs. I hollered, "Whose McDonald's pickle barrels you stole?" When he turned to answer me, his face was as gorgeous as his legs. Veronica and I glimpsed at each other, acknowledging "dude is fi-ine!"

"Mine," he answered, continuing, "And how you know they're from McDonald's?"

"Because I'm a lifelong employee," I chuckled.

He invited Veronica and I on his boat, and we took a spin. He was very charming and at least twenty years older than me. When he brought us back, he and I exchanged telephone numbers. He didn't waste any time reaching out. Within a week, I was back on his boat. At first, I thought how glamorous it was to be dating a McDonald's owner. I had what I call, *"Pretty Woman Syndrome"*—when a wealthy man who picks you up to fuck would whisk you off your feet, and you live happily ever after. In reality, when a man seeks you out to fuck, that's exactly what he intends to do.

By the time I learned that he was married with a family, I was already in it. He would be my first married man, but not my last. At eighteen, my brain didn't default to some moral compass. I just responded to the fact that he wanted me. There was no doubt I was trying to fill the emptiness inside of me. Interestingly, even back then, I wasn't under some illusion that he would leave his wife for me, nor did I want him to. He was an adventure. I enjoyed his company and the sex. That summer, he would gain my trust and violate it in the worst of ways.

One day when I arrived at his boat, to my surprise, another man who also owned a McDonald's was with him. We sat around talking and then my friend made his move on me. It hit me like a ton of bricks that we were getting ready to have a threesome. I didn't really know how to handle the situation, so I just went along. I didn't enjoy his friend and I certainly didn't enjoy my friend watching. To me, this was a terrible breach, and it gave me a moment of pause; I stopped calling him. Then he caught me one day when I answered the telephone. I told him dude couldn't fuck as my way of telling him that I didn't want to have sex with his friend. He just laughed it off. I asked if it was going to be only the two of us; when he said yes, I acquiesced. He regained my trust after I backed off; however, the next time, I looked up and his friend was back—and with a woman. They tried to get she and I to engage, but neither one of us was having it. On another day, it turned into a different mix with more men and more women. Sometimes I'd walk into what I thought was a social gathering, only to learn that I was the end game. Sure, I knew boat dude expected to have sex with me and, by the same token, I expected to have sex with him. Then I'd look up in the middle of having sex with him, and he would offer me to someone else. I never could fight the pressure of being put on the spot, so I gave in.

That's how it went; on and off for about a year, until I got the power to walk away. When he invited another girl about a couple of years older than me and she brought a friend, I was knocked back to reality. After his friend performed oral sex on me, the other girl slipped in her spot, and it triggered me back to Aunt Betty and her girlfriend. That would be the last time I laid eyes on him. Looking back, I can see how easy it is for a girl to fall into the trap of sex trafficking because I did. It's not always about physical violence or domination, but predatory behavior is always about coercion, manipulation, and sexual violence.

The summer of 1980, I thought I was the shit because I could pull a man who owned a McDonald's. The irony is I was living on minimum wage at another McDonald's and telling myself I was living my best life. By the middle of the summer, I was tired of the commute to Skokie and began working at a McDonald's closer to my house. It was the first franchise store I ever worked for, and I didn't like working there much. By then, I knew every bit about McDonald's, and the nuances in the franchise operation left me a little discombobulated. I figured I could take the good with the bad; at least I no longer had that long commute.

One day, the manager on duty asked me to go to the office because the store owner wanted to speak with me. *What, now?* I thought. On the way to his office, I prayed I wouldn't lose my job. Lord knows, I needed that minimum wage. I stuck my head in the door meekly and was stunned by the man staring back. My God, he was handsome about six-foot-three-inches tall with wavy salt-and-pepper hair and caramel skin. *Damn, he's fine!* I thought. He was sharp as a tack, dressed in a blue wool blazer, a dress shirt, well-fitted slacks, and a pair of fine Italian loafers. I came back to earth when he started talking. He asked me if I would like to represent the store on the Black McDonald's Operators Association float for the Bud Billiken Parade. My eyes grew wide. "Yes!" came out of my mouth faster than I could think. I was honored. Bud Billiken had been a landmark back-to-school parade since before I could remember. It was started in 1929 by Chicago's Black-owned newspaper, *The Chicago Defender.* The parade's participants read like a who's who in Black America.

He asked me to wear a swimsuit, which I didn't own, and he gave me a crisp one-hundred-dollar bill to buy one. Never one to disappoint, I found a red, orange, and white two-piece. You couldn't tell me I wasn't looking fabulous, matching Ronald McDonald. It was exciting to be on the float with other girls and some of the Black owners of Chicago-area McDonald's. I felt so much pride waving to thousands of onlookers for the two-mile stretch down Dr. Martin Luther King Jr. Drive.

After the parade, the owners treated all the girls to lunch at a rooftop Chinese restaurant named House of Bing, located in Chicago's South Shore community that borders the lake to the south of downtown Chicago. It was such a beautiful day, we sat outside on the patio. I could see Lake Michigan for miles across the South Shore Country Club lawn. *So, this is how rich people live*, I thought. They seemed to order some of every kind of food on the menu and set it before us like we were royalty. I didn't know what I had done to deserve that day, but I felt like a princess. The afternoon came to a close and my store owner drove me home. A few blocks before he reached my house, he pulled over on a side street so we could talk. He got straight to the point. He said he had singled me out for that day, and that he had been watching me at work. I hadn't seen this coming. I had noticed a little heat coming from him at lunch, but I dismissed it as my imagination. So, here I sat in my store owner's Mercedes after the parade, believing that I was hip to the game. Boat guy hadn't yet tainted my worldview, but he had certainly broadened my horizon. Dude eased his hand on my thigh as he outlined his proposal that we hook up occasionally, and he would help me financially. The other McDonald's owner, boat dude, never offered to help me financially the entire time I was with him. In hindsight, that's probably why I never equated the nature of our relationship to something more sinister, which it was.

At the time, I felt like I had been chosen. Out of all the girls he could have asked, he chose me. I thought I was special. In reality, he chose me because something in my behavior told him I was the perfect target, not because I was special. Then he lured me with the biggest prize in my eighteen years of life—the Bud Billiken Parade. He slid in with perfect ease, as predators often do, and I didn't have a clue. If you had told me back then that he was a predator, I would have told you to go fuck yourself. I took such pride getting out of his Mercedes every time he dropped me off. That he was offering to help me was secondary to my decision to whore myself out. I liked that he liked me.

I went into this arrangement thinking he would be easy-breezy. He was fifty-two and, by now, I knew what I was doing between the sheets. *At his age*, I asked myself, *how crazy could it get?* Well, let me tell you, he was over the top in a way that I had never experienced and never would after him. It was nothing short of unadulterated raw sex.

He treated me like I was his real-life sex toy. I was over it before it began. Within the first month, I was fired from his store because my drawer was short. Having a short drawer had been a pattern with me since I worked at McDonald's with Randy. This was prior to all the technology that told you how much change to give back. I think my problem with miscounting was that I always moved too fast. Randy knew I wasn't a thief, so he would fuss at me to take my time and replace whatever was short. In this instance, I thought the owner would intervene on my behalf as Randy had done, but I was wrong. Instead, after he told me the manager had to let me go he said, "It is better this way." I felt stuck with the little money he was giving to me. The truth is, he never laid out any large amounts of money at one time. There were no big-ass paydays like I had imagined. Clearly, I had watched way too much television. He was a sugar daddy all right, but it certainly wasn't a cupful, and I was lucky if I got more than a few spoonfuls. I continued to see him because I was struggling financially, and the little he gave me fed me for another week.

I also continued to do as he requested sexually until I couldn't take it anymore. I think the worst it ever got was when he asked me to shave off my pubic hair. I was a little hesitant, but I thought, *What could it hurt?* Pat asked me, "Girl, what is all this hair doing in the tub. You shave your coochie or something?" I was too embarrassed to tell the truth.

"Girl, no," I said instantly. However, there was so much hair left in the tub I knew I had to say *something* that sounded believable. To shut her up I told her I had shaved my legs and panty line.

The next time he and I got together, he went apeshit on me! He grabbed my clitoris and held it in his mouth like it was a penis or something. *What the FUCK was all this?* Sure, I was no stranger to oral sex, but Randy had never, ever been rough. He and I experienced and explored the boundaries of traditional sex, but at no time did he physically hurt me. This was more than I could handle. I thought dude had lost his fucking mind! He was sucking and biting like a dog with a fresh bone. I kept saying, "That's enough, baby. I'm good." At first, I thought that he had mistaken my pleas to mean I was enjoying him, because he kept gnawing and biting. I tried to relax and let him get his pleasure on, but when I had more than I could take, I tried to push his head away. He grabbed my hands and held them down. When he had finished orally, he jumped on top of me quicker than a lion on his prey. I didn't have half a second to regroup before he penetrated. He went deep fast and hard, jamming himself into me over and over. He had one of the largest penises I had ever encountered or ever would. It felt like he was tearing me open. Added to the agony was his pubic hair rubbing against my bare skin like steel wool. I tried my best to match his moves to get that shit over with.

When he rolled off of me, I went to the bathroom to regain myself. I got dressed and rode home in silence. After he dropped me off, I took a warm bath and tried to figure out my next move. That little voice inside of me asked that same old question again: *What the fuck are you doing, girl?* And still, I didn't have an answer. Nothing was what I thought it would be going into this arrangement. I was unhappy with how the whole situation made me feel. I think about it now, and all I can say is that my hurt was as wide as a sea and tall as a mountain.

I started to feel like I had lost parts of myself. Before Mama put me out, I went to church religiously. It was the one thing that kept me level and gave me hope. I couldn't believe that I had not been to church since I left Mama's house ten months ago. I stopped participating in PAGE because of the obvious—I no longer had that kind of leisure time. I had to put food on my table. I missed going to church and thought maybe it was the answer to my life's problems. I was too embarrassed to attend in Evanston because I hadn't graduated. I decided I would go to Grandmamma Julia's church. At least I wouldn't have to answer questions. Plus, I hadn't been there in years or laid eyes on her since right after I moved to her neighborhood. I figured I needed to face her again sometime, and the church was a better place than any. Grandmamma was happy to see me, and I was happy to see her. I left, promising to come back. I was disappointed to learn that Pastor Anderson had left Old Ship of Zion and was now leading a larger church, Cathedral Baptist, down the street. Still, it had been a good day and I was pleased. The choir lifted my spirits, for sure. But nothing was more soothing than hearing Grandmamma Julia's voice. I believed returning to the church was a move in the right direction.

I walked up 47th Street to the train station with a peacefulness that I hadn't had in a long time. The station had had a fire of some sort in the stairway that separated the southbound trains from the northbound. It was dark and dingy, with burned wood and a single light hanging, but I hadn't given it any thought that morning when I came through because it was still in full operation. After I paid, I walked up the stairs away from the agent. When I made it to the spot that divided the north and south stairs to reach the elevated trains, a man was standing there. He was as dark as a moonless, starless sky, and dressed in a light-colored three-piece suit. He had processed hair styled in finger waves. My first thought was that he was a character out of a 1920s movie. As I approached to pass him, he pulled a knife from under his suit jacket, which hung over his arm.

"Give me your money," he ordered. I was scared out of my mind.

"I don't have any," I said, which was the truth. My heart started to palpitate, and I felt faint.

"Then give me those chains around your neck," he demanded.

"Please, don't take them; it's all I got. Please," I cried. I loved my gold chains. I had purchased one with my hard-earned money before Mama put me out. I had purchased the other two I was wearing within the past year. I had sacrificed and gone without so I could buy them. Layering gold chains was all the craze back then, and being fashionable was always important to me. I thought I could talk him out of taking them.

"Give them to me," he ordered, moving closer. Suddenly, I could feel the knife in my side, and he said, "Walk." He put his right arm around me and held the knife close to my side as we walked out of the train station into the hot summer sun. I could feel sweat dripping under my clothes. We walked in silence with the knife pinned to my side. I was so frozen with fear that I couldn't even think to pray. We walked west on 47th Street, and he nudged me to turn when we approached Calumet Street. As we approached an abandoned building, he nudged me to go inside. We must have walked about three blocks. I was too disoriented to figure out exactly how far.

"Take your panties off." I hesitated, and he pushed the tip of the knife into my side so I could feel the blade.

"I said, take that shit off," he said. I pulled my stockings and panties down to one ankle, and he ordered me to lay on the ground. *This man on this day is going to rape me. Brave up, girl*, I resolved, and laid on the ground. I watched in a daze when he unzipped his pants, pulled out his penis, and laid on top of me. He smelled like spicy cheap cologne. When he shifted my thighs apart, his penis was already hard, and he jabbed it into my dry vagina. In the first few minutes, I was paralyzed. He jabbed harder and harder. The more he grew inside me, the more it hurt. I wanted it over. Then it occurred to me: make him cum so he could leave me be. I started to gyrate my pelvis.

"I knew a pretty yellow-ass like you would like it," he said.

Get it done, Rae, I coached. *You know how to satisfy a man. Make him happy so he won't hurt you. Get it over with.* And with those thoughts swirling in my head, I matched his moves until he had an orgasm and collapsed on top of me. I wanted to push him up to signal he was done and to get off me, but I was too afraid. After a few seconds he sprung up and zipped up his pants. He looked down at me and smiled. I turned my head in disgust. I was completely brain-locked; I had no idea where he had put the knife while he was on top of me. I didn't see it anymore now that he was standing. My only focus was to survive. I refused to look at him. I just lay there with my dress pulled up around my waist and my panties and stockings around my ankle, humiliated.

"Give me that gold chain around your neck," he demanded. I sat up and reached behind my neck with my hands to take off one of the chains. He instructed me to give him the thicker, longer one. When I held it up, he reached down and snatched it out of my hand.

"Stay here for thirty minutes," he said. "If I see you come out, I'm going to kill you." He pulled the knife from the pocket of his suit jacket that he had picked up from the ground. After he left, I took my panties and stockings that were hanging from my ankle and wiped his semen from between my legs and set them by my side. I couldn't bring myself to put them back on. I didn't shed one tear. I just sat there, wondering what had gone wrong. I thought about church and how I had felt God's presence just a short while ago. I knew with all my heart that God was up there somewhere, but it just didn't feel like it then. I waited.

Eventually, I got up from the ground and peeked out at the ruins that were once a building. When I didn't see him, I walked the opposite direction from the 47th Street station until I reached the 43rd Street station. I sat on the train fighting back the tears. Station after station, the train stopped, let people off and started again. I could smell him all over me, and it made me sick to my stomach. *Be strong girl*, I encouraged. All of a sudden, I felt a painful tightness around my neck. As the train started to take off, my neck jerked, and my dress ripped around my shoulder that was closest to the window. I hadn't noticed that my dress had gotten ripped during the attack and was still disheveled. Tears gushed down my cheeks like the Niger River. It hit me all at once. I had been raped trying to hold onto my gold chains, and now they were all gone. I couldn't move. I couldn't think. I just cried with my dress torn and my bra showing. An African American woman, about mid-to-late forties, came over to see if I was okay. Her voice brought me to the realization that my body was partially exposed. I brought the ripped part of my dress up and held it there.

"I don't know why those kids keep snatching people's gold chains," she said angrily. The chain-snatching robberies had been happening all summer in Chicago. The robber would time it perfectly—just as the train started moving—so they didn't get caught.

"I was just raped," I told her.

"They're going to hurt someone one of these days," she said, still reasoning I'd only had my gold chain snatched. She dug into her handbag and handed me a safety pin to close my dress.

"I was just raped," I repeated, and it finally hit her what I had been trying to tell her.

"Aw, honey, I'm so sorry," she said, and she reached down and gave me a hug. She sat beside me, but that's it. I don't think she knew what else to say or do. We rode in silence until we reached the end of the line at 63rd and Ashland, which was the stop for both of us. As we exited, she asked if I was going to be okay. I told her that I would, and we went our separate ways. When I got down to the street level, I was too afraid to get on the bus, so I walked the eight blocks home. I thought about the sequence of events on my walk home. What had been the point trying to talk the rapist out of robbing me when, in the end, I was raped *and* robbed. Maybe I should have just kept my mouth closed and given him my chains in the first place.

When I came through the door, Pat and Ethel were in the living room. "I was just raped," I announced.

"Stop playing, girl," Pat said. I went straight to the bathroom and turned on the water in the tub. Pat came in after me and realized that I was serious and stopped me from taking a bath. Someone called the police. They came and took me to the hospital, where the doctor collected evidence by performing a rape kit on me. At that point, I was too numb to care that a male doctor was conducting the exam. I just wanted to go home and wash the rapist's smell from my body. Detectives came to the hospital and took a statement. Afterward, they drove me to the 51st Street police station to look at mug shots. He was not among any of the criminals in the ten books I reviewed.

For days, I cried and bathed while listening to Tramaine Hawkins. On one of those nights, my cousin Kenny was on leave from the army and came over. He sat with me most of the night, and I cried in his arms. On another night, I heard Ethel ask Pat if they should stop me from taking so many baths.

"Just leave her alone," Pat said. "She'll be okay." Ethel and Pat had no idea what to do for me, but they did the best they could. I needed something I still cannot fully describe. Maybe it was the reassurance that someone cared about me. Maybe I needed a mother. I called Mama. I made myself believe, in a crisis situation, she would rise to the occasion. I was projecting what I wanted to believe about Mama instead of the hard facts about her that I continued to face. On the phone call I told her that I had been raped, and she told me to come out to the house. I saw this as another good sign. I accepted her offer and went to visit. She cooked a big meal, and I ate my misery away. She didn't say much. That was fine with me; I was simply happy that she hadn't turned me away. At some point, we went across the street to visit Ms. Virginia. We were all sitting around the dining room table and, out of nowhere, Ms. Virginia said, "Your Mama told me that you were raped." At first, it was awkward. I was a tad taken aback that Mama had told her, but I dismissed it, thinking that maybe she needed to talk about it. I mean, it is kind of heavy to hear that your daughter has been raped.

"Yes," I responded, confirming this truth. I relaxed, thinking that it was nice to have someone else concerned about me. Then she said, "You should go and find him so I can get me some." They both started laughing. I didn't respond. I just got up from the table and walked out. As I walked out of the door, I heard her saying, "Don't go. I was just playing." I didn't turn back.

After that, I didn't know who to talk to. I was too ashamed to bring it up again to Pat and Ethel. I believed they had always viewed me as smart even when I knew that I was faking it. I couldn't face their questions about how I could have let this happen. Of course, this was only a supposition rooted in my own low self-esteem. I blamed myself. Veronica was back at college, and I didn't have the money to call her. Our phone had been disconnected so I was mostly using the pay phone a block from the house up on Ashland Avenue. Coré was someone who I could at least confide in who would keep it in confidence, and I made a daily trip to the pay phone up the street to call her. Talking to her didn't make me feel any better. After a while, what more could she say other than, "It will be okay." One day, walking home from my daily call, this neighborhood guy stopped to speak. I could not remember his name, but I knew he was a friend of Ethel's boyfriend, Earl.

"You always look so sad," he told me, then asked, "You want to talk?" Every time he saw me, he asked me the same thing, and I always declined. Then one day, I gave in. What did I have to lose? He was nice to me and seemed concerned. Standing right there on the corner, I told him I had been raped. He lived on the same street north of our house and suggested we go to his house so we could talk. He had been so sympathetic and concerned about me in the past weeks that I trusted him. Once we got relaxed in his basement, he said to me,

"Now show me how you do it." He spoke softly, trying to be all sexy and shit.

"I don't want to have sex with you," I said as I jumped up. "I'll just go."
He whistled, and his two Dobermans came and sat down right in front of us. He sat down on his sofa bed and signaled for me to sit next to him, saying, "I bet you won't get past my dogs."

For a split second, I thought he was joking, but his face said, *Try me.* I undressed and laid on the sofa bed. He raped me. When he finished, he got off of me, put his pants back on, and then called his dogs to sit at his side. I got dressed and left. I reached our door and went straight to the bathroom and made a hot bath. The water was as hot as I could stand it. I immersed my body from head to toe. It burned, but the pain to my body couldn't match the pain in my heart. I never told. About a week later, Ethel came to me and asked if I had sex with him. Dude had been telling his boys that he had scored with me.

"Hell, no," I said. "What I want with a nigga like that?" I was too ashamed to tell her he raped me. How stupid could I have been to fall prey to him after I had just been raped? She believed me. "I told Earl you don't mess around with guys like that." After that, I pushed it out of my head and went on with my life.

That September, I started night school at ETHS with a newfound commitment. I didn't miss one class or assignment. It had been just a month short of a year since

I was put out of Mama's house. I had lived a lifetime in those eleven months. There had been so much betrayal, failure, and disappointment. I believed that finishing school would be some kind of redemption for me.

By the end of October, Chicago was getting cold earlier than usual. The commute to school every evening was kicking my tail—especially waiting in the cold for public transportation wearing a raggedy winter coat. I hadn't gotten a new coat since a couple of years before I left Mama's. It was time for something new and warmer, but I couldn't afford to buy one. By the time school began I was still unemployed, and my Social Security was all I had coming in. Between the commute to school, food, lunch, and my share of the expenses, I hardly had money to make ends meet. I had gone to Marshall Field's to look around and get an idea of what a new coat would cost and fell in love with this bad-ass Bill Blass full-length down coat. I coveted that coat so much I would get off the train on my way to school every week to see if it had gone on sale. I needed to figure something out because the Chicago Hawk was not playing with me. I hadn't seen my cheap-ass sugar daddy since he dropped me off that day, but I figured he was the only way. I knew he wouldn't straight-out give me the amount that I really wanted. He would string me along. I concocted a scheme to get that coat. I called and told him that I was pregnant and needed money for an abortion. The first thing he said was, "I thought that you were on birth control?"

"I was, but I missed a few pills and doubled up when we first started talking," I replied. It was the truth, just not *his* truth. I figured the closer to a truth that I could get would be best. I told him that I was roughly two months, which coincided with the last time I'd seen him. He bought it hook, line and sinker, saying he would need a couple of days. He picked me up and drove to a hotel. I knew he expected me to put out, and I gave him the show of my life. I *"yes-daddy'd"* him straight to an orgasm. He gave me five hundred dollars in loose bills like he had robbed one of his cash registers. When he dropped me off at home, I took a long hot bath and washed him off of my body and out of my life. I went down to Marshall Field's department store wearing a sweater and I walked out with my first designer coat. With that said and done, I decided to take a break from men.

I placed all of my energy into graduating. That November, I received a letter of admittance to the University of Arkansas at Pine Bluff! That previous spring, before I flunked out, I had applied to the University of Arkansas at Pine Bluff, with Mr. Perrin's help. I never knew Mr. Perrin's position at ETHS—only that he always had an office full of students. He also had a relationship with recruiters at historically Black colleges and universities. I arrived at school earlier than usual one day and went to say hello. A recruiter from the University of Arkansas at Pine Bluff was there chatting with Mr. Perrin. I told him I had applied the previous spring, and he vowed to look up my application when he got back to Arkansas. Acceptance would be a dream come true. I knew I didn't have the grades to get into anyone's college, so I dropped it and stayed focused on getting my diploma.

I was admitted through a special program the school had for struggling graduates. God, I was grateful. I felt redeemed. Around the same time, a guy named Larry Thurmond—who knew Patricia and used to hang out at our house from time to time—volunteered to pick me up from school some nights. Larry was nice, and I knew he liked me. I was not the least bit interested in him, and that made me hesitant about accepting his offer. He assured me there would be no strings attached, so I agreed. After a while, I started to feel guilty, I think, in part because he lived even farther south than I did. It was a lot to drive all the way to Evanston, pick me up, and then turn around and drive all the way south again. I finally gave in to a sexual relationship that took on a life of its own. I knew I was leaving in January to go to school, and that would be my way out.

Twenty-Seven

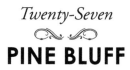

PINE BLUFF

"
The more things change, the more they stay the same."
—Jean-Baptiste Alphonse Karr

The moment I stepped off of that Greyhound bus in Pine Bluff, I was attacked by a stench in the air. *What the hell is that smell?* I wondered, as I made my way to campus with all my worldly possessions inside my blue trunk. That smell followed me to the registration office and then to my dorm room. I later learned there were six paper mills in Arkansas, and the one in Pine Bluff accounted for the foul odor. I woke up to the stink of it every single morning, and I hated it with a passion. Unfortunately, that would be only one grievance in a whole list of complaints I had at the University of Arkansas at Pine Bluff (UAPB).

I had heard so much about the importance of historically Black colleges and universities (HBCUs) in the shaping of young Black minds that I was actually excited UABP had given me a chance. I remembered watching those Lou Rawls Parade of Stars/United Negro College Fund marathons to help raise money for Black students at HBCUs. I loved every minute of it—the performers and the speeches. The motto "A Mind Is a Terrible Thing to Waste" was imprinted on my brain, and it made the reality of the school an even bigger letdown. Founded in 1873, the University of Arkansas at Pine Bluff is the second oldest public school and the oldest HBCU in the state. When I arrived, the school was in a financial crisis, having just come out of a mismanagement scandal involving school funds with the past administration. The school was in disarray from the rooter to the tooter. The newer buildings didn't make up for the older buildings that were in disrepair. A hundred-year-old building didn't give me the feeling of history or nostalgia but of being rundown and in immediate need of tuck pointing. In hindsight, with the internal problems it was having with the mismanagement of funds, the school was symptomatic of the lack of investment in infrastructure that has plagued HBCUs for decades.

After being my grown-ass self for almost two years, dorm life was an imposition on my way of life. I didn't need to be out of the dorm after 10:00 p.m., but I sure as heck wanted the freedom to do whatever I wanted, and whenever I wanted to do it. Curfew was 10:00 p.m. To make matters worse, all the dorms were segregated by gender, and the opposite sex was not permitted beyond the lobby in any dorm at any time for any reason. This rule was strictly enforced. If any of us were caught, we would be expelled. It didn't stop me or others from sneaking. One morning, I walked out of my room to go to the toilet, and some dude was easing out of a girl's room. I wasn't bold enough to risk getting caught with a guy in my room; however, I did my fair share of sneaking into the football dorm to see my new boo, Thaddeus. He was a dark chocolate cutie, just like the little boy I took under the porch. The one relief was that I didn't have a roommate in my two-bed dorm room. But I didn't have a phone, toilet, or shower, either. Instead, there was one pay phone at the end of the hall, and the bathrooms were shared by all the girls on our floor—like in gym class, for crying out loud. I had the hardest time adjusting.

I was never one to be ashamed of my body, thanks to the revolution Stevie started in me back in high school. I was my carefree self. Each morning on my way to the shower, I wore a big towel wrapped around my body and that always got me a side-eye. Some of the other girls wore bulky bathrobes. I didn't even own a bathrobe. One time, I was on my way to the bathroom in an oversized T-shirt and a girl asked me, "Do you *ever* put on clothes?" I just rolled my eyes. I refused to let her policing of my body change the positive awareness I felt about it. That Southern-girl respectability was as much annoying as it was contradictory, with all the sneaking I witnessed. I wasn't so much bothered by the body policing as I was about the condition of the bathroom. There was mold in the showers, with cracked walls and peeling paint. The cleaning crews would have earned a C, at best. If you didn't make it to the bathroom early for your morning hygiene routine, you were operating in the downright nasty zone. I hated I had to wear flip-flops to take a shower and that anyone in the bathroom knew when I had to poop, like in airport bathrooms.

Inside the dorm, I hated the school; outside the dorm, I hated the city of Pine Bluff. It was reminiscent of going down South with Mama to visit her family. It was fine for a visit, but I didn't want to live there. My city-girl sensibilities didn't adapt well to country life. The train tracks went through the middle of downtown, and the main road by the school. Every time I walked on the unpaved road next to my dorm, the sandy dirt covered my socks and shoes. I didn't have much, but I was still trying to be a diva, and that town worked against me every way I turned. Pine Bluff didn't even have a mall—just a downtown that reminded me of Mayberry on The Andy Griffith Show. If you wanted anything significant, you had to go to Little Rock, which is about forty-five miles away. There was a McDonald's, a nasty rib joint and a small convenience store by the campus. I was over Pine Bluff the day I got off the bus.

As grown as I thought I was, I spent many evenings in the lobby sulking. I met my first friend, Sheila Henderson, because she caught me crying in the lobby and stopped to talk to me. Sheila would have easily been a full-figured model by today's standards. She had big beautiful deep-set eyes and the most unblemished, deep rich brown skin I had ever seen. A junior from Memphis, Tennessee, Sheila wore her hair short and fly, and every single time she stepped out of our dorm, her ensemble for the day was as fly as her hair. Her roommate, Rita Lewis, was also a junior, and as fine and fly as Sheila. Rita was about my complexion, with thick long wavy black hair. The two of them were my only friends on campus. Everyone knew Sheila, which meant, through hanging out with her, I would eventually know everyone.

It was with them that I went to my first sorority social. Both Sheila and Rita wanted to be members of Delta Sigma Theta Sorority, Inc., and would eventually pledge. I remember tagging along that day to a meet-and-greet. I walked away with a stellar impression of the sorority. I wrote in my book, *The Politics of Respectability,* that it was the members of the UAPB chapter of Delta Sigma Theta who first made me want to be a part of the sorority. We would lose and regain contact over the years and, each time, we'd pick up where we left off. Two decades later, they would both reach out and congratulate me on my induction into Delta Sigma Theta Sorority, Inc. as an honorary member. I was inducted 2001 for "lifetime achievement to help improve the human condition." By the time my membership was rescinded some twelve years after my induction, we had lost contact. However, I have never forgotten either of them or their kindness towards me which reflects the epitome of how Black women should treat each other.

When I really think about it, UABP wasn't all bad. I loved being in a classroom with other young African Americans, especially having come from predominantly white middle and high schools. The camaraderie among the students was an unspoken cultural understanding that floated in the atmosphere. Unlike the predominantly white universities I would later attend, I never felt like I had to defend my Blackness. I was placed in English and math classes designed for below-average students and they were still difficult. For the first time, I wondered if I was cut out for college. I had developed no study habits. I still couldn't get focused, and I had insomnia. I'd wake up tired, which made sitting through classes drudgery. I could barely get anything accomplished. I had to read a paragraph over and over to make it stick. It wasn't that I didn't comprehend, it's just the information would come into my mind—but then it would leave within seconds. It was a brutal hit to my self-esteem. Some days I felt like I was pretending to be a college student. Looking back, I know now that my behavior reflected how depression manifested in me. I had such a hard time concentrating and even getting started on a project. It looks like procrastination to most people, but it's really more about the physical effort than about delay. Just opening a book some days felt as if I had the weight of the world in my hands. But then, it hadn't been a good six months since I had been raped back to back. Not to mention, kicked out the house, sex trafficked, betrayed by the love of my life and then the abortion, all within seventeen months. I just took my lickings and kept right on ticking, the pain had to show up in my life and it did, as soon as I sat still in Pine Bluff. I wanted to stick it out because I believed it was the best route to becoming successful, which meant stability in my eyes. Living in Evanston had taught me that education was the best route to prepare for the future. Everyone made it appear to be a critical factor in how well one lived when becoming an adult. I wanted the same kind of success and stability I had seen in the adults at Second Baptist Church.

In the end, I think the conditions of the school became an excuse for me to leave. It came on Valentine's Day when I entered the cafeteria, and a stinky smell was competing with all the beautiful decorations. On one hand I thought, *Oh, wow—how pretty!* On the other, I thought, *Oh, wow—what is that smell?* This time, it was not the paper mill. Come to find out, we were having chitterlings (chitlins) for dinner. "Aw, hell naw!" I mumbled. I turned my ass back around and left. When I called Mama about staying with her on spring break, she said I could. However, in her own way, she meant that if I hated Pine Bluff as much as I conveyed in my previous calls, then why didn't I just come on home? And that's precisely what I did. For spring break, I packed my shit and went home.

The week I got back to Chicago, I went from store to store in Water Tower Place, on the Magnificent Mile, and filled out applications. I must say, no matter what was going on in my life, I had an incredible work ethic, and I was never going to be without a job.

I also rekindled my relationship with Larry Thurmond and, the next thing I knew, we were engaged. I will admit that it was exciting going to C.D. Peacock, to pick out a beautiful one-quarter-carat diamond ring. Unfortunately for Larry, that was all the excitement I felt. One day we were looking at apartments, and I realized I didn't want to spend the rest of my life with him. I knew I wanted more for myself, even if I couldn't name it. Equally important, I couldn't conjure love where there was none. I broke off the engagement and kept the ring; Larry was crushed. He was kind to me, and I honestly didn't want to hurt him. It I didn't know quite what I was doing. I didn't know what I wanted to do with my life. I still believed God had a plan, but She sure hadn't let me in on it. I felt like I was wandering in the wilderness.

Twenty-Eight

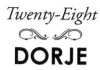

DORJE

"When you have this much hurt for this long, particularly when a bond so sacred as the mother-child bond is broken, it's a slow walk to healing."
—Iyanla Vanzant

I could hear Mama moving around in the kitchen, and I hadn't opened my eyes yet. The smell of coffee was in the air, and I knew she was about to make breakfast. I lay there and soaked in all the familiar sounds of the best part of Mama — making magic in the kitchen. Of all the places I imagined I would be, you could not have paid me to believe it would have been back at home with Mama, but here I was.

Still lying in bed, I imagined her every move—from the sink to the refrigerator and back, and from the sink to the stove and back—with precision. In so many ways, she was the same old Mama, but she was also different. She was easygoing and treated me more like an adult. The only rules she laid out were financial. I had to pay the light bill and half the telephone bill. For the most part, everything was going fine. Listening to Mama cooking, I started to doze off again. I heard the telephone ring and Mama move through the dining room to get it. Then there was silence, and sleep took over.

"Rae, telephone!" I thought I was dreaming.

"Girl, go get the phone," she said from the living room. I hadn't heard it ring again and I couldn't imagine who she'd been talking to all this time who now wanted to speak to me. I wiped the sleep out of my eyes as I made my way into the living room and sat on the sofa. Mama went into the kitchen to finish cooking breakfast.

"Hello," I said in a curious tone.

"Hello, Rae. This is your mother," the voice on the other end said.

My mother? My mother. My mo-ther. I was trying to wrap my brain around those words.

"I'm Judy, your mother." She paused, and said, "But I've changed my name to Dorje now." (It's pronounced, *Door-jah.*) My eyes teared up and my stomach fluttered. I never thought this would happen in a thousand years. As far as I knew, my mother was still a drug addict somewhere.

"Rae, my mother forwarded your information to me."

I was dumbfounded. My grandmother, Florence, had finally come through. She had stopped calling me long ago; then, I started calling her once a year on Christmas. She was my grandmother after all, whether she wanted to be or not. I was not ready to admit defeat—period. Talking to my mother now, my last call to my grandmother—on Dec. 25, 1979—came to mind. A young girl answered the telephone who I would learn was my cousin, Juli—the daughter of my mother's sister, Toni Rae. (I'm named after Toni Rae and my parental grandmother, Jane Clara.) I can hear Julie like it was yesterday: "Grandmother, you have a phone call." I could vaguely hear a voice in the background, asking who was on the telephone.

"May I ask who is calling?" She was poised and polite.

"This is Rae, her granddaughter," I said proudly.

Julie paused a moment, and then I heard her say, "Someone named Rae. She says she's your granddaughter." A few moments later, Julie came back to the telephone. "She can't come to the phone right now." I didn't know how to respond. I hung up the phone. God, it hurt. All these years, I had been clinging to a five-minute-telephone conversation and counting it as love. That Christmas Day, my grandmother's rejection opened old wounds I thought had closed. In those brief telephone conversations with her over the years, my mother was barely a topic. I asked about her and my grandmother would say only, "She's fine." Now I was feeling a certain kind of way, and it stayed with me. I hated to admit that maybe Mama had been right about my grandmother all along.

That feeling of rejection only intensified when I was pregnant, and the doctor asked me about my mother's health history. All I knew about my mother was her name and that she was a heroin addict. I had never asked my grandmother for one thing—*not one thing*. After the abortion, I decided that the least she owed me was the decency of telling me she knew something about my mother besides her being a drug addict. I wrote and asked her to connect me with my mother. It had been over a year since I sent that letter and, frankly, I had given up on hearing back.

I didn't say much but I listened intently. I didn't want to miss one word my mother said. As it turns out, she had no idea that her mother knew my whereabouts all those years.

"Even if I had known," she explained, "I was in no condition to take care of you then. I thought you were better off with Al's people."

She said, "My mother's guilt finally made her give me your letter." All I could muster was a confirmation that I had written my grandmother and asked her to connect us. I assumed she ended up calling Mama's house because Mama never changed her telephone number, ever. I listened in a daze—hearing, yet not hearing. It felt like an out-of-body experience. My body was there sitting on the sofa, but it was a hollow shell. Everything else had left and gone to some faraway place. I don't remember much of what I said to her. However, I walked away with the key points: She had changed her name to Dorje because she converted to Buddhism after her last stay in prison. She was remarried, to a Jewish man named Michael Levin. They lived in Boulder, Colorado. At some point, she asked if I would like to visit her. I agreed, and we said our goodbyes.

After I hung up the telephone, I continued to sit in a daze. Mama brought me back to reality. She stepped in the doorway of the living room when she heard me hang up the phone.

"What did she say?"

"She asked if I wanted to come and meet her," I answered. Mama didn't pursue it further.

Dorje didn't disappoint me. She called back to chat several times. It was slow going, but it was a start. When she called with my flight arrangements, I was beside myself. She met me at the airport baggage claim in Denver, about an hour outside of Boulder. Michael stayed near the car to give us a chance to break the ice. I didn't know what to expect. She looked like a leftover hippie, with long blonde hair that was turning salt and pepper, and it was thick and straggly. Her skin was pale white, and I could see that I had her chin and those dark piercing eyes. She was wearing a blue pullover top that had some kind of floral pattern. It was big and loose with a V-neck that had two tasseled strings hanging down. I swear it looked like something a flower child of the sixties would have worn. Her gray slouchy pants hung carelessly from her body. She wasn't obese but she was thick, maybe a size sixteen. I would later learn she didn't care much about clothing and rarely dressed up. She absolutely hated wearing any shoes that confined her feet, so she wore Birkenstock sandals and moccasins. On the day we first met; she was wearing moccasins.

"You are so beautiful," was the first thing that came out of her mouth. Then she drew me into her arms and kept me there for what seemed like hours. I wanted this for as long as I could remember, and I soaked in every bit of the love she had for me. I knew deep in my soul that it was her love for me that made her let me go all those years ago. There was no need to ask why. We walked hand in hand to the car.

Without a doubt, Michael was a computer nerd. He was an MIT graduate and taught computer science at the University of Colorado at Colorado Springs. Michael was shorter than Dorje, with thick brown curly hair. He wore khakis all the time. He had a nerdy nervousness about him, along with a dry humor, but he easily accepted me. They lived in a fabulous two-level house with three bedrooms and a bay window that looked out at the mountains. It reminded me of those Ridge Street homes I had admired while growing up in Evanston. I was never clear when my mother stopped using drugs, or when she met Michael and landed in Boulder. They were both devout Buddhists, with a shrine in the house. I was curious and peeped into the room, but I never intruded on the space. I didn't understand Buddhism, but it certainly felt sacred.

It was one exciting week. We went on a long drive through the mountains. Michael and I went hiking. We had dinner at a Japanese restaurant, and when Michael ordered sushi, Dorje and I said, "Yuck" at the same time. We all started laughing hysterically. It appeared that she and I actually had some things in common. It was a feel-good experience, and I thought it was an excellent start.

When I came home from that visit, I saw a shift in Mama. I was so wrapped up in the euphoria of meeting my mother, I had forgotten how petty Mama was—and that was a big mistake. I tried to tell her about my visit, and all I could get from her was "humph."

In hindsight, I can see how those experiences seemed like a threat to her position in my life. I loved Mama, and she was all I had known—good, bad, or indifferent. I don't think I was capable of trading her in. Her hold on me was powerful and remained so until the day she died. By the same token, she could never be my mother and that was a scientific fact. I could see myself in Dorje: her outspokenness and candor, her dislike for bullshit, her love of books and the fact that she had no couth whatsoever. She didn't care who you were; she said the first thing that came to her mind. It was interesting that Mama had some of these qualities, too, so I definitely got it honestly. However, there was a slight difference: Mama's candor was always self-serving, while Dorje had this compassionate undertone that extended beyond her circumstances. That part reflects who I am.

The tension grew, and it felt more like the old days of living with her. I swear she must have said to me "you think you white" more in that short time than she had during my whole life—which was a lot, even back then. I started to realize that I had become too comfortable at 802 Seward. Hanging out with old friends, walking the streets of Evanston without any fear, and not having to worry about rent or my next meal had caused me to forget all the reasons I hated living with Mama. I knew it was going to come to a head at some point; I just didn't know how. I decided to bide my time by staying out of the house as much as I could. I went to work, participated in PAGE rehearsals and gigs, and spent my other free time hanging out with Veronica, who was also home from college. I often stayed with her on weekends and went to work from her house. Mama was a ticking time bomb.

One evening, before I reached the house, I was met up the street by the daughter of one of Mama's girlfriends who was staying with us for a couple of weeks to get her out of the city. Katrina, thirteen, had been waiting to catch me before I got home. She told me I had gotten a big check from Social Security, and that it was for some sort of back pay. Katrina said Mama had opened it and worked out a scheme to get it from me. She told me because she didn't want me to fall for Mama's okey-doke.

When I walked into the apartment, the first thing Mama said was that she needed some money to go down South. She was waiting on me to say that I didn't have any to give her, so she could pop that check out. I played her like a violin until, finally, she got tired and gave me the check. The amount was around twenty-three hundred dollars and some change. After she gave it to me, I packed a bag for a previously planned girl's weekend at Veronica's. It was payday and I had gone shopping, and to hurry up I stuffed everything into a bag and got the heck out of Dodge. That Sunday, I had to work, and I left the girls while they were still having breakfast. When I arrived home, I dumped everything on my bed, including the clothes that I had purchased that Friday. Mama came into the dining room, and her eyes went straight to the price tags. She reached down to get a closer look, asking, "Oh, you big-time now, but you can't give me no money?"

I planned to give her a chunk. I hadn't because I was still trying to determine how much and, honestly, I hadn't been home and this was the last thing on my mind. I had no clue that she would go apeshit crazy.

"Mama, I plan on giving you some of this money," I said. I turned to her, adding, "I haven't been home."

She was going on about how this entire check belonged to her because I had switched the check into my name. Of course, she didn't mention the fact that I needed the money to take care of myself after SHE put me out. I imagined that when she opened the Social Security envelope and saw the check, she claimed it as her own payday. I knew she wasn't going to let up, and with what I understood about her sense of entitlement, I also knew this argument was going to a place of no return. I didn't have time for this; I had to get ready for work. I changed my clothes for work and repacked my overnight bag. I tossed in some of what I had just purchased and added more clothes so I could go back over to Veronica's after work to give Mama some space.

Mama was sitting in the living room, smoking a cigarette in her favorite spot. When I walked in with my bag, she asked where I was going. I told her, "to work, and then back over to Veronica's." That's when all hell broke loose.

"Bitch, get your shit and get out of my house!" she said.

I opened my mouth, but not a word came out. I was dumbfounded. She, on the other hand, showed her *natural Black ass.*

"You ungrateful, lowdown bitch!"

I finally got, "But Mama!" out of my mouth. But she wasn't trying to hear one thing I had to say.

"All I done for you, and you can't give me that money?" she wailed.

I resolved that I had two choices: give her the money or leave. What if I gave her the money? I would still have to live with how she was berating me. I got a nervous wrench in the middle of my stomach. The days of her dictatorship were over. I was nineteen years old, and I'd rather live in the streets than deal with this madness again. *How could I have been so stupid to fall right into this trap?* I didn't have a choice when my grandfather died, but I would be damned if I stayed there another day. I called Veronica to ask her mom if I could stay over to their house until I figured it out. Sherry said yes, and the girls headed over to pick me up. I pulled out my blue trunk and started packing everything I owned. Mama was sitting calmly on the sofa with another cigarette hanging out of her mouth. The doorbell rang, and I went to buzz them in as Mama went into the back. Veronica arrived first. I handed her some of my things on hangers and she started back down the stairs. As soon as my girlfriend Leslie Priest stepped in the doorway, Mama came charging at her with a butcher knife.

"Get your motherfucking ass out of my house!" she hollered.

"MAMA, STOP IT!" I screamed.

Leslie's eyes went wild, yelling, "SHE'S CRAZY!"

Veronica heard the commotion, handed the clothes off to Sharon Williams, and came

178

back up the stairs. Leslie moved so fast she practically jumped down the stairs to the next level, and Mama was standing in the doorway waving the knife. I was behind her in the foyer, pleading for her to stop. She wasn't paying me any attention. She had an audience, and she performed her ass off.

"I'm going to kill you motherfuckers if you try to take one more thing out of my house!" she said, waving the butcher knife at them. She turned to me, yelling, "You can't take another motherfucking thing out of here until you give me some money!"

"You lowdown dirty bitch!" she hollered in my face.

Veronica yelled upstairs to me, "Call the police, Rae."

"I don't give a fuck who she call," Mama said, waving the knife down toward Leslie and Veronica. I left her standing in the doorway with the knife and called the police. They came and negotiated between us. It was her apartment, and since my name wasn't on the lease, I needed to pay. I ended up giving her five hundred dollars, and they left after I got my last belongings down the stairs. I shut that front room door and reconciled that I was done with her ass completely, this time.

When we made it to Veronica's, we sat around laughing about how crazy my mother was, and it helped to ease the pain—at least, for a moment. But I knew that I was homeless again and needed to figure my next move. I had only a couple of weeks before Veronica went back to school. I decided to go back to UAPB, of all places. When I called, I learned that I was still in good standing, and there was a dorm room for me. It all seemed like a miracle right before my eyes. I packed all my possessions and headed down to the paper-mill capital of the United States.

I was determined to make it work. But about a week later, just like Mama, school officials told me to pay or leave. My Pell Grant had only been processed since I arrived, and I didn't have enough to pay the portion required until it was approved. I was homeless again. I had no clue. I certainly couldn't go back to Mama's. I thought about Ethel, but she was getting on with her life. Her boyfriend Earl had moved in, and Pat had moved to California with her husband. Veronica suggested I ask my mother. I had already told Dorje about my life with Mama when I visited her, but I just didn't know how she would respond to this request. While she had a lot of remorse about my upbringing, she also had some gratitude because Mama kept a roof over my head for many years, even in the madness. She never took that part away from Mama.

I stood at the pay phone with dread. I was actually ashamed I couldn't make it on my own, and even more ashamed of how it had unfolded between Mama and I this time around. I was a nervous wreck trying to figure out how Dorje would respond. But I was in dire straits. I had to brave up and get it done. When she answered the telephone, I felt like a five-year-old explaining what happened. A whirlwind of emotions flooded me as I stood in the hall with the phone to my ear. It was surreal explaining to my biological mother why my mother who had raised me kicked me out of her house, and praying that she—the woman who had given birth to me—would take me in. The craziest thing of all was that I didn't think about how crazy it was. Figuring out how to survive was my normal, as were my feelings of rejection.

Dorje looked at me with awe and pride because I had been able to make it, in spite of all the obstacles. A part of me was afraid she would think less of me now. I wondered if she would even believe me because the story was so crazy. Dorje was silent as she listened to the story of how I became homeless. I remember pleading and begging with my tone, "Please take me in." I had too much pride to beg outright, and her silence gave me no assurance. When I finally quieted down, Dorje reassured me that I had done nothing wrong. I let out a big sigh. She told me she didn't mind, but she had to speak with Michael first. She was a stay-at-home wife, and Michael was the sole financial support of their household.

Michael's concern was drugs and alcohol. It was hard as hell trying to explain to a recovering addict and her husband that, at nineteen, I had never tried drugs. I also told them I had only had a couple of ice cream drinks with the girls—heavy on the ice cream—because I didn't like the taste of alcohol. We went over it again and again. She must have worked on him because he eventually gave in, but I was duly warned: no drugs in their home. The downside was they were planning to move out of the country in December, and I would have to find a new place to live by then. Michael had accepted a teaching position at the University of Nova Scotia and had already started the immigration process. Dorje said there was a whole community of Buddhists that had moved there, and they were going to give it a try.

The first thing I did upon my arrival was look for a job. I landed the seasonal holiday job from heaven. It was at a chic female-owned boutique in the historic Pearl Street Mall in downtown Boulder. Everyone was super-cool. I loved helping to dress the women, and the clothes in the boutique were to die for. I even thought about going into a career of fashion merchandising. I could see myself as a buyer for fabulous clothing stores like I. Magnin & Company, Bonwit Teller and, of course, Marshall Field's. Pearl Street was another thing I loved about work. It had a nostalgic feel about it, with its cobblestone sidewalks, exclusive boutiques, bookstores, and restaurants surrounded by the Flatirons. On my lunch break, I would grab a sandwich from the deli across the way with my favorite drink its signature beverage called *half and half*: half black tea and half lemonade. Then I'd sit on a bench in the middle of the square and look at the wonders of God's creation.

I loved living with them because it was easy. Nothing was asked of me except respect for their home, and they respected me in return. It was the first time in my life that I lived in such peace. All I had to do when I was with them was to just *be*. Waking up to the mountains was the most beautiful feeling. There was something magical that came over me each morning, as if God were sitting by my bedside. Michael and I went hiking on the weekends after we had a breakfast of bagels with cream cheese, lox, and tea. I loved it, even his nerdy awkwardness. I could always count on him to explain as we walked. I was always intrigued. I often thought that I would buy a small retirement house in the middle of the mountains, whereas most people who relocated after retiring headed for warmth and water. I don't know if it was the height and size of mountains that always made me feel God's presence, or the magic of snow with streams of water running through it.

Dorje was not a hiker, and our best moments together were browsing used bookstores and finding gems. I didn't know anyone else who got as excited about books the way she and I did. It was our thing. When she was on her deathbed, I went to Buffalo to see about her and handle her affairs. The day I went to her apartment, the manager told me that she was rolled out of the building on a stretcher, reading a book. *Only Dorje*, I thought.

Books were my only entertainment in Boulder because Dorje and Michael didn't have a television—some hippie shit that I didn't understand. Still, in the end, it was cool. We had dinner together often. My mother was a great cook. Then after dinner, she and I would pick a spot in the living room, grab a cup of tea, and read. Every now and then she would laugh aloud. I loved to hear her laugh because there was so much sorrow underneath her skin. I wanted her to have some happiness. There was a part of her that I would never know—a dark side she sealed tightly. Drugs had taken their toll on her. If you looked closely, you could see she was once a pretty woman.

She still wouldn't talk about her past—only bits and pieces of what her and my father's life was like. This became even clearer one Saturday morning when I came down for breakfast. Michael asked, grinning from ear to ear, "Who's that on the refrigerator?"

"Awwww, ain't she a cute little baby?" I said, as I went to turn the teakettle on.

"You don't know her?" Michael asked. "Look again," he insisted.

I studied the pictures and saw there was something familiar about the baby. I kept looking at it. Dorje had come into the kitchen by then. They were both looking at me intently. I knew I was missing *something*. I couldn't figure it out for a whole thirty seconds. "Oh My God! That's me!" I shouted with glee.

Her mother had sent the pictures. Prior to this day, I had only seen that one picture Aunt Lula Mae gave me of my father holding me when I was three months old. But that day, I discovered I had lived with my mother and father in Buffalo for at least a year before my grandfather took me away from them, refuting Mama's insistence that I came as a newborn baby. One picture was of me sitting in front of my homemade birthday cake with one candle on it. There was also a picture of my mother sitting next to me in a black turtleneck with her very blonde hair up in one of those 1960s beehive styles that was popular back then. Just as I had known, she had been a pretty woman. When I came back into the kitchen later that day, the picture of her and me was gone. I asked about it. She told me she burned it because she didn't want any memories of her drug days around, and that was the end of it.

I remember her frustration about repeatedly having to do blood work for Canadian immigration when preparing to get her visa. Canada had and still has socialized medicine, and authorities wanted to be sure she was no longer an addict before they awarded her a visa. Having to repeat blood work was tough on her, and it was a trigger. She would come home angry and humiliated because they had to draw blood from her thighs. The veins in her arms were shot to hell from years of injecting heroin. Years later, when I started to receive HIV care at an AIDS clinic, I thought about her when I was having blood work done. Often there would be a woman in recovery from drug addiction with the same frustration that my mother had, because her veins were hard to find. I never failed to stop and thank God that my mother stopped using before the AIDS pandemic. Nonetheless, it hurt me to see my mother in such distress, but she pushed through all the paper work for the sake of her marriage.

About a month into my stay in Boulder, my vagina started itching so bad I wanted to rip it out of my body. I hadn't had sex and couldn't imagine what it could be. I stuck my finger inside my vagina to try and figure out what was wrong, and all this white, cottage-cheese-looking stuff was up inside there. I tried everything to get rid of the itch and white stuff. I bathed repeatedly. I even douched, which only made me red and raw, adding to the itching and burning.

After all the shaming at the hands of Mama, I dreaded having to tell Dorje because I couldn't predict her response. I also started to think that whatever was going on, I needed to see a doctor. I gave in and told her my vagina was itching and I couldn't figure out what was wrong. She asked if I had a discharge and what it looked like. When I told her it looked like cottage cheese, she started laughing hysterically. I didn't know what to make out of it. But I was immediately taken back to Mama and Ms. Virginia, and I felt like I had swallowed a cherry pit or two right then. I folded my hands across my chest and waited with dread for whatever was going to come out of her mouth next. After she regained her composure, she explained that I probably had a yeast infection. I had never heard of such a thing, and I didn't want to feel stupid, so I just looked at her. My facial expression must have said it all.

"You've never had a yeast infection?" she asked. I shook my head. She went on to explain that it was no big deal, saying something about the natural balance of my vagina being off. I looked at her with doubt and she reassured me. "Women get them all the time. It's very natural, Rae. But you do need to see a doctor," she said. She explained that it was a common fungal infection that wasn't like a sexually transmitted disease, and that you could get it even if you were still a virgin. It was moments like these when I knew I had been cheated out of a mother.

Twenty-Nine

COUSINS

"Family is suppose to be our safe haven. Very often,
its the place where we find the deepest heartache.**"**

—Iyanla Vanzant

I came back to Chicago right before Christmas 1981. Michael was leaving soon for Nova Scotia to begin the winter semester at his new job. Dorje would be joining him after their house was sold and everything was settled. I hated to leave my mother as much as I hated to leave Boulder. I loved the spirit of the city, but I never thought about trying to make a go at it on my own. Instinctively, I went back to the life I knew best, with one exception: I was going to live with my cousin Eleanor, Kenneth's mother. When she offered to rent me a room in her home, I jumped at the chance for a few reasons. For one thing, it was easiest for me—I wouldn't have to look for a place to stay all the way from Boulder. The other thing was that I liked Eleanor. She spoke to Mama on my behalf when I had to get my clothes from her and I was more than confident that she had my best interest at heart. I had some kind of idealistic belief that going from my birth mother to another biological family member would be just as peaceful as it had been at my mothers.

While living in Boulder, I thought I had prepared well for this phase of my life at nineteen. After my seasonal job at the boutique ended, I worked two ho-hum jobs. From 7:00 a.m. to 3:00 p.m., I worked at a magazine mail clearinghouse; and on evenings and weekends, I worked at the newly opened Swensen's Ice Cream Parlor. I had saved some money, minus my new wardrobe. The boutique gave us a whopping forty percent-off discount, and I made sure that I had something of everything there. I came back to Chicago with a new wardrobe and money in my pocket. Dorje had even written me check and asked me not to mention it to Michael.

I really didn't need another thing, but I told myself I needed to buy makeup. Old folks would have said money was burning a hole in my pocket. The first week of my return to Chicago, I went to Marshall Field's to get the works at the Fashion Fair cosmetic counter. Boulder didn't have any Black girl makeup, and I told myself that I was long overdue. There were no Black hair-care products in Boulder, either, but Dorje and Michael took me into Denver to a Black-owned beauty supply store we found in the *Yellow Pages*. Now back in Chicago, I was in desperate need of a hairdo, so the second thing I did was go out to Evanston to visit Coré and get my hair done. I hadn't seen her in well over a year. She was home from Spelman College trying to decide her next move. At the time, I didn't feel so bad about my issues with UAPB because she didn't much like Spelman, either. Angela, who was also a member of PAGE, had become really close with Coré and she was living with them, doing hair on the side. She worked magic on a head of hair.

When I came back to Eleanor's, my hair was *l-a-i-d!* But little old me went seeking approval. Eleanor made some remark about it not being *all that*. Her comment offended me. Then she said, in a deliberately catty way, "It needs some hair oil, if you ask me."

This was the era when Black girls had stopped using so much grease on our hair as well as retired the hot comb and roller sets for the softer, blow-dry look. I loved it. I knew my hair was fly, and her disapproval should not have fazed me. It should have, however, been my first sign that living with her may be a problem. Instead, I took my wounded ego to my room looking for hair oil. I would soon learn that Eleanor always had something negative to say, and I began to doubt my decision to stay with her. Prior to this, she had been nothing but kind to me. Now, I was witnessing a side of her I had not seen before.

It was freezing cold in Chicago, and I was stuck in the house spending most of my time in my room, away from Eleanor. Then Kenneth came home on leave from the army for the holidays, and he saved me. Every time he picked up the car keys, he asked if I wanted to "roll" with him. I didn't have to think about it twice; I'd do anything to keep me out of his mother's firing line. It was like living with Mama, but in a different way. Eleanor was a minister and didn't cuss or raise her voice or cut the fool like Mama but, good Lord, she could make me feel like shit, leaving me asking, *What just happened?*

Kenneth was everything, in my eyes. He was only two years older than me, but I looked up to him. He came across as older and more mature. He was wise beyond his years and spoke with authority, so I believed in him. He was a cool dude—laid-back and easygoing—and we had fun together. We laughed and talked about anything and everything. I felt close to him from the first time we met in Michigan at our great Aunt Geraldine's funeral. After I was raped and he sat with me for most of the night, my love and appreciation for his place in my life were sealed. He wasn't just my third cousin; he was also my friend. His mother and my father had spent their childhoods together, and their mothers were sisters. I felt like we were carrying on tradition.

One afternoon, on one of our outings, we were sitting in Burger King on 95th Street, close to their house. Somehow, we got onto the subject of dating and sex. It eventually shifted from generalities to our own sexual prowess and experiences. We were having fun talking all kinds of shit about how good we were in bed. The next evening, we went out to dinner with his mother and one of her friends. I was having a good time. Kenny and I were whispering and laughing like two schoolchildren. After I finished eating, I touched up my lipstick and Eleanor lit into me about proper etiquette. She just had to ruin the evening. The irony of her reading me the riot act about proper etiquette during dinner just went right over her head. Kenneth gave her a look and she stopped. He pushed my knee with his knee, and I smiled. He leaned in close and whispered, "If you're that good in bed, you should show me." I shook my head and gave him a side-eye. If this was his way of trying to lighten the moment and make me laugh, I wasn't participating. After we got home, I went to my room to lick my wounds. When Eleanor turned in for the night, I came back downstairs to hang out with Kenneth. He resumed the topic about the two of us having sex. I thought he had been kidding at dinner but, nope, he was serious. I was shocked.

"Kenny, we are cousins, boy-y-y!" I said.

He came back with, "So what? Cousins marry."

I knew that, in some cultures, this was true; however, in the African American tradition, it was taboo. Black folks talked about children being crazy because of family interbreeding. He wasn't proposing babies, but he was dead serious about the sex. I listened as he explained that we undoubtedly had chemistry. I couldn't deny that fact. I knew this entire conversation was problematic, but he had my attention. From the beginning, I was caught up in the thrill of the back-and-forth game of sexual intrigue between us. Banter had long been a problem for me, and I should have stopped myself on day one. Now, we were on day two, and I listened to his mack with a curiosity that would eventually need to be fed. Maybe my self-esteem needed to be fed, too. After all the hits I had taken from his mother, perhaps I needed to prove my worth the best way I knew how: between the sheets. Whatever got me to that place of considering his proposal happened when he said, "The way I see it, if you are as good as you *say* you are, and I'm as good as I *know* I am, it sounds like some great sex."

"Ohhhh, I'm good!" I defended my sexual prowess.

"Action speaks louder than words," he said with that gorgeous smile of his plastered all over his face.

"We'll see," I said, and went upstairs to bed.

The next day he started again. I gave him a playful hit. "Stop it," I said, "It's not going to happen." He leaned closer to me on the sofa and cooed, "Can't nobody lick you the way I can." I hit him playfully again but my coochie said, *Aw-ww— shit*, and twitched a little. The next thing coming out of my mouth was "Proof is in the pudding." We had gone too far, and neither one of us put on the brakes. Next thing I knew, we were in the basement on the sofa bed. The sex was *un-freaking believable*. It got so good to us that we threw caution to the wind and hooked up the next night, and the next. If he wasn't concerned about his mother, I wasn't, either. The third night, in the midst of our hookup, I heard a voice say, "Stop it." At first, I thought I was imagining things because the voice was barely audible. My legs were wrapped around Kenneth's neck and his face was buried right in-between them.

"Kenneth, I said, stop it." This time, the voice was a little more forceful, but never raised above a deafening calm. We were both buck naked. Kenneth got off me as calmly as his mother's request and put his robe on like it was no big deal. He stood by the sofa bed, looking at his mother, who was standing at the foot of the stairs glaring at me. The tension in the room was so thick it swallowed all the air. I wanted to get up, but I felt as small and nasty as those rotten green peas Mama made me eat when I was a little girl. Kenneth didn't say anything to his mother. He just stood looking at her with an air of defiance. He had no response, no shame and no apology. NOTHING. It was like his mother hadn't just caught him performing oral sex on his third cousin with her legs wrapped around his back in pure ecstasy. I grabbed the sheet to cover my naked body. "Put some clothes on, Rae, and go upstairs," Eleanor said. I hated to have to get up in front of her, but there I was. *Ain't no point in being ashamed now. I wasn't ashamed when we were doing that thang.* Eleanor did not turn away. She watched me get out of the sofa bed and reach down to get my robe and put it on. I wanted to say I was sorry, but no one else was talking. I decided maybe it was best to keep my mouth shut, too. I walked past her and went up to my room. They stayed downstairs, I assumed, to talk. I was sure she would come up to my room to speak with me, but she didn't. The next morning when I came downstairs, Kenneth was gone. Eleanor said, "Good morning." That's it. I opened my mouth to apologize, and she put her hand up to stop me. I felt like shit with vomit on top.

What made it downright bizarre was that Kenneth had no intention of stopping our sexual relationship. But I had enough. I said to him one night, "Stop asking. Your mother caught us once."

"I got this under control," he said, like he was the boss of his mother *and* me, or something. Well, I really had it under control. I knew when to call it quits. I didn't understand their relationship. Kenneth seemed unbothered and continued to undress me with his eyes, with Eleanor mean-mugging me every time I moved.

A few days passed, but you wouldn't know it because the house was still pulsing with tension like the night when she caught me wrapped around him. It was too weird and stressful for me, and I went to visit Veronica who was home from college for the holidays. When I got back, Eleanor announced she was going to California with Kenneth to visit the military base, and that I was to move in with her sister, Ann. I didn't know what to think. I waited for Kenneth to intervene or even talk to me about the situation, but it never happened. I was so mad at him that I could see red. If, like he said, he had it under control, then why was I being displaced? I was taking all the hits when it had taken two of us to tango. He got to go back to California with his mother like everything was hunky-dory, and I got punished by having to move. I asked her if I could stay at her house on my own. After all, I *was* grown. She said something about not being sure how long she would be gone; therefore, she didn't want me there. It was plain that she was alluding to my behavior instead of saying it outright. That passive-aggressive game she and her son were playing left a bad taste in my mouth.

Living at Ann's was a nightmare. Her smile said that everything was fine, but the tension and tone of her voice reflected the opposite. I assumed Eleanor told her I seduced Kenneth. I never knew the arrangement Eleanor made for me to live there and I didn't ask; I didn't want to rock the boat. In the scheme of things, Eleanor could have thrown me out of her house outright after she caught Kenneth and me but she didn't.

I had to purchase my own food and make my own meals, which I didn't mind, but all the religious rules were a pain in the butt. If you recall, Ann was the cousin whose church I visited with Aunt Lula Mae. She was a devout Seventh Day Adventist, and they followed the kosher rules that God laid out to the Jews in the book of Leviticus. They don't eat unclean meat like pork and shellfish, and some are vegetarian. Ann ate a lot of meat substitutes, which had an odd smell when she cooked it. I hated to put my food in the refrigerator because that smell sometimes transferred into it. I could not cook pork in her house, either. They also followed the Sabbath, which begins on Friday at sundown and ends Saturday at sundown, and I was expected to follow this custom. I couldn't even iron a blouse after the sun went down on Friday. I could do nothing that was considered labor. I was thankful, at least, that she didn't make me go to church with her. The real pain in the neck was where she lived. Morgan Park was a public transportation nightmare in the early eighties. I couldn't look for a job because it was so far from the center of Chicago. The Chicago winter vortex didn't make it any better, and I felt isolated. One day I felt that if I didn't get out of there, I was going to lose my mind. I didn't really have a planned destination, so I set out on the bus for *anywhere*. When I transferred to the train, I decided to keep on going to Evanston, which is about thirty miles north of where Ann lived. I didn't know who I was going to visit, except that it sure as heck wasn't going to be Mama.

I was feeling a little nostalgic and decided to drop in and chat with the owners of Selig's clothing store. When I stepped out of the train at the Davis Street stop in downtown Evanston (in my cute boots), I slipped on some ice. When I picked myself up off the platform, I knew something was wrong with my ankle. I should have turned around right then, but *n-o-o-o*, I stuck to my decision. I hopped to the store, and they had me put my ankle up. I hung out there for a couple of hours shooting the breeze. When they closed the store at six, my ankle had swollen to the size of a baseball. Outside there was a full-fledged winter storm in effect. Making it back to Ann's took over three hours. When I arrived, I got some ice and put my foot up. Ann asked what was wrong, and I told her what happened. Her response was no response: We were in the middle of Sabbath, and she pulled out her Bible and sat down to read. There was not a further question or comment about my ankle.

I was in so much pain I called Veronica to see if she could come get me. She couldn't drive to get me because the weather was so bad, and she lived all the way back by Evanston. I eventually broke down and called Ethel. She and her boyfriend, Earl, came and took me to the hospital, waited with me, and brought me back to Ann's. The doctor told me I had a bad ankle sprain and instructed me and to stay off it for a few days. I was in so much pain I could barely do anything. I couldn't stand up long enough to cook. Ann offered me no relief or support. I knew I had to get out of that house. I already hated her stares and all the freaking religious rules. Now, with my ankle in bad shape, I really wanted out.

The next day I spoke to Veronica and told her I needed to quickly find a place to live. It turned out her great-aunt Sara was looking for a temporary boarder. She spoke with her on my behalf, and the next day, she picked me up and I moved in. Ann wasn't home when I moved. I left a note saying I had found a new place to live, and "Thanks." Once my ankle was better, I started looking for a job. Unfortunately, McDonald's was all I could find. I wasn't trying to make McDonald's a career, but I needed income. Those first two weeks back in Chicago, I had spent more money than I should have on even more clothes I didn't need. I also had to pay rent again once I moved in with Veronica's aunt. McDonald's would have to do while I continued to look for something better.

Eleanor was gone for a good month. I had phoned and left messages, and she never called me back. I wanted to get the rest of my belongings from her house. I had only packed some of my things for Ann's, believing that I was coming back to Eleanor's when she came home from California. It took a couple of months for me to catch her at home. We set up a time for me to pick up the rest of my clothes, and a friend from McDonald's drove me there. When I arrived, she asked for storage fees plus interest for the length of time my things were at her house. I had given her a three-month advance. She said she had given that money to Ann, and when I left Ann's, I forfeited the money. She said I should have gotten all of my things out of her house when I moved to Ann's. I knew this was bullshit. Eleanor was talking like it was me who initiated my move. She never told me to take all of my belongings and gave me the impression I could come back when she returned. Everything happened so quickly, and I was so jumbled. I didn't have the money to give her that day because I had given Aunt Sara an advance for a few months. Without her storage fees I couldn't take my clothes that day, and they would continue to accrue until I removed them. This was her payback. I had to suck it up.

After I scraped together the money to pay her and collect my things, I noticed she had gone through my trunk. I felt as violated as she must have felt catching me sexing her son in her home. When I looked inside one of my diaries, this long-ass letter well over five pages handwritten on yellow legal paper fell out. It was clear she had read every one of my diaries. Being a minister and all, in the letter, she quoted a lot of scriptures. The gist of the letter was her prophecy that I was "possessed by a sex demon." She then gave me guidance on cleansing myself. A part of me thought she was mad crazy. *And who gave her the right to judge me?* I was HOT MAD from reading her letter. Yet, another part of me wondered if she was right.

Everything that had transpired would end my relationships with these relatives from my paternal grandmother's father's side of the family. I took my portion of the blame and retreated. The most difficult admission for me was that I had no remorse whatsoever about having sex with Kenneth at the time. I only regretted doing it in her house. Violating Eleanor's home troubled me. I asked myself, *What could have made me have sex in this woman's house?* I had no answer, and I didn't have a defense. I was wrong. I would never have violated Mama's house in this way.

In time, however, the sexual act itself became the most disturbing for me—especially after I was diagnosed with my first sexually transmitted disease. I piled this incident on top of the others and looked at them as proof that something was deeply wrong with me. For the longest time, I held onto the letter to remind me how fucked up I was. When I lost my diaries shuffling from place to place, I also lost the letter—and a part of me was happy that I didn't have its energy hanging around. I hoped my diaries and the letter were floating somewhere in Lake Michigan, and not lying somewhere in the basement of someone's home. In this moment, I just thank God I have been liberated from the bondage of my secrets.

Thirty

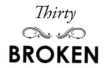

BROKEN

" A history of trauma teaches you to figure out what you did wrong to make people
mistreat you. A history of trauma teaches you to apologize for your wounds.
Healing is about unlearning the lies."
—Dr. Thema Bryant-Davis

I was sure I was broken, and pieces of me were scattered about. Worse, I had no fucking
idea how to put myself back together again. How many times had I already asked:
Girl, what the fuck is wrong with you? Now, here I was estranged from my father's
family, displaced, missing my mother, and asking the same damn question yet again.

I wanted to fix my situation. I even wanted to fix me, but I didn't have a clue how
to begin. What I had was a deep yearning to be back in Boulder with my mother again.
I craved it every single day. It had been the first break from chaos that I could recall in
my nineteen years of living. It was as different as night and day compared to any other
time in my life. I wanted that life again. That reprieve had done a lot for my self-esteem.
Without all the chaos and noise that had shaped my life prior to that point, I felt good
about myself. I even started to believe I had been fixed in some way. I hadn't made any
jacked-up decisions living in Boulder. Life was as normal as it could be for a nineteen-
year-old, but then, I didn't have any responsibility other than to just *be*. I believed that,
moving forward, my life would be different. I had come back to Chicago thinking I could
handle living on my own this time around. The reality was I was still nineteen years old
and responsible for every crumb of food I put in my mouth. Yet, somehow, I thought I
was on track. I was sure I could make better choices. I felt changed, but I wasn't. Three
months of living in an environment with no trauma could not erase the impact of living
with trauma for so many years.

Now that I was back in Chicago, life had become completely convoluted for me.
Nothing I thought was real, and the things that were real held me hostage. All I had left
from my time in Boulder were the memories of what it was like to live in peace and a
trunk full of beautiful clothes, with barely a place to hang them. The time I spent in
Boulder began to feel like fatting the cow before the slaughter. I even envisioned myself
walking toward the slaughterhouse. It hurt to the core of me to be so far off base from
what I wanted for myself. I thought if they had only taken me with them to Nova Scotia,
I wouldn't be in this mess. I wanted to go but I never dared to ask; but I hoped they
would. With no understanding of how complicated it was to move to another country; I
assumed the worst: They didn't want me.

My issues with rejection were bubbling over—not only with my mother but with
my cousins. I didn't understand why Eleanor never sat Kenneth and me down together
to talk about what occurred. The entire scene was dysfunctional and left me unsettled. I
felt as if I had been punished and Kenneth just walked away without a scratch. I tell you
what: If it had been Mama who found us in that compromising position, she would have
beat Kenneth off my ass and then beat me—but we would have understood our actions
were as wrong as a right shoe on a left foot. I could understand why Eleanor didn't want
me in her house anymore, but the fact that Kenneth had just thrown me away hurt the

most. How it all went down was disconcerting and started to cancel the residual calm I had felt from living with my mother. I would have given anything to be back in Dorje and Michael's living room reading a book and sipping on a cup of strong black tea—but I wasn't. I was out in the world again trying to be an adult.

Living with Veronica's Aunt Sara, I thought long and hard about my current situation. I needed to get my life together. Now that I was away from that environment and left to contend with my own conscience, I admitted to myself that I had fucked up again. Having sex with my cousin became one more thing added to my list of atrocities that seemingly substantiated I was the problem. I hadn't been fixed at all. I was broken. The problem was that I couldn't figure out how to change myself.

I couldn't compare this situation with any other thing that I had done, then or after. It was in a category all by itself and added an even heavier weight on my spirit. I would wear the stain in my soul like a scarlet letter for decades. I didn't dare divulge what Kenneth and I had done to a living soul. As usual, I felt the course of events was my own fault—and there was the problem. *No one told you to open your legs* became my mantra after each screwup with a man. I used it as a weapon against my soul. Why I let everyone else off the hook is still beyond my understanding. It was one thing to accept my own culpability, but to internalize the blame as all my own was beyond damaging.

I didn't think much of myself. Worse, I could not pull myself out of the slump of disappointment. I was at a loss when I landed at Sara Frazier's bungalow on South Jeffery Boulevard. All I could really think to do was pray, which I did—a lot. I even prayed that the prayer I had just said would help me. I hadn't given up on God like I had given up on myself, and I hoped God hadn't given up on me. Little did I know God was already working on my behalf.

I came to live with Aunt Sara out of what I considered desperation. In retrospect, I ended up exactly where I was supposed to be. I believe my emotional state was critically fragile during this time and Aunt Sara was exactly the remedy I needed. That, I believe, was the *God factor*. Just like the angels who were placed in my path when I was younger, it was happening again. At that point in my life, it was vital to live in a space that could counteract my low self-esteem. At Aunt Sara's home I was never judged—not with actions, mannerisms, or words. She worked on me against the negative noise inside my head that was holding me captive. She continually encouraged me and made practical suggestions about what I could do next. When our paths crossed—always in the dining room—we sat at the table and she gave me advice as if I were her niece, and I gave her my full attention. Sometimes she repeated what she said earlier in the same conversation, but in a different way, and she always used my name: "*Rae*, I think you can do anything you set your mind to do. *Rae*, it is never too late. *Rae*, everyone has *something* they can do." She said my name in an endearing way and the very sound of it held a kind of validation that lifted me and made me pay attention. She suggested that I enroll in Olive Harvey Community College because it was near her home, and I did. I was grateful for the one bus ride straight to Olive Harvey because that January was one of the coldest that I could ever recall living in Chicago, with wind chills of minus seventy degrees Fahrenheit. When I started school, I spent most of my time hanging out on campus. I would get there for my first class and hang out in the cafeteria, studying in between classes. About the second week of classes, I became friends with a girl about my age who was a fly-ass dresser. We had a class together, and one day she came over to me in the cafeteria. I think we bonded over clothes. I can't remember her name for the life of me, but for a few months she was my running buddy. It is crazy, though, to note the little things you remember.

I will never forget that she was of the Apostolic faith and attended a popular church: Monument of Faith, with Pastor Richard Henton. We'd be chatting in the cafeteria, and every single time the Luther Vandross song, *A House is Not a Home* came on the radio, she would stop dead in her tracks and start singing. She would then abruptly stop and say something like, "Lord, forgive me. I know I'm not supposed to listen to secular music, but I LOVE this song!" Then she went back to singing with Luther. I hadn't even heard of Luther Vandross at the time. He had just come on the scene, and with me having lived in Boulder—a primarily white community—in a house that didn't have a television meant I had missed out on Black culture.

It was with this girlfriend that I met the first guy I dated after my return from Boulder. Now mind you, I had decided to stay the heck away from men after the fiasco with Kenneth. However, this decision to put men on hold lasted until five minutes after she and I stepped into the school gymnasium to watch the guys at basketball practice. My eyes locked with this man's eyes, and that was all she wrote. I couldn't just lock eyes with one of the players my age; it had to be the freaking athletic director/basketball coach, who was thirteen years my senior. While my friend had her eyes on the starting player, I had mine on the coach. I don't know what I was thinking or even if I was thinking at all. I responded to what was familiar: dating older men.

From the get-go, my relationship with Gil was going nowhere fast. He was a nice and smooth man in the scheme of things. We had some good times—or, should I say, some good sex—in his Hyde Park apartment. Then one day it hit me like a ton of bricks: no matter how good a fuck I was, it was not going to go in my favor. In all fairness, he never promised me a fairy tale; I just had it floating somewhere in my head. From the start, I always had unrealistic expectations. I was the woman to pick out the wedding dress in my head and didn't even know the guy's middle name, or if he had one.

In this regard, dating was never how I imagined going into my relationships. I wanted the fairy tale of living happily ever after; I just didn't know how to go about getting it. I never tried to force a commitment. I was too insecure and afraid that if I insisted, he would walk away, leaving me with nothing. Call me naive, stupid or in denial, but I honestly went with the flow and hoped it would develop into something deep and meaningful. It rarely did. My ideas about dating were haphazard at best—sometimes learning along the way, other times repeatedly making the same mistakes until the lesson was finally learned. "We repeat what we don't repair" was a way of life for me. Psychologists call this "repetitive compulsion," when a person unconsciously places herself in situations where past traumatic events are likely to occur again. People are creatures of habit, and I was no different, seeking what was most familiar and what brought me comfort until it turned sour. The failed relationship would wreck my already damaged self-esteem even more.

I should add that I picked up my dating clues from society, Mama, and my history as a survivor of childhood sexual abuse. Society told me I wasn't complete without a man, so I was always searching. Mama created the tension in me between normal sexual maturation and respectability, and I never learned what healthy relationships were supposed to look like. My abusers taught me that sex was the only way someone could love me. So, I reasoned if I were exceptional in bed, it would seal the deal. As a result, I told myself to give him time and keep on pleasing him until he saw the light. This was another pattern, and when things went no further than sex, I would start to feel unloved, unlovable, and used. Only then would I begin easing my way out of the relationship. After a while, I started to avoid Gil. It was easier for me to quit by default rather than face the painful reality that I meant nothing to him.

I was also having a hard time keeping up with my classes. Just like at UAPB, I could not focus on work long enough to study or get through a page of reading without my mind wandering off to nowhere. By spring break, I faced the fact that I wasn't cutting it, and I withdrew to avoid the financial penalty. When I withdrew from Olive Harvey, the distance helped me get Gil out of my system. "Out of sight, out of mind," was as much power as I could muster. He went in the fuck-up column, right beside school.

After I stopped seeing Gil, I started dating a fellow co-worker at McDonald's who was only a few years older than me. We became friends right away. He was the person who had taken me to get my clothes from Eleanor's house. Eventually, we started flirting and chatted on the phone, which was the standard for "courting" back in the day (plus dinner and a movie, of course). I was going to do everything right this time around and I told myself, I could at least fix something.

For a while it was going great. Then it went downhill the night I finally agreed to take it further. I started to have doubts when we arrived at his apartment. He lived in a rundown building that had been made into a boarding house. His room was small and untidy. I tried not to be judgmental, but the next morning I could see that his room was more than untidy; it was dirty. The bathroom down the hall was shared by the residents on that floor. The smell of urine assaulted my nostrils the moment I opened the door. There was dried urine on the floor and droplets all over the toilet. Men! Thank God, Grandmamma Julia had taught me to squat. I wanted to wash my hands but took a pass on the sink that clearly hadn't been cleaned since—oh, I don't know—maybe forever? I didn't even bother to look at the shower; I was too grossed out about everything else. When I came back to the room, he went to take a shower, like the filth was no big deal. I got dressed and sat on the side of the bed with my coat in my lap. I didn't want morning sex or to cuddle. I wanted to go home. I couldn't figure out what was worse: screwing around with a man who I could never spend the night with or waking up after a night of great sex to learn that the only toilet was a shared one down the hall—and filthier than the Chicago subway. His lifestyle was depressing. That day I learned you never really know someone until you see how that person lives. This was especially true back then, if you followed the rules of courting and waited to have sex like I had done. I knew I wanted more than he had to offer. My life wasn't all that but, hell, at least I was clean. This relationship also reiterated why I had decided earlier to no longer date a co-worker. I couldn't tell you why I had reneged on that decision. It became incredibly uncomfortable to wiggle out of a relationship when I had to see the person every day. Well, I got fired—again—from another franchise and the problem of that relationship was solved. Like with Gil, my latest fuck-up took on the mantra of "Out of sight, out of mind."

I could run, but I couldn't hide from myself. Trying to make sense of dating rules added another layer of misery. I was damned if I did and damned if I didn't. I had been in and out of relationships that included sex more than I wanted to admit even to myself. Somewhere deep within, I knew there was a problem. I knew in my gut that the way it played out was not how it should be—not the sex, per se, or the partners, but how they each played out in my life. For sure that rat-a-tat-tat-tat I spoke of in the introduction had started to peck away at my soul, but did nothing to relieve my misery. This feeling however, wouldn't let me give up or stop searching for a better way to live. Thank God for my authentic self for trying to climb out of the rumble of trauma that had trampled over what God had intended for my life.

A unt Sara continued to be a blessing to me during this time. She repeatedly gave me little nuggets that pushed me to think and lift my spirits at the same time. One day she said to me, "You are one tough cookie, Rae." Her words reminded me that I had always thought of myself as tough, even if I didn't feel that way in that moment.

"Rae, you've done admirably, considering your circumstances," she told me one day. While I saw myself as tough, I had never viewed any part of my life as a success. I was always in survival mode. Coping was normal for me. When I was in the thick of it, I didn't celebrate—not even a small victory. A hit was a hit, no matter how big or small it was, and no matter how I patched my wounds, it still hurt. Instead of celebrating myself, I absorbed the pain and kept moving. I had never gotten the kind of praise I received from Aunt Sara—not even from my peers. I think they were accustomed to my calamities and often viewed me as a drama queen. Now, hearing from Aunt Sara that I had done well was like manna from heaven. It was an *aha moment* for me when I realized that I had done the best as I could for myself, considering my circumstances.

Veronica was also pushing me to move forward, just like her great-aunt had. Their persistence ran in the family, and, in the end, I learned to appreciate it. When she suggested that I apply to Southern Illinois University at Carbondale (SIU-C), where she had gone her first year, I replied, "Yeah, right—like they gon' take me." By this time, I thought my academic life was a complete failure and I didn't think I could cut it. I had withdrawn from two colleges. My high school grades and ACT scores were following me everywhere, and there was no one to intervene on my behalf at SIU-C like the recruiter from UAPB had, who recommended me for that school's special admissions program. Regardless of my outward doubts about my abilities, I wanted more than anything to complete my education. I just didn't want to risk being rejected. Veronica kept pushing me. I can still hear her saying, "Well, Rae," pausing in her dramatic manner before continuing, "How do *you know* they won't accept you?" She had a point, even if I had more evidence to prove that I was unworthy. Thank God she was known for going on and on when she had a point to prove. I eventually got tired of her badgering me about it and applied. When I received my letter of acceptance all I could say was, "but God!" Veronica said, "See, I told you."

I was admitted to SIU for the fall of 1982 through a program like the one at UAPB, for students with below-average ACT scores. This acceptance went a long way to help bring me back to the Rae I had been when I first moved to Evanston: the one who believed she could do the impossible against all the odds. It put me back on track. I completed my financial aid applications because I wanted nothing to interfere with me beginning school in the fall. I can see today how it all started to line up for me. Even my financial situation, or the lack thereof, came together. I was still desperately looking for a new job when another small miracle happened. Mama and I made up again and that was nothing but God, for real.

On Memorial Day, I visited Grandmamma Julia. When I walked through the door, I walked right into Mama's face and was sucked into her vortex. It was the first time I had seen her in nearly a year, and she carried on like she hadn't thrown me the heck out of her house for no reason and pulled a butcher knife on my friends. All I could do was shake my head. When I told her I was going back to college in the fall, she explained she was lonely and thought I should come back home and save my money until I went off to school.

Mama had this way about her that was irresistible. My repetitive compulsion took on a life of its own one way or another when it came to Mama. I wanted to hate her as much as I wanted to love her. As crazy as it sounds, some part of me missed her, too, and another part of me felt sorry for her. I accepted her offer. Not having to pay rent for a few months wasn't a bad deal, either. I eventually found a job and was able to start saving for college. Miraculously, Mama and I made it through the summer without any significant incidents.

Thirty-One

❧

COLLEGE LIFE

"Forgive yourself for not knowing what you didn't know before you learned it."
—Maya Angelou

I took Amtrak to Carbondale, Illinois in late August 1982 to begin my first year at Southern Illinois University at Carbondale (SIU). I had just turned twenty. I had a roof over my head and three meals a day; to my surprise, the cafeteria food wasn't that bad! I got a work-study job as a clerk at the Student Center information desk, and my Social Security checks came again because I was back in school. I thought I was at a good place in my life.

It had been one long year from the last time Mama put me out. There was my blip of a stay at Veronica's; my time at UAPB; onward to Boulder with my mother; back to Chicago and my cousin Eleanor's place; to her sister Ann's home; to Veronica's aunt Sara's place; and then, back to Mama's. I had lived at eight places in one year. My God—just thinking about it is exhausting. It's no wonder I was a wreck. God had seen me through insurmountable odds that year, yet again.

I viewed Carbondale as a chance to start over. I took a taxi with all my possessions in that blue trunk from the train station to Neely Hall, where I would be living. There, I met my first friend and my first suitor, Tommy, and his fraternity brother Mickey after they offered to help take my trunk to my room. I would learn that Tommy was full of shit and Mickey would remain a lifelong friend.

If you were twenty-one or younger, you were required to live in the dorms. Veronica told me to ask for Neely Hall in my housing application. It was one of three dorms, along with Mae Smith, and Schneider that we called The Towers, which were popular among Black students. I liked living in Neely. The Towers were modern seventeen-story buildings with alternating floors for males and females, and great amenities. Each room had a sink, and we shared the bathroom and shower with the students in the adjoining room. Each floor had a laundry room and a lounge with a television. There was also a resident assistant who handled any issues students had and helped to maintain decorum. Best of all, there was no freaking curfew or restrictions on who could visit your room like at UAPB.

Carbondale sits on the southern tip of Illinois. There were a mall and tons of fast-food restaurants within walking distance from campus. In fact, Main Street, referred to as The Strip, was the epicenter of campus social life, with restaurants and bars that catered to the twenty-thousand-plus students who attended the university.

I had a full-time first-year schedule of four classes. I also had to take an additional mandatory four-week classes for below-average students. I hated those required general study classes often taught by a teacher's assistant, trying to do the job of the professor. They were too large, impersonal, boring, and they failed to motivate me, which made it harder for me to stay focused. The problem of staying focused had followed me my entire academic life. It was at SIU where I began to acknowledge that I had some undefined issues that made school difficult. There were no excuses that I could make this time around. I felt helpless because I didn't know what to think or how to address whatever

I was lacking to be academically successful. In most of my classes, I was holding on by a thread of sheer determination. I went to class. I read the books, and I tried to take notes on lectures with teachers who talked faster than I could write. But the lectures never seemed to connect to the readings. In the middle of a lecture, sometimes I asked myself, *What the heck is he talking about?* I wanted to learn, and I knew I was capable, as I exhibited in my smaller classes that had more interaction. I excelled in those classes. I loved my Black studies professors because they didn't mind repeating themselves, and it seemed like they valued class participation, which allowed me to digest the lectures and readings.

Despite being hyper and talkative, it had always been natural for me to be by myself. I always realized that I was much more of an introvert, even if I seemed like an extrovert from the outside. I took discovery walks on SIU's sprawling campus, like I had done in Evanston and Boulder. I loved to walk over by the communications building, which was off the beaten path and surrounded by a beautiful, wooded area. Otherwise, I walked up The Strip and browsed around. Dairy Queen was always my first stop, even in cooler weather. In the warm months, I got a banana split, sat on the curb in front of the store to savor each spoonful and people-watched.

My absolute favorite place in Carbondale was a used bookstore on The Strip that I dropped into a few times a week. It was small and stuffy and had a generous selection of Black authors. Unlike when I browsed my favorite boutique on The Strip, which provided an adrenaline rush from trying on clothes, the bookstore was a nurturing and familiar space. I loved that earthy-vanilla smell of old books that is only found in used bookstores. It was a welcoming smell of comfort that said I belonged. Just like I took on Mama's obsession with clothes, I did a similar thing with Dorje and books. The difference was that clothes filled my space and made me feel loved, while books filled my soul. Before I met my mother, I was already an avid reader and books had developed a special place in my life. I have an enormous book collection that I began while living with Dorje. It was because of her that I first entered used bookstores. She helped to expand my reading experience, and the bookstores gave us places to bond. Now in Carbondale, I missed those days of us browsing used bookstores, meeting at the register with armfuls of books and laughing at our indulgence, but I could still experience the pleasure that perusing a bookstore brought to me when I was living with her.

While I spent a lot of time alone and sought spaces that made me feel the most at ease, I did enjoy the student center parties. It was one of the many spaces Black students carved out for themselves. Black students were roughly ten percent of the student population at SIU, and there was little socializing among Black and white students when I attended. While Black students patronized The Strip, it was not our primary hangout. Instead, we carved a cultural and social space we could call our own through Black organizations and campus-sponsored events. We had Alpha Phi Alpha fraternity, Miss Black and Gold Pageant, and other fraternities and sororities held events. The Black Fire Dancers held a performance every year and the Black Affairs Council (our version of student government) sponsored lectures featuring prominent African Americans. There were also small off-campus gatherings within the safety of people's apartments where we mostly played spades and bid whist. Black folks take playing cards very seriously, and I sorely lacked card-playing skills, so I usually passed. I found my niche at the student center parties sponsored by Black student organization. I liked the parties because there were no alcohol or drugs. They were often packed, affording me the freedom to be me with no pretense. I'd slide on a pair of Levi's 501 jeans, an Izod button-down Oxford shirt and penny loafers, and head to the student center to dance the night away. House music was on the rise and the most popular disc jockey team—DJ Inc., which consisted of Norman Powell, Erik Rye *aka* Freaky Bert, and my friend Reggie Pruitt—had perfected their method of continuous tunes that were the cornerstone of house music. A round of music would begin with one song, for example, *"Let No Man Put Asunder,"* and without a break transition to another song, *"Love Sensation,"* then to *"Dr. Love,"* and on to *"Let's Go Dancing"* and would end with *"Walk the Night."* The music never stopped and right before the last song in one cycle finished, they began the next round of songs that fit together perfectly. Those nights were magical: the music, my feet on the dance floor and freedom. When I was dancing, I felt like I had been sprinkled with fairy dust and transported to a wonderland. After the party, I went back to my room still floating from the energy I had worked up on the dance floor. Back at the dorm, I would sometimes shoot the breeze with Donna Ford, who was my closest friend at SIU, and order a pizza. Other times, I turned on the cassette player and listened to one of the tapes Reggie had given me and lay in bed, bopping my head to the beat until I fell asleep.

Donna and I met the second day I moved into the dorm. She lived just down the hall from my room in Neely Hall. She was a first-year student with a larger-than-life personality and who had a lot more friends than I. She was well-dressed always matchy-matchy from head to toe. She had long beautiful hair with blond highlights. One night, she and I bonded over hair, and the rest is history, as the saying goes. She knocked on my door to see if I had any hair conditioner. When I saw her jar of Revlon hair relaxer in one hand and regular shampoo in the other, I had a flashback to my perm disaster and asked if she had neutralizing shampoo. She was just as oblivious as I had been, so I helped a sista out. I told her about my near disaster from putting in my own perm without using neutralizing shampoo. I cautioned her and pulled out my neutralizing shampoo and handed it to her. After that night we became friends. We still laugh about me saving her beautiful hair. We spent most of our time together eating. We often walked to get a burger at Burt's, a popular place on The Strip. On weekends, we'd put our funds together and order pizza and chill.

My other close friend was Reginald "Reggie" Pruitt. I met Reggie because he worked at the mailroom in the lobby of the cafeteria where I had my meals. After I bumped into him that first time in the mailroom, I regularly stopped to chat at dinnertime when he was working. I had met his roommate, Phillip, during freshman orientation. He must have seen stupid written across my forehead because he wasted no time. Now, here I was, accustomed to dating older guys and thinking I was all savvy and shit, but Phillip immediately made me swoon and I fell into the freshman-upperclassmen trap. He had a girlfriend. When Reggie realized that Phillip was double-dipping, he tried to warn me, but I was already caught up in Phillip's web. One day purely by accident, I saw them on campus holding hands—and that was that. I immediately made my exit. I felt like a plum fool. It just so happened that by the time I learned that Phillip was a cheater, Reggie and I were becoming fast friends; neither one of us saw a reason why we shouldn't. He was smart and funny, and we slipped into a mutual friendship with ease. He became my confidante.

Partying was one thing; sex and dating were something different altogether. Everyone I knew was having sex. The freedom away from home took on a life of its own—like with my first roommate, who was always entertaining some guy she'd brought home from a bar. I'd wake up to the sound of sex moans. *WHAT THE HELL?!* My problem was more about them having sex while I was in the room. I believed it was disrespectful. I never did it and I certainly don't want to hear someone else having sex if I can avoid it. I told my roommate she had lost her freaking mind if she thought it was all right to bring strange dudes to our room in the middle of the night, or something to that effect. Anyway, before the semester was over, the saga of *My Roommate and The Strange Men* resolved itself. She was a white girl from Springfield, Illinois and, apparently, her father didn't like Black people, and he made her put in for a room transfer. I was delighted when the school assigned her to a new room.

Hormones were raging! We were all doing it, but admitting it was another thing. Respectability ruled and Black girls protected their reputations. Not a single one of us considered herself promiscuous, and we would have fought your ass to the ground for calling us a *hoe*. I never understood the policing of Black women's bodies while men were given passes. It was hypocrisy, at best: Men judged women and even other women judged other women. Of course, all these beliefs were wrapped in the self-hating and woman-shaming respectability-related values that were part of my upbringing at home and in my community. It only made us uptight and hypervigilant about rules that didn't have any real value on sex and dating, in the end. No matter how well I thought I curated my sex life, there was bound to be a man I wished I had never slid between the sheets with. Back then, the best way for a girl to guard her reputation was to get a boyfriend as quickly as possible and pray the guy you were hooking up with would be discreet. I didn't have a boyfriend during my first semester, so I prayed for discretion.

There was no shortage of suitors. I had more guys in one environment hitting on me than I ever had in my life. I also had a shortage of discernment skills and a room to myself, which made it easy to hook up. In retrospect, one would have thought my ass had been locked up in a nunnery and had not even lived on my own. All the attention was exciting but also caused constant tension between finding the right guy, maintaining a stellar reputation, and coming to terms with my own sexual identity. I have a big confession to make—I liked sex and the freedom to explore sexual boundaries. Back then, however, I would have never dared admit such a thing not to a girlfriend and not even to myself. That would come later. The girl who admitted that she liked sex was a "freak," and that label stayed with her. Yet, at the same time, I secretly rejected this idea that sex was wrong or dirty, but I didn't have a clue on what healthy sex was. It was during this time I began to think more about these values and where they fit into my life, even if I didn't resolve anything.

It was at SIU that I contracted my first two sexually transmitted diseases. And, before you ask, no, I was not using condoms. I've already mentioned that my generation believed that pregnancy out of wedlock was the greatest sin a girl could commit. To escape that fate, we took birth control pills or other contraceptives and guys, for the most part, relied on us. By and large, STDs were a secondary thought if they were a thought at all. Now, let's get back to my first two sexually transmitted diseases. There was this guy I had been friendly with the entire semester. The chemistry between us was sizzling like steaks on a grill. Every single time we saw each other, the talk got hot and heavy. I'm not even going to tell you that I saw him as boyfriend material; it was more curiosity and intrigue than anything. By the end of the semester, all the shit-talking led to a hookup. I look back on that night and ask, *What in God's name was I doing and why was it so important for me to prove to a man whose name I can't even remember that I was good in bed?* I was too impulsive, and once I was headed in one direction, I rarely stepped on the brakes. Let me digress for a moment: I'm not placing any moral judgment on this decision. Maybe I did at that time, but not today. I have come to a place where I believe that women of the age to consent should have the freedom to make choices about their own bodies, just like men. The problem for me was that I made decisions from an unhealthy, and often-distorted lens that created its own set of problems. I entered into relationships for the wrong reasons, and sometimes the outcome was brutal.

I can remember most of the details from that cold winter night of passion. I can even remember his physical appearance—like that beautiful dark chocolate skin and his Jheri curl hairdo—like it was yesterday. But I blocked dude's name out of my memory soon after I left SIU because remembering was an unwanted reminder of the outcome. That night, he was good, I was good, and the sex was everything we had promised each other it would be. When I left his room, I was satisfied and smug. I took a shower noticing that I was a little sore between my legs but didn't give it much thought because we had gone a couple of rounds. The next morning, I was still sore and a little itchy down there. I dismissed it again because the itching wasn't exactly between my legs, but around my pubic hair. *Whatever,* I thought, *maybe I am having a reaction to the soap or my lotion.* Sitting in class, the itching would not let up, and I was wilding out trying to scratch myself through my jeans on the down low. It was maddening—listening to a lecture and taking notes with an itchy coochie. I felt like I was going to lose my freaking mind. In between each class, I went to the bathroom and scratched and rubbed until I was red, but nothing helped. It felt like a slew of mosquito bites right between my legs. When I returned to my room, I took another shower and when that didn't help, I laid a warm towel compress on my pubic hair and then between my legs for a few minutes, refreshed the towel and repeated the process, but that did not ease the itching. I got dressed and went to the store to pick up some Ivory soap, made famous for its claim to be gentle. I was praying that it would help because I was out of ideas. But nothing quelled the itching or the soreness. I put some Vaseline on my red vagina and my pubic hair area and slept my blues away. The second day of itching was crazy, and I cut my day short. I skipped a class, ate lunch, and came back to my room. I was sore, irritable, and frustrated. I undressed and went to sleep. Later that night I had another round of warm compresses, took some Tylenol, and went back to sleep. The next morning, pain took up camp smack dab in the middle of my vagina. I lay there thinking, *what the hell was going on and how the hell was I going to get out of whatever the heck it was.* When I finally rolled out of bed to use the bathroom, I could barely walk because of the pain. I sat on the toilet and the urine trickling down my raw vagina felt like I had poured alcohol in-between my legs. I took some more Tylenol and went back to bed. By lunch, my tummy was talking to me. I had missed dinner and breakfast, and I knew it was time to go eat and face the world. Then water became my enemy, too. When I showered, that stung, and the Ivory soap burned like hell. Combined with the itching, I felt like I was on fire. I had never experienced anything like this, and I was shaken by it.

To get a better look at what was going on, I sat on the toilet with a make-up mirror and positioned it between my legs. The top of my vulva was fiery red and raw. I shifted the mirror down and attempted to pull the lips of my vagina apart. It was painful to touch but I followed through. I was shocked at what I saw. The insides of my vagina looked as if I had taken a razor and cut the top layer of my skin completely off. I had no clue what could have caused this. I thought about the yeast infection I had when I lived with Dorje. I tried to put my finger inside my vagina to see if I had the same cottage-cheese-like discharge, but it was too painful. As I continued to look down into the mirror, it appeared as if something was crawling around. I jerked the mirror back thinking it was on the mirror, but nothing was there. I moved my fingers through my hair and sure enough these little things were crawling around in my pubic hairs! *WHAT THE FUCK?!* I was scared out of my mind. I jumped my tail off that toilet and went straight to student health services.

When the doctor walked in, I wanted to disappear into thin air. I promise you, there is no shame worse than having to tell a middle-aged white man that you think something is crawling around in your pubic hair—unless you get caught sexing your cousin, that is. I wanted to leave, but I was so scared that something was seriously wrong with me. Also, the itching and burning were unbearable. I figured it was better to know than not to know.

The doctor listened with a poker face as I explained my problem. When I finished, he asked me to undress from the bottom down and get on the table, and he stepped out of the room. When he came back, he positioned himself between my legs to conduct the vaginal exam. I wanted to curl up and die. *Woman up, girl,* I told myself, and took a deep breath. I laid back and placed my feet in the stirrups. The doctor jammed that speculum into my raw vagina, and the pain shot through my body so fast I wanted to jump out of my skin. I clenched my thighs together so I wouldn't scream. *Oh, God—Oh, God*. I moaned silently, taking deep breaths to calm my nerves as he scraped my cervix. When he pulled the speculum out, I saw blood, and my eyes teared up. I sighed with relief when he turned around and slid the stool to swab the specimen slide. After that, he slid the stool back toward me, continuing the examination. I braced myself for whatever was coming next. He adjusted the light, shifting it upward to shine on my pubic hairs. Once the light was positioned, it only took seconds for him to focus on the area, stand up, snap off his gloves, wash his hands and instruct me to get dressed as he left the room. *Damn*, I thought. *I would have preferred more pain because now I feel like shit—a whole pile of it.*

When the doctor returned, I was sitting in the chair with my head down. I was already deflated by our interaction, and I didn't know how much more I could take. He got right to it. The little "things" crawling around in my pubic hair were a parasite commonly referred to as *crabs* because they are similar in appearance. He handed me a pamphlet. I had heard people talk about crabs but didn't know what they were. I asked him to explain, and he was cold as he rattled off what he felt I needed to know. Basically, crabs are a sexually transmitted disease. The doctor instructed me to clean my dorm room and wash all my clothes. Although rare, you could also transmit crabs through clothes, towels, and bed linen. He prescribed a chalky-like shampoo to kill the parasite. From the pamphlet, I learned that crabs are a form of pubic louse, with the scientific name *Pthirus pubis*—not to be confused with body or head lice.

After he finished that little bit on crabs, he moved on. I had also contracted the *herpes virus*. Like with crabs, I vaguely recalled hearing that term, but I couldn't say where. At the time, gonorrhea and syphilis were the only two STDs I had learned about in high school health class. I always thought I would know if a guy had either off these STD's because he would have a discharge coming from the head of his penis. Quite frankly, I wouldn't have known a discharge from an STD, from droplets of semen, if they were staring me in the face. Now that I had contracted not one but two STDs, I felt stupid. I didn't know as much as I believed I did about STDs. When the doctor told me there was no cure or treatment for herpes, I thought, *just shoot me now and get it over with*. Then he told me I wasn't going to die from it, and I thought, *well, it can't be that bad*. I had a thousand questions, but the doctor was impatient and condescending. I didn't know how to phrase the questions and felt even more stupid by the minute. I gave up. The doctor stood up to signal the end. As I was putting on my coat, he called out to me, "Young lady." I turned to face him, and he said, "You should watch who you have sex with." I gave him my *no-shit* look and walked out. I didn't need a lecture; I needed to be educated on how to care for myself and maneuver life—and, maybe, just a tad of compassion.

I walked out of the health center with the basics about herpes: There was no cure or treatment, and it will come back again. He didn't know how often it would come back, but he said I could infect someone else if I had sex during an outbreak. On my walk back to the dorm, my brain was in overdrive trying to remember where I had heard about herpes. Then it hit me: Dorje had sent me an article about the rise of herpes on college campuses across the United States. She was still in Nova Scotia and we had become pen pals. When I arrived back to my room, I shampooed away the crabs. I changed the sheets, washed every piece of my clothes and linens, and went digging for the letter with the article my mother had sent to me. *Well, now, lookey here: I had already been warned.* There was no internet or Google then; thus, I devoured the article looking for clues on what to do next. It was mostly about prevention, and it was too late for that.

I didn't say anything to Jheri-curl dude for a couple of reasons. First, I was afraid that it would get out. I had beat the rumor mill in high school, but this was a whole other level. I asked myself, *What if I tell him and he blabs to the whole freaking school. Then what?* Second, I wasn't sure that he was the person who infected me. *What if he denies it? Then I'm the one with egg on my face.* In the scheme of things, I weighed out what I knew. The virus is predictable in that it takes two to twenty days after exposure to have your first outbreak. It was true that I had never had an outbreak prior to having sex with him, but I still felt like I didn't know enough about the virus to make that kind of assessment. I could only deduce that it had to be him. I decided to move on, thinking, *I should have kept my legs closed.*

With everything I know now, I would have taken a chance to confront Jheri-curl dude because I hadn't had sex with anyone other than him in a couple of months, but I didn't understand herpes back then. I wanted to talk to another doctor about it, but there was no way I would go back to the student health center. Instead, I reassured myself with what I knew at the time—mainly, it was not going to kill me, and I could not infect my sexual partner unless I was having an outbreak. That, to me, was the most important information that I needed to know. I called myself locking my secret deep within, and it was eating away at me. I started sleeping through my morning classes. I could barely focus anymore and started falling behind in my readings. I brushed it off and crammed during finals, hoping I would at least pass. At Christmas break, I went to Mama's and slept most of the vacation away. I'm sure I was depressed, but I had no idea what depression looked like. I was so accustomed to handling things on my own, I just went on about life until I decided to reach out to my ex-fiancé, Larry. I don't know what I was thinking; I guess I was looking for a shoulder to cry on. It was a big mistake. He turned right around and told everyone he could. Ethel called to tell me that Larry was going around telling people I had herpes and that I wanted him to have sex with me because I couldn't get anyone else. I kept it simple and flat-out denied it. I was so embarrassed. I certainly hadn't been seeking sex. I was seeking advice and an opinion, I guess, on how he thought a man would respond if I disclosed my status. I was so angry at him that I never contacted him again.

Thirty-Two

TURNING POINT

"
I have planned it all out—plans to take care of you,
not abandon you, plans to give you the future you hope for.**"**
—Jeremiah 29:11

When I came back to school for spring semester, I knew that I had to make a change. The first order of business was to stay the hell away from men. I didn't need any more distractions and men were distractions, all day long. My inner voice told me, *If I had stayed away from men, I wouldn't have herpes or be on academic probation.* Yes, I said academic probation. I received my grades right before Christmas break was over, and my heart dropped to the pit of my stomach. I was already struggling and after I got herpes I started falling behind, but never had I thought I was in this much trouble. Being diagnosed with herpes had affected me more than I understood—and to the degree that I did understand, more than I admitted. When things really got bad, I put my emotions into a box and left them to suffocate. The fact is, I was too ashamed to talk to anyone about having herpes. In the weeks following my diagnosis, I slept my blues away. I barely went to class. When I arrived back at SIU, I was still in denial. Not being a morning person then, I blamed my bad grades on morning classes and my poor judgment with men. I changed my class schedule as soon as I got back to make sure it didn't work against me. During the first couple weeks I managed to keep up, and I planned to keep it that way. I gave myself a pep talk. God had made a way for me to come to SIU and I felt as if I had squandered the blessing. I had to do better. I just needed to stay focused.

I also had a new roommate. I had agreed to let this other girl move into my room because she was having roommate issues. She didn't talk very much, and we never really bonded. I figured she thought the worst of me because I was always half-naked. It was my custom to strip down to my panties as soon as I hit the door and throw on an oversized T-shirt. Other times, I lost the panties altogether and let my coochie breathe free. She, on the other hand, was as respectable as they get. I watched her every night in amazement as she placed her nightgown over her top, slipped her arms out and pull down her gown. The only parts of her body that I ever saw where her arms and legs. She was cool, though, and we never had any disagreements; however, we never had one real conversation. At least she wasn't bringing guys to the room, like my previous roommate, and her pious presence helped me to have more balance when it came to male company.

About two weeks into the semester, while sitting in the lobby of my dorm, a good-looking guy in a black suit and crisp white shirt with French cuffs started walking toward me. *Stay the fuck away from men,* I cautioned. When dude got closer, I gave him a look that said, *I'm not interested.* I was sure I had seen him on campus, looking dapper from head to toe like a Nation of Islam brother, but I didn't know his name. *I don't give a shit who he is; I'm sticking to my guns. No distractions good-looking or not.* He stopped directly in front of me with a big, beautiful smile.

"Hi," he said. "My name is Karriem Shariati." He stuck out his hand. "I'm the president of the Black Affairs Council." I looked at him like, *So what?* and cautiously shook his hand. Before I could open my mouth, he was making his pitch.

199

"I've been watching you around campus. You have a lot of energy," he said. I had that *O-kayyy—so what, negro?* type of attitude scrolled across my face. If he noticed, he didn't address it.

"How would you like to be the chairperson for our Campus and Community Affairs Committee?" It took a minute to sink in. I had to make a 180-degree turn because I had already prepared the "no" in my head. *Okay—so he's not trying to hook up.* I didn't know whether to be happy or sad. I mean, I at least wanted the chance to say no.

"I think that you will be perfect to head up Campus and Community Affairs for the BAC," he reiterated.

"To do what?" I asked with caution. I just knew there had to be a catch to it. I hadn't had a guy approach me since I came to SIU who wasn't self-serving. As Karriem explained the responsibilities, I began to relax. I was impressed and impressing me was not easy. Karriem appeared to be a little older and much more mature than the average student I encountered. He was intelligent and charismatic, and his passion for Black folks reflected in every word that came out of his mouth. I was thinking fast as he talked. If I accepted the offer, I would be responsible for coordinating social-justice activities that affected the African American student population at SIU and anything else that connected us to the community in Carbondale. It was a lofty project he was offering to me. It took me back to the Operation PUSH community forums I attended when Reverend Jackson called on the audience to serve, and I had the same emotional reaction: I was in — hook, line, and sinker.

My first assignment for the BAC was to conduct an absentee ballot drive among the African American students from Chicago to help swing the vote in favor of Congressman Harold Washington, who was running for mayor of Chicago. The first African American candidate, Congressman Washington had won the primary against the incumbent mayor, Jane Byrne, and candidate Richard M. Daley, son of the late Mayor Richard J. Daley. Thanks to the massive voter registration and Get Out the Vote spearheaded by African American leaders such as Lutrelle "Lu" Palmer, a journalist, activist, and founder of Black United Communities, which focused on increasing the Black vote, and Reverend Jesse L. Jackson, Sr. and Operation PUSH. They were joined by a host of other progressive organizations and Washington was now the Democratic candidate. Washington was in an historic battle with the Republican nominee, Bernard Epton.

I went to work on this project immediately. The excitement among African Americans in Chicago had spread like wildfire and it spilled over to our campus and made my task easy. I carried absentee ballot forms with me all the time. I was that girl, and everyone knew it. I wasn't letting anyone off the hook. Monday through Friday, I hung out in the student center for the unofficial Black social hour, collecting forms so that I could send them to the Chicago Board of Elections—even if it meant missing a class or two. My African American professors gave me tons of leeway, but I also excelled in their classes because they kept my interest.

Then in February, Karriem gave me an additional assignment after Reverend Tyrone Crider challenged us to help with Get Out the Vote on Election Day. Reverend Crider was the national youth director for Operation PUSH and one of our featured Black History Month speakers on campus. He was electrifying as he called on our generation to step up. He informed us that the Washington campaign would provide as many buses as we could fill for students who wanted to come back to Chicago on Election Day to help. This assignment was more difficult than collecting absentee ballots. Carbondale is three hundred and sixty miles south of Chicago, and the six-hour, one-way bus ride was not attractive to many students. I had a little less than two months to get it done. I was not going to be defeated. I didn't give a lot of thought about my role or title; it was about the work. I was content doing my part to help Harold Washington make history. I heard the call and responded with all my heart. I went at it as if my life depended on it. At dinner, instead of eating, I went from table to table, recruiting. At parties, instead of dancing, I recruited students. On nights I should have been studying, I was making appearances at the meetings of Black organizations on campus, appealing to students to sign up. I was focused, passionate and, most importantly, convincing.

What I was doing was second nature to me. I felt like I was meant to be here at this place and time doing exactly this. It was the most alive I had ever felt. Working on these two projects was my introduction to political organizing, although I didn't know it at the time. This was the beginning of what would become my future for the next ten years. I felt good doing my part for the Washington campaign and I wished that I could feel like this always—but that was not the case.

Every time I made it back to my room, my energy dropped, and my sleep was restless. I was still struggling with my herpes diagnosis, and it left a knot in the pit of my stomach. When I was on campus in the mix of things, recruiting students to make the trek to Chicago, I didn't have any space left to think about it. But once I returned to my room and stilled myself, I could think of nothing else. I knew that I needed someone that I could talk to, but after the fiasco with Larry, I was afraid that my trust would be violated again. I was thankful I hadn't had an outbreak since I was originally diagnosed before winter break, but that didn't erase the emotional baggage that came with having the disease. I was afraid of having another outbreak. Just the thought of it sent a chill up my spine. I was afraid of infecting someone and I was scared shitless of the news getting out on campus. Like always, I was good at masking the pain. If you had seen me on campus, you would have thought that I had it all together. I was *Ms. Politics*, but inside I was suffering.

One day when I was talking to Reggie about dating, I told him I had herpes. It just came out. I even surprised myself. I didn't intend to tell him, but ever since we met, he had been my confidante. He was understanding and didn't judge me. I felt a sigh of relief that I could count on him to cheer me up. Now that the cat was out of the bag, I confessed I was afraid that no one would want to date me. One day, I was really beating up on myself, having a big old fat pity party a *woe is me* moment. All of a sudden, Reggie said he would date me, even with herpes. This admission led to another one I didn't see coming. He confessed that he had been attracted to me all along but had never said anything because we had the uncomfortable fact between us that I used to be in a relationship with his former roommate. He explained that he didn't want me to think he was trying to take advantage of me because of the fiasco with his roommate. I was attracted to him as well, but I didn't want him to think I was a hoe because I had been with his roommate. We talked it out and the truth was that my relationship with his roommate began and ended within a span of a few weeks, so why should it have meant anything to either of us? His roommate had graduated and was no longer a part of our everyday lives. After our discussion, we became an item. He was the first and only guy I dated who had a connection to a former lover. He was also my first official boyfriend at SIU. I felt good about us. We spent a lot of time together. For a while, life was good, and we were good—really good. I felt like I had it all. My role in BAC was going exceptionally well. I was becoming more popular on campus because of my activism. I loved what I was doing, and I loved that I had a man on my arm. Everything was peachy-keen except that I was struggling academically. The classes I liked I did well, but everything else was a struggle. Not all classes were equal, and I just couldn't pinpoint how to overcome my areas of weakness. I wanted more than anything to be successful, but looking back, I didn't have the skills or the resources necessary to excel. In some ways it was easier for me to give my energy to my BAC projects than face the difficulty I came up against academically.

By spring break my life started to unravel—first, with Reggie. I didn't go home to

Mama's; instead, I stayed with Reggie. By now, our relationship had really heated up. We were spending more time together, and this week was going to be some romantic thing we had cooked up in our heads. I don't know if it was because we'd hit that three-month mark, or some other reason. From out of nowhere, Reggie flipped. One afternoon while we were having sex, he asked if he could tie me to the bedpost. I had seen it on television and thought, *What the hell? Go for it*. It was at once kinky, exhilarating, and scary to surrender my control in this way. When the sex was over, Reggie got up to go to the bathroom. After he came out of the bathroom, he went into the living room and left me tied to the post. After three minutes or so, I called out to him, and he didn't answer. I kept calling him and, still, he did not answer. I panicked! I tried to free myself from the ties by wriggling my wrists to no avail. I didn't know what was going on. My anxiety increased. *Why the fuck would he do this?*

"Okay, Reggie," I called out. "Stop playing and come untie me," I yelled into the living room. Still, he would not answer me. I went into full panic mode, calling him repeatedly.

"Please, Reggie," I whined. I felt utterly helpless and violated. My memory drew me back to the night I spent with Randy after our breakup.

I had been adamant about not seeing Randy again when he walked out of my house in the wee hours of the morning. He, on the other hand, kept pleading with me to see him. Eventually, I gave in and spent a night with him at his apartment. I think his woman was out of town. We had just finished having sex and were cuddling. I was hugged up under him, with his arm loosely around the back of my neck. In one move he shifted his arm lower and placed me in a neck hold. His grip got tighter, and it scared the shit out of me. I pushed up on his arm and it didn't budge.

"Randy," I whispered. "Let me go."

"I told you if I couldn't have you, no one could," he said, in a chilling voice that I will never forget, and he tightened his grip around my neck even more.

"Randy," I said, pushing his arm again. "Let me go." He ignored me like I never opened my mouth.

"I could break your neck right now and no one would know." Sweat started to drip under my breasts. I was scared out of my mind. I tried not to freak out, but my voice cracked, as I pleaded again, "Randy, pleassse—let me go."

"I could snap your neck and my brothers would help me bury you," he kept talking, ignoring my pleas. He was right. I hadn't told a soul that I was spending the night with him because I didn't want to hear the flak. I continued pleading with him as he gripped me a little tighter and, for a second, I felt like I couldn't breathe. I really thought that he was going to kill me. Then, suddenly, he loosened his grip, but left his arm around my shoulders. I pushed his arm up and slipped from under him. "I have to go to the bathroom," I said. After I used the toilet, I remained seated there to get myself together. I wanted to go home but it was the middle of the night, and I was somewhere in Chicago's West Side, which I knew nothing about. When I got back in the bed, he pulled me close into him. "You know that I would never hurt you?" he asked. It was a statement, but he asked it like it was a question. He then said, "Girl, I will never stop loving you; you will always be mine." It was the last thing he said before he fell into a deep sleep. I was too scared to sleep, so I lay in his arms, with my eyes wide open, until the morning. It would take a couple of decades before I saw him alone again. After that incident, I would never go anywhere with a man without someone knowing where I was. I hadn't even thought about that night in the last few years.

Now, tied to Reggie's bedpost, those same feelings of desperation, helplessness, and panic rushed through me like they did that night with Randy. My friends knew I was staying at Reggie's for the week. However, what good was that going to be if something happened to me? Reggie had never threatened to hurt me, but Jesus Christ! I didn't know what to think. He had never acted this way before. I was crazed out of my mind. I was tied up for at least ten minutes. Whatever he was up to, the damage was done. I felt betrayed, and that devastated me. I was smack-dab back where I started; I didn't know who or what I could trust anymore. Reggie came back into the bedroom, smiling. I didn't think anything was funny. I waited until he untied me before I went the fuck off. I was yelling at him, and he was like, *Aww, stop trippin.' It ain't all that...* a typical explanation from a man.

"FUCK YOU!" I said to him; then, I packed my shit and left. I might have been stupid and naive about a lot of things, but I did not fuck around with a man who took away my physical freedom. I felt like my power had been taken away from me, and that was where I drew the line with Randy and Reggie and all the men that came after them. Thank God the dorms reopened the same day. I spent the weekend alone, sulking, and eating Ritz Crackers and Cheez Whiz from a jar because the cafeteria didn't reopen until that Sunday evening. I was pretty freaked out about the whole incident. It made me take a deeper look at my choices in men. Every little bump in my life was a major crisis for me and I always came back to the same conclusion: I was flawed. I kept thinking, *Why can't I pick a good man?* I acknowledged Reggie had betrayed me and our relationship; however, I was even madder at myself for allowing it to happen. I didn't focus so much on what Reggie had done to me. I just felt as if I had opened the door to his antics by allowing him to tie me up. We broke up behind the incident, but eventually we became friends again. Monday, when classes resumed, I went back to my old routine. I wouldn't allow myself to think about the hurt. Instead, I focused increasingly on recruiting students for Harold Washington's Election Day activity.

At midnight on the day of the election, the BAC loaded seven charter buses full of students to make the twelve-hour round trip to Chicago. We arrived at Operation PUSH on April 12, 1983, at seven in the morning. Operation PUSH was used as the disbursement headquarters for college students who volunteered for the campaign. By nine in the morning, there were at least a few thousand students from various college campuses throughout Illinois. My school had the most significant representation of all the schools combined. I looked out over that auditorium and felt nothing but pride. With the largest delegation, I was thrust into a leadership position. Karriem was with Reverend Crider most of the day, doing what the bigwigs do. My role, along with Mark Allen and James Anyike, was to help coordinate the Get Out the Vote among college students. It was exciting to organize the day's activities of dispatching students to various polling places and making sure they were supplied with campaign literature, and lunch. I was in my element. If asked, I could tell you which students from which schools were at which polling place within seconds. I was a natural.

That evening, after the polls closed and the students were boarding the buses to go back to their respective schools, I was standing at the front of the auditorium making sure everyone was out when Reverend Crider walked in and asked to speak with me. I was awed that he wanted to have a conversation with me. In my mind, he was one step down from talking to Reverend Jackson himself. We sat on the stairs leading to the platform of the auditorium. He placed his arm around me, and I froze. In my head I was screaming, *HELL, NAW!* Like with Karriem, I had thought he was making an advance toward me. I would later learn this was just his way. He was a touchy-feely kind of guy, much like President Joe Biden has been criticized for in this age of #MeToo. It was never anything sexual, but my own history with men made me clam up in those first few seconds. Further, I fully recognize today that this kind of affectionate gesturing is a liberty men are more inclined to take with women and girls than women and girls will take with men. When I first heard the sexual harassment complaints about then-Vice President Joe Biden, I flashed back to my friendship with Tyrone. While the intent may have been pure, the action itself reduces a woman's agency of her own body. I was glad that Mr. Biden acknowledged this fact and tried to correct it. As a young woman, I didn't have the language or the power to express what I felt. I always guarded myself until I was sure that any man who I had to be in close contact with was safe. I'd had so many bad experiences by now, I was wary when it came to men. Reverend Crider began talking and I began to relax.

"Look, Rae, you did an incredible job today," he said. I didn't know what to say, so I let his words sink in. "I'm not sure if I could have done this without your help." I was hearing but not believing. This was *the* Reverend Tyrone Crider telling me that I was all that and a bag of chips. "You really stepped up to the plate," he added. "I would like to offer you an internship in the summer." I couldn't believe he thought that highly of me. I didn't see my worth, although I had done one heck of a job. He handed me his business card and walked me to the bus. All the way back to Carbondale, I wondered if there was a trick to it. It seemed too good to be true. Until I met Karriem, no man had ever given me a damn thing that wouldn't cost me my dignity. Now, Tyrone was offering more of what I had at BAC with Karriem. I was stunned, to say the least.

When we arrived back to campus in the middle of the night, sleepy and tired, we learned Harold Washington won the election. The next day the campus was bursting with energy. African American students were jubilant, proudly walking around campus wearing Washington paraphernalia. The students who made the trip felt as if they were a part of history, and rightly so. There was praise all around for Karriem and me. He already had a lot of respect among Black students and our efforts made him shine even more. This brought my popularity to an all-time high. I was known among African American students as the *radical girl* on campus. I was in the know about all things Black, especially if it was about advancing the cause of Black folks.

During this time, an African American student, Stephanie Jackson, was running for vice president of student government. Black students were still fired up by Washington's victory, and that energy spilled over into campus politics and her campaign. Stephanie was our girl, and Washington's win made us fearless. Most people I knew supported her. She won, becoming the first African American to hold the position at SIU. After her victory, I was sure I had found my calling. The combination of my work on the Washington campaign and my support of Stephanie's campaign took me back to Reverend Jackson's Easter Sunday sermon at Second Baptist Church. The more I thought about it, the more it made sense to me. I was sure that being a servant for my people was what God wanted for my life. Who better to help the rejected and locked-out than someone who had known rejection her whole life? Now, almost five years later, I was at a crossroads of my life. I didn't know how it would come together, but I had decided Tyrone Crider would be the first person I called when I got back to Chicago.

With popularity came even more attention from men, and I took it all in. Reggie was the last thing on my mind. He lost me by acting a fool. I forgot (again) that I was supposed to stay the fuck away from men. Child, you couldn't tell me nothin'. I was back on top of the world. I was still somewhat apprehensive, though. Herpes was still something I had to think about when it came to sex. I hadn't had an outbreak since the initial one back in December, and my next one wouldn't happen until the following September—some nine months after I left SIU. I was torn about disclosing and weighed it out. I was clear that I would never have sex during an outbreak. I would never deliberately infect someone. Plus, herpes was painful. I couldn't understand how someone could have sex during an outbreak. Granted, the first outbreak after exposure is the worst, but in all these years, I have never had an outbreak that wasn't painful. In the end, I decided to use the science I had at the time to inform my behavior.

I was captivated with Rayvon from day one. It wasn't so much about his well-sculpted body as it was his easygoing personality, and those freaking dimples endeared him to me. He didn't come across as conceited—just as a nice guy who happened to be good-looking. He had undeniable charisma and sex appeal that followed him like a shadow.

It began with a lot of flirting that quickly moved to sex. I followed that same old pattern of wanting and hoping for more and never asking for it. I hadn't told anyone on campus about our relationship because deep down, I knew that what we had was a plain ole booty-call thing and I didn't want to be judged. It was an easy relationship to conceal because he and I were very friendly on campus, and we were both big flirts with each other as well as with other people. No one was the wiser, or so I believed. One day, he shocked the shit out of me when he said he had told his boy how good I was in bed. I still hadn't told anyone and was uneasy about his confession, and I told him, "Oka-ay…. glad you like it but, um-m-m, please don't talk about me to your friends." Kiss-and-tell was always a turnoff for me. Then another time he said, "You know, my boy really likes you." Annoyed again, I rolled my eyes to signify he should stop it, and he shut the fuck up. All this talk about his boy liking me really started to make me feel a certain way. For sure, it helped me to see a bit more clearly that all I was and would ever be to him was a fuck. It hadn't escaped me, either, that he never said to me that he told his boy to back off. I figured it was time to cut my losses, and I began easing myself out of the relationship. I stopped calling and initiating. Still, I had a hard time saying no when he put the pressure on. Doing the typical, avoidance was my easiest route to no. I tried to stay out of his sight, but that was hard with a small Black population. Honestly, whenever he said to me, "You know you want to," he was not wrong; I did want to. He was good between the sheets and worth every single lay, and I would give in.

One night right after we finished having sex, he started that shit about his boy again. He said, "You know, he wants to try this out." Now I was pissed. Was he really offering me up? *Aww, HELL NAW!*

"Ray-von! It ain't gonna happen! Stop it!" I might have moved on from one to another without a lot of space between them but hooking up with two men at the same time was not pleasurable for me. I certainly didn't want to be passed around. Those days were over. I believed if a man even suggested such a thing, he didn't respect you. Even if I was just a lay, I didn't want to feel like one. I had learned that lesson the hard way from McDonald's dude, with his depraved tendency for group sex.

Rayvon dropped the subject and eased out the bed to go to the bathroom. Unlike my dorm, Boomer Hall—an older, all-male dorm—had bathrooms that were outside the rooms. I lay in the dark, waiting on him to return. When he opened the door to come back into the bedroom, I was still a little irritated, but figured, "Why not? Maybe round two." He lay on top of me and immediately felt different. Skinnier. Longer. Panic rushed through me like a race car going two hundred miles an hour.

"Rayvon told me how good you are in bed," he whispered in my ear. I was in shock. *This cannot be,* I thought. *What had Rayvon done to me?*

"I just wanted to see for myself," he declared.

"You don't mind?" he half-assed asked, as he proceeded to effectively rape me. *NOOOOO, DON'T DO THIS!!!!* I was screaming in my head—only it never came out of my mouth. My heart was thumping, and my mind was racing. I was jumbled and couldn't make sense out of what was happening. *What had Rayvon told him?* He shifted and pushed my thighs open and guided his hard penis inside of me. There was no pretense. No foreplay. He was ready. My body went limp as he pounded into me. I heard him say, "Damn, this is some good pussy." The last thing I heard was him moaning. I don't know how long he was on top of me, but it seemed like an eternity. After he climaxed, he got off me and left in the same dark silence through which he had entered. Every part of me shut down. I lay there like a wounded animal. It took everything I had to get out of that bed. I was overcome with grief. Then I was overcome with fear. I told myself to get the hell up. I rolled out of the bed and scrambled around the floor in the dark, feeling for my clothes. After I finally got my jeans on, it hit me that I was still in the room alone.

Where the fuck was Rayvon?

When I made it to the door, I was afraid to walk out. In desperation, I thought that maybe someone else was waiting. I slowly opened the dorm room door and peered outside, looking both ways, before I sprinted down the hall and out the building.

The moment I walked into my dorm room, I started shedding my clothes. I left each piece where it fell, turned on the shower and watched it until steam rose to the ceiling. When I was sure it was hot, I stepped in and let the water cascade down my back, then my hair, face, and chest. I lathered and scrubbed my body over and over. Once finished, I dried off and crawled in bed and cried. I didn't leave my room for two days. Shame and self-loathing settled in: *How could I have let this happen? Why didn't I scream? Why didn't I tell him to get up? I should have beaten his back until he got the fuck off me. Why didn't I say NOOOO!?* I told myself, *You simply lay there, limp, like a fucking fool. Rayvon had been hinting at this all the time. How stupid can you be?* My gut had told me something was off-center and away from the norm, but not in my wildest imagination could I have known I would end up at this place.

I didn't approach Rayvon about what happened because I was so ashamed to have fallen victim to their sick scheme. Just like the dude and the dog in his basement, I kept my distance, and so did he. He knew that shit was wrong, and so did his friend. Neither of them could look at me after that. One part of me wanted to report them, but report what? A part of me didn't even see all of it as rape. I know that seems like a contradiction but, honest to God, I had these thoughts simultaneously. Having sex with Rayvon was consensual. However, I didn't want to have sex with his "boy"— but because I didn't push him off, I blamed myself. While I knew Rayvon had clearly orchestrated all of this, I was torn about getting him in trouble. I know that sounds crazy, but I still considered him a friend and didn't really want to see him hurt even though he had hurt me. I knew I couldn't turn one in without the other. So, I pushed Rayvon's friend out of my mind to the point that I cannot even recall his name. Today, however, I believe I could identify him from a photo taken back at that time. Years ago, I even asked a mutual friend when I was trying to put a name with that face, which I had long ago forgotten.

I was also protecting myself from the scrutiny that comes when females name their rapists. I thought long and hard about the questions people would ask, especially since, technically, Rayvon wasn't my boyfriend. Like I said earlier, sex with a boyfriend was more acceptable; anything else was whoring around, and only a few people defended *loose women*. I didn't have a name then for rape-shaming, but I understood the culture where girls were sometimes blamed for their own rapes and scrutinized for everything. I didn't want to be one of those women because I dared to have sex without a commitment. I had enough of that living with Mama. I could hear it now: *What was she doing in Rayvon's dorm room? Why didn't she fight [Rayvon's "boy"] off of her?* I didn't see how reporting the rape would turn out in my favor, so I let it go. After being locked away in my room for two days, I emerged. I pushed the sexual assault to the back of my mind and continued my new assignment with the BAC. I buried myself in my work; it was a salve for my soul. When I wasn't working on BAC projects, I was sleeping. The semester ended and I was placed on academic suspension—another one for the fuck-up column.

I didn't have sex with Rayvon anymore that school year, but I did when I came back to SIU after sitting out a year. One night he came over to my apartment from out of nowhere. Other people were over that night. He and I went into the back to my bedroom and had an intense quickie; we didn't even get in the bed. When it was over, we came up front like nothing had happened. After everyone was gone that night, the memory of Rayvon and his friend rushed through me like a freight train. True to form, I asked myself, yet again, *What is wrong with you, girl?* Also, true to form, I didn't have the answer to the question. But this time, remembering the pain gave me a reason to pause. I told myself then and there I would never have sex with Rayvon again. About seven years after I left SIU, I saw Rayvon at one of the SIU Black alumni picnics. A group of us was standing around and he asked me for my telephone number. As soon as we exchanged numbers, I regretted it. About two weeks later, he called about one o'clock in the morning. At the time, I had just transitioned to AIDS, and I was in therapy. It was clear he was not my friend. I hung up the phone. It had taken facing death to begin the journey of taking back my power.

Thirty-Three

BECOMING

> " The whole point of being alive is to become the person you were intended to be; to grow out of and into yourself again and again."
> — Oprah Winfrey

I officially began my first assignment as a volunteer at Operation PUSH, under the leadership of Reverend Jesse Louis Jackson Sr. and the tutelage of Reverend Tyrone Crider, within a week of arriving back in Chicago from Carbondale. At the time, Tyrone wore two hats at PUSH: He was the national youth director and the national executive director of PUSH for Excellence, the educational arm of the organization. He kept his word to me, and my paid summer internship began a few weeks later at the beginning of June 1983. I had just turned twenty-one. I knew that my future was somehow connected to what I was doing; I just didn't know exactly how. It was a gut feeling that I could not let go. Talk about a faith walk: That was my truth. I prayed that God would continue to make a path for me.

It was nothing short of a miracle to work for the organization founded by the very person, Reverend Jackson, who had sparked the flame of service inside me at Second Baptist Church six years earlier. His sermon that Easter morning helped me to see beyond my own pain. Only God could craft such perfection in the midst of so much imperfection that had filled my life up to that point. I knew that I wanted a life beyond what I had. I was never afraid to try new things. If something didn't work out, I accepted it, but I would never stop trying. My work with PUSH was another effort to head in the direction I believe God had planned for me. In retrospect, I see how my life had already been headed in this direction and how seeds were planted along the way. I intuitively followed this path when it kept showing up in different ways: a socially conscious eighth-grade homeroom teacher, pastor, and a church youth director who introduced me to the NAACP, which led me into a leadership mindset that made my participation in my high school student council a natural fit. Then, it would be attending PUSH with Coré and her mother, that made me receptive to Karriem's proposition and my work with the Black Affairs Council, that opened the door for my internship at PUSH, where the seeds started to bloom. That is how God works, but you must be willing to put yourself out there.

Once I began my first assignment it was second nature, just like it had been at SIU. I was asked to identify African American student leaders who could attend a student leadership conference Tyrone was planning for the fall. He gave me a list of HBCUs and instructed me to identify the Student Government Association (SGA) presidents on the list. Each day, I made telephone calls to student activities offices to get the names of the presidents. With their names in tow, I made cold calls to every SGA president. After I introduced myself and pitched the conference, I sent an official letter and then made follow-up calls. I stayed on top of things so that the conference would be a success. I spoke with everyone on my list at least once a week—sometimes twice or three times. I knew who, what, and when regarding each person. Tyrone gave me his full confidence to grow, nurture and maintain the network. I directed every ounce of my energy toward the project. With the phone receiver in hand, I stood, sat, and squatted until every call was made and the number of student leaders grew. When I reported back, Tyrone never said I was talking too fast, or that my mannerisms or the volume of my voice were too much for the office. He embraced me just as I was, which gave me even more confidence. I pushed any remaining doubt out of my head and continued to work my tail off. During the week, I spent anywhere from nine to twelve hours a day at PUSH. I commuted an hour on public transportation each way. I didn't have much of a personal life, and I think my breakneck schedule was a buffer for me living with Mama. We didn't have any incidents that summer, although she did ask once, "What kind of job you got over there with PUSH?" I explained what I was doing, but it was over her head. Every now and then, I would hear her mention me to someone on the telephone, saying something like, "She call herself doing something over there with Jesse Jackson." Then, she laughed. It felt like she was insinuating I was lying, but I didn't let it faze me. I knew that if I let her get into my head, it would disrupt the flow I had created in my life. I also knew I needed a place to lie my head. I couldn't afford to be put out. I didn't want anyone at PUSH to know about my childhood and the madness I had already gone through, so I talked very little about my family or my past. I wanted to be normal. To keep the peace, I gave Mama some money out of my meager paycheck every two weeks and gave my energy to PUSH.

Within a month, I developed a network of over a hundred student leaders around the country who also had networks I could tap into. My task was made easier because Reverend Jackson's name preceded him, and I had no problem using it to help get me through the door. Once I had a student leader on the phone, the rest was up to me—and I could talk them to heaven and back. One example was William Allen, who was the youngest Carter-Mondale delegate at the Democratic National Convention in 1980, and very much connected in New York. William then introduced me to Melvin Lowe, who was the chairman of the citywide network for the student government associations within the City University of New York system. With Melvin on board, I had access to a point person in every city college in New York. It went like this across the country. We could then tap into a network in almost every major city to help with the work we were doing. What originally began to increase attendees for the conference became a network of student leaders across the country that we would utilize on other projects for the youth division of Operation PUSH.

The first major political action I oversaw that summer was the youth role in the boycott of Anheuser-Busch products and the summer music festivals it sponsored. PUSH was boycotting because African Americans comprised over fifty percent of its consumers, and the company's investment into the African American community didn't match the patronage. The youth focus of the boycott was the Anheuser-Busch Super Summer Festivals that used Black entertainers, but did not use Black promoters, vendors, or public relations firms. I organized student activists to picket and distribute leaflets in every place a festival was held. We demanded economic reciprocity with our picket-line battle cry: "Bud is a dud; don't drink those suds." We had such a tremendous showing of young people boycotting the festivals that we were able to decrease the sales of tickets; and in a couple of cases, shows were canceled. Our protests helped to force Anheuser-Busch to the table to negotiate.

My life was changing before my eyes. Working to make life better for others became a mission for me. I was becoming a young woman with a purpose. My political activism took me out of myself and my problems and placed me in the middle of the world's problems. Without a doubt, working for PUSH was the best decision I could have made.

PUSH had a staff of over thirty, and I was one among twenty interns that summer assigned to the various departments. April Branch, another intern, became Tyrone's administrative assistant and we were a team. I didn't have a title and I didn't care; I was just honored to be in the fold. The first week, interns were assigned to read *Why We Can't Wait*, by Dr. Martin Luther King Jr. I don't know whose decision it was to assign the reading, but Tyrone told me the book would help me to understand the foundation of the work we were doing at PUSH. He told me to go outside and look at the sign posted over the entrance to the building. It read, "Dr. King's Workshop." He said I would have to understand Dr. King's work to understand PUSH's work, and I *got it*. PUSH began as Operation Breadbasket, which was the economic arm of the Southern Christian Leadership Conference (SCLC). Dr. King appointed Reverend Jackson to head Breadbasket and lead the work of challenging white corporate America to reciprocate financially into the Black community. After King's death, Jackson founded Operation PUSH and the activism expanded.

What struck me the most in *Why We Can't Wait* were the parallels between what PUSH was currently doing regarding voting rights. PUSH had just launched a massive voter registration drive in the South. The Southern Crusade. Reverend Jackson and the staff traveled throughout the Southern states that summer, partnering with local PUSH chapters, churches, community leaders and elected officials to register African Americans to vote. They would register 150,000 people.

The ways that white people were still able to disenfranchise Black people—twenty years after Dr. King had written *Why We Can't Wait,* and eighteen years after the Voting Rights Act of 1965 was passed—was an eye-opener for me, and that's stating it mildly. In some states, Reverend Jackson requested that the U.S. Department of Justice intervene because many of these laws violated the Voting Rights Act and were clearly extensions of Jim Crow laws that had historically disenfranchised African Americans. These laws were mostly in areas with predominantly Black populations and some of them required a person to register in the town and the county in which that person lived. The problem was that a county registrar's office could be as far as sixty to ninety miles away from his or her home. If you were poor, didn't have a car or couldn't take off from work, then you didn't get to register, which meant you didn't get to vote. If you didn't vote, you had no voice in government. Until I became involved in Mayor Harold Washington's campaign, I had never thought about voting. In fact, the 1983 presidential primary was the first time I voted. Likewise, I hadn't given any thought to electoral politics. Now, I was having a personal awakening that flowed outward. The political disenfranchisement of African Americans was disconcerting to me.

The exposure to so many brilliant people was one of the best things about being at PUSH. It not only helped me to become a better organizer, but it broadened my knowledge on issues and helped to shape my intellectual discourse. The Saturday morning community forums were mandatory for staff, and I never knew what giant of a person would show up. One Saturday, it could be a president of an African country; another Saturday, it could be New York Congresswoman Shirley Chisholm or Gary, Indiana, Mayor Richard Hatchett. Then there were the civil-rights leaders who were in and out of PUSH, and around Reverend Jackson. It was one thing to read about Reverend Hosea Williams, a lead organizer for SCLC, but it was another thing altogether to sit and talk with him. My favorite of the bunch was Reverend Dr. C. T. Vivian, who would receive the Presidential Medal of Freedom from President Barack Obama in 2013 for his work in the civil-rights movement. Reverend Vivian will always be known for that rainy day on Feb. 15, 1965, when he went toe to toe with Sheriff Jim Clark on the steps of the Dallas County Courthouse in Selma, Alabama. After Sheriff Clark knocked Vivian down, he jumped back up and asked, "What kind of people *are* you?" I loved to talk with Dr. Vivian because he could illuminate the moral dilemma of racism like no other. Whenever I saw him—whether on the road or in the office—he was willing to engage with me, and it was never just a monologue. He wanted to know what I was doing and why. He gave me even more context for the work activists had done in the early days of the SCLC, which gave me more perspective on my current work.

PUSH staff also helped to shape my worldview. I listened intently to the elders and sat with the ones who had an open-door policy, such as Reverend Edward Riddick. He was an historian and there was no topic he could not explain. Reverend Frank Watkins was the only white person on the staff; he was Reverend Jackson's speechwriter, and he headed the press department. He was a seminarian who had joined Reverend Jackson in the Breadbasket days. Frank was a consummate strategist who had an uncanny ability to explain an issue in a way that made it crystal-clear in my head. We were a serious bunch and we often talked strategy all day and into the night. Other young adults in and out of PUSH with brilliant minds, like Sheldon King, kept the dialogue going in our office, with Tyrone in the center.

Why We Can't Wait was only the tip of the iceberg when it came to book recommendations and I read like a hungry animal. Until this point, mostly fictional books—such as *Black Boy* and *Native Son*, both by Richard Wright; *The Invisible Man,* by Ralph Ellison; and a slew of writings by Langston Hughes—had informed my understanding of racism in America. Now, another genre—nonfiction literature—would influence my intellectual growth. There was never a shortage of people to recommend a book, and never a shortage of books to recommend. Books like Stokely Carmichael's *Black Power,* James Baldwin's *The Fire Next Time* and W.E.B. DuBois' *The Souls of Black Folks* were invaluable in shaping my societal and political worldviews.

Everything was new and fascinating. The internship was life-changing for me; it placed me in another world. The more I learned at PUSH that summer the more I wanted to learn. I can't even begin to measure the breadth or the depth of my experience within such a short time. Imagine: The year before this, I was unemployed and living in the lion's den, holding on by a thread and a prayer. It couldn't get any better than this. Interns were even included in staff meetings. We were treated with the utmost respect and given assignments that helped us to grow.

The first time I attended a staff meeting, sitting in the little chapel waiting for the meeting to begin, Reverend Jackson walked in—I couldn't believe it. *Did he really just walk in here?* I asked myself. To say that I was surprised is a gross understatement, and that he ran the meetings; that was mind-blowing. At the time, Reverend Jackson was larger than life to me. He was often on television and on the covers of magazines, and the possibility of him running for president was the primary discussion in American politics that summer. Headlines everywhere read, *Should A Black Man Run for President?*—and everyone had a point of view. The sheer boldness of the topic was empowering to African Americans. Staff meetings were educational and informational, and sometimes they were Saturday morning mini-forums. This was especially true after Reverend Jackson had just come off the road. He would report back to the staff everything that had taken place, including the number of new voters they registered. He was always fired up, and I hung on to his every word.

Reverend Jackson was profound, measured, and thoughtful in staff meetings, while Reverend Willie Taplin Barrow, the vice president of PUSH was always bubbling over. Everything that came out of her mouth sounded like a pep rally. You had to listen closely, or you might miss a jewel that dropped from her mouth. It was in a staff meeting, listening to her, where I first learned that the work I was doing was called *organizing*. Remember, I had no idea that what I was doing was a real thing—a job with a title—I was just doing it. One day in the staff meeting, Reverend Barrow commented, "Tyrone and those young people working with him are organizing other young people and doing an awesome job." She said it with so much pride. I was in awe. *Wow,* I said to myself, *I'm an organizer.* I liked the sound of that. From that day forward, I called myself a *political organizer* and went about establishing that as a career path. God had answered my prayer.

Reverend Barrow had a profound influence on me. She had a rich history as a union organizer and had also been at PUSH since Breadbasket. They called her the Little Warrior because she stood no taller than five foot one, but when she opened her mouth, you would have thought she was six feet tall. She had a larger-than-life personality that made her seem unapproachable. She talked with her hands, and she talked fast. *Finally,* I thought. *Someone who speaks faster than me.* She would continue to influence my growth—especially being a female among the male-dominated leadership. I watched her maneuver and make a space for her voice. She fought against the subtle ways in which women were excluded, sometimes on purpose and sometimes through implication. She was the first feminist or womanist who I ever met; Mrs. Jacqueline Jackson, Reverend Jackson's wife, was the second. Watching them navigate helped me to shape my own path as a young woman involved in social justice—a field dominated by men. There were so many other women on staff. Lucille Loman was the chief financial officer and there were also Janice Bell, Daisy Camps, Theresa Fambro Hooks and Attorney Jeanette Wilson ran the Legal Clinic. Joyce Dorsey Kenner was Tyrone's Deputy Director for PUSH Excel. Sharon Robinson, the daughter of famed baseball great Jackie Robinson, was a member of PUSH Excel's board of directors, whom I got to know well.

It would be through Reverend Barrow that I would also have my first glimpse into the ugliness of Acquired Immune Deficiency Syndrome (AIDS). At the close of each staff meeting, Reverend Jackson said, "Let's keep Keith in our prayers." There were nods of agreement and somber amens. One day, I leaned over and asked Tyrone, "Who is Keith?" He shushed me. Later, he explained that Keith Barrow was Reverend Barrow's son and he had AIDS. Keith was twenty-eight years old and an amazing R&B recording artist. He would become one of many well-known African American men to succumb to the disease in the early years.

I had seen news reports on television about HIV/AIDS. The disease was portrayed in a way that made me believe it only affected white gay men. Having learned about Keith Barrow, I now knew that it also affected Black men. I was around Reverend Barrow in the months leading to Keith's death. It was heartbreaking to see this jubilant woman struggle as she watched her only child die a horrible death as the medical community scrounged for knowledge and the masses watched in fear, shame, and denial. My first glimpse of Keith was one day at the Saturday community forum, when Reverend Jackson introduced him. He was frail but it had never occurred to me he was dying. The next time I saw him was the day of his funeral. I would be forever bonded to him because of his death that summer.

The 20th Anniversary of the March on Washington for Jobs and Freedom would be another defining moment in my life and a glimpse into the future that I would claim for myself. It was held in Washington, D.C. on Aug. 28, 1983, to commemorate the 1963 March on Washington. April and I flew to Washington with Tyrone the week going into the march to network with student leaders arriving from around the country. This event opened more doors for me to expand our student network beyond HBCUs to other African American student leaders at predominantly white institutions. I had no idea what to expect going into the march. I had a narrow view of its purpose, which was officially to demand a national holiday to commemorate the work and life of Dr. Martin Luther King Jr. By now I had heard firsthand the various stories about the civil-rights movement and the 1963 March on Washington from many of its participants. I believed that the success of the original march was out of a sense of urgency to change Jim Crow laws that infringed upon the civil liberties of African Americans.

What I learned on the ground was that people had shown up for Dr. King, but they also came to protest the policies under the Reagan administration. Ronald Reagan was one of the most conservative presidents in history. His policies benefited the rich and the massive military buildup under his administration happened at the expense of social programs. And his main policy, trickle-down economics left people, especially African Americans, worse off. Reagan was the king of dog whistles. To have lived both in the Trump and Reagan eras, I have always taken offense to the Never Trumpers who use Reagan as the litmus test for Trump because Reagan was just a different version of the same thing. One author compared Trump and Reagan this way, "Trump is to Reagan much like crack is to cocaine: faster-acting and less glamorous. Still, in their essence they are the same, I wholeheartedly agree. In comparison, Trump referred to African countries as "shit holes," while Reagan referred to African diplomats as "monkeys" in a phone conversation with Richard Nixon. In fact, Reagan canonized the term "Welfare Queen" by suggesting that Black women were shiftless con artists scheming the government. He might not have been as vulgar as Donald Trump but his repeated stereotypical references to Black women was just as insidious, oppressive, and effective in disparaging their collective character. The march gave people a voice and, at the same time, it gave life to a new level of awareness among African Americans. And so, people came *en masse* for Dr. King and to protest Ronald Reagan.

A couple days leading up to the march, Tyrone introduced me to the coordinator. In his typical fashion, he always explained who a person was prior to an introduction, especially if the person were someone he admired and thought I could learn from. He pointed to a woman, asking me, "Remember when I told you that my friend Donna Brazile was the person organizing the march?"

I nodded in confirmation. He said, "That's Donna. Let me introduce you."

"So-o...." I asked Tyrone. "Did she organize the who-ole march?" He nodded his head affirmatively.

"Like, not just the students?" I asked.

Still nodding affirmatively, he said, "She's BAD!"

"Really?" I mumbled.

Tyrone had already told me Donna was hand-picked by Mrs. Coretta Scott King, the wife of the late Dr. King, to coordinate the march. Years later, I learned from reading Donna's memoir, *Cooking with Grease: Stirring the Pots in American Politics,* that there had been opposition among the Black leadership, including Mrs. King, to give Donna the title of national coordinator for the March on Washington because of her age. In fact, the first office space for the march came by way of Reverend Jackson, who allowed Donna to share our D.C. office with Jack O'Dell. By the time they officially appointed her, she had done the work and the march was headed for success. As we approached Donna, I noticed that she wasn't wearing an ounce of makeup. *Lord, help this woman,* I thought. Lip gloss was a must, as far as I was concerned. She was friendly and down to earth, but her sharp Southern accent made me think, *Badass, my ass.* Back then, I hadn't considered how unfair and sexist it was to judge Donna in that split second based on her appearance. I'm sure if she had been a young man—casual, with his sleeves rolled up to work—I would have probably been thinking, *He's working his tail off.* It was a double standard that I learned from society.

The day of the march, however, my opinions and stereotypical thinking changed completely. I was caught in the excitement as the thousands of students left our starting point from Howard University to join the larger march in the direction of the Lincoln Memorial. I was on the front line of the student march with Tyrone on one side of me and Elijah Smiley, the president of the Florida Statewide Student Association, on the other. I don't know how close we were to the Lincoln Memorial when we stopped. No matter which way I turned; I saw nothing but people. I took it all in; the speeches, the energy, the diversity of the people—Black, white, young, and old. I did a complete turn and looked out over the three-hundred-thousand-plus people gathered at the Lincoln Memorial, and I thought about Donna. I had to give it to her. She had done it, lip gloss or not. She was only three years older than me—my contemporary in age. There was no doubt in my mind now that Donna was a badass. And I decided that one day, I was going to be a badass too, just like her. From Tyrone, I had been given an opportunity. From Reverend Barrow, I had my title; and, through Donna, I began to see the possibilities for my future. I left the march not only inspired but committed. After that day, I continued to watch Donna's rise as a political operative, and she would remain my inspiration until I retired from politics in 1992.

After the march, I assessed my life. In three months, I had taken a basic internship and transformed it into a promising career. If I added the four months of organizing work I did at SIU, I had come a long way in a short time. With my work at PUSH, I had already started to gain a reputation as a national organizer as well as the go-to person for youth and students for Operation PUSH.

As the summer ended, there was more and more in-house discussion about the possibility of Reverend Jackson running for president. Tyrone had hinted at the possibility of me and April staying on beyond the internship in our current roles and transitioning to work on the campaign if he decided to run, and I was praying it would happen. God knows I had no idea what was next for me. As other interns began talking about their next move—going back to college or starting a job—it started to sink in that I was facing the possibility of being stuck at Mama's with no job. I certainly couldn't go back to SIU.

The executive director, Mr. Sam Tidmore approved the plan, however, some staff members were unhappy, claiming it to be favoritism. *Favoritism, my ass!* It was absolutely not true. I had worked my ass off, and the results were evident in project after project. Unbeknownst to me, rumors about Tyrone and me had already been circulating. Rumors like why he and I were so close, Why I was given all the best projects, Why I had flown to D.C. for the March on Washington and the rest of the staff had taken the chartered bus. Come to find out, Tyrone had shielded me from all the gossip. I was SO very pissed. This had been one of the first times in my life I had kept my freaking legs closed. I certainly felt the brunt of the old adage *Damned if I do, damned if I don't*. No one at PUSH knew how deeply I had been affected by the hurtful rumors. Looking back, it was sexism at its best. If I had been a male intern, no one would have given it a second thought. As I was being unfairly judged, I could see more clearly how unfairly I had judged Donna.

Tyrone had foreshadowed this possibility and given me a big brother lecture my first week at PUSH. While he never made an advance, he believed other men might. He said I had a bright future and not to mess it up by screwing around. "If you start," he said, "they will use you and pass you on until you are used up." Finally, he said, "And people *will* talk." I took Tyrone's advice. And, for the record, not one man at PUSH made a pass at me that summer. However, I did meet a couple of guys my age who volunteered at PUSH and went on a few dates, but there were no lifetime matches. I had a crush on Abe Thompson, who was an executive at WGCI Radio. He was eleven years my senior and friends with Tyrone. Because he didn't work at PUSH, I saw him as fair game. Abe never bit. When I was writing this memoir, I asked him why he never made a move on me. He said he knew I was interested but he felt if he reciprocated, he would be taking advantage of me, and he didn't want that on his conscience. I was left speechless. Abe was the epitome of what I wished all men could be.

Over the years, I've seen how quickly we label young women and blame them for the behavior of men, especially men in power. On one end, it sends the message that women are responsible for men's behavior; on the other, it sends the message that male sexual prowess is so powerful that they cannot control themselves. Neither is true. I know also that I was so messed up then, if Abe had reciprocated my flirtations, I would not have given it a second thought. My bright future and all that came with it would have sunk because women are held to a different standard than men. I can truly thank God for placing a couple of men in my life who saw my worth beyond my vagina, and their worth beyond their penises.

Thirty-Four

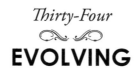

EVOLVING

" Trust yourself enough to let go, shift, uproot, give yourself permission to shed who you used to be. You are allowed to start over and find new ways to bloom into your best self."
— Alex Elle

October 31, 1983. I walked into the "Jackson for President" national campaign headquarters at 2100 M Street NW, in Washington, D.C., molting my old skin and making room for the new one. On the outside, I was evolving into a different me and better self; on the inside, I was still a wounded little girl. I skillfully layered my success on top of my pain and kept it moving. Relocating to D.C. was a bold move. I was twenty-one. I didn't know a single soul beyond the few who had also transitioned from PUSH. For the first couple of days, I stayed at the Howard Inn and was looking for permanent housing.

The Howard Inn was owned and operated by Howard University, and it was our "official unofficial" residence. Almost everyone affiliated with the campaign had either stayed or lived there at some point during the campaign, including Rev. Jesse and Mrs. Jacqueline Jackson. About a week later, I moved into the home of Dr. Cynthia Sadler, a physician in the medical residency program at Howard University Medical School, who was seeking a roommate.

I continued to work under Tyrone, who held the same function he had at PUSH: the national youth director. He continued to be the figurehead and primary strategist for our department. I was appointed to be the deputy national youth director and continued to serve as the point person. I was tasked with implementing the ten-point plan for youth engagement. I achieved a lot in a short time, and it felt good. One month into the job, I walked into my office and found my first box of business cards on my desk. I pulled out a card, laid it in front of me and rubbed my fingers over my name. It read, "Rae C. Lewis—Deputy National Youth Director." I wore my pride like a badge of honor. It was a surreal moment.

My first assignment helped bring in youth and student leaders for Reverend Jackson's official announcement to run for president. I began organizing for the announcement before I arrived in D.C. The week we planned to move, Keith Barrow died and the PUSH people transitioning to the campaign stayed in Chicago for the funeral. That Sunday night, Steve Jeffries picked me up from Mama's with all my belongings, and we started on the twelve-hour car ride to Washington, D.C. to begin a new chapter in our lives. Steve was a young person from PUSH who would be working as Reverend Jackson's traveling aide. He drove through the night except for bathroom breaks, food stops and an occasional Pac-Man game, and I kept him company. I arrived at the office, tired as dirt, and I got right to work. Everyone was knee-deep in the trenches to help make the announcement a success. Anita Bonds—a seasoned political strategist and campaign manager for Marion Barry's mayoral bids—was already in place as the national field director. Donna Brazile had also been hired; she and Anita spearheaded Reverend Jackson's official announcement. Tyrone instructed me to invite our network, focusing on student leaders from states that were the closest to D.C. and, more likely to make the trek. With three more days left until the announcement, I was back on the phones. About twenty-five student leaders from our network made the trip and brought with them up to five members of their student government cabinets. However, the ones who delivered the busloads of young people were Norman Nixon, who was an integral part of Mayor Barry's youth network; and Warren Green, who was the SGA president for the University of the District of Columbia as well as youth and student campaign coordinator for D.C.

On November 3, 1983, at the D.C. Convention Center, Reverend Jackson announced his bid to run for the Democratic nomination for the president of the United States. After many speeches from leaders and elected officials across the Rainbow Coalition, Congresswoman Shirley Chisholm made her way to the microphone. She was nothing short of amazing as she introduced Reverend Jackson. In 1972, Congresswoman Chisholm had been the first woman and Black person to run for the Democratic nomination for president. Ten years earlier, she had done her best with very little support. That race began with thirteen candidates. Chisholm came in fourth, winning twenty-eight delegates to the Democratic Convention. Bringing Reverend Jackson to the podium, she said, "As part of the continuity, a new day for national politics unfolds at this very moment." The moment Reverend Jackson began his speech. I knew I was in the right place at the right time in history. Those first few sentences of his speech illuminated the work I believed God had called me to do.

We are here to heed the call of this nation's highest and noblest principles that we might fulfill our mission to defend the poor, make welcome the outcast, deliver the needy and be a source of hope for the people yearning to be free everywhere.

Tears welled in the corner of my eye because God had placed me, Rae Clara Lewis—the little girl who had been told every day from age six to sixteen that she had no worth—smack-dab in the middle of such a noble work. My heart was full of gratitude. April Branch and I were the youngest staff persons working in the national headquarters. April worked in the press office assisting Eric Easter and Florence Tate. The next youngest would have been Donna Brazile and Tyrone Crider, but they had already been exposed to Black leaders of this magnitude—Donna through her work on the March on Washington, and Tyrone because of his position at PUSH. Working in the national campaign headquarters was just as exciting for me as it had been working at Operation PUSH. It was not unusual to see any number of senior campaign advisors in the office. One day it could be Ernie Green of the Little Rock Nine or Reverend Dr. Benjamin "Ben" Chavis, Jr. of the Wilmington Ten, both whom I got to know quite well.

Watching the women navigate in this political space was especially meaningful—they were a sort of road map for me. The one thing that can be said about Reverend Jackson is that he surrounded himself with powerful, brilliant women, and he respected their counsel. One day, it was Alexis Herman, who would become the secretary of labor in the Clinton administration. On another day, it could be Leslie Baskerville, C. Delores Tucker, Maxine Waters, Dorothy Height or Jewel Jackson McCabe. Black elected officials were in and out, too, such as Mayor Marion Barry; and Mayor Richard Hatcher, our campaign chair; or any number of Black Congressional representatives who supported the campaign, including John Conyers, Ronald Dellums and Gus Savage. Every day in the office was like a who's who in Black politics.

Minister Louis Farrakhan, the leader of the Nation of Islam (the Nation), walked through the doors one day. He already provided security for Reverend Jackson with the Fruit of Islam, the Nation's elite security outfit, until the Secret Service took over. Reverend Jackson had so many death threats that the minister stepped in. He had a remarkable presence. Before the campaign I had only seen him on television, and I had never heard him speak. In a bold and historical move, Minister Farrakhan reversed the Nation's long-standing policy of no involvement in electoral politics and endorsed Reverend Jackson.

A month into the campaign, Minister Farrakhan and other religious leaders—Reverend Wyatt T. Walker and Reverend William Howard Jr., the former president of New York Theological Seminary—accompanied Reverend Jackson to Syria to gain the release of Lt. Robert Goodman, an African American Navy pilot shot down during a bombing raid over Lebanon. The night of their return, the campaign held a rally at a church in Washington, D.C. I was mesmerized as Minister Farrakhan described the meetings and negotiations that had taken place to gain Lt. Goodman's release. He was brilliant and eloquent as he methodically walked us through each moment in the dialogue between Syrian President Hafez al-Assad, Syrian religious leaders, and Reverend Jackson and his American delegation of religious leaders. That night stayed with me, just as that morning's arrival at the airport with other staffers to cheer for Reverend Jackson's return. I watched intently and with pride as the United States Air Force VC-13 landed just before the break of dawn. The plane door opened, and Reverend Jackson emerged like a superhero, with Lt. Goodman by his side. It was moments of history like those I experienced during Jackson's 1983 campaign that became a notebook of lessons that helped shape my advocacy work. The campaign placed me on the trajectory that would inform my life's work in social justice from electoral politics to my work as an AIDS activist. This revelation wouldn't come to me until years later. Back then, while I was in it, I simply felt privileged.

Every step of the way was new territory for me. At the top of my learning curve was a practical understanding of coalition-building. Reverend Jackson wanted a coalition of people and issues whose disenfranchisement bound us all together—and together, he believed we could win the White House. I had spent months arguing why a Black man should run for president. Now I was adjusting to this concept, which took time and an open mind. One of those adjustments meant embracing the diverse composition of the campaign staff. Our campaign was a melting pot in the truest sense. Reverend Jackson wanted staff to reflect the coalition we were trying to build to win the election. Political scientist and campaign senior policy advisor Dr. Ronald Walters asserts in his book, *Black Presidential Politics in America*, "Care was taken to assure that the coalition was comprised of three categories of representatives: male and female, ethnic/racial, and issue representation." We had an impressive bunch of diverse people: Black, White, Latina, Jewish and Arab.

In the beginning, I didn't know what to think about all the white people in the coalition. I had a genuine distrust that grew out of my readings on race over the years. Furthermore, I had spent the summer reading Stokely Carmichael and James Baldwin as well as making the Black power sign every Saturday at the PUSH forum. Now, all of a sudden, there I was in a room with white folks, and I was supposed to believe that their support of a Black man matched mine? No, my only solace came from one fact: the higher up the staff chain, the blacker the campaign was. At least Black people were running things. At the helm was Arnold Pinkney, an Ohio businessman and political strategist who, more than fifty years ago, ran the successful Stokes brothers' campaigns: Carl for mayor of Cleveland, and Louis for Congress. We had some phenomenal Black women in leadership, such as Chief Operating Officer Barbara Williams-Skinner, finance chair Emma Chapel and field director Anita Bonds.

The broad section of staff assigned to organize around social justice issues like equality for women and the right to choose, LGBTQ rights, unfair labor, environmentalism, migrant farm workers and Native American rights helped to broaden my understanding of social-justice work. I was learning about issues that had nothing to do with me or the people with whom I identified. For example, there was the plight of migrant farmworkers in Ohio, and why I boycotted the Campbell Soup Company. In the scheme of things, switching my brand of soup was easy. I had already learned the effectiveness of boycotts to leverage a political agenda at PUSH. By the same token, it was a personal choice that cost me nothing. The challenge, however, was standing toe to toe for someone else's cause and taking a hit for it. A candidate's platform on paper was one thing, but defending it publicly was something else.

My first lesson came hard and fast. Our campaign received a request from a private school for boys in Maryland to send a representative from the campaign to participate in a panel discussion with other candidates' representatives and their students. Tyrone passed it to me. Prior to that day, I had not done any public speaking and I didn't see myself as a speaker. I was a flat-footed organizer, but I figured, *How bad could it be?* The day of the program, I was a little anxious. However, I started to relax once we began. A teacher introduced each panelist, and then each campaign representative made a short presentation, including me. There were at least five of us. I thought I had done a good job, even a tad better than the others. The teacher came back up front and opened the forum for questions. I immediately noticed that the questions from these young people were pretty sophisticated, but I was handling myself pretty well. When the questions became a little more complex, I thought, *Why on earth are these kids asking about foreign policy and taxes when they can't even vote?* This was a middle school, mind you—grades six through nine. I got a little nervous and tried to brush it off. I knew that I could talk about the campaign in broad strokes. I was an expert on why a Black man should run for president and the overall message of why Jackson was running. The problem was I had not studied all of the campaign's position papers. Steve Cobble, our issues person, pushed them out quickly but I was not reading them with the same urgency; nor was I paying attention to the details in the ones I had read. The best answers to the students' questions were in the details of the position papers. In a flash, the program went downhill and tumbled right on my head. A young man stood up to ask me a question I have never forgotten.

"How could Reverend Jackson support murderers like the Palestinians?" Every eye turned to me. I wanted to crawl under the chair I was sitting in. He didn't stop there. He said something else about *killing someone with a knife,* and *bare hands,* and *how could you?* and finally, *the Jackson campaign...* I didn't hear the rest because I stopped listening. I had to come up with an answer that didn't make me look like a fool. I took a deep breath to reassure myself. I had read the campaign's position paper on the Middle East and the Jewish-Arab conflict. I knew my candidate supported the right of Palestinian people to have a homeland. It was a controversial position that made Reverend Jackson the enemy of some Jewish people. The day of the announcement, an organization called *Jews Against Jackson* interrupted his speech. It was a wild circus, and it went on for all of five minutes. The protesters shouted down Reverend Jackson, and the predominantly Black audience shouted down the protesters as the police escorted them out of the room before they got a collective beatdown. Black folks were not having it—not on that day, and not at that moment.

My flashback to the *Jews Against Jackson* disruption offered me no defense that day in any shape, form, or fashion; no one was there to help me. I was not prepared to defend myself or my candidate. I was not savvy enough to have this debate; still, I would have to do my best based on my understanding of why Reverend Jackson supported a Palestinian homeland. However, there was a deeper history and even deeper wounds between the Jews and Palestinians that I had no idea how to address. And if I thought it couldn't get any worse, I was wrong. That young man had started something that had become a whole other thing. One after another, the students hit me with questions, as if the other candidate's representatives weren't sitting there. I couldn't think fast enough to answer their questions. I kept trying to explain our position. It wasn't flying. Nope! The program had reached a point of no return. I kept waiting for a teacher or any administrator to intervene. No one did, and I wanted it to be over. I had never been so happy to hear a school bell ringing. I stood up with a quickness and said goodbye to the other panelists.

A mixture of sympathy and glee in their eyes silently articulated, *Poor you ... glad it wasn't me.* The boys surrounded me with even more questions, so I told them my ride was waiting. I wasn't trying to answer any more questions. When I finally made my way out of the room, a young man met me in the hall. I thought, *Boy, you better take your ass up out of my face!* I was not going to have that debate anymore today.

"Miss," he called to me. I slowed my pace and turned to him. "Thank you," he said. I was confused, but relieved he was not hostile, even if I didn't know why he was thanking me. I stopped and he walked closer to me.

"This is the first time that the Palestinian side has ever been heard in this school," he said. "I will never forget you as long as I live. You made me feel proud to be a Palestinian." I didn't know what to say so I reached out and gave him a hug. He leaned into me, and I tighten my grip. I didn't have all the facts, but my gut told me this young man was the difference in our campaign. This was the kind of inclusion for which we were fighting. We were making room for those who had been locked out, ignored and rejected. It was becoming clear to me that even if Reverend Jackson didn't win, the landscape would never be the same. It reminded me of a quote from Dr. King: "The ultimate measure of a man is not where he stands in moments of convenience, but where he stands in times of challenge and controversy." While issues that affected Black people would always be my number one priority I was coming to terms with the intersection of suffering among all races. Dr. King was right about another thing, too: *No one is free until we are all free.*

After that day I promised myself that I would NEVER EVER speak publicly again. Period. I much preferred one on one, two by two, or three by three, whether in-person or with a phone in my hand. Drop me off in a cornfield on Monday and ask me to fill it by Saturday, but do not ask me to speak on a program. I also decided I would never again go into a setting unprepared. As soon as I made it back to the campaign office, I immediately sought our Middle East coordinator and Lisa Levine, our Jewish coordinator, to learn everything I could about the Israeli-Palestinian conflict. I started to engage other experts. Every time I saw Dr. James Zogby, the founder of the Arab American Institute and a senior advisor to the campaign on the Middle East, I asked him questions. He was another one of my favorite people to chat with about current affairs and was always willing to impart knowledge. I realized it was time to understand this rainbow rather than resent it, so I began to make it a point to learn from all of the field staff on our campaign. Carolyn Kazdin, for example, worked on women's rights and farm issues. She explained that some of the same farmers who had supported Reagan were suffering under his policies. It wasn't always about party affiliation, but also policies that created an intersection where we joined together to achieve a common goal. I went down the list. Jack O'Dell would have one of the greatest impacts on my intellectual growth involving social justice issues.

Jack was a senior advisor in economics and foreign policy for the campaign. He was a brilliant scholar and strategist who had served as a senior advisor to Dr. Martin Luther King Jr. during the civil rights movement. Two weeks before the March on Washington, President Kennedy asked Dr. King to sever his ties with Jack because of his ties to the Communist Party. Whenever I talked to Jack, he would weigh in on a topic and analyze it from an entirely different vantage point than everyone else. When I told him what happened at the school, his starting point wasn't the Palestinian-Israeli homeland debate, but the Black-Jewish relationship that began to fracture in the civil-rights movement of the 1950s and 1960s; our brutal disagreements around affirmative action in the 1970s; and Israel's support for the apartheid government of South Africa. Israel supported South Africa's military with the sale of weapons that were used against Black South Africans to help maintain apartheid. He gave me the human-rights argument that lifted both Jews' and Palestinians' right to live and thrive. Jack pushed me and he liked the fact that I was a critical thinker. He helped me shape that skill.

Dr. Ronald Walters had a similar influence on me. In addition to being the senior policy advisor to the campaign, he was the chair of the political science department at Howard University. Dr. Walters was in and out of the office and always willing to impart knowledge my way. It was because of him that I first considered a Ph.D. in political science. After every conversation with Dr. Walters, I wanted to know more about political theories and how they worked. The sum total of working on the campaign was my political coming of age. I was profoundly influenced by Reverend Jackson's agenda and the people I was exposed to during this period. I was forced to think deeper. As the campaign progressed, it became clear that I would have to gain my voice. I had to figure out what I believed and why I believed it. I was evolving in ways I did not anticipate.

I spent almost every waking moment pushing the ten-point plan Tyrone created that was the foundation for how youth and students operated within the campaign. I think every generation can point to young adults who tried to make a difference in their era, from SNCC in the sixties to the Black Lives Matter movement today. My generation was no different. We had some of the brightest and most fearless young adults in the country working with us. As the go-to person for all things related to youth and students, I continued to be amazed at their brilliance. Reverend Jackson had been preaching the narrative that Black people should run for elected office, even for dog catcher. Our plan encouraged young people to run as Jackson delegates, and they took us to heart. Two of our statewide student and youth coordinators, Mabel Thomas and Cleo Fields, ran as Jackson delegates and won. They would use their victories to launch their own political careers. Mabel ran for the Georgia House of Representatives and won. Cleo would follow her three years later to become the youngest state senator in Louisiana at the age of twenty-four, and then serve two terms in Congress by the age of thirty.

When I compare my generation with the ones after me, I am encouraged that young African Americans continue to make their mark. There are millennials like Bakari Sellers, who, in 2006 at the age of twenty-two, defeated a twenty-six-year incumbent to become the youngest state representative in South Carolina. Malcolm Kenyatta became the first openly gay person to be elected to the Pennsylvania House of Representatives in 2018, at the age of twenty-eight; Congresswoman Lauren Underwood, from the suburbs of Chicago, who won a seat in the U.S. House of Representative seat in 2019, at age thirty-three; and Generation Z's Haley Taylor Schlitz, who, at seventeen, ran as a delegate to the Democratic Convention for now-President Joe Biden and won, becoming the youngest delegate for 2020.

The network of young adults I worked with would be classified today as mostly Baby Boomers and the older individuals of Gen X. Many of us would make our mark in history after the campaign, but some were already influential at the time. Attorney Starlett "Star" Jones comes to mind. She is best known as one of the original co-hosts of the daytime talk show *The View*. During the campaign, Star served as the statewide youth and student coordinator for the campaign in Texas. She was also the international second vice president of Alpha Kappa Alpha Sorority Inc., one of the largest African American Greek-letter sororities in the United States. My exposure to Star inspired me to keep pushing to be the best woman I could be. My growth as a young adult was a product of all of these people converging in my life at the same time. My exposure to seasoned activists and nationally recognized people was a benefit, without a doubt. But it was a whole other thing to sit in meetings and talk regularly to other like-minded young adults who were my peers. They included Brenda Davenport, who was the national youth director for SCLC. Despite the SCLC leadership supporting Walter Mondale, Brenda gave us her support. There was Reverend Cynthia Jefferson—who was the Pennsylvania statewide youth and student coordinator and the SGA president at Cheyney University of Pennsylvania—who also ran as a Jackson delegate; and Julie Henderson, was the campaign's point person on all things Native American; she was Black and Native American, and influential in the Native American community and invaluable to our youth and student work. I never thought that I was capable of holding my own in the middle of greatness, but here I was holding my space.

There were also accomplished young men in the network. Hilary Shelton, who currently serves as the senior vice president for advocacy and policy at the NAACP, served with his brother Craig as our state youth and student co-coordinators for Missouri. At the time, Hilary was also the president of the National Organization of Black University and College Students. Gregory Moore, the former deputy national political director for the Democratic National Committee, was the newly elected president of the United States Student Association (USSA) and the first African American to hold that position in its thirty-six-year history. Tyrone and I met him at the March on Washington and started to nurture a relationship with him. By the midpoint of the campaign, he helped open doors among other student leaders across the country. Likewise, Keith Jennings, an international human-rights leader, was also at USSA. He had just replaced Donna Brazile as the chair of the Third World Student Coalition and was instrumental in opening doors with non-African American people of color. These are just a fraction of the young people who were involved in the campaign. We were a cutting-edge group, and I was proud to work with them.

I was anxious to get on the road and Tyrone encouraged me to put together a plan he could present to Arnold Pinkney. It was my first time writing a strategic plan. I was confident in my ability and grateful for the chance to go solo. I took everything I had learned in the last six months, pulled out my list of contacts, a map, and made tons of phone calls to Greyhound. It was the cheapest mode of travel at the time, and I didn't want cost to interfere with my plan being approved. We were headed into Super Tuesday—a five-state contest that included Massachusetts, Rhode Island, Alabama, Georgia and Florida. I thought I would be most effective and physically safe as a young woman traveling alone in the states where I already had strong networks; in those states would also be the greatest possibility to expand on the work our department had already done. I chose Alabama, Georgia and Florida; collectively, those three states had over twenty-five Black colleges and universities, and some fairly large white institutions. My proposal was approved. I prearranged as many meetings as I could with both the student leaders who were already committed to the campaign, as well as those who were interested but not yet onboard. I was given a modest food allowance and the funds I requested to purchase bus tickets from city to city.

In early February, with a hundred Xeroxed copies of the *Students for Jackson Plan* in tow, I hit the road in my three-inch heels on a Greyhound bus. I traveled to a different city each day, alternating between Alabama, Georgia and Florida every three days. It was grueling work, and I loved every minute of it. My schedule was pretty tight; sometimes I even changed my clothes in the bus station. I would leave my luggage where I could as I made my rounds. I slept wherever I could find a bed. Sometimes, one of the local campaign people provided me with a place to stay; other times, I stayed with one of our student coordinators. Reginald Holt, the Alabama statewide youth and student coordinator, let me bunk on the sofa in his trailer-apartment for one night. In Tallahassee, Florida I spent the night with the *Students for Jackson* campus coordinator in his off-campus apartment. Dale was also the SGA president of Florida A&M University; I met him during the youth conference that September at PUSH. He was good-looking and charming, and we had already flirted back in Chicago. That night, one thing led to another, and there you have it. I didn't regret it, but I put myself back in check. For the most part, I tried to keep my personal life away from the campaign. The majority of our network were young men, and I wanted nothing to undercut my place of authority in the world of double standards.

The most magical moments for me on the road happened when I crossed paths with the campaign entourage for a campaign rally with Reverend Jackson. It was a rock concert/church revival hybrid, and I had a front-row seat. The audience was always filled to the rafters, with hundreds of people; sometimes people were standing outside, hoping to get in the door. You couldn't help but get caught up. It was always a reunion with the press corps I got to know, and other national staff and advisors floating around the venue. Any given night, a prominent civil-rights leader or elected official would share the podium with Reverend Jackson and some noted gospel singers. My favorite was Reverend Wintley Phipps. When he performed the song "*Ordinary People*," it touched right down to the core of my soul. It is a simple song, but it packs so much power in the lyrics:

> *Just ordinary people, I'm so glad God uses, ordinary people. He uses people, just*
> *like you and me who are willing to do as he commands.*
> *God uses people who will give their all,*
> *it doesn't matter how small your all may seem to you,*
> *because little becomes much, when placed in the master's hand.*

Each time he came to the podium, I would find a spot and get still. By the time he reached the second stanza, my tears would be quietly falling. I believed God was using Reverend Phipps to tell me, *Keep going, my daughter; I have even more work for you.* I kept that song on replay for the next ten years of my life until cassettes became outdated. After Reverend Phipps finished singing, Reverend Jackson started his famous call-and-response: *I am somebody!* The audience repeated after him: *I am somebody! From the outhouse to the White House, I am somebody.* Toward the end of his speech, he challenged the audience to run for office. He said, "If you don't run, you're guaranteed to lose. If you do run, you might lose." The audience always responded with *Win! Jesse! Win!* and it ignited like a wildfire. At the end of each day, I gathered these experiences into myself, and they gave me hope to carry on.

It was on the road campaigning that my relationship with Mrs. Jacqueline Jackson began to blossom. She was one of the most impactful people in my life from my time on the campaign into my thirties. Every time she came into the campaign headquarters, I would walk out of my office to be in her presence. I was surprised to see her out there campaigning as hard as her husband. She was a popular surrogate for the campaign and always packed the room. We crossed paths sometimes in the local campaign headquarters, and other times at Reverend Jackson's rallies. Whenever she saw me during the Super Tuesday campaigning, we had the same conversation, or so it seemed to me:

"Baby, what are you doing here by yourself?" she asked.

"Trying to get your husband elected president," I answered enthusiastically. "Be careful out here trying to get Jesse Jackson elected president," she retorted, then gave me a hug. It always made me feel good that she was concerned about my well-being. I loved chatting with Ms. J, as I began to call her. She was a brilliant critical thinker who was equal to her husband. I connected with her uncanny ability to critique an issue: It was a skill I also had, but she could illuminate that issue for any given audience. She didn't mince words. I listened to her being interviewed as often as I could, and she did not allow a reporter to reduce her or place her in a box. She was gracious in public, and everyone seemed to matter to her. When an unfamiliar person approached Ms. J, she paused what she was doing and chatted with him or her like she knew that person her entire life. Afterward, she turned to me and said, "Always be gracious, Rae. People don't have to like you." I took her philosophy as my own, especially when I became a public figure. Those times hanging out with Ms. J helped influence my public persona. Another thing she told me more than once was, "Be careful what you do in public; people are always watching." After a few times of bumping into Ms. J on the road, she asked, "Baby, how are you getting to all these different cities?"

"The Greyhound bus," I replied, swelling with pride like I was flying in a private jet.

"Really?" she asked with surprise. I nodded.

"You be careful out here, baby, on the Greyhound bus," she chuckled. I just smiled and, if there was time, I sat with her until it was time for her to go.

I loved, loved, loved talking to Ms. Jackson, about clothes. I admired her style and poise from the first day I laid eyes on her at PUSH. People always asked me how I came to be put together so well. Well, it was due to my time with Jacqueline Jackson. She represented Black women in a space where we had not been included — as the wife of a presidential candidate—and she did so with style and grace. Unbeknownst to her, she became my style muse. I took mental notes every time I asked her about an ensemble she was wearing. She was always so gracious. She took any opportunity to teach. As I've mentioned, I already had an eye for the finer things, but she was the person who taught me about fabric, designers and quality. With her advice, I started to define my look: classic, with an edge.

The first time I copied Ms. J was with the purchase of a handbag. I coveted her large Louis Vuitton Speedy Bandouliere handbag and, one day, asked her opinion about me purchasing one. After she had given me a history lesson on Louis Vuitton, explaining that he was one of the finest and oldest bag designers in the world. She advised me to start with a smaller version of her iconic Speedy. She said it would give me something to appreciate as I matured. I took her sage advice to heart. I thought I was rich at the time. I was making more money than I ever had in my life—a whopping one thousand dollars a month! I gave Cynthia three hundred dollars monthly for rent and purchased my own food; I had no other expenses so, yeah, I thought I was rich. It was my third or fourth paycheck; I marched down to the Louis Vuitton store on Connecticut Avenue and asked to see the twenty-five-inch Speedy. I examined every inch of that bag before I decided to take the leap.

"I love it!" I declared to the salesperson, who nodded his approval.

"Can I put it on layaway?" I asked, gleefully. You should have seen the look on his face. He stopped smiling and became dignified, acquiring one of those snobbish looks that salespeople sometimes give certain customers in high-end stores.

"Ma-dam," he said, meticulously. "We don't have layaway at Louis Vuitton." I left the store deflated, but undeterred. At the time, the bag cost five-hundred-fifty bucks. I saved a hundred bucks out of my paycheck every two weeks for three months and marched my tail right back to the Louis Vuitton store, and I walked out with my first designer bag. It was my travel companion for the entire campaign. Every time Mrs. Jackson saw me with my *Louie,* she asked, "Are you enjoying it?" You would have thought I had just won a beauty contest the way I smiled. I still own that bag out of sentiment, even though it is no longer a part of my wardrobe.

I was in Miami to advance Reverend Jackson's speech to the Florida State Student Association and bumped into Ms. J in the hotel lobby. It seemed to me that everyone in the national campaign office converged on Miami that weekend.

"What in the world are you doing all the way in Miami, and how did you get here?" she asked. I explained how I had taken a bus from Tallahassee to Pensacola, where I met with student leaders at West Pensacola University, and that Tyrone had arranged my lodging and a ride to Miami. She just shook her head at my tenacity.

Elijah Smiley, was now the Florida statewide youth and student coordinator for the campaign and the president of the FSSA, and had arranged for Reverend Jackson to speak at the conference. Being asked to work in the larger campaign apparatus on the road for the very first time confirmed in my eyes that the higher-ups, not just Tyrone, had faith in my ability to get the job done. This was a pivotal moment for me to show my skills and shine outside of Tyrone's shadow. I was responsible for the venue walkthrough with the Secret Service and briefing Reverend Jackson before his speech. You talk about being a nervous wreck—my God! Until then, I had opened my mouth only to say, "Hello, Reverend," before scurrying away with anxiety. The magnitude of it was overwhelming, but I had done my due diligence. Florida was a critical state, and a big one. We needed to get more student leaders onboard outside of the historically Black colleges and universities that we had already recruited.

That day we gained the endorsement of the statewide student association and picked up support from many more student leaders throughout the state, including white ones. We were starting to build a rainbow coalition. Later, in the lobby, I crossed paths with Reverend Jackson, and he stopped and said, "Good job!" You would have thought he had just handed me a million dollars in that one second of praise. Mr. Pinkney, standing next to him, gave me a nod of approval, too. Moments like these helped me gain more confidence. I started to see myself through the lens of others who saw the best in me. I still had a distance to go, but at least I began to see concrete examples that contradicted Mama's narrative that I was never going to amount to anything.

When it was time to leave Florida, I was given an airplane ticket and taken off the Greyhound bus permanently. Mr. Pinkney told me that Mrs. Jackson demanded that he—and I quote—"Get that baby off the damn bus!" I was grateful to travel by plane, but I would have been happy to continue by bus. What meant the most to me was that Mrs. Jackson cared enough about me to take me off the bus.

After Super Tuesday, I came to Chicago to work the Illinois primary. I was proud of myself. The Saturday before election day, I went to visit Mama. Her girlfriend Mary and her adult daughters were over, visiting from Ohio. From the moment I walked in, all the attention went straight to me. Everyone but Mama wanted the Jackson scoop. By this time, the campaign was one of the most talked-about subjects in the African American community. The contest for the Democratic nomination had begun with eight contenders: Sens. John Glenn, Alan Cranston and Ernest Hollings and former Govs. Rubin Askew and George McGovern. Now, there were only three men standing: Vice President Walter Mondale, Sen. Gary Hart and Rev. Jesse L. Jackson. The Black community had done the math and Jackson had made it further than five white men in the race. Pride swelled. Debate parties sprung up all over the country and families gathered around the television to watch a Black man compete on the national stage that had been reserved for white men.

That day at Mama's, Mary and her daughters were aware I was in the middle of an important moment in Black history, and they told me so. They wanted to know what it was like for me to be a part of it all. One after the other, they fired questions my way. *What is it like to be on the campaign? What is Reverend Jackson like? Where have you traveled? What are his chances of winning?* My heart was leaping with joy and excitement. One of Mary's daughters said, "Rae, you should be proud." And I was—not just because I was a part of the campaign, but because this was the first time any of Mama's friends saw me outside of her lens, and it felt good. Mama shuffled between the kitchen and the front room. She would listen for a while and then go back into the kitchen. Finally, she came and stood in the living room doorway with a cigarette hanging out the side of her mouth and a drink in her hand. The last thing I remember someone saying before Mama opened her mouth was, "This is the opportunity of a lifetime for you, Rae." Mama took her cigarette out of her mouth and wailed, "That bitch ain't working for Jesse Jackson!" Everyone got quiet. My stomach sank, and despair took over. Eyes shifted from me to Mama and back to me. I looked at Mama with dread and waited for the next thing to come out of her mouth.

"She ain't working for no damn Jesse Jackson," she repeated.

"She's fucking him!" she said, all smug-like. I was shrinking by the minute. My mind was racing. *How could she embarrass me like this? How could she even part her damn lips to say such a thing?* She had everyone's attention now.

"Yeah," she twirled her hand with the cigarette in the air to make her point, "She's FUCK-ING him. That's the only reason he's keeping her around!"

WHAT THE FUCK IS THIS?! screamed in my head. I heard someone say, "Rae, don't no one believe that crazy shit but Georgia." I looked at Mama, and she was waiting on my response with fire in her eyes. I fought back the tears.

"Mama, why can't you just be proud of me?" I asked, my voice cracking. I wanted to defend myself and Reverend Jackson. I looked up to Reverend Jackson, and that accusation hurt me to the very core. I looked at her, standing there puffed-up. She reached back and placed her drink on the dresser. With a hand on one hip and the cigarette dangling in the other, she waited for me to defend myself. I knew any defense would be futile and would escalate into an argument at a fever pitch. She would tell me how *fast* I had always been, starting with the little boy under the porch when I was six years old.

"Huh, Mama? Why can't you just be proud of me?" I asked again. I waited on her answer as she waited for more of a reaction from me. I heard someone say, "Aww, Georgia—stop it." That was her cue, and she went berserk. She yelled, "You sitting up here talking about what you doing. You doing this, and you doing that. You ain't doing shit but fucking!" She said it with so much hatred and bitterness that I got up and grabbed my coat.

"Sit back down, Rae," her girlfriend Mary said to me. "You know how Georgia is." I heard someone else say, "Georgia, you ought to quit." I fought back the tears as I put my coat on and walked to the door. Her friends pleaded with me: "You don't have to go. Sit back down. Don't let Georgia ruin everything." Mama was silent. When I reached the door, I turned to look at Mama. She was defiant. I looked at her friends and their pleading faces and mumbled, "I really do have to go." I left the apartment, and my first tear dropped.

"If she that mad, let that bitch go!" Mama shouted. As I made my way back to my hotel by way of public transportation on that chilly March day, a thousand questions ran through my head. *Why couldn't she be proud of me just once in my life? Was Mama ever going to change? Could I ever do anything that would meet her approval?* I knew those answers weren't coming soon so I pushed Mama from my mind and focused my attention on the primary that was coming in a couple of days.

D isappointments kept coming—this time, in politics—but they also forced growth. Actually, growing pains might be more accurate. I had always taken certain things very personally. When I learned that Mayor Harold Washington ran a slate of delegates to the Democratic Convention who were committed to him as the "favorite son of Illinois" rather than to Jackson, I was mad as hell. This would cause me to have my first "coming to Jesus" moment between politics and politicians.

I was already looking at Mayor Washington with a side-eye because he had endorsed Charles Hayes over Lutrelle "Lu" Palmer to replace his vacant Congressional seat. Now here we were again, with what I viewed as a betrayal of both men. Of course, I didn't know any of the nuances that affected Washington's decision in either case, but I understood loyalty. I knew that it was Reverend Jackson and Lu Palmer who had led a coalition of Black and Hispanic leaders to ask Washington to run for mayor. Washington was not sold on the idea and told them that if they registered 50,000 new voters and raised $100,000, he would consider running. Within six months, they raised the money and registered 275,000 new voters. They did that and so much more to help ensure Washington's victory. It was also Lu Palmer who coined Washington's campaign slogan: "We Shall See in '83." So, damn right, I thought Washington should have supported both of them; if not, then he should have at least stayed the hell out of the way. I never viewed Mayor Washington in the same way again. If I were nothing else, I was principled and loyal—even to a fault. As you can imagine, negative critiques of Washington were a very unpopular position back then; he was Black Chicago's superhero. Washington was my first candidate and my first campaign, and he and Jackson were intertwined, in my mind. I could not shake how I felt despite that Harold Washington wasn't the only African American mayor who didn't support Jackson. Wilson Goode, Tom Bradley and Coleman Young were also on the list. In retrospect, maybe the other mayors' disapproval didn't bother me as much because I was not connected to them.

I wasn't sure I was cut out for cutthroat politics. I was so damn self-righteous and loyal. I believed there was a certain order to things, and it reflected in an ideology I thought was pure. Washington had shaken that ideology. I remained self-righteous and loyal, but Washington's lack of support for Jackson forced me to see the world as it really is; I learned that backroom deals do happen. By the end of the campaign, I knew I would never run for office. I saw politics as a vehicle to help make life better for people as a means to an end. My challenge was hanging onto my idealism and not allowing the ugliness to taint me or make me bitter.

The New York primary was exhilarating. It was the most exciting primary that I worked on during the '84 race. New York was very different from working in the South. It was fast-paced and constantly moving, which demanded quick decision-making. The New York Students for Jackson, headed by Melvin Lowe, was in full force. As I've mentioned earlier, Melvin was the chair of the CUNY Student Association, and he used the extent of his power and resources for the campaign. We had three students running on the ballot as Jackson delegates, Anthony Gant, William Allen and Esther Mitchell and two would win. Reverend Jackson held a big rally at the City College of New York, with Melvin and William by his side. New York was the first time I put in fifteen-hour days. I was running on adrenaline until the very end. One night I arrived back to my hotel room at about two in the morning. I planned to sleep in because Reverend Jackson was going to participate in a Puerto Rican parade, and I was not needed. I was grateful when my head hit that pillow.

When the phone rang a few hours later, I sat straight up in the bed, looked at the clock and picked up the phone. It was six in the morning and I thought, *Whoever it is has lost their freaking mind*—until I heard Tyrone's voice on the other end. I had new instructions. Reverend Jackson wanted to emphasize poverty on the parade route, and I was supposed to make it happen. I called Melvin and William to explain. Thirty minutes later, Melvin swooped me up from the hotel with an area already in mind, which made my life easier; William joined us later. In the days before cellphones, this was one crazy assignment. I had to accomplish this mission before Reverend Jackson left the hotel for the day so that the Secret Service could advance and approve the spot. By 7:45 a.m., we had found the perfect place: a vacant house on the parade route, with dead rats and all. I found a pay phone and called Tyrone to let him know I had located a site for Reverend Jackson. I was instructed to wait for the Secret Service to conduct the walk-through. Melvin, William and I waited and waited, and waited some more. By noon, the Secret Service arrived; then, we waited some more for the parade to arrive. As they neared us two hours later, Reverend Jackson deviated from the route with the media and their camera crews in tow. It took all of ten minutes for what had been seven hours of work. I was relieved we had no hiccups. When Reverend Jackson started to move back into the parade, somehow, I was pushed into the flow of movement and, before I knew it, I had walked the length of the parade in a suit and three-inch heels. You talkin' 'bout one feet-hurting, tired-tail, Black woman? That was me—and I would not have taken a million dollars in exchange for that moment.

After New York, I worked the Pennsylvania, District of Columbia and Ohio primaries. Sometime after the Ohio primary, Tyrone walked away from the campaign. He just quit. He gave me no warning whatsoever. I learned about it from Sylvia Branch. There were no cellphones I could pick up right then to ask him why but, soon enough, he reached out. The best conclusion I could draw from the conversation was that Tyrone wanted his independence. He and Reverend Jackson bumped heads and he walked away from the campaign. He left me, and I was hurt; we were a team. I felt abandoned.

After his departure, I was not given any tangible instructions except to continue doing what I had been doing, and I started reporting to Anita Bonds. I liked Anita. She was easygoing. I gave her my weekly reports and she didn't interfere with my work. Nonetheless, the campaign structure was changing. Funds were running low, and I didn't go back out on the road. Honestly, there was no need for me to travel. The youth and student department didn't have an extensive student network on the West Coast, where the remaining contests were held. I spent my time back in my office making cold calls, plugging students into the local campaign offices and sending them *The Students for Jackson Plan*. Being in the office with only half the work I had previously done was not a good thing for me. I look back at times like these and understand now why I was a workaholic and kept a breakneck schedule: I needed to keep my mind occupied because sitting with myself and my thoughts left me vulnerable to self-doubt, low self-esteem and memories of my childhood, which would seep into my brain like carbon dioxide into an airtight car with the engine running. With no smell and no warning, by the time the negativity consumed me, I was so far in that coming back out was a fight for my life. Men were one of those battles.

I had done so well with my dating and sex life since I began working with PUSH and on through the campaign. Even though I had a lot of would-be suitors, I was slow to act and thoughtful about my decisions. On the campaign, I had one relationship with a reporter who was a permanent member of the traveling press corps. Sylvester Monroe, who worked at *Newsweek,* pulled up on me a few times, and I always took a pass. I didn't want to get caught up in some bullshit, particularly since Ms. J had taken me under her wing. Sylvester was persistent. When we first arrived in New York, he asked me to dinner and an off-Broadway play at the New York Negro Ensemble Theater. Technically, he didn't work for the campaign. Still, it was a bit murky. After New York, Sylvester and I discreetly met whenever we were in the same city. Those moments away from the madness of the campaign turned into a friendship that has lasted decades.

Back in the campaign headquarters and away from the breakneck schedule and the intimate moments with Sylvester—I was again a loose cannon. I first noticed this handsome guy stuffing envelopes in the outer office. He was about six-foot-three, brown-skinned with wavy black hair that was cut close. On top of that, he had a beautiful smile. I asked Thomas Atkins, the volunteer coordinator and office manager who knew everything about everybody and everything, who the heck this guy was. Thomas gave me that look, noting, *He's fine, ain't he?* I gave it right back: *Damn straight!* It turned out he had just gotten out of the military, and both he and his father were volunteering. *How nice*, I thought. A week later, Thomas brought Greg to my office and introduced him. Greg eventually asked me to lunch, which turned into more lunches and visits to my house. He was so charming, and such a gentleman; he even opened doors for me. We laughed a lot and had great conversations about politics. He was the consummate renaissance man, and husband material. The chemistry in bed was mind-blowing and I thought I had found the love of my life. He, his brother and father were devout Muslims. I was a devout Christian, and my first mistake was changing my life to align with his religious beliefs—right down to the food I ate and the pans I used to cook the food. Greg didn't want pork near anything he ate, and I complied. I even celebrated Ramadan with him. Imagine: me fasting for something that I didn't believe in. This man had my nose so wide open.

As the campaign started to wind down, I spent more time with Greg because I had no other friends in D.C. Everyone I knew was affiliated with the campaign in one way or another. At first, somewhere in my dream world, Greg was the one who was going to sweep me off my feet and we would live happily ever after. Then reality started to set in. I didn't know Greg as well as I thought. But, then again, how do you know anybody in only a couple of months? The red flags started popping up all over the place. He had a lot of free time and a lot of money, but no job. He told me he was an entrepreneur trying to get his business off the ground—but I could never pinpoint what exactly he was doing. When I asked again, it was always vague; he'd say something like, *a little of this, a little of that.* I knew in my heart that it wasn't adding up. I dismissed anything shady because it was easier. Besides, he didn't meet any stereotypical images of a hustler. He was not a flashy dresser, he drove a very old car, he didn't have people in and out of his home that he shared with his brother. For Christ's sake, I met him while he was stuffing envelopes.

One night, everything changed. We were in bed messing around and he asked me if I wanted to try some cocaine. I was shocked. This was the first time he had ever mentioned drugs to me. I thought he was strait-laced as you could get, like me. He didn't drink or smoke. I asked him about it, and he told me that he occasionally snorted cocaine. This was the early eighties, on the cusp of the crack-cocaine crisis. Among my peers, marijuana was the drug of choice. Cocaine was viewed as the high-class drug mainly used by those who had money to spare. I had heard about fancy parties where cocaine was generously laid out for the guests. I had even heard that cocaine and sex made the ultimate combination. The master of manipulation—that's exactly where Greg went.

"You know, cocaine will give you the orgasm of a lifetime," he said. I didn't want to have this discussion. I had already told him I did not use drugs, and all I could think about was how to get out of his proposition.

"I already have great orgasms," I said, with sass. "I don't need drugs to make me come; all I need is you." But he was persistent, and he was wearing me down—and he knew it. He got out of the bed.

"Let me just go get it. If you do not like it, I will never ask you again," he said. I sighed and gave him a pathetic shrug. He crawled back into the bed with the cocaine already on a book and a razor blade in his hand. I had only seen this done on television, and I watched in amazement as he chopped the white powdery substance until it was as fine as sifted flour. He then divided the drug into four straight lines. He reached into a drawer on the bedside stand and took out this short little straw—almost like a coffee stirrer—and he told me, "Watch me." He bent down to the book and sucked the cocaine into his nose through the straw. He wiggled his nose again with his hand and took another hit. It was my turn. I had an adrenaline rush; I couldn't believe that I was really going to do it. As he held the book in his lap, I took the straw and reached down to take a hit. I could feel him watching. My mind was racing. I didn't want to lose him, but all I could think about were the few conversations I had with my mother about her and my father's drug use. By now, my heart was pounding. In those seconds, I replayed my childhood through my mother's words, and I froze: "We were a big fucking mess— an interracial couple living in Buffalo, New York in the sixties and strung out on drugs with our Black baby. Our life was plain old crazy. We loved you Rae, but we were unable to take care of you."

I had lost so much because of drugs. Now here I was about to go down the same path. I knew in my heart this was the beginning of the end. I bent down further, but then I couldn't. I could hear Dorje as clear as day saying, "We were two junkies getting together." I wanted Greg, but my hatred of drugs was more potent than my love for him.

Their drug addiction had left me in a world filled with abuse. This was not a life I wanted for myself. I sat up. "I don't want to." I said.

"Are you sure?" he asked. I nodded yes. I was sitting on pins and needles waiting on his acceptance. He took a couple more hits. "That's okay, baby," he said, pulling me into his arms. I breathed a sigh of relief. We had sex the way he wanted, which was an all-night marathon. I figured it was a small price to pay for his acceptance of my decision, sore vagina and all. After that night, things about Greg started to add up for me. But I gave him credit that he had shielded whatever the hell he was doing from me, but that night had created a shift within me. In a small way, he was introducing me to my future with him—and I got the message, loud and clear. He and I were going in two different directions. I didn't bother to have that conversation; I just started plotting my exit.

Now what? That was the hundred-thousand-dollar question. After Tyrone left, I didn't process what it meant for me or my future. Instead, I buried it like it didn't happen or have any consequences for me. I was at a loss. Before his departure, Tyrone and I were on the road all the time, often in different cities, which meant we no longer had the long talks like we had at PUSH. He had mostly done the figuring for me during those past fourteen months. I had been focused on my work and hadn't thought about looking for my next project. Now, he was gone and I was handicapped. I had all these big dreams to be a national organizer and save the world, and didn't have a clue how to proceed. I had never once thought about what was supposed to happen at the end of a presidential campaign. I knew the Democratic Convention was going to be held in San Francisco, but I didn't know how it worked. No one had mentioned it to me, and I couldn't ask what I didn't know. I tried to talk to staff that was still around, but I got the impression people had placed me in a box. I was the student and youth organizer, period. Sure, many of them knew I had talent, but they didn't see *me* doing the work *they* were doing. Everyone assumed that I was headed back to school, like April. When I talked about my dreams, I always got the, *Yes, but finish school first* pushback. I wanted to finish school more than ever. I had been inspired by Dr. Walters, but I also flunked out a year earlier. Going back wasn't that simple. In a pinch, I'm sure Mama would've allow me to come back to live with her, but at what cost? I had called to check in on her here and there after I walked out of her house that Saturday back in March, and I knew there would be a price to pay.

I was confident that I had mad skills, but I had no clue how to launch them into my next project or even what kind of project I could create to use my skills. At the same time, I knew I needed to get away from Greg. He didn't approach me about drugs again; still, I was over Casanova. He would disappear even the times I was at his house in his bed waiting for him to return. There were endless women calling. The inconsistencies and lies piled up. I finally broke down and called SIU to see if there was a way I could come back. Admissions told me I would have to petition for readmission. In response, I wrote a letter about my growth in the last year and my work on the campaign. I asked Sylvia if I could get a letter of recommendation from Reverend Jackson; along with my letter, it sealed the deal. Afterward, when people asked about my next move and I said I was going back to school, I got the nod of approval. In the meantime, I was still stuck with Greg to take care of my basic needs. You don't *even* need to ask if I was saving my money. My over-the-top spending would become a mistake I would repeat in different ways well into my forties. That aspect of my behavior would not change for me until I began to deconstruct the reason behind my spending and break the cycle. I wanted to tell Mrs. Jackson I needed help with moving back to Chicago, but couldn't. I was too embarrassed. I was afraid she would throw me away if I had told her about that ugly part of my life. Instead, I asked her if I could go to the Democratic Convention. She promised to make it happen.

Reverend Jackson won 3.5 million votes; 41 Congressional districts; and the Democratic primaries in Louisiana, South Carolina, Mississippi and the District of Columbia. It was predicted that Jackson would only win between 175 to 200 delegates; instead, he won 465. The Jackson would have won double that number if the Democratic party rules weren't stacked against us and were distributed based on the popular vote.

Mrs. Jackson kept her word to me. My plane landed in San Francisco the Sunday before the convention began. They lost my luggage, which meant I got to shop with my per diem and the extra money Greg had given to me. In the day, I volunteered in the hotel campaign office and was given guest credentials in the evening to watch the convention. On the night of Reverend Jackson's speech, I had a prime seat on the convention floor. I stood on my chair the entire fifty-two minutes, glued to every single word that came out of his mouth. We had made it, and that was satisfying to my soul. Reverend Jackson was electrifying, profound and spiritual. I fought back the flood of tears during the entire speech. Then Wintley Phipps began singing "*Ordinary People.*" Tears rushed out my eyes like the Niger River running its course to the Atlantic Ocean, and I cried myself ugly.

Thirty-Five

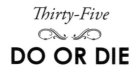

DO OR DIE

"
"You may encounter many defeats, but you must not be defeated."
— Maya Angelou

I came back to Carbondale in late August 1984 to begin fall classes at SIU, but my heart was back in Washington, D.C., with my dream of becoming a national organizer. Coming back was the only choice I believed I had at the time. Now back in Carbondale, I asked, where was that brave young woman who moved to D.C. without even a place to live? I wondered how the heck I had spent an entire year listening to Reverend Jackson talk about taking chances while I had been afraid to take another risk. Every time I stepped out of my trailer apartment onto the gravel road adjacent to it, I thought, "I came back to this—for what, again?" The only thing that made Carbondale remotely tolerable was that Veronica had transferred back to SIU and we were reunited.

My political work on campus kept me sane. I ran for assistant coordinator of the Black Affairs Council. However, I really wanted to run for the top position of coordinator, but the members of Alpha Phi Alpha Fraternity wanted one of the fraternity brothers to have the position. They made it perfectly clear to me that I would lose if I went up against them. I weighed my chances. Sure, I already had a reputation on campus for my work on Harold Washington's mayoral campaign. People knew I could get the job done. I also had some newfound popularity because I worked on Reverend Jackson's presidential campaign. On the surface my chances seemed good, but the Alphas were extremely popular, and their network was large. They even had more Alpha Angels on campus than Alphas, and they were very popular in their own right. Some of the brothers came to me and offered a deal. If I ran for assistant coordinator instead of coordinator, they would support me. As a Black woman going up against a Black fraternity, I knew the backlash would be swift, so I agreed. I had made my first backroom deal. I didn't like the heavy-handedness, but I thought it was a good tradeoff. If I ran and lost, I would have no official role; however, if I accepted their deal, at least I would still have an integral role within the organization. I had a lot of ideas, and I wanted to be in a position to see them implemented. I told myself it was about the work, not the title. In reality, I just didn't have enough confidence to go up against the Alpha's popularity and influence on campus. I struggled to be a team-player the first couple of weeks. My feelings were hurt that the Alphas had bum-rushed me. I had considered many of them my friends, but this ordeal left a bitterness that I forced to the back of my heart so that I could face them on campus.

I bounced back quickly, though. I remembered Reverend C.T. Vivian telling me you should do the work wherever it is needed. I stopped feeding my ego and got to work. The Free South Africa Movement had sprung up like wildflowers on college campuses across the globe. Students were demanding their universities divest all monies from companies that invested in South Africa. With SIU, the investment portfolio was often funneled through university foundations, so the targets were both the school and the school's foundation. I created a Free South Africa Committee under the BAC banner. My main co-conspirator was Stephen Shaw, the assistant editor of the BAC newspaper.

We recruited students, made signs, and picketed in front of the University Foundation building a few times a week. Some days it was just little old me in front of the office, chanting, "DIVEST NOW!" If I was nothing else, I was determined. Other days, we had a crowd. We never had hundreds of students join the protests, like on some of the other college campuses across the country. Nevertheless, at various times that semester, our protests picked up steam. We even made the evening news and had features in both the school and local newspapers. This went a long way in forcing the University Foundation to respond.

I became somewhat disillusioned with Black students and their priorities. I was in revolutionary mode all the time and wanted everyone else to to embrace my sentiments, but that was not the case. College students also wanted to party, and part of my job as the assistant coordinator was to arrange party dates for the campus Black organizations with the student center. Well, my failure to efficiently execute this assignment was my biggest blip.

I knew the student center parties were important to Black students because they were our primary social events. I somehow mistakenly double-booked another organization's party date with the Black Fire Dancers event. Honestly, I don't know how I messed up so badly. All I can remember is the craziness that followed. The Black Fire Dancers were so pissed that they wanted to physically fight me over those damn party dates. To say the least, my failure at this task was embarrassing, and everybody had an opinion. I was told, in no uncertain terms, to watch my back. Lord, I was scared shitless! I viewed it as a frivolous mess, but I didn't voice my disapproval because I didn't want to get beaten up. I certainly thought about the triviality of it, compared to real-world problems. In my worldview, their priorities were in the wrong place. The separation of the races in South Africa was unconscionable. Black South Africans lived in deplorable conditions— stacked on top of each other in townships with no running water, electricity or toilets, and limited education. *FUCK party dates!* I emotionally punched out. I don't remember how the issue was resolved, only that the members rolled their eyes at me every time we crossed paths the entire freaking school year. In the end, all I could do was take ownership of my mistake and continue my duties with the BAC. Yet again, my idealism didn't match my reality.

Beyond my Free South Africa work, SIU just didn't excite me. In the classes I liked, I attended and excelled. I even received some A's both semesters. The classes I struggled with the most were ones I gave less of a priority, and I did less and less work. In those classes, my grades stalled between C's and F's. I was repeating the pattern of my first year at SIU. I really wanted to finish college, but my determination was not enough to push me through at this juncture of my life. How the hell was I supposed to make it through college algebra when I had barely made it through freshman algebra in high school? I also had legitimate deterrents that contributed to my poor outcomes. They were perfect distractions that helped me to avoid rather than face my academic failures. That school year, when I wasn't protesting, I worked odd jobs to keep a roof over my head and food on my table. I worked at a pizza parlor, at the corn-dog stand in the mall, waited tables in a pub on The Strip and posed nude for upper-level art classes. Posing nude was the highest-paid student job on campus, and I jumped at the opportunity. When I wasn't working, I was on the phone arguing with Greg—yes, Greg, the boyfriend back in Washington, D.C. I had told myself it was over when I boarded that airplane; I just never told him. After the cocaine incident, I decided to hang in there until I came back to SIU. I thought it was because I needed the financial help, for which I had already paid a hefty price. While that may have been true, the other truth was I was so emotionally attached to him that I couldn't let go.

Holding on would cost me not only my emotional health; it would cost me my physical health, too. When I was still living in D.C., the day I returned from the Democratic National Convention, Greg picked me up from the airport; we then went straight to his house and had some badass, I-missed-you sex. Later that night, I answered his telephone when he was out. It was a girl whose name I had heard before. I took it upon myself to set her straight. How crazy was that? Granted, I was moving out of town. Still, I had to set her straight. It was me at my low point, trying to keep a man that I knew in my heart was never going to treat me with the respect I deserved.

"Stop calling my motherfucking man!" I demanded.

"You need to tell him to leave me alone," she said to me in a smug tone.

"Girl, Greg don't want your ass," I hollered through the telephone.

"Well, he wanted my ass when you were out of town," she said curtly. Sitting on the side of the bed, my mind raced like a greyhound—fast and hard. I asked myself, *How did she know I was out of town?* She broke the silence.

"If you don't believe me, ask him," she said, cool as a cucumber. I didn't know how to respond, so I said nothing. She knew she had my attention and went on to tell me Greg wasn't shit and all she was doing was playing him for money.

"Did he tell you I gave him gonorrhea when you were away at the convention?" she asked.

"Greg don't have gonorrhea" came out of my mouth before I could even think. But I knew it was true the moment she said "convention."

"Ask him," she insisted and hung up.

This is where dumb gets dumber. Earlier that day, I was coming out of the bathroom and caught Greg taking some medication. I asked him and he told me he had pulled a muscle lifting weights. When he came back home that night, I confronted him about my conversation with her and he stuck to his story. I wasn't convinced—not really. I knew in my heart he was lying but, to make sure, I wrote the name of the medication— tetracycline—and asked my roommate, Dr. Sadler, what it was used to treat. Instead of telling me my man wasn't shit, she had me look it up in her medication book to draw my own conclusion. I must have read it a dozen times. It confirmed he had an infection— maybe an STD. I was a glutton for more punishment. I accepted Greg's lie with some crazy rationalization that the drug could be used for more than an STD. With age and experience, I've come to understand that sometimes I didn't want the truth because it would force me to make decisions I was not emotionally prepared to make. About a week later, Greg confessed to having gonorrhea. He explained that the girl seduced him. He didn't admit to it originally because he didn't want to hurt me and he was sure he had taken enough medication to fix the situation before I returned, but he hadn't. Consequently, Greg infected me with gonorrhea and continued his medication, and it cleared up; however, I re-infected him, and that is the only reason he finally confessed. I only had a couple more weeks before I left for Carbondale, and I told myself I needed to stick it out because he was the person financing my return to SIU. I told myself that once I left, I'd be done with him.

When I first arrived back in Carbondale, I tried to get him out of my system. Reggie and I flirted—yes, the same Reggie I had broken up with the year before. I had reached out to him to help me find an apartment and a job, and he came through on both. But we couldn't make it work. He was in an out with another girl and I was all tangled with Greg. Greg just kept calling and I kept giving in. That October, he sent me a train ticket to meet him and his family in New Orleans for the World's Fair. After that, he came to visit me. At first, it was like old times: I cooked his favorite foods and we had lots of sex; then, like old times, it went downhill. The final straw was the showdown I had with him and the woman he had been dating for many years—not to be confused with the woman who gave him gonorrhea. His longtime girlfriend called my house and asked if Greg was with me. I told her he was. She proceeded to explain how long they had been together, and blah blah, blah. Every time I tried to explain it away, she had an answer, and I knew it was the truth. When he got in that taxi to go back to the airport, I was done.

Greg was out of my life, but I still had to deal with the fallout from his whoring. I was talking on the phone to Dorje one day, and I told her about this nagging low abdominal pain that wouldn't go away. I loved the simple fact that I could talk to her about anything without fear of judgment. She told me it sounded like I may have a sexually transmitted disease. I didn't see how that could be and I shared that Greg had given me gonorrhea, and that I had already been treated. Her response was, "Fucking bastard!" I loved that I was so much my mother's child. Her DNA was all over me, with simple things that could have been classic Rae reactions, too. Eventually, she ran across a newspaper article about chlamydia and sent it to me. The article stated that dual infections of chlamydia and gonorrhea were on the rise. There was a concern that women were being treated exclusively for gonorrhea with penicillin, which does not treat chlamydia. Sure enough, I had received a shot of penicillin in my ass to treat the gonorrhea. I hadn't even been tested because I told the doctor I knew for sure my boyfriend had given me gonorrhea. When I first noticed the pain, I dreaded going to the student health services after my experience with herpes the year before. I hated to do it, but with this new information I knew that I needed to get tested quickly. They diagnosed me with chlamydia and treated me with the same medication Greg had taken: tetracycline. At last count, I had contracted four STDs: herpes, pubic lice, gonorrhea, and chlamydia. I thought I had learned my lesson with the first two. It just didn't seem right or fair that I would get the second two from someone I loved and who I thought loved me. I had at least expected him to protect me—to keep me safe. I wished now that Greg and I had used condoms. I told him I had herpes and gave him a choice, and he chose not to. I wasn't quite empowered yet to mandate condom use. I didn't want to rock the boat, so I followed the man's lead. I just didn't understand why dating had to always be so damn hard.

Lamont Lucas brought honor back into dating for me. He was good friends with my friend and BAC comrade Stephen, who played matchmaker. He courted me, and I loved every minute of it. We had lots of fun, great conversations, and amazing sex. At the start, we had an honest conversation about dating and sex as well as what they meant for us as a couple. Neither of us was looking to fall in love but we were looking for companionship that was rooted in fidelity, and that is exactly what we had. I didn't have any drama with Lamont but, Lord, my roommate was a handful.

Zoe was a young lady whom I met through Veronica and her family. When Veronica presented me with the idea of her moving in, I thought it was a good one. I had a two-bedroom trailer, and I wasn't exactly rolling in the dough. It worked out well, at first. Then her dog got fleas. There were fleas everywhere—in my bed, hopping on me while using the bathroom. It wasn't until the fleas bit her that she agreed to cover half the cost to have the trailer treated. Then, baby girl started defaulting on her share of the rent. She promised to pay the back rent when she received her Pell grant-refund check; instead, she went to Florida for spring break. The eviction notice came while she was partying in Florida. I was so pissed. Lamont suggested I move in with him and Stephen. I jumped at the chance—another impulsive move. I had let my anger with Zoe rule my decision-making. Honestly, I thought I was proving a point. My attitude was, *I will show her!* In hindsight, I probably should have figured something else out because what I did was mean. My agreement with Lamont and Stephen was only for the next five weeks, until the semester ended. I hadn't thought about what I was going to do next.

When it was time for finals, I assumed I had flunked out of school again. Cramming was not going to help. I hadn't done enough work to earn me as much as a D in some classes. I was back where I began. School was ending, and I was headed for homelessness. I had come back to Carbondale so I wouldn't have to go back to Mama's; now, that cycle was destined to repeat itself. At first, I couldn't bring myself to ask Mama if I could move back home. Out of desperation, I went down to the U.S. Army recruiting office and arranged to take the test. Lamont and Stephen had served in the military, and they talked me off that ledge, thank God. They told me that my radical ass wouldn't make it through boot camp. I moved back in with Mama. This time, though, I was at the place in my life where I knew what I wanted. I also realized it was not going to be handed to me on a silver platter. I needed to do what I had to do right then, but I also needed to make some real changes if I wanted to get out of this cycle and move forward. I was either going to get off the pot or stay stuck on it.

I took a long hard look at my relationship with Mama that summer. Good, bad, or indifferent, Georgia Lee was still Mama—the only mother I had known for most of my life. It was natural that I gravitated her way. If she had done nothing else well, she had fed, clothed, and housed me more years than not. I didn't have the language for our relationship then, but today, I recognize that we were codependent. What I had was clarity that this back-and-forth with Mama was not good for me, and that living with her placed me directly in the path of her abuse. I needed to move, once and for all; only then could I develop a different relationship with her.

I started working at Operation PUSH almost as soon as I returned from SIU. Reverend Barrow was now the executive director and she hired me to be the national youth director. Nothing was happening in Chicago that excited me until some organizers came to PUSH to meet with me about this international youth conference that was being held that summer in Moscow. The festival was initially organized by the World Federation of Democratic Youth and the International Union of Students after World War II, and the event was a vehicle to help keep peace among nations by building bridges through future leaders. The *World Festival of Youth and Students* had taken place every four years since 1947. Santita Jackson, the Jacksons' eldest daughter, and her girlfriend, Michelle Robinson—later to be known to the world as Michelle Obama—represented PUSH four years earlier when the festival was held in Cuba. I wanted to be the one to represent Reverend Jackson this time. I went straight to Mrs. Jackson. She said yes, and took care of all the financial arrangements.

I boarded a plane in Chicago bound for New York, then on to Shannon, Ireland; and on to Moscow. This was 1985, at the height of the Cold War. There were no direct flights from the United States to what was then the USSR because the Reagan administration was anti-Communist and at odds with the Soviet Union.

There were over 26,000 youth leaders ranging in age from thirteen to forty who represented over 150 countries. The United States was the only Western country that didn't endorse the festival. I didn't care. *Whatever!* This was an opportunity of a lifetime for me. I only had one moment of hesitation, right after the opening ceremony. There was a statement issued by the U.S. State Department saying that attending the festival was against national security. The *New York Times* further reported that the U.S. delegation fought among ourselves about carrying the American flag upside down in the opening ceremony. A Vietnam veteran was supposed to have ended the debate by agreeing to take the flag. That report was a bald-faced lie; it was propaganda. There had been no such debate, and my friend Keith Jennings carried the flag the entire ceremony. We had 750 of the best and brightest in progressive politics in our delegation, including Bernice King, the youngest daughter of Dr. Martin Luther King Jr., attending the conference. Each delegation had a hotel. The larger delegations also had clubhouses and were free to invite others to talk. We stayed at the Cosmonaut Hotel, one of the newest hotels in the city, and it doubled as our clubhouse.

Right off the bat, I became friendly with Lisa Williamson, another young woman in our delegation. She was a student leader from Rutgers University, in New Jersey, who would later become a *New York Times* best-selling author and the hip-hop artist known as

Sister Souljah. Once we connected, I spent most of my time hanging out with her. Lisa and I tried to visit every African clubhouse and hotel we could, often debating politics for hours at some of the most radical delegates' clubhouses.

After hours of dialogue with delegates from African countries, I could see how capitalism and bigotry were symptomatic of a sickness that disenfranchised people of color worldwide. Black people in America were simply one part of the whole story. Slavery, The Black Codes and Jim Crow laws had been tools rooted in bigotry to advance capitalism in America the way colonialism had been used to build Europe—at the expense of African people and their resources.

There were so many wonderful moments. One afternoon I walked into our hotel restaurant, and everyone was buzzing: *That's Angela Davis!* To us radical leftists, Angela Davis was God herself. I bullied my way to the front to get a look but wasn't brave enough to say hello to her. I was frozen in that space, thinking, *That really is Angela Davis!* Seeing the Russian Ballet perform Swan Lake in the middle of a lake was another magical moment at the festival. The large events, including the opening and closing the Soviets' performances were just magnificent. Mikhail Gorbachev had just come into power as the general secretary of the Communist Party, and he was impressive. He spoke to the full conference and when he finished, many of us in the American delegation believed he was going to bring change. Less than ten years later, the USSR, as we knew it, dissolved. The day the Berlin Wall came tumbling down, I thought about the conference and Gorbachev, and was glad to have witnessed the beginning of his journey.

Apartheid in South Africa was one of the hottest topics at the festival, and the African National Congress was the most sought-after delegation. When our delegation finally met with that group, the faith and courage the Black South African people exhibited were beyond anything I had ever witnessed. Their first-hand accounts of the horrors of apartheid held us spellbound. They confirmed, for me, the urgency to bring national attention to apartheid, like when I began at SIU. I was proud of the work we had done at SIU; however small, it was still a part of the equation leading to their human rights. They ended the meeting with the famous *Toyi-toyi* song and freedom dance. When they finished, there was not a dry eye in the clubhouse.

I finally gained my voice being at this conference and hanging out with Lisa Williamson. While I firmly believed people should take one side or the other, I still hadn't developed the boldness to share my personal views publicly, especially on controversial issues. Lisa changed that for me. Before meeting her, I had met a lot of young people—my contemporaries—working for social change. But, Lisa was dynamite that had already been lit. She was bold and uncensored. I was impressed with the fact that she took a side, let everyone know it and didn't blink an eye—and she didn't backtrack, either.

One morning at breakfast, it was announced that the Palestinian Liberation Organization (PLO) delegation wanted to have an official meeting with the U.S. delegates. While many from our delegation claimed to support the right of a Palestinian homeland, few of us were willing to say it publicly. I guess the optics weren't a good look. I understood because I had watched lighter fluid thrown on our campaign and a match lit to it because of Jackson's stand on Palestine and the "Hymietown" controversy. Even before that, Andrew Young, the first Black U.S. ambassador, was forced to resign from the United Nations because he met with PLO Chair Yasser Arafat. I was so disappointed with my so-called "radical" comrades in the delegation, but I certainly understood why they declined.

Later that day, Lisa grabbed my hand in the lobby. "Come go with me," she said. I didn't think twice. After we jumped in a taxi, I asked her where we were going. "To a rally," she said, adding, "I promised some people that I would speak." When we arrived, the crowd was thick. Lisa turned to me and explained she was already late and needed to get to the front. Getting to the front seemed hopeless, but I grabbed her hand and pushed our way through the crowd to the front and over to the side of the stage. Lisa kept saying, "I'm from the U.S. delegation." The next thing I knew, she was being whisked on stage to speak. I took a breather. We had made it! I hadn't thought to see where we were because the focus had been to get her up front to speak. Standing on the side of the stage, I listened to the woman introducing Lisa in a language I didn't recognize; then, the intro was repeated in English. I didn't think much of it until Lisa started talking. She said something to the effect that we stand in solidarity with the Palestinian people. I looked around. Almost everyone was wearing a keffiyeh scarf representative of the PLO. *Oh, my God!* I thought. *We are really at a rally in support of the PLO.* I just shook my head in amazement and continued listening to Lisa speak. Of all the people in our delegation who thought it was unfair to deny the PLO's request to meet with us it was Lisa who was willing to take the chance. On the way to our next stop, while wrapping the keffiyeh that had been gifted to us around my neck, I said to her, "I can't believe you did that." In a matter-of-fact tone, she said, "Rae, if you don't take a stand, what's the point?" I nodded my head as I listened to her explain what it took to be a change agent. She was right. Going along to get along would not help bring about change. Ever since that day, even when I'm sometimes afraid, I take a stand.

The morning our delegation was to head to the airport, I took my first bold stand. It was announced at breakfast that the Israeli delegation wanted to meet with the U.S. delegation. I would have liked to hear what that group had to say but I also wanted to hear what the PLO had to say. It would have been intriguing as an outsider looking in— to lay these discussions side by side and deconstruct them. At the same time, I didn't see meeting with one delegation and not the other as fair. I argued right along with others that our delegation should say no. In the end, the delegation was split. Some chose to go meet with the Israeli delegation. I stuck to my priniple and decided to say goodbye to my friend Joao.

I met Joao while hanging out with Lisa. He was a part of the delegation from Guinea-Bissau. He spoke three languages and told me his father was the president or prime minister of his country or something like that. I was, like, *Yeah, right.* I gathered he was at least a diplomat because he had security. He was incredibly intelligent, soft-spoken, and absolutely handsome. When he changed into his beautiful traditional African attire in the evenings, I said to myself, *Take me home, Jesus, before I do something I regret.* He was never aggressive, but he certainly let me know he was attracted to me. When I tell you that I wanted to give him the best sex of his life, I am not lying. I thought about it at least twice—maybe even five times. But I also thought about Mrs. Jackson. She had trusted me to represent them and be aboveboard. A part of me rationalized that she would never know. But it would be just my luck that something stupid would happen, and I'd have to go back to Chicago and face her. By the same token, Joao would go back to Guinea-Bissau with no repercussions. I declined. But I told him, "If you ever come to the U.S., I will gladly spend the night with you."

I came back to Chicago on a high. I was inspired and wanted to get back on track. With every beat of my heart, I wanted to help bring about change. I wanted to do it beyond PUSH, beyond Chicago, beyond Mama. I started chatting with my political friends in D.C. to get an idea of what was happening and see how I could get back to the action and away from Mama. Fuck being ashamed of needing and asking for help. I took a page out of Veronica's playbook this time around and networked, networked, and networked some more. It was up to me to make it happen. Mama had been trippin' all summer, but when I came back from Moscow, the tension became extra thick. She made snide comments to me about my trip and talked about me on the telephone to her friends loud enough so I could hear. It was the same old crap: "She think she something" and blah, blah, blah. I was not biting this time. I just stayed out of her way as well as I could and kept making calls. I had just gotten off the telephone with my friend Julie Henderson talking about what I needed to do to get back in the loop. Julie and I had struck up a friendship from working on the campaign.

No sooner than I hung up the phone, Mama and I argued. I don't remember what it was about. I just remember thinking; *This is some stupid shit.* I decided that maybe I needed to give her some air. Julie had suggested I come to D.C. for a few days. I had enough credit on my Carson Pirie Scott credit card and could have booked a flight through its travel agency, but I had spent all my money in Moscow. Julie said it didn't matter, that she would feed me, but I still passed. After Mama started cursing me out— *bitch this, bitch that*—I reconsidered Julie's offer. I called her back and told her I was coming. Then I told Mama I was going away for a few days. She told me, "If you leave, take all of your shit with you!" I called Julie back and asked if I could stay with her for about a month until I worked out permanent arrangements. She said yes. I packed every single thing I owned into that same blue trunk that I had since I first went to UAPB, and never looked back.

Thirty-Six

SHE'S READY

" I believe luck is when preparation meets opportunity. If you hadn't been prepared when the opportunity came along, you wouldn't have been lucky."

— Oprah Winfrey

When I arrived in Washington D.C., in August 1985, I had twenty bucks to my name. I needed a job. My first stop was the Rainbow Coalition. I had hoped to be hired as the national youth director, but that position had been filled by this dude named Craig Kirby. When Sylvia Branch told me, I asked, "Craig who?" In fact, there were a lot of new faces in the office, and I was thankful for the few that I knew like Sylvia, and Jack O'Dell. When Craig walked into the office, Sylvia shot her head toward me to let me know it was him, and then introduced us. As soon as he walked out, I rolled my eyes. My first thought was, *Who hired this Black boy who sounded like he had been white all his life?* It turned out the new executive director, Yolanda Caraway, had hired him. I saw her at the Democratic Convention in San Francisco looking important and elegant, but I didn't know she would be the one to run the newly formed Rainbow Coalition. Sylvia introduced me to her. *Whatever!* All I wanted to know was why Craig Kirby had *my position.* I took an immediate dislike to both of them and dismissed Craig's qualifications. He was pretty impressive but, I was not going to feed his ego. He had been the first African American president of the American Student Association. I gave him the third degree, asking where he had been during the campaign.

I felt shafted. If the Rainbow was going to bring in a young person, then, I didn't have to move to Carbondale in the first freaking place. Why wasn't the job offered to *me*—the one who had traveled for the campaign by Greyhound for a whole month? I was mad as hell! I wanted him fired so I could have the job that was supposed to have been mine. I went straight to Mrs. Jackson. She said, "Now, Rae, we can't just fire the boy." My feelings were hurt, and it took months for me to warm up to Craig. Every time I came into the office and saw him walking around like he didn't have a care in the world, I rolled my eyes. He even had the nerve to ask me for my contacts. *What balls,* I thought. I told him, "Hell to the NO! Get your own." Besides, any good organizer in her right mind would never, ever, give up her black book. Child, that is your lifeline and your meal ticket. I had learned at least that much. Eventually, his clueless and unassuming demeanor would grow on me and win me over; we would even date for a while.

I was on a mission. If I couldn't have Craig's job, then I certainly had to get a job. By the end of the week, I had been hired in the call center of a large medical insurance company that was housed in the 2100 M Street office building. The manager had befriended many of us in the campaign. At lunch from the call center, I stayed in the Rainbow office. I never knew who I might bump into who could open a door for a new job. I had to stay on that grind. My job in the call center was temporary and paid extremely well, affording an opportunity for me to save money in the interim. There was no shopping this time around; I needed to hold onto everything I had. Time was ticking. The first month I lived with Julie, commuting into the city from her Alexandria

Virginia, apartment. I was grateful for her hospitality, but her large studio apartment was getting smaller by the minute with both of us living there. I put out feelers for permanent housing. I was networking my tail off to make D.C. work for me this time around. My friend Thomas Blanton, who had helped organize law students for the campaign, came through for me. He; his wife, Marsha Lillie-Blanton; and their pre-teen daughter, Jamehl lived in a three-bedroom house at 2nd and P streets NW. They were looking to rent a room in their home to undercut expenses while Marsha was working on her Ph.D. at Johns Hopkins University. I settled into the Blanton's small guest room with my blue trunk that had carried my worldly possessions for the past four years. I didn't even have sheets for the twin bed that rested against the wall, but I knew without one doubt that I had made a smart decision by leaving Mama's.

My first night at the Blantons, I promised myself I would never, ever live with Mama again. My gut told me if I continued to go back to Mama, she would kill everything good inside of me. It was clear that in the past two years, God had given me a glimpse into what I had been called to do with my life. This time, I was going to use every tool I could to actualize my dream. I didn't know how it would show up, but I knew it would.

Once I settled in, I caught up with friends I had met in Moscow. I had become pen pals with both Lisa and my African prince. Lisa and I were finally reunited in person that October, at the Congressional Black Caucus Foundation (CBCF) Annual Legislative Conference. Back in the day, the CBCF Conference was the Black political event of the year. The Washington Hilton Hotel was the hangout for the who's who in the Black liberation movement across the country. It was a networking heaven. Lisa and I met at the youth brain trust on Capital Hill where she was a speaker. Afterward, we sat in on the hot topic workshops with noted speakers. The South African brain trust had prominent Black leaders on the panel, the TransAfrica Forum's Randall Robinson and Congressman Walter Fauntroy. But it was Lisa, sitting in the audience next to me, who stole the show that day. I watched in amazement as she took both Mrs. Coretta Scott King and Reverend Jackson to task for accepting donations from the Coca-Cola company because they had investments in South Africa. Mrs. King looked startled that she had been challenged and rambled for much of her response. Reverend Jackson always had a response, and he and Lisa went a couple of rounds. Lisa was sure-footed, going toe to toe with Reverend. Congressman Fauntroy tried to shut her up with something about respecting her elders— and she retorted, *You get respect when you earn it.* Everyone was like, whoa! She kept blowing me away with her ability to bring it on those issues that were important to her. She was more than talk. In the end, she led the Rutgers University Coalition for Total Divestment and has been credited as the force behind the university's 3.6-million-dollar divestment of financial holdings from companies that had investments in South Africa. I admired her ability to articulate coherently and debate point to point. Not like Lisa. I had grown tremendously since I began my political work with the Harold Washington campaign, but I was convinced God had not gifted me with that ability like Lisa. (Nine years later, God would prove me wrong.) Maybe my strength came from my own tragedy, or maybe God was preparing me for a moment and time in history, and Lisa was one block in my building. Either way, I have never forgotten her.

After the CBCF, I was more determined to find a job that involved organizing. Unfortunately, by the time my job ended at the insurance company, not one prospect for a political job had come my way. I started knocking on doors. I was never going to be without a job or homeless again. In the midst of job-searching, I had a shocking surprise. Late one afternoon the doorbell rang; when I opened it, my African prince was standing there looking like, well, an African prince. He was in Washington, D.C., for the 40th-anniversary celebration of the United Nations. He was in town for one night before leaving for New York to attend an event at the United Nations. Later that evening, we met for dinner and a wonderful night of distraction. The next day, I was back on the grind looking for a job.

I ended up at the Hecht Company department store in Landover, Maryland. I hated the long commute on public transportation, especially because it was only part-time but, hey, any job will do when there are no other prospects. However, I loved being assigned to the Black-owned, Fashion Fair makeup counter. I had personally used Fashion Fair since I was sixteen and I was hyped for the new experience. After a while, the regional manager for Elizabeth Arden approached me about working for that company. It was a promotion on many levels. I would become a representative exclusively for Elizabeth Arden, with full training and sales commission in addition to the minimum wage the Hecht Company paid. It was a great offer, but I also knew the regional manager had approached me because of my skin color. She never said that, but it wasn't rocket science, either. The luxury makeup brands in department stores across the country rarely, if ever, hired Black women other than for Fashion Fair and Flori Roberts. A few years earlier, Veronica wanted a makeup counter job and unsuccessfully tried her best to break into the industry. It was a hard trade for Black women to break into, especially those darker than me. I wasn't confused that Elizabeth Arden needed a Black girl for the mall that had transitioned to serving a mostly Black patronage—certainly triggered by the historical white flight patterns in Prince George's County, like in other American suburbs—as areas closer to cities had more Black people. However, they needed their token Black woman to look more white than Black. I didn't like it, but I accepted the position because of the benefits and, most importantly, the money. I had always loved playing in makeup, and this was an opportunity to have professional training. It was a skill I would carry with me forever.

The best thing about working at Hecht's was Ruth Miner, a woman who worked at the fragrance counter. She was one of the highest-ranking salespersons in the department. She had a demeanor and smile that said *YOU matter*. Ruth took me under her wing. I will never forget when I transitioned to Elizabeth Arden, I overheard some of the other representatives saying, "Who does that bitch think she is?" I kept my cool because I had a job to keep. Ruth cut the hating with a sharp knife, telling one woman, "If they wanted you, they had every opportunity to hire you since you've been here a whole lot longer than Rae has." She told me, "Baby, don't pay them no attention; they just jealous."

Ruth invited me over for Sunday dinner, and that day was the beginning of a lifelong friendship. She was divorced with three sons— Darnell (who we called Reggie) Rick, and Ronnie—and one daughter, Joyce. Everyone lived at home but the oldest, Rick. She talked openly about leaving her husband. She told me one day, "He call himself gonna hit on me." She was my first understanding of what domestic violence looked like. Ruth took her children, moved into an apartment, and left him in the house. The children still had a relationship with their father, but I think *he* would have gotten *his* ass whipped if she had stayed with him any longer. Ruth talked slowly and with a North Carolina drawl; she could quote the Bible with the best of the preachers. We believed she had missed her calling to preach. Whether a woman could be a preacher was always a topic of debate in her house. The boys were about as traditional and sexist as they could be, and Ruth was a womanist without the language. Ten years later she married again to a pastor of a church; I flew in for the wedding. She didn't settle for the title of "first lady." Almost twenty years after we first met, we both accepted our call into ministry around the same time. I was already in seminary working on my Master of Divinity degree when she preached her first sermon.

I enjoyed every minute of every hour each time I was with her family. They were an example of the old saying "We didn't have much, but we had each other." I felt their love. Ruth's faith in me never faltered. When I was first diagnosed with HIV, I was too ashamed to tell her. Then I moved back to Chicago and felt I didn't need to disclose it to her. As life got crazy, Ruth and I lost contact, but she found me after I appeared on the cover of *Essence* magazine. Again, she would be my biggest cheerleader. She knew every preacher in the Washington, D.C. area and made sure I had as many speaking engagements as possible. Reggie, who was the second oldest and a year older than me, became my running buddy. He was my *dude*. Ruth and her family became my family. For the three and a half years I lived in D.C., I spent my holidays with them, from Thanksgiving to Labor Day. She freely shared her life with me. Looking back on our relationship, Ruth was another bright star shining over me. I will never tire of saying and showing the many ways God worked in my life—always filling the voids and gluing my broken pieces back together. I cannot express this enough: Yes, I was determined to keep going, but I did not do it alone.

My first break came by way of Donna Brazile. I bumped into Donna somewhere I can't recall and didn't waste any time asking her if she could help me find a job. To my surprise, she called me a couple of days later with a tentative interview in the office of Congresswoman Barbara Mikulski of Maryland. The position was for a receptionist, and I didn't care I just needed to get my foot in the door. I was interviewed by Gerri Houston, the office manager. That afternoon she called me back to say the congresswoman wanted to fill the position with someone from her district. I knew that was typical, but I was still bummed. Later that day, Donna called to see how my interview had gone and I told her I had not been hired. I know I sounded pitiful. I told her if anything else came across her desk to *pleassse* keep me in mind. She seemed surprised and said she would call me right back. About thirty minutes after we hung up, I received a telephone call from Nikki Heidepriem, Mikulski's chief of staff. She told me they had originally wanted someone from the district but reconsidered on Donna's recommendation and that I could start on Monday. Donna called me back to make sure I had been notified about the job. You're talking about being blown away? That, my readers, was a master class in Influence. I was just glad to be on the receiving end.

The first week, I wasn't sure how long I would last. I wasn't qualified to handle the secretarial part of the position. I flunked typing in high school. I hated the class, and I hated that Mama made me take it. During my entire education, typing was the only subject she ever asked me to take. She said something about being a secretary—a career that I had no intention of ever pursuing. Well, that came back to bite me in the ass; also, my spelling was atrocious. Other than that, the job was a breeze. I had all the personality in the world to handle the front desk, the telephone calls, the constituent visits, and requests for services. You better believe I was trying my darnedest to make it work. I was sure that not even Donna could keep me in a job where I simply couldn't perform my duties with excellence. The typing assignments were small, usually letters with envelopes to constituents with White House and U.S. Capitol tour dates. But still, sometimes I had so many errors that I had more correction fluid (or Wite-Out) on a letter than I had typing. This was in the days of electric typewriters, and Wite-Out was a typist's best friend. If it had not been for the office manager, Gerri Houston, I would have been out on my ass.

Gerri was an African American woman who had worked on the Hill for over half my life; she was known to help an office get its act together and work efficiently. She took me to lunch in the Capitol restaurant to have that *Auntie* talk with me. "Look, girl, I'm going to help you get it together." The first advice she gave me were pointers on how to dress for the front office. Capitol Hill was a little more conservative than what I was accustomed to, and stockings were mandatory. I put a safety pin in my shirt at the breast to minimize cleavage, got some Hanes Ultra Sheer stockings from Hecht's and fell in line with the dress code on the Hill. She gave me different samples of business letters that were my responsibility and had me to practice until I got them right. Gerri was not playing with me; when the office was slow, I practiced. I wasn't playing, either; I needed this job and did everything I had to do to make it work. A Black woman got me in the door and a Black woman kept me in the door.

I liked Congresswoman Barbara Mikulski—that is, when I wasn't scared of her. She stood all of 4-foot-11 but, Lord, she had this booming voice that sent chills up my spine. She was a progressive congresswoman who represented the 3rd Congressional District in Maryland, including Baltimore and the predominantley Black Prince George's County. At the time—in 1987—she was also running to replace retiring Sen. Charles Mathias. After I left, Congresswoman Mikulski would make history and become the first Democratic female elected to the U.S. Senate. But, Lord, working in her office was stressful. The rumor mill on the Hill ran better than Congress some days, and I was duly warned that the turnover in her office was one of the highest among her colleagues. I was advised to walk lightly. Even as a senator, Barbara Mikulski's reputation preceded her. In 2007, a former aide was quoted in a *Politico* article saying that the senator "changes staff like most people change their underwear." I learned to stay the heck out of her way when she was in a funky mood. The worst days were when she was on a diet—which, to me, seemed like all the time. You had better pray she didn't smell your lunch in the office because there would be hell to pay. A couple of people quit within the same week during my tenure, but I was on a mission and determined to stick it out. I occasionally had lunch with a quiet legislative aide by the name of Lori Lightfoot—yes, the same Lori Lightfoot for whom I would proudly cast my vote some thirty years later for mayor of Chicago. She was hired after me, and I was delighted to see another sister other than Gerri and me in the office.

Now that I was working an 8-to-5 job, I had to use my time on the Hill wisely. On one thing I was clear: I had not come back to D.C. to be a receptionist; I came back to organize. I didn't have any one particular job in mind; I was open to all the possibilities. I had come to a point in my life where my dreams had become bigger than my brokenness. Ruth often said to me, "Baby, if you take one step, God will take two; that's for sure." I took her words to heart and stepped down those hallways of the Rayburn House Office Building into every office where someone worked and with whom I had any kind of personal relationship. There were many Black congressmen who had supported Reverend Jackson's 1984 campaign and I knew all of them. I developed a friendly relationship with Congressman Ronald Dellums' chief of staff, Carlotta Scott. After I bumped into Carlotta in the hallway and was given an open invitation, her office was my go-to for lunch. Sometimes I even stopped over after my office closed; she was always working.

My turning point came sooner than I expected—and in the least expected way. It had a lot of moving parts that began with Congressman Dellums. As a Black congressman, he was uncharacteristically and heavily involved in peace and disarmament issues. While most Black congressmen focused on apartheid in South Africa, Dellums was arguing against nuclear testing and the military-industrial complex that had grown significantly during the Reagan administration and apartheid. He also happened to be on the board of directors of the National Committee for a Sane Nuclear Policy (SANE). SANE was the oldest and one of the largest peace and disarmament organizations in the country. Carlotta often attended the meetings on Congressman Dellums' behalf. One day I walked into her office and plopped down in the chair in front of her desk, and she handed me a job announcement to see if I wanted to apply. I scrolled down with a quickness and looked back up with a smile that said, *Hell, yeah, I want to apply!*

SANE was looking to diversify the senior staff for the first time in the thirty-year history of the organization. I was qualified and I used every networking tool I had to give me an advantage. I already had Carlotta's support. I went to Jack O'Dell who was also on the board of directors of SANE and was highly respected in the peace community. However, it was Susana Cepeda who was my ace in the hole. Susana previously worked at SANE as its first Latina hire and was also very good friends with the executive director, David Cortright. Now, she worked at the Rainbow Coalition and had become close to Mrs. Jackson. The icing on the cake had come months earlier—prior to David taking on the status quo in his charge for a more diverse SANE. I had a chance to chat with him on the very topic one day in the café lobby of the Howard Inn. Mrs. Jackson had told me that people were always watching, and I am glad I took her advice to heart. It just so happened that I went over to see Mrs. Jackson; Susana was with her when I arrived. Later, David arrived to pick up Susana. Instead of leaving right away, he sat down. There was a lot of chatter around the table and, somehow, David and I started talking about his work at SANE. We had a profound discussion about the need for diversity in the peace movement. He told me he wanted to make changes at SANE. I didn't know it at the time, but he had been impressed by what I said during our chat. Gerri Houston helped me get my resume together, and my village went to bat for me.

I had a couple rounds of interviews with some of the department heads, who included the director of organizing, the director of the canvassing department and the deputy director of the organization. It was democracy with a small "d," where everyone was included in the decision-making process. To make it friendly, we were positioned in a circle like we were at a campfire, but it didn't feel friendly to me and seemed to defeat the purpose of diversity—that is, putting a Black woman in front of a group of white people who fired questions to her one after the other. I put on my big-girl panties and shrugged it off. I knew that if I could do nothing else, I could organize and talk my ass off. *Keep on hitting me with questions,* I thought. *I can organize rings around this room.* My second interview came a week later with the political director, Daniel Houston, who was himself a new hire and the first African American in that position in the organization's history. When I walked out of Dan's office and headed back to the Hill to finish my day in the congresswoman's office, I knew I had the job. In June 1986, I joined SANE's staff as the national field coordinator for the southeast region. It had taken me ten months to make my dream come true, but I was on my way.

Thirty-Seven

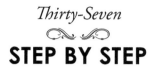

STEP BY STEP

"The secret of change is to focus all of your energy,
not on fighting the old, but building the new."

— Socrates

In the summer of 1986, at age twenty-four, I was finally living my dream. I was a national organizer in a prominent organization. My new job as the Southeast regional coordinator for SANE was a major achievement in my career. My position helped broaden my organizing skills and build my resume. It also allowed me to achieve the stability and financial independence I always wanted.

The weekend before I started, I moved out of the Blanton's home into a place of my own. I had an amazing basement apartment in a beautiful four-story brownstone a couple of blocks off Logan Circle that I found purely by accident. Sometimes after work, I went to Kramer Books & Afterwords: A café—a combination bookstore and cafe in Dupont Circle—to peruse the shelves and people-watch. Afterward, I would walk the fourteen blocks to the Blanton's. I loved walking and exploring the neighborhoods, admiring the architecture and those coveted brownstone homes that lined the streets around Dupont Circle. On one of those evenings, I noticed a stunning four-story brownstone with a "for rent" sign in the basement window. The owner, Dorothea Nelson, was a widow and a member of the Washington, D.C. upper crust. I loved the magnificent crystal chandelier that hung in her hall; it was nothing short of breathtaking. When she reviewed my application and saw I had worked on Reverend Jackson's presidential campaign, she approved me on the spot. Beautiful azaleas lined the well-manicured front yard. Rosewood shutters adorned the windows. I had a large two-room apartment with high ceilings, stunning parquet floors, and a wood-burning fireplace. There were nights I walked through my two rooms naked just because I could. For the first time living on my own, I felt relief. My life was finally coming together, seven long years after Mama had first thrown me out of her house.

I moved into my apartment with just my clothes, and a mattress and box spring that sat on the bedroom floor until I was able to purchase a bed frame. I was starting from scratch. I needed linen, dishes, and furniture the whole works. However, I was in no rush to fill my place with things. I wanted to take my time decorating so I could create the perfect space for myself. I was also trying my best to live in a fiscally responsible manner and didn't want to spend every dime I had right away on furniture. I had decided to go for that Ashley Stewart, shabby-chic look. My first major purchases were these cute wicker and white wood bar stools for my kitchen island, and they were perfect. I spotted them at a quaint shop in Georgetown and pleaded with my new friend Barry to take me to pick them up. I met Barry Saunders during the Congressional Black Caucus weekend. He had been a classmate of Jonathan and Jesse Jackson Jr. at North Carolina A&T University. One afternoon we were all sitting around the lobby of the Hilton hotel shooting the breeze, and Barry and I struck a conversation that led to a friendship. Barry would become my closest and single most important friend for fifteen years until his death from lung cancer in 2001. He was the person to walk me down the aisle at my wedding and the same person who wanted to come to Chicago to whip my ex-husband's ass when things got bad. Barry seemed to know everyone. He was the ultimate connecter and had more female friends than any woman on the planet. His friends were your friends, and most new people who came into my life typically came because of him. I was still tight with Ruth's son, Reggie, too, and most of my time spent with him and Barry involved meals. Houston's Restaurant in Georgetown became my go-to place. But home was my safe space, and I preferred curling up in front of my fireplace with a cup of tea and a book to any other activity. I was at a good place in my life.

For the first time in a long while, I thought it was time to go back to church. I hadn't been to one since I was raped leaving Grandmamma Julia's church. Every now and then, I thought about going, and only thinking about the process paralyzed me. Getting dressed, traveling to church, and walking through the door was all fine with me; the problem was that I couldn't attend church without having to eventually come back home. The thought of traveling back home had such a powerful hold on me.

How could life be so brutal? I lamented. *Where the fuck was God?* Then after the other rapes, I didn't know what or whom to trust anymore—or even if I could trust going to church again on my own. While I couldn't explain *why* I was raped, I had continued to talk to God every single day. I even felt that God talked back to me, when I took walks with the sun shining down on me.

Without question, this rape broke off another piece of me I wasn't sure could ever be repaired, but I was still standing. I reasoned that if I hadn't allowed the rape to diminish my faith in God, why allow it to take away what had always brought me joy: worshipping with fellow Christians in the place we symbolically called God's House? When I looked over the breadth of my life up to this point, I knew that something bigger than me—something infallible—had gotten me here. I had a couple of choices to make; I could allow the fear of tragedy to have power over me or I could take my power back.

I ended up at Springfield Baptist Church about ten blocks from my house. Springfield was a traditional Baptist church with all the bells and whistles. It was large like Second Baptist with an abundance of programs and ministries. The pastor and the worship service reminded me of Reverend Anderson and the Old Ship of Zion. I felt like Little Rae was back at home, and I became a member. I joined the young adult ministry and volunteered to work with teenagers. I remembered how broken I had been when I attended Second Baptist in Evanston, and how the people and programs enriched my life. I wanted to give back some of what had been given to me. My fondest memory was when I volunteered to provide my newly acquired make-up artist skills for the young adult fashion show. When I wasn't on the road for SANE, I was at some church activity. I was trying my best to live a balanced life socially, spiritually, and professionally.

My primary responsibilities at SANE were to help develop new local chapters in the Southeast region of the United States and help existing chapters grow. The overlapping area of responsibility for my region was the political action committee (PAC), which gave me a chance to work in electoral politics and grassroots lobbying. Although SANE had a full-time lobbyist, regional coordinators were responsible for implementing grassroots lobby campaigns in support of its legislative agenda. Even though SANE's primary focus was to end nuclear testing in the United States, over the years it expanded from this single issue to broader peace work. I settled into this new work experience, excited to be a part of the changes David Cortright was making within the organization. I hadn't considered how the role would unfold for me as the first African American to hold the position. I learned that my friend Thomas Atkins, with whom I had worked on the Jackson campaign, was Daniel's administrative assistant. I walked away assuming David's efforts to bridge the color gap at SANE had more cheerleaders than critics. This was two decades after the civil rights movement, and SANE was a "liberal" organization. It had taken them twenty-five years but, in my opinion, they had ushered in a new era.

After I started the job, I realized David had not only made the organization more diverse, but he had also bulldozed it. When the white male lobby director departed, he was replaced by an African American man named Aubrey McCutcheon. Shortly after I came onboard, Ana Culian, a Latino woman was hired as the Southwest regional coordinator. Ana and I had no experience in the peace movement *per se*, but we were both great organizers. On the other hand, the new Northeast and Northwest regional coordinators were white men, and the director of the organizing department was a white Southern woman. All of them had a history in the peace movement, which was a badge of honor. The culture among peace activists was toxic and it made me as a newcomer, feel like I was an uninvited guest at best. Sometimes Ana and I locked eyes in staff meetings to signify, *Did I just hear what I thought I heard?* In the end, people of color outnumbered our white counterparts five to three among the programming team, and it made for a tense work environment. SANE would become my first lesson in white privilege and the hypocrisy among white liberals when that privilege is threatened. In all fairness, no one ever said to me directly that I or any of my colleagues of color were not welcome. However, actions sometimes speak louder than words.

On a daily basis, individually and collectively, my colleagues of color and I endured snide comments and patronizing responses regarding our ideas. If we pushed back on a topic, we were made to look overly aggressive. Language was used to contain us. It might be suggested that I just didn't quite understand how things were done in the peace movement, or that I wasn't open to new ideas. In actuality, I *was* a new idea, and so were my other coworkers of color. Here's the thing: We brought not only our Black and Brown bodies to work every day but our experiences and culture, too, and the pushback was insidious. The critiques were coming from the organization's original paradigm, which illustrated an unwillingness to embrace the idea of diversity. Ana and I whispered back and forth throughout the day, and when Thomas took a cigarette break, I walked with him and talked about the dynamics of our situation.

Interrelations were so bad that the board of directors hired consultants to address the "communication problem" among the staff. I don't think it resolved anything, because the problem was not about how we communicated with each other, but that the language was no longer homogeneous. The changes were hard, and the pushback was felt every day. Nevertheless, I continued to do my job. The Southeast region had the most African Americans and I was expected to bring progressive African Americans into the fold, just as Ana was expected to bring in the Latino/Hispanic demographic from the Southwest. Mind you, this task was not expected of our white counterparts, as if there were no Blacks and Latinos in other parts of the country. The burden of color was placed solely in the laps of the two organizers of color.

At first, I was very optimistic about my ability to deliver on what had been asked of me. In most of my meetings with SANE's local leadership, I was told not only were Black people welcome but, in some chapters, the Black leadership in the city was already extended an invitation—but with no response. Any insight I could provide to help bridge the gap was welcomed because not much headway had been made over the years. I used my Jackson contacts to arrange meetings with local African American leaders throughout my region to help inform me on how to tackle the issue of inclusion. For sure, more African American activists were focused on bread-and-butter issues that affected them, like fair housing, better schools, and health care. Stopping nuclear testing was not viewed as an issue that would help to put bread on the table. On the other end of the spectrum, I learned that part of the problem was rooted deeply in culture differences. In one city, for example, the SANE chapter was pretty well-established and doing excellent work. When I met with African American activists in that city, I was told there was an interest in collaboration; however, the problem was the location of the meetings. Apparently, SANE held its monthly meeting at a local church that was historically associated with the Ku Klux Klan in the city. Black folks didn't care if Jesus hosted the meeting; they were not going to step one foot inside that church. When I went back to SANE's leaders to explain the history, they didn't have a clue. They explained to me that this particular church had been chosen because it was centrally located downtown and provided free parking. They had no intention of changing what in their eyes was a great location.

Let me be clear: I'm not saying that the white people I encountered through SANE were a bunch of bigots. It wasn't as simple as that. In fact, many believed themselves to be morally superior to openly racist white people. I didn't have a term for white privilege back then; that would come decades later. In the meantime, the best description I could come up with to describe them was that they were hypocritical. For sure, their pushback had a daily impact on what it felt like to be a Black woman working in this space.

In spite of the pitfalls of working at SANE, I was able to see the upside of my job, which was a sign that I really was maturing. I had moved away from the desperation that characterized so much of my young adult life. I had much more confidence in myself knowing how hard I worked to get to this place in my career. I was sure of my skills, and I knew I could take myself and my talents out of SANE's door at any time and find another job. The space was uncomfortable at times, but I saw no reason to run. I agreed ideologically with the mission of the organization. Equally as important, I respected and agreed with Congressman Dellums' efforts around issues of concern. He was once quoted as saying:

> How are we going to deal with the problems of education, housing, health care, guaranteed annual income—all other issues that need to be addressed in this country—so long as we spend fifty and sixty and seventy and 100 billion dollars a year killing other human beings, most of them black or brown or poor people?

I was grateful for the door his chief of staff, Carlotta, had opened for me literally and figuratively and I wanted to live up to her expectations. I also understood that I was in a unique position to help educate African Americans about nuclear testing, war, and military proliferation. I was doing what I could with what I had at the time.

Thirty-Eight

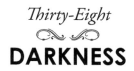

DARKNESS

Help me to shatter this darkness,
To smash this night,
To break this shadow
Into a thousand lights of sun,
Into a thousand whirling dreams
Of sun!
— Langston Hughes

The decision to leave Chicago was a smart one. Even smarter was the distance I maintained between Mama and me this time around. I had speculated, and was correct, that distance was the only way to break the dysfunctional cycle and her hold over me. It was as much emotional distance as it was physical distance that I had to maintain. As hard as it was, it was the only way to shift the paradigm. I checked on her at least a couple times a month to make sure she was good. If at any point she started talking crazy, I'd politely end the conversation. *I was just checking in, Mama,* I'd say, *I'll talk to you later.* Sometimes, I straight up told her that respect should flow both ways. It always got me a good cursing-out and sometimes a hang-up. I owed her my respect, but I didn't owe her my soul. Mama rarely called me; when she did, it was because she wanted something. So, on the day she called to tell me she was going to be baptized, I dropped everything and flew to Chicago. This was something I had to see for myself. Grandmamma Julia and I both cried tears of joy that Sunday morning, and I returned to D.C. that evening. Getting religion didn't outwardly change anything about Mama; she was the person that she had always been. I couldn't change who she was, but I could change how I responded to her, and that became my superpower over how she treated me.

At the same time, I was redefining my relationship with Mama, the woman who raised me, I was trying to define my relationship with my biological mother, Dorje. Like Mama, she was a complicated woman. Whatever darkness had shaped both of them affected who they were and how they operated in the world. By the time I moved to D.C., Dorje and Michael were back in the States and living in Boston. In her letters, she had told me that she hated living in Nova Scotia. It was a tight-knit Catholic community that didn't take kindly to the migration of people of the Buddhist faith. Once they came back stateside, Michael decided he wanted children and asked her for a divorce. Dorje was totally caught off-guard. Before they were married, Michael was well aware she couldn't have children. She told me she had complications when she was pregnant with me, and that my premature birth ended her child-bearing days.

She and I went from writing letters to talking on the telephone regularly— sometimes, even a couple of times a week. I was ready for us to pick up where we left off in Boulder and give our relationship a chance to flourish. That summer, we were off to a good start. One weekend, I took the Amtrak train up to Boston for a visit. We had a blast! We went to the movies, walked in the famous Harvard Square, browsed used bookstores, had ice cream, and laughed—a lot. That Saturday night back at her place, we had a cup of tea and talked. She felt Michael had thrown her away. Dorje had gone from a drug addict to a housewife; now, she was trying to figure out what was next. She had a one-bedroom apartment in Lynn, a suburb about nine miles from the center of Boston. She had her faith; a shrine was set up in her bedroom. She had her Buddhist community in Boston, and she had me.

That night when we were preparing for bed, I came into her bedroom. I can't remember for what—only that I saw the most beautiful strand of pearls on her dresser.

"These are beautiful, Dorje," I said. "Can I pick them up? She looked over to where I was standing by her dresser to see what I was talking about.

"Oh," she said nonchalantly. "Oh yeah, go ahead."

"Are they real?" I asked, picking them up.

"Yes, they belonged to Michael's mother. She gave them to me as a wedding gift."

"Nice," I sighed, realizing that I had started an unpleasant topic for her.

"Yeah, they're the nicest thing I've ever owned," she chuckled.

"Well, they certainly are beautiful," I said with a smile, realizing that she was still light-hearted about the topic.

"Take them," she told me. "Where the hell am I ever going to wear them?"

"No, I can't; they were a special gift for you." She walked over to the dresser, picked them up and placed them in my hand. "I want you to have something special from me," she said. I hugged her, resting my head on her shoulder.

"Thank you so much," I said, all choked up. "I will always cherish them."

"You deserve them, and so much more," she said while pulling her pajamas off the hook behind her door. From then on, I would wear them almost every day, and the pearl became my favorite gemstone. I left my mother that Sunday with plans to get back together after I came off the road traveling for SANE. I had a weeklong trip planned for Atlanta. SANE was considering whether to open a Southern regional office and I went there to do some groundwork.

When I returned to D.C., I repeatedly called Dorje and could never seem to catch her. After a while, I started to worry. I understood she spent a good portion of her days meditating and reading, and I knew she sometimes went on weeklong Buddhist retreats, but I had spoken with her a couple of times before I left to go to Atlanta, and she hadn't mentioned plans to go out of town. I started calling her like a stalker, day and night, to no avail. I didn't have Michael's telephone number. The only other person I could think to call was her mother—my grandmother—Mrs. Wilson. In the six years since I met my mother, my grandmother continued to keep her distance from me. I had started back sending her Christmas cards after I met mother, but she hadn't sent one back. I wanted to call before, but I didn't think I could handle the rejection, so I let it go. Now just thinking about my grandmother created a whole lot of anxiety. Every day I came into the office, I sat at my desk agonizing over whether I should call. For a couple of days, I picked the telephone receiver up and slammed it back down. On the bus going to work one morning, I told myself I was being ridiculous. I had given this woman power over me, and she had no right.

By the time I arrived at work, the lining of my skirt was stuck to my thighs, and I kept fanning my breezy summer top that I wore over a tank top. It was another hot and humid August day in D.C. On the two-block walk from the Metro, my curls had become an afro. I was cute, though, with tan pumps to match my tan skirt and the pearls my mother had given me. As soon as I arrived at SANE, I went straight to the bathroom to wipe the dampness from my body. God, I hated those summer days that felt exactly like I was living over the swamp that rested beneath D.C. After I pulled my hair back into a ponytail, I stood over my work desk and phoned my grandmother before I lost my nerve. When I heard her voice, I got straight to the point. All in one breath I said, "Hello, Mrs. Wilson; this is Rae. I've been trying to reach my mother, but I can't seem to catch her. Do you know where she's at?" I could hear her breathing heavily as I waited for her answer.

"Your mother is in the hospital," she finally said. I plopped down in my chair to brace myself. The word H-O-S-P-I-T-A-L flashed in my mind like a neon sign advertising a hotel vacancy on the side of a road. I started firing questions at her. How long? What hospital? What's wrong? Why didn't anyone call me? I could feel the perspiration building under my shirt again and I pulled at my bra to give me a little relief. My grandmother still hadn't responded to any of my questions.

"Mrs. Wilson?" I asked. I could hear her breathing, and her silence was making me crazy.

"It's not that kind of sick," my grandmother finally said. "She tried to hurt herself." She went dead silent again. Her statement *she tried to hurt herself* hung in the air like thick smoke. I repeated it in my head, and then echoed, "She tried to hurt herself?"

"She's in a mental institution."

I was speechless. My grandmother broke the silence: "You should call Michael; he can tell you more." She gave me his information and hung up. I immediately called him. Michael—with his straight-to-the-point, no-nonsense nerdy self—gave me the details all in one scoop. "Dorje tried to kill herself. It's a wonder that she is alive. She spent hours cutting on her body. The only reason she did not bleed to death was because a neighbor found her." Apparently, Dorje had stepped outside of her apartment into the hall covered in blood at the same time her neighbor was locking her door, and she called the ambulance. The story sounded unbelievable. *Her poor neighbor,* I thought. "At least she survived," was all I could manage. Michael encouraged me to call Dorje's psychiatrist. He gave me the name and number, and we ended the call.

With the receiver still in my hand, I stood to stretch my body and my mind. I knew she had been struggling since the divorce but, Lord, I couldn't understand how she could have gone as far as to hurt herself. I thought back to the time I tried to kill myself. The moment I started to feel sick, I ran for help. I couldn't even fathom what Michael told me. I took a deep breath and dialed the doctor's number, sitting back down as I waited for that person to come to the phone. If I'm to be honest, I don't remember most of the conversation with the psychiatrist, but the parts I do remember I have carried with me for over thirty years. Dorje had been hospitalized for a couple of weeks. This meant she must have done this not long after I left to go to Atlanta. I thought Michael had prepared me and the doctor sufficiently warned me it was bad, but I shrugged it off. I wanted details so that I could figure out how to help her get on with our lives. That was wishful thinking.

"She cut off both of her breasts," was the first thing he told me. I reached for my own trying to picture what he had just said and calculating the size of her breasts as I remembered them by measuring my own.

SHE - CUT - OFF - BOTH - OF - HER – BREASTS? screamed in my head right beside my rough estimate that Dorje wore at least a 42- or 44-D sized bra.

"Dear God," I mumbled. "Why the fuck would she do that?" The doctor heard me and said, "She is a very sick woman." Tears streamed down my face as I listened. "She sliced up and down her body," he said and then paused.

"She took an iron and burned a hole in her head." *An iron?* I said to myself, trying to figure out how she could have done that. He said, "We had to shave her head," and I gently touched my head and thought about her beautiful thick, salt-and-pepper shoulder-length hair. I started to visualize her with no hair, imagining what had taken place. I could see my mother plugging the iron and pressing it on her head until her hair burned, and her skin fell off, revealing a gaping hole in her head. "Oh, God…." came out of my mouth a sorrowful moan.

"She is a very lucky lady," the doctor said. I inhaled a deep breath to take it all in. He continued to talk about her care. When he finished, I asked, "How can I help her?" My office mate Ana slipped some Kleenex in front of me, and I wiped the tears from my stained face. She didn't know that one small gesture of kindness initiated an internal signal that it was time to stop crying and shift into action. It was time to go take care of my mother, as Ana had just taken care of me.

"What can I do?" I asked again. "Can I see her?" I was ready to drop every single thing and come to Boston; this was my mother. The doctor explained that Dorje had repressed some of her memories from that night. They wanted to release her for an overnight visit to her apartment to see if it would help recover those missing parts. I have no idea what I was thinking, but I said yes. We finished our conversation, and I hung up the telephone and told Ana, "My mother tried to kill herself." She came over, held me in her arms and rubbed my back. I could feel everyone watching us, but I didn't care. Ana was the balm I needed at that moment.

When I arrived in Boston, I went shopping to make Dorje a beautiful basket of goodies. I had paperbacks of her favorite genre, exquisite chocolates, fresh flowers, tea, and a bunch of other little delights. I trucked out to the sanitarium, and they let me visit for about fifteen minutes. She was happy to see me, and I was trying my best to put on a happy face. After I talked to the doctor, I went to check out her apartment. Michael had told me the apartment was a mess and he had hired someone to clean it but hadn't been back to check it out. When I walked into that apartment, I was so glad I had followed my first mind to double-check the condition it was in for myself. I can't imagine what it must have looked like before it was cleaned because the aftermath was not a pretty sight. I didn't even catch my breath; I rolled up my sleeves and got to work. There was no way in hell I was going to let my mother walk into a half-cleaned mess. I went to the nearest store to get supplies, and then I tackled the walls first. There were still small blood splatters on the wall throughout the living room. The walls in her bedroom looked like someone had smeared a mixture of blood residue and water, turning some areas a musty brown color. I cleaned the walls of her apartment with elbow power and a mixture of bleach and Comet that kept my eyes watering and had me stepping away to clear my airways. After the walls were done, I set about cleaning the entire apartment that was visible to the eye, dusting and refreshing the bathroom and kitchen. The mattress had blood splatters, so I covered them up with clean linen and made her bed nicely. I tried to clean the dried blood embedded in the fabric of the sofa and rug, but it was futile. The best I could do was to arrange a sheet and blanket on the sofa for me to sleep on as a ruse to hide the stains.

The hardest part was throwing away the knives she had used to mutilate her body. Whoever had cleaned the house washed the knives—big knives, steak knives and even butter knives—and scissors, and placed them in a pile on the kitchen counter. It was a chilling scene, like something out of *Criminal Minds*. I examined each knife, trying to imagine how she had used it. It was inconceivable she'd taken these knives to her body. I held the largest butcher knife in my hand the longest, rubbing my fingertips along the sharp edge. It sent chills up my spine. This was some morbid-ass shit and it made me doubt my decision to spend the night with her. I shook it off and began the hour-and-a-half-long trip on public transportation to the sanitarium.

I picked up Dorje late on Saturday late evening and we went to dinner. When we sat down, my eyes went straight to her chest. She had on a loose hospital gown at the sanitarium, obstructing my ability to see. But now, in street clothes, I was able to have a better look. I didn't want to make her uncomfortable but, for a few seconds, I stared. I was tormented by the fact that she had cut her breasts completely off. We ate dinner and I replayed the course of events over in my head — what the doctor told me, cleaning the house, and dealing with the fact that my grandmother hadn't thought enough of me to call.

I didn't know what to say or how to console her. I thought about my own life and how I had a lot of dark moments and persevered, and caught myself right before sinking into the bottomless pit. Even in the times when I felt like I had hit rock bottom, I always found a way to climb out of the gutter. This—what my mother had done—I didn't understand. Finally, she said, "I look a mess, don't I?"

I managed, "It's okay, Dorje." Actually, she looked like a wounded animal. There was no life in her that I could immediately find. Her skin was paler than white, and her head was wrapped in a scarf. She had lost weight and looked tattered and out of it. It broke my heart. I kept searching for the mother I had left weeks ago, sipping tea, and laughing hysterically, but she was nowhere to be found. She didn't talk much, and I didn't force her. I wanted to ask why, but I kept that to myself. She was incredibly apologetic to have brought this pain to my doorstep. Her shame was embarrassing, and I just wanted to wrap her in my arms and keep her safe. When she asked how I learned about her situation, I confessed that I'd been so worried about her that I called her mother.

"Oh God," she burst out laughing. "How did that go?"

"She was a sourpuss." I told her, and we both laughed hysterically; then, we fell silent again. She told me that night that her mother was "being a bitch." I let it hang in the air, trying to make sense of their relationship. It irked me that my grandmother could be mean to my mother at a time like this.

We arrived to Dorje's apartment around nine o'clock that night. I asked if she wanted a cup of tea. She mumbled something that was not intelligible and went into her bedroom and shut the door. I laid on the blood-stained sofa and tried to force myself to sleep. I tossed and turned, wondering what she was doing in her bedroom. My mind started playing tricks on me. *What the heck had I signed up for?* I couldn't shut my thoughts down, no matter how hard I tried. Lord, I couldn't believe that I had agreed to do this without any consideration to my own well-being. Shit—maybe I was just as crazy as she was. My mind was jumping around like a jackrabbit with my crazy ass mother sequestered in her room. *What if she tries to kill me?* I thought— And Lord I didn't have anything to protect myself, because I had thrown away all the knives. My ass hadn't even asked the doctor if she was a danger to me. I assumed he wouldn't have released Dorje into my care if she posed a threat. Now I wasn't so sure.

My thoughts were so dark and disturbing that I felt sick to my stomach. I ran to the bathroom thinking I was going to throw up, but only tears flowed down my flushed face. I was too afraid to close my eyes that night, so I prayed that God would take away my crazy thoughts and lift my mother out of this darkness. And then, I said the same prayer over and over, like a Buddhist mantra, until the break of dawn: *Lord, keep me safe. Lord, please keep me safe.* The next morning, when Dorje emerged from the bedroom, I was dressed and waiting. I had been too afraid to knock on her door. We went back to the hospital in silence. After I dropped her off, I boarded an Amtrak for D.C.

A couple of days after my return, I wrote my grandmother a two-and-a-half-page letter. I couldn't stop thinking about Dorje telling me her mother was being a bitch to her. I had no idea what I thought I would accomplish. In my letter, I informed her I had visited my mother, and she was recovering just fine.

I don't know who the hell I was trying to convince—my grandmother or myself. What's clear today is that I was trying to hold onto what little family I had. It was more of a rallying cry to band together than anything. I write:

I love my mother in spite of my childhood. I have put the past behind me. I am just happy that she is a part of my life now. Help her stay a part of my life. Don't let the pain kill you or her. All of my life I have wanted a family. Now that I have one, let's pull together and make it good for us all.

My grandmother never responded. I pushed her to the back of my mind so that I could focus on the most important thing: my mother. I was not giving up on her or us.

Work was a perfect tool of avoidance to keep my mind free of the darkness that had consumed my life in the aftermath of my mother mutilating her body and I kept myself as busy as I could. We were moving fast into the mid-term election season, and I was asked to identify political candidates in my region that our PAC could support. I was still traveling for work, and during a trip to North Carolina I met with an African American staffer named Wyatt Close, who was working on David Price's campaign in the 4th Congressional District in North Carolina. I was able to secure a PAC donation from SANE that was credited to his efforts on behalf of the candidate. Price won the election, rendering SANE as a friend in Congress; Wyatt came to work in the Capitol Hill office, where we became friends.

More than anything, I wanted to help Black folks in any way I could while at SANE. The Congressional race that I was most proud of was for Mike Espy. He was one of the hottest new faces in the 1986 electoral season. Mike had been the assistant attorney general of Mississippi and was running for the congressional seat in the Mississippi Delta. His grandfather, Thomas J. Huddleston, was a successful entrepreneur and prominent civic leader in the Black community. Born at the end of Reconstruction into an era of Jim Crow laws, terrorism and restrictions forced on Black people, Huddleston was able to succeed against immense odds. In 1928, he built and ran the Afro-American Hospital in Yazoo, Mississippi, providing healthcare to Black people for over forty years. Many of us viewed his grandson as an extension of his family's legacy of Black excellence. SANE didn't have a chapter in Mississippi but I didn't care; I went to bat for him. Mississippi was in my region, and I argued SANE should be nurturing relationships with congressional candidates of color. I pushed to have Espy lead one of our brown-bag discussions with staff, which went extremely well. Espy was impressive, and this talk opened the door for me to assist his campaign in other ways. Our PAC followed with a generous financial contribution to his campaign and co-sponsored a D.C. fundraiser on his behalf. The fundraiser was the brainchild of mine and my former housemate Marsha Lillie-Blanton. One day, I bumped into Marsha at a political event and, somehow, we started talking about Espy's campaign. She knew other people who wanted to help, and we got together and planned a fundraiser. Marsha pulled from her resources within the city political elite, and I pulled from SANE. We had an impressive list of co-chairs, Mayor Marion Barry; Congressman Walter Fauntroy; D.C. Councilmember Hilda Manson; and William Winpisinger, the national president of the Machinists Union and the chairman of SANE's board. Mike Espy's campaign placed me in the center of the work I enjoyed best: electoral politics. This fundraiser kept me busy and shielded me from my doggone mind. Thoughts of what my mother had done gave me some sleepless nights and raising funds for Espy helped keep me distracted. I'd stay at work well past office hours, making calls to members of our board of directors to ask for donations. We raised $19,000. I was proud of our efforts. By today's standards that was small potatoes, but back then we felt like we'd struck gold. I was counting the days until I could travel again and wrap myself in my work. I convinced SANE to loan me out for in-kind services to Mike Espy's campaign. The last two weeks of October, I went to Humphreys County, Mississippi, to work in the local campaign headquarters to help coordinate the "Get Out the Vote" efforts. When I boarded the plane to head back to D.C., I was humbled to have made my contribution in a small way to help elect Mike Espy—and make history as the first Black person elected to Congress since Reconstruction.

Dorje was released from the mental institution in early October. I called often to check on her, but all the laughter and camaraderie we shared was gone. The calls were emotionally painful and became harder and harder for me to make. I continued, though—I think, out of a sense of duty as her daughter. If I could call and check on Mama after everything she had done to me, I could certainly do the same for the woman who had given me life.

Thanksgiving was approaching and I asked Dorje to come to D.C. Holidays are supposed to be spent with family. Plus, I wanted to see her for myself to assess how she was *really* doing. After prodding her, she gave in. I met her at the bus station, and she looked as tattered as she had when I last saw her. We went to dinner someplace close to my apartment. Other than looking like she had lived through a hurricane, she seemed like herself again. We laughed and talked. I was hopeful for her—and us. Afterward, we walked back to my apartment, sat at my little kitchen island, and ended the night with a cup of tea. It was just like old times. A sense of relief came over me and I started to relax. We continued laughing and talking until our eyelids started to droop. I hadn't purchased a sofa yet, so I gave her my bed and made a pallet on the floor for myself. When I came out of the bathroom, she was sitting on the side of my bed crying.

"I don't deserve to sleep in a bed," she whined. I stopped in my tracks and turned to her.

"I didn't do anything for you," she said, "I'm a horrible person." I didn't know what to say to her. I just stood there, looking dumbfounded.

"I'm going to sleep on the floor," she said. "You take the bed."

"No, you will not!" I snapped back. *What in God's name is this?* I thought. My heart started to beat fast. In a split second, our lovely evening had turned into some crazy ass shit I didn't understand. I took a deep breath, trying to get myself to stay calm.

"Dorje," I said. "I don't care what you did or didn't do. No mother of mine is going to sleep on the floor when there is a bed that she can sleep in."

"I don't deserve to," she responded, crying.

I sat beside her, overwhelmed, and trying to find the words to say. All I really wanted to do was go to sleep. I had worked all day, and I was spent. Finally, I said, "You are still my mother. I don't care about that other crap. You have done the best for me that you could." She stopped whining. I got up from the bed and started walking toward the living room. Turning to her, I said, "You're sleeping in the bed and I'm sleeping on the floor." I cut the ceiling light off and left her sitting on the side of the bed with the lamp still on. I was done with that foolishness. After a while, she finally turned the lamp off. I had a restless night; when I got up, I felt like I hadn't been to sleep at all. When I made her breakfast, she started the same conversation again—about how she didn't deserve me, and on and on. She had a deep sense of guilt because of my crazy childhood. I tried to explain to her that it didn't matter anymore. None of it could be undone. Mama had done what she did, and everyone had to live with that fact.

"We have each other now; let's make the best out of the mess that we are," I told her.

She persisted, and after a while, I stopped feeding whatever this thing was and just let her talk. Thank God, she eventually shut the heck up. She sat at the island sipping her tea and looked on as I prepared our Thanksgiving dinner. Later, when dinner was ready, we ate in silence. When it came time for dessert, I pulled out a rice pudding.

"I don't like rice pudding," she said.

"Didn't you tell me that it was your favorite?" I asked her.

"No. Rice pudding is nasty," she said, almost child-like. "I like bread pudding."

I had made a mistake. The funny thing was I didn't like rice pudding either and loved bread pudding, too, and I told her so. We laughed so hard. We ended up having sweet potato pie and tea. I was relieved; we had made it through most of the day. Then she started crying again. I didn't know what to do for her. When she stopped crying, she told me she was tired, and we prepared to call it an early night. When she started back on the sleeping-on-the-floor thing again, I just didn't have any more fight in me. I said, "Okay," and went to bed. However, I didn't sleep. The next morning, she said she wanted to leave. I was so damned relieved.

My mother was not well. I didn't understand why she had been released from the hospital. In time, I would connect the dots to public policy. In 1981, President Ronald Reagan reversed most of the landmark Mental Health Systems Act that was ushered in during President Jimmy Carter's administration. By signing into law, the Omnibus Budget Reconciliation Act, Reagan gutted federal funds for state mental institutions, leaving mental health in the care of the states. This reversal of community mental health would have a profound impact on the well-being and care of the mentally ill. In the '80s, about forty-thousand beds were eliminated in state mental institutions, and people were released from the facilities without getting the care needed to help integrate them back into society. Many of them never recovered, ending up homeless and on the streets. My mother would be one of those people who never recovered.

Thirty-Nine

TROUBLED WATERS

" I found that I could not climb my way up to God in a blaze of doing and performing. Rather, I had to descend into the depths of myself and find God in the darkness of troubled waters."

—Sue Monk Kidd

On Dec. 31, 1986, I washed all my dirty clothes and mopped and waxed my floors, changed the sheets on my bed, cleaned the bathroom and shopped for groceries. *Never bring in the new year with dirty clothes and an empty refrigerator* had been the rule in Mama's house, and it was a part of her that never left me.

Late in the evening, I piled a bunch of pillows and blankets in front of the fireplace, fixed me a cup of tea and sat down and thought about all the glorious milestones of 1986: a new job filled with new experiences, a new church, and a place to call my own. I was beyond pleased with myself. There had been only one dark moment—Dorje's suicide attempt. While it was painful, at least the drama wasn't my own making. At midnight, with a grateful heart, I got on my knees like Grandmamma Julia had taught me right after Granddaddy passed away, and I prayed. I thanked God for the clarity that had guided me and the determination to follow through. I had laser-like focus since being back in D.C., and it paid off. I didn't know what was ahead for me in 1987, so I asked for God's continued guidance and strength to persevere, no matter what came my way. When I got up, I put my favorite Tramaine Hawkins album in the cassette player with the volume on low. The last thing I heard before I drifted off to sleep was Tramaine singing, *A change, a change has come over me.*

At SANE, I was mobilizing for the "Boycott South Africa-Not Nicaragua March" that was going to be held in Washington, D.C. on April 26. SANE had joined the fight to change the United States' policies toward South Africa and Nicaragua, and all hands were on deck. In the two years since I'd led the South Africa divestment campaign at SIU, the Free South Africa Movement had spread like wildfire across the country. College campuses had imploded with the demands of divestment.

I had just started at SANE when the Anti-Apartheid Act bill introduced by U.S. Reps. Ronald Dellums and William Gray—both members of the Congressional Black Caucus—passed in the House. The bill applied sanctions against South Africa that—among other things—prohibited farm products, iron, steel, coal, and textiles, and banned new U.S. loans and corporate investments in the country. The bill made it to the Senate. It became my first grassroots lobbying campaign, by activating phone-banking and letter-writing campaigns in support of the legislation in my region. It was good old-fashioned organizing work—making calls to people who would then make calls locally, and so on, flooding Congress with the message to pass the Anti-Apartheid Act. The bill passed the Senate, but President Reagan was adamantly opposed to sanctions against South Africa and vetoed it. Now in his second term, Reagan had done nothing to indicate he would favor Black people at home or abroad.

After the veto we activated the grassroots campaign again, and pressure continued to mount. Celebrities and politicians escalated civil disobedience at the South African embassy. The pressure worked and, in an historic move, Congress overrode Reagan's veto making it the first defeat of a United States president foreign-policy agenda in the twentieth century. We celebrated and went right back to organizing for the march. Reagan's veto sent the message loud and clear that his heart was not in the fight against apartheid. We wanted to ensure the bill's implementation. The march progressed as planned.

Similarly, we wanted to apply pressure and bring national attention to Reagan's policies in Nicaragua. Under Reagan, the United States provided military and financial aid to assist the contras, a counterrevolutionary group actively trying to overthrow the legitimate Marxist Sandinista government of Nicaragua. In doing so, the United States helped enable the contras' drug trade which placed drugs in Black communities in the United States. The irony was that Nancy Reagan, the president's wife, had launched her infamous *War on Drugs Campaign* that targeted Black people—with the slogan "Just Say No"—at the same time, her husband was illegally trading drugs for guns to destabilize a legitimate government. As a result, I was in the trenches working my tail off.

I rarely ended my day at five because I needed the distraction. My mother's suicide attempt still weighed heavily on my heart. I was glad she had moved from Boston to Buffalo, leaving all those horrible memories. However, her temporary move with her mother created a tense situation for me. The first time I called my mother, I didn't know how I should address my grandmother. I had always referred to her as "Mrs. Wilson," and now that my mother was living with her, I wondered if I could drop the formality. The tone of her voice, however, made it clear she wanted to keep our relationship formal. At first, I thought that maybe I was overreacting or being presumptuous about my grandmother's cool tone. A couple times I tried to engage her, but she was short and cut me off: "I'll get your mother." At least she acknowledged that much. My attempts were pitiful and equally as futile. I always heard her calling my mother: "Judy, telephone!" I don't know what irked me the most: that my grandmother would never call my mother Dorje, which had a spiritual meaning, or that she totally disregarded me. It never occurred to me that if she had no regard for her own daughter, why would she have any for me? I wasn't going to keep getting my feelings hurt for her to say only, "Oh, hold on." Like, *Oh, it's you again.* I kept it simple, asking, "Hi, this is Rae. Is my mother available?" She never greeted me; she just said, "Oh, hold on." It was painful to be rejected outright.

I finally asked Dorje why my grandmother was so cold to me. She explained that she still blamed my father for her addiction despite the fact she was using before she met him, and my father had been dead twenty-one years. It was batshit crazy that the burden of my mother's action had been transferred to me, especially since neither of her daughters was capable of raising their own daughters. In my opinion, whatever happened to my mother started and ended with that bloodline. Period. Back then, I hadn't put it all together. I just desperately wanted a family. My solace was the thought that maybe one day she would come around. For decades, I clung to this idea. With every accomplishment, I asked Dorje if she told my grandmother. I asked when I finally graduated from college and entered graduate school. I asked after the *Essence* magazine cover. I even asked after I received an Emmy for the series of first-person news reports on my life. In all the times I asked Dorje to mention an achievement to my grandmother, she only gave me feedback from my grandmother one time. After the *Nightline* special on my life in 1996, Dorje told me that my grandmother said, "She [meaning me] is impressive, and very pretty." That one compliment had taken her thirty-four years after I was born and sixteen years after I met my mother.

Acouple of weeks into the new year, I decided to organize a blood drive at SANE. The idea came to me after a horrific Amtrak accident and an appeal for people to donate blood. On January 4, 1987, Amtrak Train 94—the Colonial, from Washington, D.C.—headed to Boston and crashed at 1:04 p.m. in Chevy Chase, Maryland. Fourteen passengers were killed as well as the Amtrak engineer and lounge car attendant. I couldn't imagine what these families were going through.

In the days immediately following the accident, news reports continued to mention that the Red Cross was in dire need of blood. I was shocked to learn that donations had decreased because people actually believed they could somehow contract HIV from donating blood. I simply don't understand how people allow their imaginations to run wild when it comes to science. Six years into the AIDS pandemic, the fear of HIV/AIDS was still rampant. In this time, I had seen innumerable news reports about AIDS discrimination fueled mostly by fear and ignorance. I understood to some degree that people were afraid of what they did not know; however, by then, we knew you could not contract HIV from clean needles. It hadn't been a full year since Surgeon General E. Everett Koop sent his controversial report on HIV/AIDS to every household in the United States; I read it, and everyone should have. It was clear on the different ways people could contract HIV. I also knew a little something about donating blood. Remember, I had volunteered at our high school blood drives and donated each year. Likewise, I donated my first year at SIU. I knew from my own experience that the Red Cross used all new equipment for each person, from the needle to the bag that held the blood. It was fear—and propaganda—that clouded logic more than anything. I took this assault on blood donation personally. I was outraged by the sheer ignorance of this type of thinking. I had already been influenced in small ways by the pandemic. Keith Barrow's death had deeply affected the people I had come to love at PUSH, and their heartache made my heart ache. Working for Reverend Jackson and rooting for people living with AIDS and the LGBTQ community was an eyeopener. I had also been shaken by the photos from the Amtrak accident. I asked for permission to have a blood drive at SANE. I figured between the programmatic staff and the canvassers, we were good for about twenty to thirty people. After I was given the go-ahead, I contacted the Red Cross and arranged for the agency to come to our office. I made fliers and distributed them to the staff. On my lunch break, I went from office to office and desk to desk signing people up to donate. I don't do anything halfway.

On Martin Luther King Day—January 17, 1987—SANE's programmatic staff joined the canvassers and collected canned goods and money for the homeless community. We had the day off, but I thought it was a cool idea and a perfect way to celebrate Dr. King's birthday through service. Later that night, I almost choked on my own spit when I saw a news report that civil-rights activist, Reverend Hosea Williams had been attacked while leading a "brotherhood anti-intimidation march" with about seventy-five people. It happened in an all-white town about forty-six miles outside of Atlanta, Georgia. I had never heard of Forsyth County but, apparently, in 1912 white residents ran the Black residents out of the county, similarly to what occurred in Tulsa, Oklahoma, in 1921.

In Forsyth, the terror campaign of 1912, led by Night Riders, was sparked after the attacks and rapes of two white women, in separate incidents; one died. All of the alleged suspects were Black, one of whom never made it to trial—he was pulled out of jail and hanged by a lynch mob of white men. The other two were Black teenagers who were found guilty after a short trial; they were hanged in a public execution. Still, that wasn't enough justice for the white community of Forsyth County. In the months that followed, the entire Black population of about eleven hundred residents was terrorized and forced out of the county, leaving their property and valuables behind.

In the six decades that followed the race riots of 1912, there were very few Black people who lived in Forsyth County, and the white residents planned to keep it that way. As gatekeepers of whiteness, they used various tactics over the years to intimidate nonwhite persons who dared to venture to the county for any reason. They posted signs around the county with the words, "Nigger Don't Let the Sun Set on You in Forsyth County." Black truck drivers making deliveries had to be escorted by the Georgia Bureau of Investigation. Over the years, there were also incidents around Lake Lanier, a popular getaway spot in Forsyth frequented by people from Atlanta. Ten Black boys and counselors on a camping trip were told to leave Forsyth or be carried out "feet first." A Black firefighter from Atlanta was shot in the eighties while driving near Lake Lanier. The list of atrocities went on and on. Reverend Williams organized and led the march in response to the ongoing intimidation of Black people in the Forsyth area.

I watched the news reports of the attacks on Reverend Williams and the protesters in horror. The scene was reminiscent of old civil rights footage of protests in the sixties. When Reverend Williams and the marchers arrived in Cummings, Georgia, they were met by approximately five hundred hostile counterprotesters waving Confederate flags; throwing bottles and rocks; and chanting, "Nigger, go home!" In a flash, everything escalated—the counter protesters broke through the line of state troopers and local police and attacked the civil-rights marchers. Reverend Williams was hit in the head with a rock. *What in God's name is wrong with this world?* I didn't believe what I was seeing. The attack on Williams and the marchers made it around the world at warp speed and SCLC organized a do-over march for the following week.

On January 24, 1987, well over two-hundred buses loaded in the early morning at the King Center and headed to Forsyth County. SCLC had expected about five thousand people, but the outrage brought around thirty thousand—including me. SANE footed my bill, but I would have paid my own way if I had to. I remembered listening to the stories back at PUSH from both Reverend Williams and Reverend C.T. Vivian from their days marching with Dr. King. Reverend Vivian had talked about how marching for civil rights was God's work. He and Reverend Williams had both been part of the Selma march, where they were attacked on the Edmund Pettus Bridge. Now it was my turn. This was my Edmund Pettus Bridge, and I was proud to serve.

The motorcade from the King Center started later than expected because of the sheer volume of participants. In addition to the buses, there were God only knows how many cars filled with people. On the bus, we sang freedom songs and discussed the horrible stories about Forsyth County. I struck up a conversation with a girl, her boyfriend, and his best friend. Lo and behold, the best friend, Paul, lived in D.C. and had also flown to Atlanta for the march. We were immediately attracted to each other, and, in between freedom songs, we flirted all the way to Forsyth. Time idly slipped by. The trip, which should've taken about one hour, had taken more than three. The meeting point of the march was a shopping center outside of Cummings, Georgia, but our bus never made it that far. There were so many people and so much gridlock that buses stopped on the side of the road and let people unload.

The march down Route 9 toward Cummings had white counter protesters on the hills of both sides of the road, some in Klansman robes. We chanted, "Hey, hey/ho, ho/the KKK has got to go!" and they shouted back, "The KKK is here to stay!" The atmosphere felt frenzied and crazed. As we marched into Cummings, we were met by a couple of thousand angry white counter protesters—a combination of white-supremacist groups, sympathizers and the KKK. We were divided by barricades and protected by seventeen hundred National Guard soldiers and members of the Georgia Bureau of Investigation wore riot helmets and were holding billy clubs; and other law enforcement personnel—sheriffs, local police, and the Georgia Highway Patrol—were present. Helicopters circled overhead. A section of the area was cordoned off near the speakers' stage for the press and news outlets.

Counter protesters didn't give a hoot about the press, or the protection afforded us. They unapologetically showed their asses. With contorted faces they yelled NIGGERS! at us, and when they spotted the droves of white marchers they screamed, Nigger lovers! Nigger lovers!

I hadn't realized the number of people participating in the march until we were all moving together. No matter which way I looked, I saw a sea of people—in front of me, behind me and on either side of me. Blacks, whites and Latinos chanted, "Forsyth County! Have you heard? This is not Johannesburg!" It was a perfect chant that drew a parallel between fighting the decades of apartheid in South Africa and our own version of apartheid that we thought had been rooted out decades earlier. As people from other buses merged into the massive crowd and the program began, of all people, I spotted Jesse Jackson Jr. trying to get through the crowd. "Jesse!" I yelled over the chanting to get his attention. I kept calling until he heard his name and spotted me. We pushed toward each other and hugged.

"Rae-Rae, girl, what are you doing here?" he asked.

"Representing, like you," I said, smiling. He looked out over the crowd, "Rae, I'm supposed to be up there speaking in about ten minutes," he said, looking down at his watch.

"I know if anybody can get me up there, you can," he said. I grabbed Jesse Jr.'s hand, reminiscent of that day back in Moscow with Sister Souljah and pushed our way to the staging area. By the time I made my way back to my new friends, Jesse Jr. was being introduced. They started jiving around with me about how I knew Jesse Jr.

"Look at you, girl. How do you know Jesse Jr.?" I told them I worked on Reverend Jackson's campaign.

"Girl, you lying. For real?" Paul asked.

"Yep," I said, "For real, for real."

I was trying to concentrate on the illustrious speakers, but my heart was beating like I was watching a horror movie—anticipating the next move and fearing it all at the same time. I was on edge the entire time. In between speeches, counter protesters chanted, "Nigger, go home! Nigger, go home!" And we'd drown them out chanting, "Forsyth County! Have you heard? This is not Johannesburg!" Then, suddenly, another speaker would talk, and we'd stop the chanting and listen. Every now and then, I'd see people ducking ahead of where we were standing, and we knew that a rock or bottle had been hurled at us. Around dusk, participants in our immediate area started mumbling about being caught in Forsyth after dark. All of us had heard the message loud and clear, like the signs that had been posted in Forsyth over the years with the words, "Nigger Don't Let the Sun Set on You in Forsyth County." At some point, worry overtook me, and I tuned out the speakers. I remembered that Jesse Jr. and Bernice King spoke, but I couldn't begin to tell you what they said. I was scared out of my mind. It was getting later and later as speeches dragged on and on. The sun had set, and I think the march organizers perceived the anxiety hanging over us like fog and ended the program by singing "We Shall Overcome." For a moment, my anxiety vanished. I found comfort in holding hands, moving together, and swaying in sync—our voices of hope drowning threats of hate demanding, "Nigger Go Home!" Someone gave a closing prayer, and we began walking back to our starting point with white men, women and children taunting us. The march back to the buses and cars moved slower than a turtle. My effort to keep a happy face was getting more difficult. We were on a road that had virtually no lighting and it was getting darker by the minute. All I could think about were the KKK members I saw on the hills on the way into Cummings and the civil rights workers of the sixties who were murdered in the dark of the night all across the South. Every now and then, someone repeated the chant, "Forsyth County! Have you heard? This is not Johannesburg!" The chant rippled backward; by the time it reached my ears, I'd already joined in. Then, it had already started to die down up front as it continued to ripple its way backward. After each chant died down, we'd march in silence and my anxiety quickly escalated again. The fear was palpable.

We boarded the buses immediately; as one bus filled, it moved into the motorcade line. I sat in silence, as did everyone else on our bus waiting for us to get the hell up out of Forsyth County. Sitting next to Paul, I closed my eyes and prayed, "Lord, protect us from these crazy-ass white folks." Right as the bus started to move, someone up front asked us to join hands and pray, and we prayed one of those old-time prayers calling God to send angels and build a fence of protection around us. When we reached the highway, I could feel the tension leave my body, and I silently prayed, "Thank you, Lord." We were out of danger.

Paul and I exchanged numbers and we became an item soon after returning to D.C. I hadn't dated since the summer of 1986, when I dated a well-established man who lived in a beautiful brownstone in Georgetown—one of the most coveted addresses in D.C. I was maturing, and I could see we were going nowhere fast. I had gotten to the place where I could spot bullshit a mile away. I eased myself quickly out of the relationship before I became bitter or got hurt.

Paul was fun, and the attraction between us was exhilarating and intense. I saw him as marriage material. He had a lot going on for himself. He was a minister working on his Master of Divinity degree at a prominent university in D.C. He was good-looking, well-spoken and around my age—yep, he was husband material. In two weeks, I had become quasi-domestic. After a long day at SANE, I came home, cooked dinner and waited on him to arrive. My ass had even started doing his laundry. Dude would bring a big bag of dirty clothes on one visit, and I'd have them washed and folded by the next.

The day of the blood drive, I woke up to a freaking blizzard. *What the hell?* It was more snow than I had ever seen in all the years combined in D.C. I flipped on the news and learned that the entire northeast coast of the United States had been hit. They were calling it "Snowmageddon of 1987." My heart sank. I called the office to ask if we were still going to open. The District of Columbia was notorious for shutting down with much less snow than in the Midwest and New England states. To my surprise and delight, we were open. I got ready for work and bagged the goodies I had baked the night before for the blood drive. I slid into my Chicago snow boots and winter coat, and braved Snowmageddon. They were estimating somewhere between twelve to twenty-eight inches of snow. I was praying that other people would come to work that morning despite the weather. If I could just get through the blood drive, I wouldn't care if we shut down for days.

When I arrived to work, there was a phone message already waiting on me from the Red Cross. I called and was informed they canceled our location and rerouted us to another site a couple of blocks from our office. I was disappointed; the snow had stolen my momentum. Still, I was thankful that it was only a five-minute walk to the other site. I wrote a memo with the new location and circulated it to the staff, then placed the baked goodies in the snack room. In spite of the snow, everyone who had come to work that day made the trek to the other site to give blood. When the snow slowed down a tad, Ana and I walked over together. After they finished drawing my blood, the tech gave me a little card explaining that I could call the number in a couple of weeks and enter the private code and it would tell me if I tested positive for the HIV antibody. "Wow," I said. "When did they start doing that?" She said it had been done that way for almost two years. In early March of 1985, the FDA approved a diagnostic test to detect the HIV antibody exclusively to prevent the HIV virus transmission through blood and blood products. The Red Cross began testing all donated blood a month after FDA approval of the antibody test.

When I got back to the office, I tore up the card and threw it away. I didn't see myself in a primary risk group for HIV. Don't get me wrong: I wasn't naive or stuck on stupid, but not viewing myself to be in a primary risk group was different from believing I couldn't contract HIV. If a man could get HIV from having sex with another man, I had no reason to believe that women were exempt from contracting HIV from a man. At this time, however, the amount of men infected from heterosexual sex was minuscule, and I just didn't think I would be in a relationship with an intravenous drug user nor, a man who had sex with other men. I considered myself lucky that I had been educated on some aspects of the gay life from my friend Thomas Atkins. Living in D.C. with a large population of Black gay men, there was a lot of talk about the virus. When I moved to D.C. the first time back in 1984, I learned from him that D.C. was the capital of gay Black men. At the time, I was clueless about homosexuality. I thought gay was gay and straight was straight—until Thomas began pointing out men who I believed to be straight who were also having sex with other men. If I had my eye on a guy, Thomas knew the 4-1-1. He had given me that best advice ever: "Use a condom, because you have no idea who's zoomin' who." I took his advice to heart, so there was no need to hold on to a card because I thought I had it all figured out.

About a month after the blood drive, I came home and took a quick glance through my mail and noticed a letter from the Red Cross. I saw no urgency in opening the letter, assuming that it was a thank-you for organizing the blood drive. I tossed everything onto the counter, changed clothes, lit a fire in the fireplace and had my dinner. After dinner, I opened the letter. The only thing that sticks in my mind is the line that stated, "There is a medical problem with the blood you donated." *What in God's name?* I read it twice to make sure I had not misunderstood. My heart started pounding. I picked up the telephone and dialed the number on the letter. When I received a recording, I punched in the extension and got another recording. I hung up and dialed again. I couldn't imagine what was wrong with my blood. I called repeatedly, too hysterical to think that if I was home from work, it was after work hours at most places. My nerves were shot. I thought back to the other times I had donated blood; no one had ever mentioned anything about testing my blood for anything until this time. I replayed everything over in my head on the day I had donated: The little card the woman had given me, her instructions, and the code on the back where I could check my HIV status on my own. *Well, that little card is in a landfill somewhere by now.* I often moved too doggone fast for my own good. I mulled it over in my head until the magnificence of the sun shone through my bedroom window. I got dressed, went to the office early and watched the clock that sat on my desk, waiting for the Red Cross to open. The first time I called, I was transferred to the extension and the line was busy. I hung up and redialed several times. When a lady answered, I calmed down and gave her the best professional voice that I could and explained the letter I had received. She said she couldn't discuss it with me over the telephone. I'd have to come into the office.

"I don't understand," I said calmly. "It's my information. Why can't you tell me over the phone?"

"Miss, I'm sorry, but you will have to come into the office."

"But it's my information!" I insisted. "Tell me!"

"Miss, I'm sorry but you will have to come in." No matter what I said to her, she wouldn't bite, and she patiently repeated that I'd have to come in. Maybe there was a part of me that thought if she could've told me over the phone, then maybe it wasn't so bad.

"Tell me, please," I started to beg. "Please."

"Just come," she said, "and we can talk about it." I conceded and jotted the address down on a piece of paper, grabbed my coat, hurried outside, and flagged a taxi.

One month to the day that I donated blood, March 4, 1987, I walked into the American Red Cross building and my life changed forever. I sat down across the desk from this middle-aged white woman. She didn't waste time.

"I'm sorry, Ms. Lewis. Your blood tested positive for the HIV antibody." I thought how bizarre it was that she'd separated me from my blood, as if my blood had run away from my body and somehow contracted HIV. I sat, emotionless.

"Do you understand what I'm telling you?" she asked.

"Yes," and I repeated what she had told me. "My blood tested positive for the HIV antibody. I guess you are saying that I have HIV?"

"Yes," she said, "But you only have HIV."

"You may never get AIDS," she explained. At the mention of "AIDS," I thought about Keith Barrow and felt faint. I unbuttoned my coat because I was hot all over. If I had been standing, I think I would have collapsed. I closed my eyes and took several deep breaths to center myself. I mentally told myself, *You are not Keith; you do not have AIDS.* I continued to listen as she explained that HIV is the virus that causes AIDS and, so far, not everyone that had tested positive had developed AIDS. Even the surgeon general's 1986 report on HIV/AIDS said not everyone affected with HIV would develop AIDS. This disease hadn't made the ten-year mark and the medical community didn't know what they didn't know. We did know, however, that AIDS was a death sentence. Time and scientific advancement would change our understanding of both HIV and AIDS. Until then, I clung to the idea that I "may never get AIDS"—like holding onto a piece of a sinking ship hoping that I would not drown, but it wouldn't be enough to save me.

"Are you okay?" she asked.

"Yes," I said, nodding.

"Well," she hesitated. "You're so quiet." I wanted to scream, *BITCH! What am I supposed to be doing?* I hated this white woman and white people, in general, trying to tell me how I should respond to or feel about something. I got enough of that at work. I didn't know this woman from Adam, and I certainly wasn't going to spell out my life story for her.

"You do not have AIDS," she repeated, "and you may never get AIDS." I held on to her words; they were the encouragement I needed. After an awkward silence, she referred me to the National Institutes of Health, widely known as NIH. I got up from the chair and left. The entire meeting had taken less than fifteen minutes.

When I walked out of that Red Cross building, the cold and sun hit me at the same time. I bundled my coat and walked down those pretty white marble stairs and prayed, "Lord, don't ever let me get AIDS." As soon as I got to work, I called Veronica and told her what the lady at the Red Cross said. In all the years I had known Veronica, this was the first time she was at a loss for words. She said, "Call my mother." Sherry always knew what to do. I ended the call with Veronica and, with the receiver still in my hand, called Sherry. She gave me the pep talk of my life. She said something like, *Rae, you are not dying, and I don't want you to even start thinking that foolishness.* It was enough to get me through the rest of my day. I was headed out on the road for SANE the next day and had to finish preparing for the next ten days out in the field. Every time I drifted to thoughts about HIV, I reminded myself I had no energy to give it. I could not get bogged down thinking about it; I needed to stay focused and finish my work.

When I got home that night, I started packing and doing Paul's laundry at the same time. I'd promised him I would finish it before I left town. I washed and waited for his arrival. *We've been using condoms,* I reminded myself. I was doubtful he had infected me or I, him. I thought it was important, though, that I tell him. Before he took his coat off, I blurted, "I have HIV." I had to get it over with. I'd felt like I was going to explode earlier as I waited for him. I was hoping by washing his clothes and keeping our routines that things between us would stay the same. I believed that if I pretended everything was okay, then maybe it would be. There was a part of me that even hoped his faith would be his guide. I knew that we shared the same Christian values. He looked puzzled.

"What?" he asked.

"I have HIV," I repeated.

"Girl, stop playing." he said.

"I'm not playing, Paul. I donated blood and the Red Cross told me today that I have HIV." I watched as his countenance changed from disbelief to a brief moment of fear across his face.

"You're for real?" he asked.

I said, looking sheepish. "I'm sorry, Paul." I gave him the same number that had been given to me at NIH so he could get tested as a precaution. He didn't mumble a word as I handed him the number. He took the paper from my hand and looked at it and picked up his laundry. He walked toward the door, then turned back and said, "YOU BITCH!" That was the last time I saw him. After he left, I called Tyrone Crider and Coré Cotton to tell them about my diagnosis. I had no idea what the future held for me. I had already lived a lifetime in twenty-four years. I couldn't imagine a world filled with more pain. The only reassurance I had was that I had survived a brutally painful past. Maybe I would get through this, too. I couldn't believe God would bring me this far to leave me. I crawled between my sheets. I had no tears. I prayed again, "Lord, don't ever let me get AIDS."

Forty

THE WAY FORWARD IS
WITH A BROKEN HEART

"We go on because it is the thing to do. And we owe ourselves the difficulty.**"**
—Nikki Giovanni

I arrived in Asheville, North Carolina, with a kaleidoscope of emotions all crashing down on me at once. Where in God's name did I get HIV? All that calculating I had done about who could have infected me had obviously been a miscalculation. Truth be told, I hadn't used a condom with every man—at least not every single time I had sex. But I couldn't stretch my imagination far enough to think I could have had sex with a man with this virus.

I had so many questions, none of which I could answer. Why didn't I know? I guess because I didn't feel or look sick. That's why they say, "The only way to know your HIV status is to get tested." But then, that advice didn't emerge until the '90s. Thank God I had donated blood, and that all donated blood was being tested for HIV in the United States. That seemed like common sense but in France, the government decided to wait on its own test rather than use the U.S. test that was available in 1985. They believed that the U.S. had stolen their research and rushed it to paton, and didn't want to pay the U.S. for the test. As a result, approximately 1,250 hemophiliacs in France were infected from HIV-tainted blood supply. You can't make this stuff up, but that's how it was back then. We didn't have the kind of scientific collaboration like we had for COVID-19.

I was trying to be brave, but it was surreal, unnerving, and all-encompassing. On the plane, I thought maybe I should have canceled this trip and gone to the doctor's office. Like with all my road trips for SANE, I had put maximum energy into planning this two-state trip. Countless meetings had been arranged, and I couldn't figure how to gracefully cancel them, so I came to Asheville, North Carolina, my first state stop; I then continued to Black Mountain and Charlotte before leaving North Carolina and heading to Nashville. At the airport I called the National Institutes of Health and scheduled the first available appointment after I returned to D.C. Then again, if I canceled the trip I would've had to explain to my boss, and there was no way in hell I would tell another person who didn't absolutely need to know. I had told Paul, Veronica, Sherry, Coré, and Tyrone the previous day in practically one fell swoop. Now, it was on a need-to-know basis—period! I had heard too many stories about people living with HIV/AIDS who'd been ostracized, hysteria ruled over common sense.

The one story that touched me the most was that of Ryan White. A hemophiliac who contracted HIV through contaminated blood plasma from a Factor VII treatment. Ryan was thirteen years old when he was diagnosed with AIDS. The testing of blood products came a little too late for Ryan and famed tennis player Arthur Ashe, who believed he was infected with HIV during heart surgery in 1983. The chaos surrounding Ryan was nothing short of crazy, and it was cruel and disheartening. I had been watching his story closely for the last two years. The parents and teachers at Ryan's middle school had circulated a petition to keep him out of school. His mother, Jeanne White, took the school to court, but the Indiana Board of Education rescinded the local school's decision, allowing him to come to school. As a result, some parents took their children out of school. Ryan was forced to use paper utensils at lunchtime. Even some uninformed person shot a gun into their home. Now he was an AIDS activist whose story had reached international proportions.

By the time I became an AIDS Activist, Ryan had passed. However, in the years that followed, Jeanne and I have worked together. She told me people in her town spread a rumor that Ryan had AIDS because she was a poor housekeeper. Imagine being told that your child's health was connected to how well you clean your house? Across the globe, Ryan became a symbol for intolerance against people living with this disease. All parts of society exhibited intolerance. Pastors were refusing to perform funerals of people who died from AIDS. Funeral homes were refusing bodies, and nurses and doctors didn't want to care for people with the disease. Families were even abandoning babies born with HIV or children of parents who had died from AIDS. Clara Hale, better known as "Mother Hale," founded the Hale House in New York City to give these unwanted children a home. If people were cold enough to throw innocent babies away, what would they do to a woman who started having sex at thirteen? Shoot, that placed me well into the whore category, and I was not trying to make headlines. Nor was I trying to be anyone's activist, like Ryan. I had no intention of changing course. I wanted to be a political operative like Donna Brazile, and nothing would get in my way—not even HIV. I had come too freaking far against so many odds to let small minds interfere.

That afternoon I stood in the kitchen of my host, a local peace activist named Kitty Boniske, and contemplated (having told Paul already) which boyfriend I should tell next that I had HIV. I could only come up with a couple names. Saying that now sounds like a cop-out or like I was in denial, but the truth is there was no way I could've known when I became infected or by whom, because the information I had available to narrow it down was based on what we knew about HIV in 1987. I was living in the era that would write the history of HIV/AIDS for people to read decades later. We didn't know a fourth of what we know today. The same year I learned that I was HIV-positive was also a coming of age for HIV, with many milestones happening. (See the timeline, milestones for HIV/AIDS in the back of the book.)

We were six years after the CDC identified the first cases of AIDS, and even the medical community didn't know what it didn't know. Lord knows, I had no clue where to start. Later that year, the FDA declared condom use for male prevention of HIV; no one was talking about women. There were no examples of women with HIV who could guide me—and no organizations where heterosexual women were welcomed. Victoria Noe highlights this point in her book, *Fag Hags, Divas and Moms: The Legacy of Straight Women in the AIDS Community*. She writes, "HIV-positive women were acknowledged only in terms of their child-bearing ability. They became part of the conversation when they were pregnant, with the focus on the child's health." As an early volunteer, she addressed how heterosexual women were held with contempt by gay men who were part of activist organizations. The bottom line at this juncture was that, the research, the treatment, and the press nearly all the attention went to men who had sex with men.

I had no reason to believe I was infected with HIV before I moved back to Washington. It was far-fetched that I could have been infected between 1981—when AIDS was first identified—and the subsequent years, when AIDS became a gay white man's disease. Trying to figure out when I got infected and if I had infected someone was making me crazy. The only thing that made sense was to tell my most recent sexual partners.

Kitty was out running errands. This would be the best time to make the calls. Before I lost my nerve, I picked up her telephone and called Lamont.

"Hello, Lamont, this is Rae."

"What's up, girl?"

"I have something I need to tell you." I knew Lamont and I had used condoms, but he was on the list of recent sexual partners. After I left SIU, I had seen him a few times that summer before I moved to D.C. and on one visit back to Chicago.

"I donated blood about a month ago and they just told me that I have HIV." I paused but he said nothing.

"You need to go get tested," I advised.

"Damn. Girl how are you holding up?" he asked. My eyes teared.

"I don't know, I'm just hanging. I'm sorry."

"Well, it is what it is." We talked it through a little bit more and said our goodbyes. There wasn't much more to say. He needed to go get tested. He called two weeks later to tell me his test came back negative. I was relieved.

After I finished talking with Lamont, I looked out of Kitty's big picture window at the beautiful Rocky Mountains. God, how I loved nature. The mountains made me think about when I lived with my mother back in Boulder. Every morning, waking up to such beauty and then hiking with Michael and their golden retriever became the best way to start the day. Hands down, that was the easiest time of my life since my grandfather's death. And I was on top of the world before my mother tried to kill herself. Now, there was this. Things had dramatically shifted, and I wasn't so sure how I would recover. I wondered if there would ever be another time when I'd get another break even remotely similar to living with my mother. And for the first time since I learned my status, I cried. Why had life been so damn hard for me? I didn't have an answer, but I knew it was time to pick myself up and carry on like Dr. Cotton told me to do eight years earlier. I went to the sink, wet a few paper towels with cool water to make a compress and pressed it against my face. It felt so good. When I removed the compress, I looked at the mountains in all their glory and, for a moment, it felt like God was telling me it would be all right—that whatever might come my way, it would be all right.

I sat back down at the island and called Greg next. We had a brief fling after I moved into my new apartment out of loneliness and curiosity. He said he'd just gotten out of jail and that he'd been tested while he was there and was negative. I was shocked he'd been in jail. I was relieved he was negative but glad I had cut my losses with him and moved on. I thought about calling Craig Kirby and dismissed it as quickly as I'd thought about it. *What if he freaks out and tells others?* It would have been a mess. He knew way too many people I knew and I could not afford for this information to get out. We had also used condoms and that gave me some relief.

During the entire trip, I went through the motions—juggling meetings and smiling through the pain. I had little time to myself because. It was the pits. After meetings all day and often into the evening, I had to make small talk with my host. The only moment of peace I had was after I shut my bedroom door for the night. That was *my* time—just me and my mind doing flip-flops all night long. I was a ball of emotions—confused, hurt, anxious and scared. All I could do was sit with my emotions and thoughts because I couldn't get a wink of sleep.

The week I returned to Washington I had my appointment at the NIH in Bethesda, Maryland, about a forty-minute metro ride from my apartment. I had seen the NIH on television, but I had no idea of the magnitude of the campus. There were so many buildings! It was as if I had been planted into an alternate world of larger-than-life buildings looming over me. The immensity of the campus made me feel small. The metro stop was on the campus grounds, and I must have gotten lost and asked for directions at least five times before I found the right building. By the time I got on the elevator I was a nervous wreck, to put it mildly. I'd called myself looking cute dressed to impress. I wore a powder-blue cardigan with a lace collar, slacks, pumps and my pearls. I looked like I'd just stepped out of a Laura Ashley catalogue. I didn't want the doctor to think poorly of me. I had felt that Black girl respectability syndrome bad. The only women who I had heard about with HIV were prostitutes and intravenous drug users. That I was going to the doctor about a serious health issue—yet all I could think about was what she would think of me—was sad. I was embarrassed just thinking about being embarrassed.

I stood in this waiting room that had toys scattered about as well as small tables and chairs in the primary colors. It was a children's clinic in the morning and the study clinic in the afternoon. The coordinating nurse, Jackie, came into the waiting room and escorted me to an examining room. I was so damn happy she hadn't asked me to undress after taking my vitals. As I waited on the doctor, sweat dripped from under my breasts beneath my bra and between my legs. I never understood why I sweated in the most private places, and I hated it!

The doctor, Susan Leitman, was very friendly, and met me with a smile. She was the chief of the Blood Services Section in the Department of Transfusion Medicine. Dr. Leitman explained that I had been referred for an HIV study, not a doctor's visit, per se. It was an epidemiological study of HIV-positive, asymptomatic blood donors conducted collaboratively by the American National Red Cross and NIH. At first, I was a tad taken aback. I thought it was inappropriate to push me into a study rather than send me to a physician. Even being as well-read as I was, the only medical research study I had heard of was the Tuskegee Syphilis Study. It was a legitimate natural history study on syphilis and men that began prior to any known treatment. Once penicillin was determined to be a viable treatment for syphilis, those in charge of in the study made a deliberate decision to withhold treatment from the study participants, who were all African American; it compromised the lives of participants and destroyed the trust of many in the Black community. Dr. Leitman reassured me this was not a drug study, but one that looked closely at the lives of people who had learned of their HIV status through blood donation. *What the heck,* I thought, *maybe my participation would be a way for me to contribute and turn this bad thing into something good.* I would repeat this trip to Bethesda, Maryland to see Dr. Leitman, with Jackie scheduling my appointments and arranging my travel after I had moved back to Chicago, for the next ten years.

That first day Dr. Leitman took an extensive life history, digging deep into my health and my parent's health, of which I had no information. Then there was a no-holds-barred conversation about my lifestyle — drugs, alcohol, and my sex life. As soon as she asked me about drugs and alcohol, I told her flatly, "I have never used drugs. NEVER, EVER." I told her the amount of alcohol I drank in my lifetime might fill a pint, and that was stretching it. She gave me that suspect look, like, *Girl, stop lying and tell me the truth.* It was hard for people to believe I didn't drink—not even socially. "You have never had a beer or a glass of wine?" she asked. I shook my head resolutely. "Nope." I explained that the few times I drank alcohol had been with my girlfriend, Veronica, and that crew, and they had been ice-cream drinks. I had to admit, Veronica could make the heck out of a Creamsicle Cocktail—amaretto liqueur with orange juice and vanilla ice cream. Other than that, I never acquired a taste for alcohol. She asked if any boyfriends used drugs. I knew one of them had snorted cocaine. What did I know about the behavior of others outside my peripheral vision? Not a damn thing. The same was true when she asked if any of my boyfriends was bisexual. How the hell would I know such a thing unless they told me, or I saw it with my own two eyes? Neither had happened.

Dr. Leitman's questions about my partners became a moment of truth for me. Whatever I thought I knew about my partners' lives—no matter how well I *thought* I knew a person—there was *something* that I did not know. I tell women all the time, "Unless the penis is in your pocket, you have no idea what it is doing when it ain't with you." #Facts!

At one point, I thought Dr. Leitman was being a little too intrusive. *Why the fuck does she want to know about every freaking man I've dated?* I thought. After about five minutes into the interrogation about men I had had sex with, I blurted, "I am NOT a whore." At least, I had never seen myself as a whore. But in that very moment, I knew society sure would have considered me to be one.

That day, I had a gut-wrenching, *coming to Jesus' moment* that hit me like a ton of bricks. I had been in and out of sexual relationships since I was thirteen.

I'd had sex with men I thought I loved and men I thought loved me back.

I'd had sex with men who I wanted to love me.

I'd had sex with men while going into a situation thinking one thing, only to come out of it with the knowledge of a different thing.

I'd had sex with men who I made wait the proverbial three months—and, still, the relationship did not work out.

I'd had sex with men because they were the perfect specimens of fineness.

I'd had sex in a bed, on a floor, in the front and back seats of a car. To round off my torrid sexual history, I'd even had sex *in the park after dark.*

Was HIV the cost of my sexual liberation and false paradigm? That was the hundred-thousand-dollar question; my answer was that if I hadn't had sex, I wouldn't have HIV. I was my own worst enemy; with that acknowledgment, I took all the blame. That day I spilled all the details about the partners and the sex: oral, vaginal, and anal. She assured me whatever I told her would be heard without judgment and would never leave the room.

With all the questions and answers, I still hadn't come close to figuring who infected me. She told me Paul was tested and was negative. She took me through the list of risk factors. Since I was drug-free and had never had a blood transfusion, the conclusion was that I contracted HIV from having sex. I wanted to know who infected me, and she asked me some questions that were standard during that time. Had I traveled to Africa in the past year? No, I hadn't. Then she asked, "Have you had sex with a permanent resident of Africa visiting the United States?" I hesitated for a moment and slowly I said, "Yes," pausing. "I guess I have." Then I explained my rendezvous with my West African friend when he was visiting for the United Nations celebrations.

He couldn't be. I dismissed it with a quickness. *He's a diplomat!* I was stunned even at the possibility. Then I remembered in one of his letters he told me he had been having some health issues; then, the letters stopped. I had no way of verifying he was HIV-positive. It had been almost two years since we'd been together. I remembered that day he appeared at my front door, looking as fine as ever—not sick. That night, we used condoms but every single time he pulled out of me the condom was wrapped around the lower part of his large penis. It was a wild night of passion and condoms couldn't contain him. Tracing our contact in my head, *Damn!* I thought. *It fits—he infected me!* Or maybe I needed it to fit. In reality, it was a huge leap to assume he was the person who had infected me simply because he had stopped writing and the condom broke during sex, but I needed a resolution. And reconciling Dr. Leitman's question referencing regions in Africa with when I thought I *may* have gotten infected, I fixated on him. After that, I stopped worrying myself about any other sexual partners; with that unsettling truth, I moved on.

She asked me to undress, but to keep on my panties. I was relieved on the one hand because I still couldn't get that day when I was diagnosed with herpes out of my mind. But on the other hand, I was surprised. I had clearly become infected with HIV from having sex, but my vagina had no value in this study. I found it curious, but I didn't know what questions to ask, so I dropped it. After the physical exam, I had a urine test and Jackie took me to another room where they drew blood. I was shocked when I saw the bags on the hook waiting like I was getting ready to donate blood. Well, that is what I did, and they took as much as was medically possible at one time, all for research. By the time they finished, I'd given two-and-a-half of the large bags and some test tubes full. Over the years the number of questions would become shorter and the amount of blood less.

I had a lot to think about when I left Dr. Leitman that day. There was still no treatment for people living with HIV. The drug AZT had been approved around that time but only for limited "compassionate" use. I wasn't "sick," so there was no treatment for me. Dr. Leitman explained the only thing she could do was to monitor my health for disease progression. There were so many questions in March 1987 for which only time would render an answer. While we knew that HIV caused AIDS and AIDS would kill you, we still knew very little about the impact HIV would specifically have on my body. How long would it take to cause AIDS, if ever? On the metro, I thought again about Keith Barrow. I hoped I would never develop AIDS. And that became my constant prayer. *Please, Lord. Don't ever let me get AIDS.*

Forty-One

LAMENTATIONS

" We must accept finite disappointment, but we must never lose infinite hope."
—Martin Luther King Jr.

I was slipping into a dark place and doing my best to stop it. For a while, I thought my heavy workload at SANE was my savior. That April, the "Boycott Nicaragua, Not South Africa March" was a huge success. It was a rainy day, but we still had over a hundred thousand people in attendance. It would go down as one of the largest peace rallies in U.S. history. There was a list of illustrious speakers, but it was Reverend Jesse Jackson who stole the show. He was in his prime. There had been speculation he would run for president again and, after that speech, I was certain he would. I went straight to Mrs. Jackson and threw my name into the running. The Bible says, *You have not because you ask not,* so I asked to be the national youth director for the 1988 campaign.

After the march, when my workload returned to normal, I couldn't stay focused. I'd sit at my desk with papers scattered about but, by the end of the day, I hadn't done a damn thing. Once home, I made dinners I barely ate. I had started to lose weight and, before I knew it, I dropped from a size ten to an eight. By eight o'clock on most evenings, I had literally and figuratively settled into the darkness. With the lights off, the fireplace sizzling, and Wintley Phipps or Tramaine Hawkins in my cassette player, I would drift off until the warmth and light of the fireplace fizzled and left me in the cold and the dark. Then I'd get in my bed for another sleepless night. Some mornings, it took everything I had to get dressed and out the door. I started to withdraw. All that smiley-smiley shit I had been doing to make the white people at work comfortable just stopped. I did my job and I was cordial, but I didn't have the energy to pretend. I needed every ounce of whatever I had to get through this slump. I withdrew socially; work and home became my routine. Sometimes, on Friday nights I'd still go to Kramer's Books & Afterwords Café to lose myself in books and people-watch. I'd always found comfort in books, and they were the perfect distraction. I didn't even need to open one book; I could peruse the titles and be carried off to another place.

I continued to go to church but there was no joy, no celebration, no worship. I lamented with my whole body and spirit. I could hear the old folks yelling, *Talk to Him, baby. Talk to Him!* And that's just what I did.

"Why, God?" I moaned.

"Fix me, Jesus. Fix me," I cried.

"How much pain do I have to bear?" I asked.

"Answer me," I demanded.

"What's wrong with me, God?"

I'd wail until I was exhausted, and then lay bare my ultimate request—*Please, don't EVER let me get AIDS*—into the bosom of God. And just like that, I'd wipe my tears and clear all the ugly snot out of my nostrils, open my Bible and follow the sermon. There were no revelations—just the rhythm of the music soothing my soul. It was enough to get me through another week. Come Monday morning, I did what I did the best—I kept on moving.

You can do this, Rae, I reminded myself every day. I was the same person who had withstood Mama every single time. Even when she branded me like a cow, I'd stood my little self in front of the ornate mirror that I loved so much, beaten to a pulp—red, bruised and bleeding. I traced those two bloody welts covering the left side of my jaw over and over as close as I could get my fingers without touching them, wondering why Mama didn't love me. If I could withstand Mama, then certainly I could live with HIV. *Mama didn't win, and neither will HIV,* I told myself. Those scars—I could still trace them if I looked closely enough—became a symbol of what I survived that day, and a source of strength of what I could survive now. I had to draw from the strength that had gotten me this far. In the past, no matter how battered and shattered I had been, I kept moving forward. It was the only way I knew.

Why should this be any different? It wasn't that I fell or about the time it took me to get back up. It was the miracle that I got back up, every time. I needed a miracle because time had changed, and darkness had settled in.

I was pressed down by my HIV diagnosis and my mother, who hadn't made any progress mentally from her suicide attempt. Physically, she was just fine. She didn't want to reconstruct her breasts and she was wearing wigs to cover the scars on her head. The relationship I had hoped and prayed for had been undermined by her mental illness. I wouldn't have stated it that way then, but surely it was the beginning of our end. Some days it seemed there was no light in her tunnel, not at the beginning or the end. It was just dark. Every now and then during our talks, she would appear in all her fullness. We'd laugh and talk about my work, hopes and dreams. She felt like the mother I had bonded with back in Boulder. In those times I wanted to tell her I had HIV, but we were in such a good place I didn't want to ruin the moment. We had never talked about her suicide attempt—not back then when it was so fresh. So, I decided not to bring my health into the equation. When our calls ended, I thought, *Maybe next time.* Then the next time would be dark and getting more than a few words out of her was like pulling teeth with pliers. I couldn't tell her about my diagnosis when she was already in a dark place.

When Dorje finally moved out of my grandmother's house into her own apartment, I was relieved. I had enough to deal with than to subject myself to grandmother's constant rejection. While Dorje's move solved that problem for me, it didn't make her better, as I had hoped. I wanted to help her for her sake as much as ours. I was failing miserably. I knew if she didn't get the help she needed, it would be the barrier that would always block our growth. I had asked her about therapy, and she told me that the therapist she had seen in Buffalo looked down on her. I was so desperate to make her better. It was like one bleeding person taking off a shirt to tie the wound of another to stop the bleeding. We were two sad saps. The only difference was that I was a master at putting on a good face. *Just grin and bear it*—that was my specialty. Dorje, on the other hand, just didn't give a fuck that she was having a bad day, and God help us all.

I realized I was out of my league and at least had the gumption to get some help for myself to help her. I said that right. If she wasn't going to go to therapy, I thought that maybe I needed to talk to a mental-health expert to help me find a way to help her that didn't stress me the hell out. Here I was, clearly going through a situational depressive episode after being diagnosed with HIV. Yet, instead of seeking therapy solely for me, it was about her. It turned out my medical insurance provided short-term situational therapy. Retrospectively, I wish that it had been more; nonetheless, it would become the beginning of my long journey toward healing. I was asked to complete this long history about my life, and not one time did I mention that I had just been diagnosed with HIV. And not one time, in my eight therapy sessions, did "HIV" come out of my mouth. After the therapist read my history, he did, however, promise that if there were issues that came up during those eight weeks, he would put them in a box and revisit them at the end. The first thing I did in therapy was recount the horror of my mother's suicide attempt and my rescue mission. Then I told him about Thanksgiving and everything thereafter. That was the end of our fifty-five-minutes to be continued next week.

I was amazed I told everything without one bit of reluctance. Each week, after I walked out of his office, I felt like tons of bricks had been lifted off my shoulders. It must have been late spring or early summer—the weather was beautiful, and I would walk from his office in northwest D.C. between Georgetown and Dupont Circle, to my apartment in Logan Circle—a thirty-minute walk away.

One day on the walk home, I saw Jack O'Dell close to the Rainbow Coalition office at 2100 M St., and we walked and talked for six or seven blocks. I've never forgotten that day because he provided the "wise uncle" affirmation I needed. I gave him the 4-1-1 on SANE's merger talks with another peace organization, The Freeze Campaign (Freeze). I had started back on the road to be a part of what SANE called the Listening Project. They were supposed to be sessions held with both SANE and Freeze members to gather feedback on a possible merger between the two. In my opinion, they were bitching sessions on why the lily-white grassroots peace organization, Freeze, was not going to be co-opted by the lily-white upper-class peace organization, SANE.

Jack listened as I told him about it—that it was all so exhausting. He had a discerning way about him. When we stopped at the corner that would send us in different directions, he gave me some sage advice and much-needed praise. He told me he was proud of the work I was doing at SANE. He said it was brave of me to be a change agent within the organization. He told me no matter what SANE assigned me to do, my presence as a Black woman with my experience and worldview was a calling. He said, "You've been raised well by some of our political greats. When your usefulness is over at SANE, you will know it and you will move on to do more great work." He hugged me tightly and walked away. I felt like I had had another therapy session. With all that had been going on in my life with my mother, and now HIV, I hadn't stopped to think about the war I had been fighting at SANE. Every day I walked into the building; I carried the burden of my color. My work and even my body language were judged culturally in a way that my white counterparts' were not. I had heard older Black people say, *We Black people have to work twice as hard as white people.* And I had learned it was the truth at SANE.

The therapy sessions didn't change my situation, but they did change my approach—at least toward my mother. I came to understand I could not save Dorje; she had to do the emotional work herself. The therapist believed that my mother was a danger to herself and, possibly, to me. Every cut on her body was an indication that she was trying to punish herself, not kill herself. If she had not survived, her death would have been a by-product of her original intent. She was troubled. Full stop. I thought about the psychiatrist at the mental institution convincing me to take her home for an overnight visit and me agreeing to that crazy stunt. I recalled that Thanksgiving visit. It was stressful but I didn't believe she would hurt me. Then again, in the wee hours of the morning my mind started playing tricks on me, causing me to wonder if she was going to turn Norman Bates on me. In any case, I didn't have to worry about that now because I was in D.C., and she was in Buffalo. All these years I wanted a mother who would love me unconditionally, and Dorje had not disappointed me. Now, I honestly felt as if God was testing me. My prayer had been answered, but could I love and support my mother in spite of her brokenness? I had another bitching session with God. Just why did everything have to be so dang hard for me? I wondered if there would ever be a time when the good was not gift-wrapped around so much bad. I stayed on my knees during this period because with prayer came faith, and faith is the substance of things hoped for. It was all I had to keep hope alive.

Forty-Two
❧ ☙
HOT BOILING OIL

The fear of rejection stings...
more in most cases than the real thing
more than Momma's swift flick with the switch
more than the pop of boiling grease.
This fear of rejection stings...
it climbs up my spine,
closes my throat,
threatens to steal the very breath I'm holding in,
because the truth of it lives on my lips... and now in my blood.
Confused
Angry
Exhausted
and suffocating with fear of rejection.
Waiting to exhale could kill others
As surely as it is killing me
I breathe my truth
Its like balm on the wounds I delivered to myself
I breathe
and I live... my truth.
—LaToya Renae Porter

The fear of rejection rose in me like the foam of hot milk sizzling and boiling over. *Who in the hell is going to want me with HIV?* was all I could think about. I had never been rejected by a man until the day Paul walked out of my apartment. At first, I didn't give his abrupt departure a lot of thought; he had to have been as scared as I was that night. But after I learned he had tested negative and hadn't even called to check on me, my feelings were deeply hurt. I had so many questions: *When do I tell? How do I tell? Who do I tell? Would Paul be my new standard? What kind of relationship was even possible for me with HIV?*

If I was confident about nothing else, I knew I could walk into a room and have any man I wanted. Now, I was living with the one thing in my lifetime that would cause a man to balk. It wasn't that I "needed" a man to complete me; it was more about how HIV had changed my life in a blink of an eye. I now carried the burden of HIV—not just my savvy, smart, provocative self. I was literally two diametrically opposed things wrapped in one body. The thought of telling a man, *Oh, by the way: I have this virus that may one day kill me and that I could possibly give to you and one day, it might kill you too,* was overwhelming and too much to fully wrap my brain around. In the meantime, I thought it best to stay away from men until I could figure this thing out.

Life can really mess up a plan. Trouble came knocking on my door. My old friend Sylvester Monroe moved to D.C. I avoided him as I had avoided other men. I didn't accept dinner invitations and I didn't give my telephone number to new would-be suitors.

I felt like HIV was robbing me of my life. Sylvester was my friend and there was no reason I couldn't at least have a phone conversation with him. We eventually talked, and I made excuses about why we couldn't get together. One evening he caught me off guard. We were laughing and talking, and he said, "Girl, you should come on over."

"Ohhhh, Vest," I said. Before I could get the excuse out of my mouth, he jumped in.

"I don't see a problem. You're single; I'm single. Neither one of us is doing anything tonight." I was quiet, and then he said, "Rae, I really would like to see you." *Darn it*, I thought.

"Ohhhh, Vest," I said again. I really wanted to see him, but our chemistry and history said I could be headed for trouble. Sylvester had always been a perfect gentleman, but HIV was new and I didn't know if I could trust myself.

"Girl, call a taxi and come over. I'll meet you downstairs to pay for the taxi." In the meantime, he said, "I'll order Chinese."

I arrived at his apartment at the beginning of a blizzard. It would've been the perfect excuse to not come, if only I'd known it was going to snow. The moment I walked in the door; I was surprisingly relaxed. I was happy to see him. It had been a couple of years since we'd laid eyes on one another. We settled in with food and laughter. We talked about the possibility of Reverend Jackson running for president again in the '88 primaries. We reminisced about the breakneck campaign schedule in 1984. Then we laughed and joked about sneaking around back during the campaign and what would've happened if anyone had found us out. I hadn't laughed like that since before the months of my mother's suicide attempt. I was having such a great time I hadn't thought about the direction the night was going. When Sylvester reached for my hand to get off the sofa, reality set in as he began pulling out the sofa bed in his studio apartment. I started weighing my options in my head. I had all these rules about not teasing men if I wasn't going to carry through, but I never put on the breaks. By the time he had the bed out, I told myself it would be just fine. Sylvester was a condom man, and I was reassured by the fact that you could not transmit HIV if you used a latex condom. I drifted off to another place when I felt the caress of his lips on my breast. I surrendered. After the loving, I nestled in his embrace like nothing had changed.

As the endorphins waned, reality started to sink in. Something *had* changed. I had HIV! I felt flush. I started to simmer on the inside. I felt the sweat form under my breast and trickle down my stomach. I got up and went into the bathroom, dampened a towel with cold water and placed it on my face. The coolness of the towel was a wonderful contrast to the hot boiling guilt inside. "You had no right!" I scolded in a whisper. I had a rapid succession of emotions. Guilt. Shame. Unworthiness. Fear. "You had no right!" I mumbled. I sat down on the cold tile trying to figure my next move. *We had used a condom*, I reminded myself, but it did nothing for the guilt welling in me. *You have to leave*, I told myself. I came out of the bathroom and asked Sylvester to call me a taxi.

"What?" he asked, totally thrown off guard.

"I have to go home; call me a taxi," I explained. "Please." He studied me to see if I were joking, then finally asked, "Why can't you spend the night?" Sweat started to drip under my breast again. I was never good at lying and I knew I had to have been sounding crazy right about then.

"Because I didn't bring any clothes and I need to get to work early in the morning," I said. That much was true. I hadn't brought any clothes because I had planned on having a meal and going straight back to the house. *Was I in denial or something? We had a robust sex life in the past. Why would this night have been different?*

"Rae, do you realize how bad it is outside?"

"Yes, but I need to go." There was nothing he could say to change my mind. I couldn't even look him straight in the eye. He did as I asked. We waited for over an hour because of the snow. The entire time, Sylvester continued to say. "You know you can stay."

I knew he was sincere but, at that point, I was a mess—not because I thought I had given him HIV, but because I had taken away his right to choose by not disclosing. I thought about what I would want for myself if it had been the other way around. I thought about the time Greg had infected me with gonorrhea and lied about it. There was so much to think about now that I knew my HIV status. I was fighting a war inside me that night and I knew I needed to get a battle plan. It wouldn't be resolved that night or the night after. Sylvester rode down on the elevator with me. He gave me a long hug and a quick kiss on the lips. When the taxi arrived, I stepped into the brisk wintry air; the fast-blowing snow hit me hard in the face. I stood there for a moment, accepting it as punishment. When I got in the taxi, I rolled down the window so the cold air could chill the fire burning inside.

After this night with Sylvester, I was a wreck. I couldn't figure how to bring up the topic of HIV to a man. I didn't know what I would say, other than "I have HIV." The now-classic Randy Shilts book *And the Band Played On* was published that year. I didn't bother to pick it up because it was a book about white gay men dying from AIDS and being rejected and neglected by both the government and their families. As far as I was concerned, the book had nothing to do with me. I didn't have AIDS and I certainly didn't want to read about dying from it. I needed to read a book that didn't exist—*How to Live with HIV*. Being clear that a condom would prevent my sexual partner from contracting HIV just wasn't enough. HIV was not like diabetes, in that you can take your insulin, change your lifestyle, and keep it moving. From the beginning, HIV had political, social and medical implications for every person living with this virus, and everyone had an opinion about it. I believed a person dating me would have more of a burden with the stigma of HIV than he would with contracting the virus. People were so judgmental—and some were downright vicious, from pastors to politicians.

U.S. Senator Jesse Helms wanted to lock us up. Thank God it didn't happen, but he was able to get the Helms Amendment, SP 963, attached to a 1988 appropriations bill passed. The amendment prohibited the use of federal funds by the CDC for HIV educational and prevention materials that would "promote, encourage, and condone homosexuality sexual activities or intravenous use of illegal drugs." Senators Kennedy and Hatch were able to get some of the language changed but, in the end, it passed the House 358-47 and the Senate 94-2. The Gay Men Health Crisis, Helms original target, took it to court and won, but the damage was done. CDC acquiesced and swiftly altered its guidelines, prohibiting all printed material from using any genital organs and the anus. It also mandated that all materials had to warn about the dangers of IV drug use, promiscuity and promote abstinence. These changes would have a lasting negative impact on how we educated young people about STI's for years to come especially about HIV/AIDS.

I couldn't sit down with a man to tell him I had HIV with my head jumbled. I had to come, with clarity and self-confidence—neither of which I had in those months immediately following my diagnosis. How was I even supposed to talk to a man about proper condom use when a picture of a penis was prohibited on educational material?

It was an awful period in America's history—and a very stressful time for me. How the heck was anyone supposed to come to terms about living with HIV in this climate? Society was irrational, but I was supposed to think and act clearly.

"Good AIDS/Bad AIDS" was another one of those irrational things that took root. If you were infected through a blood transfusion or blood products, a child infected at birth or through breast feeding; (the child had Good AIDS and the mother had BAD AIDS) and if a woman was infected by her husband, then she had "Good AIDS." Basically, people who were perceived as a victim had Good AIDS. Everyone else had "Bad AIDS" and was going to burn in hell—and deserved that fate. I fit into that "Bad AIDS" category as a single woman who couldn't tell you who had infected me. Even if you were in the Good AIDS category, it didn't ensure that people would treat you with kindness. Ryan White was an example of how cruel people can be. People were afraid of this disease. And most people treated people with HIV and AIDS with a long-handled spoon. I don't know what I feared the most: rejection from a man or status as an outcast. I had lived my life to meet people's approval; now, I had an illness that caused mothers and fathers to abandon their own children. I didn't want judgments about my personal life to affect my career trajectory. I had worked too hard to let it all collapse because of something that had nothing to do with my ability to get the job done. I think Barry Saunders got it out of me because he had that way about him; he was so smooth and easy to talk to. Plus, he sincerely wanted to know why I was seeing a doctor at NIH, which meant whatever was going on with me was serious. I folded. After that, I even kept my visits to NIH a secret. Truth be told, I was just as ashamed as I was afraid of being thought of as a horrible person.

I had started the year with a big bang; now, it had exploded in my face. I didn't know how to get myself to a better place emotionally and I was disappointed that I didn't have the answers. After all, I was still the Miss-Know-It-All.

Being on the road to oversee the SANE/Freeze listening project in my region was the perfect distraction, and it came in the nick of time. On the road, I didn't have time to think about my personal problems because I spent all my time listening to people bitch and moan about a possible merger. Once back in D.C., the cycle of worry would start all over again. Work was going just fine, or so I thought. I was blindsided by my year-end evaluation—as if I needed one more thing to bring me down. Grandmamma Julia used to say bad news comes in threes. First there was Dorje's suicide attempt, then my HIV diagnosis and now, I had been placed on probation—all within the same year.

My boss handed me the written evaluation. I read as she watched. I don't know which was worse: having to read it in front of her watching me or reading that I was a fuck-up without any kind of reaction. By the time I finished reading the evaluation, I was mad as hot boiling oil. If I had done nothing else, I had worked my ass off. She acknowledged that some of my work had been exemplary and gave an accurate assessment of areas of weakness where I could stand improvement. The problem was the evaluation was more about my personality than my work performance. The list of transgressions she had outlined blew my mind. She had documented the fact that when I arrived in the morning, I had a cup of tea and crocheted at my desk before starting work, which was true. Mrs. Jackson was teaching me how to crochet and I'd practice before I started my day. Learning to crochet was a wonderful distraction and the only thing that kept me sane—no pun intended—during this time. Crocheting was my morning process to start the day, like my white male colleague who had his coffee and leisurely read the paper each morning. I asked her point-blank to explain the difference, and she couldn't.

She also noted that my body language in meetings signaled a lack of interest. I had to give her that much; I was easily bored. I tuned out bullshit with a quickness. I still couldn't make myself sit still like Grandmamma Julia had tried to drill into me—not even at the age of twenty-four. The scary part of the evaluation was that she had been watching me so closely while conducting meetings. WHAT THE HELL?!? It was like she was waiting on me to make a wrong move. I wanted to ask if she had been watching my colleagues the way she was watching me, but I decided that I shouldn't be a smart-ass, since I still needed to pay rent. The big whammy was her assertion that I was not a team player, and she had a list of infractions to prove it. For example, when I showed up for staff gatherings, I was disengaged. I was floored that she had been watching me at what I considered social events. For one thing, I resented that I was asked to participate in events that made me uncomfortable and had nothing to do with my job. I had told everyone at

SANE I didn't drink alcohol. "Not even wine or beer?" someone would inevitably ask. "Not even," I'd answer. I didn't blow the gatherings off. I always made an appearance and chatted a while but by the time people were on their second rounds, I'd had enough.

I found myself reading and responding to the evaluation in my head as a way to defend myself against the absurdity of being judged about things that had nothing to do with me doing my job. I knew that if I said my thoughts aloud, it would have become a full-fledged argument with the white woman trying to get the angry Black woman to calm down, adding validity to this crap. She noted I complained about the mattress on the bunk bed where I was supposed to sleep when we went on a staff retreat. *Of course, I did; they looked like they'd been gathered from an alley or some other nasty place.* I made people feel uncomfortable when I took it upon myself to clean the bathrooms. For a moment I thought, *She has got to be kidding.* The place was a pigsty. The toilets, sinks and shower hadn't been cleaned in—oh, I don't know—how about, never? My ass found some supplies and scrubbed the women's bathroom spotless. I couldn't contain myself anymore and before I knew it, I said, "The bathrooms were filthy!" She told me I was supposed to go with the flow—that we were bonding. This was some *Survivor* reality television crap years before its time. I was not down for it. I didn't understand back then how culturally biased my evaluation was, but I was certainly pissed off. I reminded her that I had helped to cook every meal the team ate that weekend. She didn't remember it the same way I did. The most hurtful part of the review was that most every place I visited in my region had reported back to her something about me that had nothing to do with my work, but everything to do with me. I was being too *Black,* too *pushy.* I was passionate about things I believed in. I took my work at SANE very seriously. If we were going to integrate SANE, my ideology was simple: *Let's do this thing and stop making excuses.* I felt betrayed because some of the critiques had come from people who I thought were sincere, and I'd trusted them. I accepted the evaluation and probation, walking out of that meeting with my head held high.

I knew that my time at SANE had come to an end, just as Jack had predicted. I had gotten all the usefulness I could out of this organization. It had been a steppingstone to more exposure and training that would diversify my portfolio. Now that I'd been placed on notice, I was watching them watch me. There was one person who I had considered a friend and trusted as sincere; her evaluation of my work in her region stung the most. She would replace me when I left. I had been pushing her to pursue a particular job and, apparently, she had her eye on my job. I doubled back to Mrs. Jackson about the campaign, and she assured me she would look out for me.

The Midwest Academy was the last training I would have at SANE. Midwest Academy is a national training institute committed to advancing the struggle for social, economic, and racial justice. I had heard that the Midwest Academy yearly conference that took place in Chicago was a must for grassroots activists and people in political organizing. SANE designed a mini-planning retreat for senior staff to be held at the conference. I looked forward to being back in Chicago. After I arrived, I called Mama to check in. I hadn't seen her since she got baptized. During the call she asked me to do a deep cleaning of her apartment, so I went over just to do that.

A day before the conference began, SANE had an all-day program planning meeting. Once the conference began, we were free to attend workshops but still had parts of our day blocked off for SANE. One night, I spotted this brother at a reception. My eyes scanned over him, and I was mesmerized with his beautiful brown skin and perfectly fitted black suit. I did a double take and, sure enough, he was still there—a *fine* Black man with beautiful brown eyes standing off to the side with a smile that said, *Welcome!* My first thought was that he had to be important because he was wearing a suit. There were two undeniable facts about Midwest Academy—white people outnumbered Black people at least three to one; and white people who professed to be liberal did not dress up, and many Black people had joined that club. On the other hand, I continued to dress my tail off and I could spot an important brother—or at least one I thought was important by the clothes he wore. Our eyes met with the acknowledgment, *I see you, boo*. And with that, I disappeared into another SANE meeting, making a mental note to find out who he was. I have to admit that I was intrigued at first sight, but I wasn't particularly looking to get involved. I had kept my distance from men since Sylvester and didn't want to tempt fate again—at least not until our eyes met that next night in the lobby and he waltzed over to where I was and introduced himself as Reverend Bill McGill. We found a spot in the lobby and ordered soft drinks. He worked at an organization for tenants' rights in Port Huron, Michigan. Thank God he lived in another state, and I could chat him up and keep on moving. I saw no harm in a friendly conversation.

Bill was charming. What impressed me the most was his passion to help people in need. He could talk that talk, and I was glued to every word. Two hours later I was still sitting in the same place, completely enamored with him. The chemistry was sizzling, and I found myself blushing; it was something I hadn't done in a long time. When he suggested that we go to his room, that little old thing called anxiety crept up on me and I could feel the moisture beneath my underwire bra. It put me on notice that I was in a tight spot before it registered to my brain. He reached for my hand, and I paused a moment before placing mine in his. I was completely in my head now. Again, I thought about that night with Sylvester. I certainly did not want a replay. I dismissed going further with a quickness. I'd just met this dude. *No way am I going to have sex with him, even if I didn't have HIV*. As we made our way to the elevator, I started to second-guess myself. Maybe this was not a good idea. But I liked this guy, and my curiosity hadn't been piqued like this in a long while, even before I found out my HIV status. *I should walk away*, I told myself; still, I kept going to his room. I sat in the chair, and he sat at the end of his bed and pulled my chair as close as he could. That first kiss told me that I wanted him. To hell with HIV. But, I had to do the right thing. *Tell him, Rae, or walk away*. I weighed my options in between kisses. If he rejected me because of the HIV, there would be no collateral damage. He was a stranger to me. He knew absolutely no one who I knew. He would go back to Michigan; I would go back to Washington and never see him again. I was thinking quickly. I knew you could not build a relationship on a lie. If I didn't tell him—even if we didn't have sex this time, and when we did have sex and used a condom—I would still have to tell him, eventually. I excused myself and went to the bathroom to pull myself together and allow things to cool down. When I came back, I said, "Bill, there is something I need to tell you before we go any further." He took my hand into his, "Whatever it is, I'm sure that it will be as fine as you." I laughed. In that split second, he had reduced all my tension and given me the space to do what I needed to do. "I have HIV," I said. And I have no idea what was said after that. He kissed me with a passion that I had never known not before him, or after him. Then we talked about it and went back to kissing. If Bill had any anxiety, I was unaware of it. He never missed a beat. That night, we were intimate but limited our moments of passion because neither of us had a condom. The next morning, I slipped out of his room and went back to mine to pack and get ready to leave. We met in the lobby and said our goodbyes.

Bill called me that night after he arrived back in Port Huron; from that moment, we were inseparable. His voice was the first one I heard each morning and the last one I heard each night. He wrote me beautiful love letters and introduced me to intimacy via the phone that helped to ease the distance. I didn't think there was anything new I could be taught in that area. Boy, was I wrong! I wanted this relationship to work, but I also knew that my history with men had not been a good one. I had never stopped believing I was broken; I had just become a master at gluing my pieces back together again. On our long talks, I told him about my childhood and how I was a mess. If he could stick it out and work through my brokenness, I believed we had a future together. I told him about my mother's suicide attempt, and about my therapy sessions and some of the things I had discovered about my behavior as a result.

At the close of those sessions, the therapist had kept his promise and suggested a couple of books for me to read. He handed me a piece of paper with two books: *The Struggle for Intimacy* and *Adult Children of Alcoholics*. After I had read the titles, I looked at him and asked, "And I should read these books, why?" He replied that growing up with an alcoholic could have a long-lasting impact on one's life. First, I didn't know who he was talking about. Dorje did not drink; she used drugs, and that was years ago. Of course, the topic of Mama had come up. I had to explain why I had two mothers and how I related to them. And, yes, I might have mentioned that Mama drank her Christian Brothers or Smirnoff or whatever her flavor of the month was, but was she an alcoholic? Alcoholics, as I understood them, were out-of-control drunks. If Mama had nothing else, she had control. She went to work every day. She never slurred her words, and she never staggered a day in her life to my knowledge. I didn't express any of this because my time was up. My eight sessions were over. He had dropped a ticking bomb in my lap and now I was supposed to go and brave the world on my own. As he closed the door behind me, he advised, "Just read the books and you'll understand." I left his office and walked over to Kramer's Bookstore, and had the store order the books for me.

The *Struggle for Intimacy*, was an eye opener. I didn't believe I would ever find love if I didn't shed some of my distorted thinking on how relationships should work versus how they really worked. I felt Bill was my chance to get it right. I sent him the two books. I placed sticky notes in those parts that I believed spoke specifically to me. I believed if I gave him a deeper look into how and why I thought a particular way that, magically, it would give us a better chance.

I didn't understand that building a relationship took more than reading a book. People often quote Maya Angelou's, "When you know better, you do better." However, what I know for certain is that knowing better is only the beginning of the solution. Change takes time and work, and more work. It would take me years of therapy, more awareness, more reading, and a desire to break the destructive cycle in dating and sex and reject what was easy, familiar, and habitual.

Bill visited me first. That weekend, we talked about the books in between the lovemaking and the meals I cooked for him. We had a glorious three days. I took him sightseeing. We laughed and talked. I was so happy—not just to have a man who accepted my HIV status, but a man who truly loved me and not just how I made him feel in bed. That Sunday, we went to church together. When my pastor asked visitors to stand, he learned that Bill was a minister and invited him to sit in the pulpit. I was so very proud. In between Bill's visits, Pastor Jones asked me how that young preacher of mine was doing, and I'd smile and say, "Very well." Bill McGill was everything I believed I wanted in a man. We shared the same faith and social consciousness, we were both ambitious, we could talk about anything and everything and the sex was magnificent.

I visited him next and, boy, did we play house. During the week, I cooked dinner and had it waiting when he came home from work. Sometimes he popped in at lunchtime and we'd have a quickie. He introduced me to many of his friends and family. I went to a big-time dinner with his civic club; we looked good together. I looked fabulous that night in a beautiful, not-so-navy-blue wool gaberdine dress that Mrs. Jackson insisted I purchase. People admired us all night, and I admired Bill for being the first Black man to join this organization that had been reserved for white men.

Everything was going so well that is, until it wasn't. In that same week, there were phone calls he didn't answer, and that caused my insecurities to well up in me. The calls were persistent, calling all hours of the night. It seemed like some female trying to find where her man had disappeared to all of a sudden. That first Saturday after I arrived a woman called, and I politely told her Bill was in the shower. I dismissed it because he dismissed it. But then the calls kept coming and none of his explanations was satisfactory to me so I went looking for answers. Eventually I'd find my answers, in this case, love letters from another woman.

Now, thirty-three years later, I can say that if your partner has given you any cause to doubt, then it is already over. Looking will only add more pain and prove to be emotionally destructive. The ironic thing is, if I had actually read the books again that I insisted Bill read, then I would have realized I had unrealistic expectations for the relationship from the beginning. It takes time to build trust, and this idea that you become each other's world instantly is pie in the sky. In reality, people need time to clean house, to be sure, and some men require more time than others. Bill was one of those men. I wanted him to love me with all of my imperfections but, at the same time, I demanded his perfection. What I had missed was that he was also broken. We were two broken people trying to love each other to the best of our ability at that place and time, but it wasn't enough. Bill would be the one man to help me understand that bad things happen to boys just as they do to girls. Boys also have mothers and fathers who degrade them, beat them, drink, use drugs and go missing; fathers beat their mothers, and there are aunts who sexually molest their nephews. Boys become men who are shaped by their childhood trauma, just like girls.

We tried to make it work, but we were both shattered. He had violated my trust and I had violated his, even if I didn't admit it then. When he said to me one night, "I don't know if I can trust you. You had no business going through my things." I was like, "Fuck you and your privacy." I'm ashamed to admit all the bickering was about us our failures to ourselves and each other. Never once did I think about the danger of infidelity within the backdrop of HIV. We had used condoms but, still, with just one misstep it could have had serious consequences. When I moved back to Chicago that November, Bill and I were still trying to figure out things, but not for long.

Forty-Three

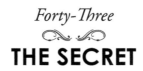

THE SECRET

"He who conceals his disease cannot expect to be cured."
—African proverb

I moved back to Chicago to join the staff of the 1988 Jesse Jackson presidential campaign a couple weeks before Mayor Harold Washington died. I was sitting at my desk on November 25, 1987, when our receptionist, Maria Perez, announced his death. Stunned, everyone in the office gathered around the television. We watched the news in shock, silence, and disbelief. The mayor's death was a devastating blow for progressive politics and Black people in Chicago. Just six months into his second term, his death would change the trajectory of Chicago politics for decades to come. A conspiracy theory that Mayor Washington had been poisoned crept through the Black community like a thief in the night. Actually, he died of a massive heart attack. He was overweight and had hypertension, high cholesterol, and an enlarged heart.

The grief that descended on Chicago in the aftermath of Washington's death was suffocating me—or maybe it seemed that way because I was living in my own private hell. On the outside, I was exquisitely put together and wore my confidence to the office every day in my fly-ass, four-inch-heel, black leather pumps. On the inside, I was still having a difficult time coming to terms with my HIV diagnosis. It had been eight months since I learned I had HIV, and I could not shake the shame. I had internalized everything I had been thinking about in my first conversation about my sex life with Dr. Leitman. It was the easiest answer to my desperate need to understand how I had ended up with HIV. I was ashamed and blamed myself solely. I securely latched onto this thinking, and it pulled me back into the carnage I had been desperately trying to crawl out of since I was a little girl. It would take years for me to stop blaming myself for contracting HIV.

Being back home in Chicago, I became paranoid that my status would be revealed and somehow weaponized against me, whether it was intended or not. While I had kept my HIV status close to the vest in D.C., I didn't have the concern of being exposed because my personal connections with the people I worked with were minimal. In Chicago, I was living and working in an environment where the lines were totally blurred. The double burden of living with HIV and keeping it a secret started to occupy space in my head. Some days, it was easy to push to the back of my mind. Other days, not so much. All it took was for me to have too long of a pause between telephone calls at work, and anxiety would consume me.

Am I going to get AIDS?

What if someone finds out?

Of all the things that could have happened to me, why this? I'd catch myself slipping at my desk and take a break, usually, a walk over to Marshall Field's just up the street from our office; I'd browse around the china section to help clear my head pick up some Frango Mints and get right back to work.

I was a master at forging ahead, even to a fault. As I had done in the past, I immersed myself in my work to shield myself from the pain of life. Work was my happy place. I was mission-driven above all else, including my pain. I told myself, *If Jesus could stay on that cross and carry out His mission, so can I.* I loved working on projects that could in some way make a difference in the lives of people, and a Jackson agenda sought to do just that. I was good at it, too, and it gave me a boost of confidence—like a shot of endorphins in the middle of the day. Looking back, I see how my work was a form of validation for me—a gold star on the board, so to speak. It gave me something I could point to that had not been tainted by all the trauma in my life. I took a lot of pride in my work; that's why I knew my boss at SANE had evaluated me on some other standard. I might not have been the social butterfly, but I worked my butt off. I was happy I'd left SANE for something more meaningful to me. Mrs. Jackson told me at Reverend Jackson's announcement on October 10, 1987, in Raleigh, North Carolina that I officially had the job.

In my first meeting with the campaign manager, Gerald "Jerry" Austin, he said, "I was told that you are going to handle the youth and students for the campaign." I smiled at the sarcasm in his statement and nodded. I felt no need to prove myself to him for a job I already had. I handed him the proposal I put together for a student leadership conference to network and help me recruit for the campaign.

The organizer in me had already begun working on my department even before leaving D.C. Unlike the 1984 campaign, I didn't have all the statewide student and youth directors and college coordinators in place, and I wanted to get ahead of it. I piggybacked off the Congressional Black Caucus Annual Legislative Conference weekend by hosting a reception at my apartment to network with young adults and student leaders who were in town for the conference. Veronica's mother, Sherry, was visiting me and helped prepare a soul-food buffet. It was a success with the who's who of Black student leaders in and out of my apartment that evening. I walked away with a busload of contacts—which, combined with my other connections—gave me a place to start. As the national youth and student coordinator for the campaign, I had a lot of early mornings and late nights with the phone receiver in my hand. Just like the good old days, I was making cold calls to recruit young leaders into the campaign. I was also pushing voter registration drives on Black college campuses. I knew, without a doubt, that if we could get Black students registered and to the polls on election day, the chances they would vote for Jesse Jackson.

The campaign manager approved my proposal. The conference was to be held at PUSH on the Martin Luther King Jr. holiday weekend. Tyrone suggested it to me, and I wasn't even mad that I hadn't thought of it first. Centering the conference around the PUSH Saturday morning forum, was a great organizing tool. An afternoon luncheon with remarks from Reverend Jackson would seal the deal for recruits to work on the campaign. I loved that Tyrone and I were working together again even if it was only to bounce around ideas every now and then. This time, he was the national ministers' coordinator pulling pastors into the campaign from all over the country.

On top of organizing a conference and getting my department up and running, I was also looking for a place to live for the duration of the campaign. I had temporary housing with the oldest of my stepsiblings, Kathy Tobler-Perkins, and her family. I was grateful, but it was a horrible commute from the western suburbs to the campaign headquarters in downtown Chicago. Working late and having to take public transportation—sometimes catching the last bus for the evening to get me closest to Kathy's house—was becoming unmanageable. I was at my wit's end looking for a place when Mrs. Jackson inquired about my housing. I gave her the rundown and she invited me to share their newly purchased second house with her two eldest sons, which was just across the street from their family home. It was my good fortune and I jumped at the opportunity. Jonathan and I were the first to move in, right after Christmas. A week later, Jesse Jr. moved in. It was a perfect arrangement. On the second floor, there were four bedrooms. Jonathan had the master bedroom with a full bath. The room I chose was a two-room spread with one entrance. I was able to create a sitting room at the entrance, and my bed and dresser were in the other room, behind the sitting room. Jesse Jr. had the third-floor attic that included two rooms and a bathroom. The two additional bedrooms at the back of the house were empty. For a while, I had the second-floor bathroom across the hall from my room to myself. We furnished our own bedrooms and Mrs. Jackson furnished the first floor we shared as a common area.

Shortly after moving in, I got a cold. My commute was only a thirty-minute bus ride but standing a stone's throw away from Lake Michigan in Chicago's winter without the proper clothes was plain cruel. I knew better, but I hadn't taken time to shop for Chicago winter clothes, which requires a whole other level of warmth than is needed for D.C. winters. I guess, between the winter weather and my breakneck schedule, my body had enough. I was still coming into the office with a hacking cough that wouldn't let up. One day I was packing up to go home a little early when Rhoda McKinney, who I was just getting to know by way of our mutual friendship with Tyrone, said to me, "Honey, I hate to be the bearer of bad news. You don't need to go home; you need to go see a doctor." Our next-door neighbor—Iris Thomas, a friend of the Jacksons who also watched over the house for Mrs. Jackson—was in the office that day and called, Dr. Cunningham, to see me right away. Rhoda volunteered to take me (I never will forget it) in her brand-new car, a maroon Volkswagen Golf GTI.

Dr. Cunningham was an internist with an established practice in Chicago's historic Bronzeville medical district. I had a fever of 101 degrees and was diagnosed with bronchitis. I was shocked I had become so sick so quickly. It had started as a cold; within the same week, it had transitioned to bronchitis. Dr. Cunningham asked if I had any health issues that could have exacerbated a cold, like asthma or some other lung disease. I had never been prone to colds. But the winter before, I learned I had HIV; I had the worst cold ever and took a week off from work. I didn't give it a lot of thought but now that I knew I had HIV, I started to wonder. I had heard about "AIDS pneumonia," but I didn't have AIDS. I wondered still if I should tell him that I had HIV, but I quickly dismissed the idea. Lord knows I was not trying to tell another soul in Chicago my secret—not even a doctor.

"No," I said, hesitating. "Not really."

The doctor didn't respond. Instead, he looked at me over his glasses for about thirty seconds that felt like hours.

"I have HIV," I blurted before I lost my nerve.

"HIV?" he asked for clarification, "Not AIDS?"

"Yes," I nodded.

If he had any hesitation, I didn't see it. He didn't miss a beat. He asked me to fill in the blanks, and I started with my donating of blood and participation in the study at NIH. He never asked how I became infected, but I volunteered that I believed I had been infected through heterosexual sex because I had never used drugs or had a blood transfusion. He explained that the severity of my illness could be related to the fact that my immune system was being attacked by HIV. It stopped me cold. I had spent so much of my time worrying about developing AIDS that I had not given one thought about what living with HIV meant for me. Dr. Cunningham had given me a lot to think about. He prescribed rest, an antibiotic, and a bronchodilator. But he did so much more: He allowed me to walk away with my dignity intact.

I filled Rhoda in as we walked to the car, minus the HIV part. She couldn't believe I had developed bronchitis so fast either and she kept asking questions—digging, like the reporter she was. (Rhoda was a staff writer for *Ebony* and *Jet* publications at the time.) I wanted to tell her what Dr. Cunningham had told me to shut her up, but I quickly remembered that loose lips sink ships. Frankly, Rhoda and I had just become friends and I didn't know if I could trust her with my secret. Dr. Cunningham was cautious about my status, having said he would keep it out of my chart to protect me. Insurance companies were doing their best to rid themselves of people with HIV/AIDS, so not having a paper trail was to my advantage. I also knew that HIV discrimination had grown exponentially and in the most unlikely of places, even among doctors. The ugly truth is that some doctors were turning people away. Just two months earlier, the American Medical Association issued a statement that doctors had an ethical obligation to treat people living with AIDS as well as those living with HIV who had no symptoms. I was relieved that Dr. Cunningham didn't shrink one bit when he learned of my HIV status—and equally pleased he would keep it between us.

Rhoda seemed so genuine that a part of me was conflicted that I didn't tell her. Keeping HIV secret was not easy. It tugged at my heart and made me feel like a liar by omission. But my fear of HIV stigma and discrimination tugged just a little bit harder and would rule for years to come. It was around this time I became strategic about who should know I had HIV, even if my calculations changed over time. I thought about how connected we are in this world—like sitting in a beauty salon and overhearing a woman talk about a friend who is messing around with someone's man whom you happen to know. It would just be my luck that my HIV status would end up with the wrong person over a fluke. I thought through every detail of how my secret could get out in any given situation. I even doubled back to Dr. Cunningham. After I left his office, I felt I could trust him, but I didn't know if I could trust everyone in his office. My mind went over the top as I imagined every detail of how my secret could have gotten out. I played out every scenario from Dr. Cunningham's connection to Mrs. Thomas to a staff person telling somebody who might know me or even the Jackson's.

The Health Insurance Portability and Accountability Act (HIPAA) wasn't signed into law until 1996. Just like you couldn't stop a friend from violating your confidence, at the time, there were no laws to protect your medical information. I had no control over an office rule broken with the juicy information that I had HIV or someone finding out about my status over some fluke. It was an emotionally heavy way to live but being back in Chicago meant I had to find any loophole through which my HIV status might be disclosed. The relief I felt with Dr. Cunningham's decision to keep my secret was a reminder of the weight of living with HIV. It also reinforced my need to keep my secret just that: a secret. Waiting on the car to warm up, eventually, Rhoda moved on to how she could help.

"Rae, you're too sick to be home alone," she said. "You're going home with me." Jesse and Jonathan were off somewhere campaigning. I protested, thinking, *This girl is being awfully bossy*. But I soon learned that even I couldn't outargue Rhoda. She paid me no attention, saying, "But first we have to stop at Treasure Island." Treasure Island was a gourmet grocery store that carried a lot of European imports. It was as fancy as Rhoda: A graduate of the acclaimed all-girl Spelman College, she put the "b" in bourgeoisie. Her father, Reverend Samuel B. McKinney, was the pastor of a prominent church in Seattle and the chair of Reverend Jackson's campaign in Washington state. I would also learn that Rhoda was as genuine as I thought her to be and had a heart of gold. In her little apartment, I had never felt so cared for in my life. The girl could cook. She made me chicken noodle soup from scratch and hot lemon toddies. Those hot lemon toddies were so good, I have made them every time I've gotten a cold for the past thirty-plus years. My fever passed and I went home. That Monday, I was back in the office with a hacking cough, though, because I had a conference to finish planning. Rhoda continued to check on me in the campaign headquarters; our friendship was sealed.

My conversation with Dr. Cunningham about HIV created even more anxiety for me. I had already become manic about protecting my housemates from me, or rather, from my HIV, a worry I didn't have living alone in D.C. I had always used bleach because Mama used it, but you would have thought I was trying to rid the house of the plague with the amounts I used to clean the bathrooms and kitchen. Even a glass got a douse of bleach before I washed it. In reality, there was no need to take these extra precautions because there was no way for me to infect any of my housemates through casual living. I knew HIV could not be transmitted through casual living, like using the same toilet, insect bites, pets, coughing, sneezing, hugging, kissing or even through saliva. I knew I was being irrational, but I just couldn't stop myself. Truth be told, living in the Jacksons' space was a big deal to me. I mean, Reverend Jackson is a civil-rights icon, and I didn't take it lightly that I had been granted the privilege to live in his space. More than anything, I didn't want to disappoint Mrs. Jackson. I didn't want any part of HIV to come back and bite me in the ass, so I constantly cleaned. In retrospect, I was modeling behavior I absolutely deplored. For God's sake, I had organized the blood drive because of irrational fears about contracting HIV. This disease kept me off balance; thinking clearly was out of the question. Some days I couldn't think at all, and other days I thought too much. I was living by trial and error based on the information that was available, and how I interpreted it and thought others would. People think I always had it together. That first year, I was a complete and total MESS!

Dr. Cunningham's explanation about my failing immune system scared the living daylights out of me. Protecting myself from anything other than the stigmas of HIV wasn't even on my bingo card; now, I was thinking about bacteria and parasites. Let me say that while it is true HIV was destroying my CD4 T cells, which ultimately would affect my immune system, it was an oversimplification of HIV at this stage in my diagnosis. However, it was the extent of knowledge I had at the time, and I ran with it. I started to look at my housemates with a side-eye and became more obsessive with cleanliness if that were even possible. I second-guessed everything I believed could become a potential threat to my immune system. I look back and wonder how the heck I did not have a nervous breakdown. I was protecting my secret of HIV from the mean world, protecting my housemates from my HIV, and trying my best to protect my immune system because of HIV. I was annoyed with them all the time and they were annoyed with me because, well, I acted like I was crazy.

Jesse Jr. was my biggest pain in the ass and threat, I believed, to my well-being. Of course, this was just as absurd as my bleach obsession; however, at the time, you couldn't have convinced me otherwise. Among other things, the dude would take showers in the bathroom on my floor because his bathroom only had a tub and dripping water would follow him out the bathroom and up the stairs. Our arguments were always heated, and sometimes we ended up across the street. For example, there was the time he kept drinking my orange juice and placing the empty carton back in the refrigerator. Men!

After one of our blowups, Jesse Jr. said, "I'm going to tell Mama that you are crazy," as he headed for the door with me on his heels every step of the way. Mrs. Jackson laughed as soon as we entered. Junior—as I often called him—said, "Mama, this is serious." We started talking at the same time, telling our sides of the story. Mrs. Jackson interjected for clarity, admonishing both of us appropriately. When we ran out of steam, Junior—who had to have the last word—asked, "Mother," all proper-like, "why do you allow that girl to live with us?"

"Whatever, Jesse," I said, taking a seat at the dining room table.

"Mama, I'm serious!" Jesse waited on a response to his question.

Inevitably, Mrs. J said, "Jesse, you're just mad that Rae won't take any shit off of you."

"MAMA! That's not true!" he insisted, and Mrs. Jackson didn't miss a beat, "And, she's the only one who pays her rent on time." I sat there gloating—that is, until it was my turn. "Rae, it doesn't pay to be so damned right all the time," Mrs. Jackson said. Looking back, I must admit Jesse Jr. and I were hilarious, and sometimes the levity of it all helped to ease my anxiety a bit. Other times, I was triggered to the max over the smallest things, and nothing could calm me. My housemates would look at me like I really was crazy, with my face full of ugly tears as I cried over something as insignificant as a dirty glass in a sink. In actuality, I didn't know what I didn't know about a failing immune system, and I wanted to control everything I thought humanly possible to help keep me alive.

One time, Jonathan, who was mostly laid-back, locked the thermostat so we couldn't change the setting. He called himself putting that MBA degree he was working on to use for a bill he wasn't paying—for a solution to a problem he hadn't been asked to solve. Everyone was cold! So we convened one of our made-for-reality-television "house meetings" to try and reason with him before taking it to Mrs. Jackson. (Also, he had the key.) He listened to us, smug-like. He wasn't budging. He even suggested we put on sweatshirts and grab extra blankets. I was over his reasoning and started hollering about the draft in that big-ass house. I was really scared, but I couldn't tell them I was trying to protect myself from another cold like the one I'd had. In my mind, revealing any of my fears might cause them to ask questions that might trip me. I would much rather have suffered in silence than reveal my secret.

When I finally disclosed my HIV status, I learned that Jesse Jr. had told Mrs. Jackson about my HIV tirade after a house meeting. At the time, no one could have imagined I was living with HIV. Mrs. Jackson assumed Jesse Jr. and I were being our overly dramatic selves and had been overreaching that day.

It all began when I had seen some special on television about AIDS. I lost control in one of our house meetings and I, in a roundabout way, told them I had HIV. I went into a tirade about some people being unable to fight off bacteria because of a weakened immune system. In the fray of things someone asked, "So, you got AIDS, now?" I jumped up from my seat and shouted, "What if I do?" and stormed off to my room. "Thank God" is all I can say. If Mrs. Jackson had taken Jesse Jr. seriously, I would not have denied it. I'm sure, however, that publicly disclosing my HIV status in 1988 would have changed the trajectory of my life and had a different impact on me than in 1994. I won't speculate on the ins and outs. I will say only that even with all the pain I endured in silence, I held onto my secret because it was what I believed to be best for me at the time.

Not looking or feeling sick helped me maintain the secret. It also kept me and those who knew I was infected in a state of quasi-denial. The saying, *Out of sight, out of mind* was a real thing with me and HIV. Those who knew I had HIV kept my secret—some of them even better than I. In a weird way, the secret became a secret inside of the secret in that none of them talked to me about how I was living and coping with HIV that first year or so after my diagnosis. Now, thinking about it, maybe it was my own silence that helped set the tone with the few people who knew. Either way, the secret fueled the silence, and the silence fueled my outward denial and helped to keep my head jumbled. Every now and then Tyrone asked me, "You good?" and I knew what he was really asking me. I'd answer, "Yep, so far." He'd hug me and say, definitively, "You gon' be okay, girl." It was the closest we had come to a conversation about HIV in the nine months since I told him. One day, he came over to my desk to grab me for a man who wanted to meet me. I didn't know what to think—or what Tyrone was thinking, for that matter. He was pretending my life was normal, and my tail was playing right along. He leaned down and said, "Rae, there's someone who would like to meet you."

"I'm busy," I said, even though I was curious. About ten minutes earlier I looked up, and this dude and his small entourage walked into the office. Our eyes locked. He was short and built like a linebacker, dressed in slacks and a blazer. There was nothing that stuck out about him, except that I couldn't shake his brown piercing eyes. My eyes followed him until he disappeared into the rear conference room.

"Rae, you would want to meet him," Tyrone said to me.

"Tyrone, I don't have time for this," I said. Whoever he was, I figured I would find out later. I just didn't have the energy. Besides, Bill and I were still arguing and holding on by a thread. I knew I had too much going on to meet a new man and complicate my life even more.

"I promise," he said. "You want to meet him." I looked at Tyrone, like, *Give me a break.*

"It's Mike Tyson, girl." With a clueless expression, I raised my outstretched hands and shrugged my shoulders, *So what?* Then asked, "Who the *hell* is Mike Tyson?" Tyrone, incredulous, just looked at me—speechless, at first. Then he laughed theatrically. "Girl, stop playing," he said.

"Tyrone, I really don't know who he is." He shook his head; by that time, Steve Jeffries had come up behind Tyrone. "Man, she *don't* know who Mike Tyson is." They looked at each other and shook their heads.

"I don't!" I laughed and threw up my hands. "Okay, I guess I'm stupid," I said.

"Rae, he's only the heavyweight champion of the world," Steve spoke sarcastically slow and methodical. Now, I was intrigued. I got up and followed them to the conference room where Mike and his entourage were sitting. "He's in town for an exhibition fight," Steve filled me in on the way. "If he offers you tickets, take them." I gave him a side-eye.

Mike Tyson was sitting on the opposite side of the conference table from the door. As soon as I walked into the room, he stood. *All sookie now,* I thought. *Chivalry ain't dead.* He held out his hand and introduced himself, "Hi, I'm Mike." He offered me a seat next to him and we started talking. Everyone else left the conference room. He was so soft-spoken—almost shy, even—that it threw me off. I was struck by the contrast of his gentle voice and subdued mannerism to the weight of his body and the power it rendered. We made small talk. He wanted to know who I was and what my role was in the campaign. I explained that I worked with college students and young people. In between his questions, there were gaps of silence and I thought, *What the hell am I doing?* I exited by telling him I needed to get back to work. Before I could get up, he asked if I would come to see him fight. I knew, if asked, I would because of Steve and Tyrone—but I told him I wasn't too keen on fights. I had never been to a fight, and I thought boxing was too violent. He explained the fight between him, and James "Quick" Tillis was an exhibition fundraiser to help rebuild Holy Angels Church, a Black Catholic church on Chicago's South Side that had been destroyed in a fire. I perked up, impressed that Mike was donating his time and name to a good cause. Tyrone, Steve, and I went to the fight, which was held at DePaul University. It was exciting, but I still didn't feel comfortable with the violence. We also went to the after-party but didn't stay long. Mike and I exchanged information.

I would be lying if I said I wasn't flattered by the attention from Mike. He was a boost to my self-esteem after Bill's whoring. His cheating had made me ask, *Why wasn't I enough?* Of course, in time I understood his cheating had nothing to do with me, but it was the perfect scenario to open the door for a rich and powerful guy to walk right in. It was also the perfect scenario to create more chaos on top of what was already going on. Honestly, I had no idea what I wanted from Mike. I just knew I didn't want to be the side chick in his on-again-off-again saga with actress Robin Givens. I really liked talking to Mike. There was something under his veneer I could not pinpoint or shake, and it drew me in. Whatever it was, he was like a magnet. Every time he called me, I dropped whatever I was doing and chatted with him. Mike and I talked and formed a friendship, while Bill and I argued profusely every damn day.

Bill and I never officially called it quits; we just accepted that the crack in our foundation could not be repaired. To avoid the bitter arguments and the nasty calls, we just stopped talking. I have no doubt that we were very much in love but the love was too young, and we were too immature and too wounded to make it work. Mike wasn't the only man showing interest; men were coming out of the woodwork like they could smell my breakup. There was a young man from New York who had come to my D. C. event with another good friend and made his interest known at the Chicago student leadership conference. Besides those two, Ken Bennett—better known today as the Rappers' Dad, father of talented rappers Chance the Rapper and Taylor Bennett—was all up in my grill. He was everything I wanted in a guy: close in age, good looking, charming, smart, conversational, and knee-deep in politics.

I met Ken in a Jackson Action Network Task Force meeting at campaign headquarters. Jackson Action, as it was called, was an *ad hoc* group of politically involved young adults that had grown out of PUSH and was led by Jesse Jackson Jr. and Minyon Moore. The members of Jackson Action were a talented group of Chicago-based young adults, all of whom went on to do great things. To name a few, there was Randy Crumpton, who became a well-known attorney as well as a mover and shaker in Chicago's arts community. Desiree Sanders became the owner of Afrocentric Bookstore that would become the premier retail center for African and African American literature in the Midwest. Michelle Reeves won an *Essence* contest for the July 1990 issue cover model. There was also, Minyon—who, at the time, worked at PUSH as Reverend Willie Taplin Barrow's executive assistant and would soon transition to the campaign. Minyon would later go on to bigger things, like the White House. Members of the group were outspoken, and we clashed right away. Ken gave me the hardest time of them all. As always, I went in like a bulldozer. I had assumed Jackson Action would be under my purview in that it was composed of young adults and students supporting the campaign. I wasn't trying to be the boss of Jackson Action, but to incorporate its work into the youth and student department. I wanted to get them invested in the overall youth and student plan I created for the campaign so that we were working on one accord. They respected my position but had no desire to be co-opted into the youth department. They wanted to contribute to the campaign and not be confined. After that was resolved, Ken and I never stopped sparring.

He would come into the office after work, looking important in his suit and tie. Every time he'd flash that beautiful smile at me, I melted; however, I would not give an inch when we had one of our heated debates. He made it seem as if I was the *bourgeoisie* of the political spectrum like I was W. E. B. Du Bois, and he was the *grassroots* of politics, like Booker T. Washington. When he learned I lived in "the house across the street," as most people in that circle called it he would not let me live it down. He was always trying to situate himself with the little man. I thought that was a crock of shit since he was an aide in Mayor Washington's office at twenty-something, and told him as much. Although Ken joked with me, he also told me more than once he thought I was brilliant. He genuinely respected me and admired my drive. I loved that about him because men his age, at that time, would much rather have complimented a woman's legs than her accomplishments. I thought equally of him. I knew his future was bright; you could see it written all over him, and he did not disappoint. After the 1988 campaign, Ken continued to work his way up the political hierarchy paying his dues the hard way: with hard work. He would go on to have an illustrious career as a campaign operative and eventually serve as deputy assistant to President Barack Obama as well as deputy director of presidential personnel. Over the years I have admired his success, and the success of his wife Lisa, of thirty years and their two children, Chance, and Taylor.

When we weren't fighting like school kids with a crush, he'd say, "When are you going to have lunch with me so I can get to know you?" Then my paranoia about disclosing my HIV status would bring me back to reality. I wasn't afraid of Ken rejecting me. Bill had made me feel lovable again and shown me that a relationship was possible with a person living with HIV. My fear was more about a future I couldn't predict or control. Let's say that Ken was fine with my HIV status and we entered a relationship— but then it didn't work like it hadn't worked with Bill, then Ken would be another person who knew my secret and that, in my mind increased the possibility for even more people to know. Ken was intricately connected to my political life and I did not want anything to destroy that.

Quite frankly, after Bill and I broke up, I should have taken a step back from all the flirting—not just because my breakup was so new and I was still hurting, but because it had placed me back in the same spot where I had been before I met Bill. Remember how I had fumbled through those first months after my diagnosis? I couldn't get my footing when it came to men and disclosure, as was obvious that night with Sylvester Monroe. I've looked back and tried to figure what was going on in my head. The hardcore Rae would say it was my ego trying to build my self-esteem—that I was acting out the "bad bitch" who could still have any man she wanted, despite having HIV. The compassionate Rae might say I was being human — seeking to be loved and seeking someone to love. Either way, living with the secret of HIV was difficult for me. One day I felt like Cinderella before her prince arrived; the next day I was wearing the ball and the chain. I muddled through all the contradictions, fears, and doubts, and was trying to hang on to how it used to be when "this is how it is" was staring me in the face. I continued to flirt and, most days, it made me feel special—until it didn't. I tried my best to keep Ken engaged and keep his attention until I was sure I could trust him with my secret. He would stop at my desk to say hello and I'd push back in my chair, slowly cross my fabulous legs and let my skirt peel open to the top of my stocking, where it connected to my garter. I took pleasure in every minute, knowing I had just stopped him in his tracks as his eyes followed my legs up to the garter. I sat close to him sometimes; even in meetings, I situated myself so he could see just a little bit of my cleavage. Yet, I still wouldn't go out to lunch with him.

Mike called one afternoon to let me know he was in town and asked if I would come over to the hotel and hang out with him. He was staying at the Ambassador West, the second tower of the historical Ambassador East Hotel in Chicago's Gold Coast Historic District. I entered Mike's hotel room and the first thing I noticed was that big-ass bed. It was my first moment of pause, but I shrugged it off. I had accepted his invitation. I wanted to spend face-to-face time with him and here I was in his room. We made small talk and got caught up until he asked if he could kiss me. I leaned into him sitting on the edge of the bed and he pulled me onto his lap. He felt good—I mean, real-ly good— and we kissed and scooted to the center of the bed. I felt his penis rise and the moisture between my legs. *Hell, yes!* I was caught all the way up. But then my head said, *Hell to the no! I didn't come here to do this.* But there I was. I felt a trickle of moisture underneath my breast—my signal that I was in dangerous territory. *Oh, God.* I thought. *I've made a mess of things yet again. When am I going to learn? WHEN?!* Mike reached for the top button of my blouse. I knew I had to stop this. I took a deep breath and said to him, "I can't."

He whispered in my ear, "I won't hurt you." Fear swelled in me. *What if he won't stop?* I understood that I had the right to say no at any point and a man should honor my position. I also knew that men get crazy when their dicks get hard. No, I am not saying today or ever that men cannot control themselves or that a woman should be responsible for a man's actions; I am saying that some men choose not to control themselves, and since I had learned I could not depend on a man to protect me, I protected myself. I had broken my cardinal rule. I typically didn't go into uncertain situations with a man. I realized I was in a vulnerable position. I actually had not come for this, but I'd be lying if I told you that had it not been for HIV, I would have been buck-naked. His tongue followed the contour of my neck back up to my mouth and I melted. He pressed his body against my thigh, and I started to surrender. When he shifted on top of me, I came back to reality.

"Mike, I'm not ready to go there," I murmured. He kissed me again and asked, softly, "Are you sure?"

"I like you, but I just can't—not right now," I said. I tried to sound a little more convincing. *Get it together, Rae,* I coached. I knew I couldn't have sex with him. In those couple of months of chatting, I was unsure whether to tell him that I had HIV. Mike was another blurry line for me. It was just like my thoughts about Mrs. Thomas everyone knew someone who knew somebody. I was still trying to assess if Mike should be placed in that category of people who were too close to the things that were important to me to know my HIV status. We didn't have any condoms, either. To move forward would have been wrong.

"I can't," I repeated. He asked one more time, "You sure?"

"Yes," I whispered, and Mike eased off my body and the bed, and sat in the chair. I sat up. Relief, shame, and guilt swept over me. I could see his penis bulge through his slacks. I moved over to the edge of the bed right in front of him.

"I'm sorry," I said emphatically. "I'm just not ready."

He grabbed my hand and said, "It's okay." I sighed with relief. "I respect you," he said. "Whenever you are ready."

"Thank you," was all I could say.

I had dodged that bullet, but reality had smacked me hard in the face. My pseudo-denial was not going to make HIV go away. I knew in my heart that I had to find a better path than the one I was traveling. But then, how was I supposed to figure out how to live with HIV in a world that was still trying to come to terms with the virus? The web of secrecy I spun around my HIV status became more complicated and had a thousand holes and contradictions. The secret became a cancer that would grow until I was brave enough to cut it out.

Forty-Four

DON'T SURRENDER!

" Don't surrender, my friends. Those who have AIDS tonight, you deserve compassion. Even with AIDS, you must not surrender.**"**
—Reverend Jesse Louis Jackson, Sr.
1988 Democratic National Convention

My first campaign assignment on the road was to work out of the Southern regional campaign office in Atlanta, and I couldn't wait to get the hell out. I think I carried a grudge against that city for years after the election. In hindsight, my dislike for Atlanta had little to do with the city and more to do with the people I interacted with daily as well as my emotional state of mind at the time. Jesse Jr. was also working in the regional office. He and I were the only two from the national headquarters, and the youngest in the office. We sometimes felt like northern interlopers. He would come into my office and plop down in a chair, and we'd chat it out and laugh it out and move on. One day, Junior peeked into my office to tell me someone was on hold to talk to me. Lo and behold, it was Mike Tyson. This was my first time talking to him since the hotel rendezvous. I was pleasantly surprised. After that, Mike's calls became bright pick-me-ups in my otherwise miserable existence in Atlanta. One week, Mike promised to come to hang out with us and help relieve our boredom but didn't show. Monday morning, Junior came into my office, saying, "Rae, Rae—Mike Tyson didn't come to hang out with us because he was busy marrying Robin Givens." I looked up from my desk with an expression that said, *Stop being ridiculous.*

"I'm not playing. Mike Tyson married Robin Givens this weekend," he said, taking his usual seat by my desk.

"Danggg!" I said, "Mike Tyson married Robin Givens." We sat in stunned silence for about thirty seconds before we said in unison, "That's crazy." Now that Mike was married, his role in keeping things upbeat was gone—but, thankfully, Junior was stuck there with me.

My lodging situation only added to my other problems. I didn't like this arrangement of staying in people's homes much, now that I knew I had HIV. I couldn't name what I felt as depression; I only knew I couldn't shake an overwhelming sadness. After having bronchitis, I was coming to understand that HIV was changing my life, and it frightened me. I was afraid of what I knew—and didn't know—about HIV. There were still not a lot of resources for heterosexual women, so I had no place to turn and no place to learn. Organizations for women like me were emerging on the East Coast, but there was nothing in Midwest cities like Chicago. Only thirteen percent of the National Institutes of Health money was dedicated to women's health issues, and information on women and AIDS was almost nonexistent. When I ran across certain articles on HIV in various magazines, I was left even more confused.

That weekend I had been home recovering from the bout of bronchitis, for example, I caught up on some of my magazines. When I made it to my *Cosmopolitan,* a headline read, "A Doctor Tells Why Most Women Are Safe From AIDS." Like a hungry animal,

I pounced on the article and devoured every word. I was horrified! The psychiatrist, Dr. Robert E. Gould, said that women with "healthy vaginas" could have unprotected vaginal sex with an HIV-positive man and not worry about contracting HIV. *WHAT THE HELL?!* I knew it was a BIG LIE, and I was living proof. When Gould claimed it was impossible to transmit HIV using the "missionary position," I felt dirty and judged. I kept coming right back to the ugly ways society judged people with HIV. How in God's name was I supposed to come to terms with it all? Were there only three types of women who contracted HIV—druggies, whores, and sex workers? I felt like I was trapped in the rubble of a collapsed building. I knew also that my life with HIV would bring more change, and I had to figure how to make peace with this new normal. My solace, however, came from knowing God could still use me, even with all my dysfunction and missteps. That was my singular reassurance that would not let me give up.

All eyes were on Super Tuesday, and Atlanta was the epicenter of our Southern strategy. Our regional operation was sophisticated—a well-oiled machine. We didn't have a regional office in the '84 campaign, and I was impressed with how focused our strategy was this time. At the helm was Dr. Ronald Daniels who was the Southern regional coordinator and deputy campaign manager. I liked Ron. He was one brilliant dashiki-wearing brother. Super Tuesday was a twenty-state contest, and ten were in the South. I didn't move around the states, as I had in 1984. I could do more in the shortest period by staying in one place.

We were going into Super Tuesday on a high. It was a five-man race between Massachusetts Governor Michael Dukakis; Congressman Richard Gephardt; U.S. Senators Al Gore and Paul Simon; and Reverend Jesse Jackson. Jackson had come in second place in the New Hampshire, Minnesota, Maine and Vermont primaries and caucuses. Victories in these states, which had small populations of Black people, clearly indicated Reverend Jackson had been able to gain a significant number of white voters who resonated ideologically with his agenda. Now, we were going into the contests where a whopping fifty-three percent of all African Americans lived in the combined ten Southern states of Super Tuesday. I was sure we would come out on top.

Super Tuesday was my biggest primary responsibility, and my goal was to make the most out of the student support at the historically Black colleges and universities in the South. With over a hundred Black colleges in that region, we had the potential for both a powerful voting bloc and workers committed for the election day "Get Out the Vote (GOTV)." Now, it was about getting young people to the polls. I used the same paradigm nationally that Tyrone and I used in the '84 campaign. State coordinators were responsible for the overall state operations, and student campus and citywide coordinators were responsible for their specific cities or campuses. Some states were organized better than others, so I was recruiting and plugging young people into the state student operations and the local campaign headquarters. I was putting in a good ten hours a day, but I still wondered if I was giving and doing enough because I couldn't shake the blues. There were some mornings I didn't want to get out of bed, and evenings that seemed to drag on. Even after I had left the office for the day and was dog-tired every night, I still couldn't shut my mind down. It was a vicious cycle: I would go nonstop at the office, eat lunch and dinner at my desk, go home tired, wake up dog-tired, and go into the office and get back at it.

The Southern regional operation paid off, as Jackson won first and second places in sixteen of the races while Dukakis won twelve, and Gore took eleven. According to the *New York Times*, Jackson received ninety-one percent of the African American vote and thirty-one percent of first-time primary voters. He also received thirty-three percent of the 18-to-29-year-old votes overall in the Super Tuesday primaries.

Jesse Jackson resonated with young voters. These voters were born after the passage of the Voting Rights Act of 1965. They had been told the stories of sacrifice and bloodshed.

I would even venture to say many of their grandparents had pictures of John F. Kennedy and Reverend Martin Luther King Jr. hanging on their walls. They had come of age in the backdrop of the Vietnam War and school desegregation in cities that had never been put back together after the riots. They were ready for Jesse Jackson—a man who looked and talked like them; for some, who had also been born to single mothers out of wedlock (like him), he *was* them. It was an exciting time—a Black man beating three white men and neck-and-neck with a fourth man for the nomination of president. In 1988, Reverend Jesse Jackson was to young Black people what Barack Obama was to them in 2008.

Over the years, I have watched critics try to erase the significance of Jackson's 1988 presidential campaign—which I take offense to, personally. To diminish Jackson means to water down my contribution and those of all the young voters who were inspired by a man who dared to rock the boat. We had a formidable campaign in 1988 and, if I had all the social media and internet tools that the Obama campaign had in 2008, I could have done even more amazing work with young voters. Think about it this way: I was using the telephone directory assistance—yes, 411—and the white pages to gather information. I would take one contact and make a hundred more and that, my friend, is good-ass organizing. We had surpassed any outcome I could have imagined, and not even HIV could squash the joy I felt helping to make history.

At the victory party, Jesse Jr. leaned over to me and said, "I'm out of here first thing in the morning." My eyes bulged. His living situation had been less than ideal, too. He had been sleeping on someone's sofa the entire time and was as ready as I was to get the hell out of Atlanta. I asked to ride with him, and we met at the campaign office early the next morning. Around nine that evening, we pulled up to the house—home, sweet home.

The victories kept coming, and they had a euphoric effect on me. If only for a short time I could bask in something other than my own pain. Two days after Super Tuesday, Reverend Jackson won the South Carolina primary as well as the Alaska and Colorado caucuses. The Democratic Party did not know what had hit them. For Christ's sake! A Black man had won Alaska and Colorado. No one saw this coming—not even me. But I never lost faith in the progressive agenda we were pushing, and now we were proving that people were willing to embrace change within the Democratic Party. The party hadn't had a transformative candidate since the McGovern-Humphrey campaign in 1972, and it was speculated that these predominately white geographical wins were a sign that Jackson was picking up McGovern and Humphrey voters. These wins placed Jackson in a tie for delegates with Mike Dukakis, and as the candidate with the most popular votes.

It was good to be back in Chicago and sleeping in my own bed for a couple of weeks. Working on a presidential campaign is grueling. You must perform. A misstep could end your job and, possibly, your career. On the road, I had the dual responsibility of making sure the youth and student operations ran smoothly across the country and doing whatever additional work was required for the primary in the state I was in. A well-put-together state operation, like the one I had in Illinois, helps ease the heavy load. Mark Allen was the Illinois statewide youth coordinator for the campaign. He and his sidekick, James Anyike, founded the Illinois Alliance of Black Student Organizations. I knew them both from Harold Washington's first campaign. They had stayed local and done the groundwork in Illinois, building a powerful statewide student network. Mark and James were also members of Jackson Action and, after the dust settled, I was able to recruit other members as college campus coordinators for some of the Chicago colleges and universities.

The overall statewide youth and student strategy and the team were solid, and the proof was in the pudding. Jackson won forty percent of the 18-to-29-year-old vote in Illinois. Overall, Jackson came in second, with thirty-two percent to Senator Paul Simon's forty-two percent. We won ninety-one percent of the Black vote in Illinois. We had done well, but I was convinced Senator Simon stayed in the race only to deliberately siphon votes from Jackson. His campaign was dead. He had done so poorly in the other primary contests he opted out of Super Tuesday but stayed in the Illinois race, only to drop out a month later. Boy, did I hate Chicago politics. It felt like anti-Jackson fuckery to me and was *déjà vu* from the 1984 campaign with Harold Washington and the delegate fiasco. Ironically, Washington redeemed himself by endorsing Jackson's '88 presidential bid a couple of months before his death. Washington was quoted as saying "Jackson's qualification for president is perseverance over a long period of time dedicated to the basic proposition of fairness in this country. No matter where you go for the past 20 years, Reverend Jesse Louis Jackson has persevered, and he's done it as a quasi-public servant." I was a whirlwind of emotions, to say the least. I had been pleased that Washington had endorsed Reverend Jackson over Senator Simon but, with his death, we had lost an important ally in Illinois. Now, here we were again, and I was mad as I was in 1984. Reverend Jackson took the high road. As quoted in the *Washington Post,* he said, "Illinois has treated both its favorite sons very well. It has brought Paul Simon back into the race, and it thrust me into leadership." On the contrary, I thought, *Fuck Paul Simon and those monkey-ass Democratic regulars.* And just like I had with Washington, I held that opinion for a long time.

In Michigan, Kim Miller was our statewide youth and student coordinator. We had established a campaign presence at all the major colleges as well as in cities like Detroit and Flint. I was assigned to work with actress Kim Fields, who had come to the state as a campaign surrogate. At the time, Kim was a sophomore at Pepperdine University and had just finished her ninth and final season in her role as Tootie on the NBC sitcom *The Facts of Life.* My first task was to take Kim shopping. Her luggage was lost in transit, and she needed to replace everything. I tagged along while she shopped in one of the large department stores. It was going great until Kim's check was declined. She was shocked, and so was I. She nicely explained to the saleslady that there must be a mistake and she should check it again. The saleslady didn't budge; she just held the check over the register waiting for Kim to take it back with a look that said, *You know you can't afford this.* I swear I wanted to shout, "DO YOU *EVEN* KNOW WHO THIS IS?" with hand claps between each word, but I held my peace following Mrs. Jackson's rules about public etiquette. For a moment, there was a standoff. Finally, Kim said something like, *I know I have more than enough money in my account to cover this purchase. You need to check it again,* waving her hand in front of the check. The saleslady said she would have to ring the entire sale again and then call to see if she could get approval. Kim told her, "We will wait" and we did, in silence. Of course, this time, Kim's check was approved. We looked at each other smugly as the saleslady bagged Kim's items. The moment we stepped out of the store, Kim said, "The nerve!" and I echoed, "Gurrl, she *tried* it!"

Jonathan Jackson, Kim, and I joined Reverend Jackson's entourage in a huge camper across the state. Being a part of the entourage was a wonderful change of pace for me. The high energy within the entourage was infectious. I couldn't help but come alive and be in the moment. In Michigan, Casey Kasem—the man known as "the voice" who hosted *American Top 40* and was the voice of Shaggy in Scooby-Doo—campaigned with us for parts of that weekend. Michigan had a large Arab American population and Casey was making appearances. I loved being around him; he was so gracious, and he was passionate about progressive issues. Congressman John Conyers was also with us for parts of the weekend. He was a class act all the time, and always happy to talk with me about politics and policy. I always felt privileged being in this space and took advantage of every moment. I may not have taken pictures with the celebrities and political giants I was exposed to, but I was never shy about a conversation. At the time, Conyers had just proposed the Universal Voter Registration Act that would establish same-day on-site voter registration to help expand the enfranchisement of voters. It was a transformative idea and Reverend Jackson made the bill one of his platform issues at the Democratic convention; it was accepted by the Dukakis campaign as well. Nonetheless, here we are today, in 2022—still fighting for access to the voting booth.

Campaigning with Reverend Jackson is an experience I will always treasure. From the moment we entered a venue until we were back in the caravan, everything was magical. Unlike in '84, Black people actually believed the White House was within our reach. That single belief created even more crowds, tears, and cheers. The church-revival atmosphere, with standing-room-only crowds, was a shot of adrenaline like drinking three Red Bulls back-to-back. Every stop, no matter how tired he was, Reverend Jackson unveiled a vision for those who were hopeless, locked out and rejected. The words "YOU MATTER" had never come out of the mouth of a presidential candidate with such conviction, and people latched onto it with their hearts and souls. I relished every second of each day we piled in the camper. The trail of elected officials, entertainers and civil rights legends was a staple in Reverend's entourage. Once back on the road and heading to the next stop, the atmosphere was light, with joking and laughing between serious conversation.

Jonathan and Kim started flirting. That was not on my bingo card, but it was fun to have a front-row seat watching young love as it unfolded. At every stop, Reverend Jackson was a magnet. People came out by the hundreds and thousands. Kim's star power was amazing. At one stop someone spotted her in the window of the camper; before we could unload, people—both young and old—swarmed the vehicle. It was another light moment. Reverend Jackson thought the crowd was waiting for him; but with Kim in tow, it was her they went running after.

Kim was the epitome of what Reverend Jackson had advocated for years through his Citizenship Educational Program, which promoted civic responsibility and electoral participation. He argued that a high school graduate should walk across the stage with a diploma in one hand and a voter registration card in the other. Being eighteen and a first-time voter, Kim had taken the bull of civic participation by the horns. Not only was she registered to vote, but she was on the campaign trail rooting for the candidate of her choice. These days, it is common for young celebrities to campaign for a candidate. In 1988, however, Kim's role as a Jackson surrogate was cutting-edge. She was emblematic of every young Black person who saw themselves in a Jackson candidacy. It was special to watch Kim at Reverend's side. He would introduce her first and she would come to the mic and talk about what it meant to her as a first-time voter to be able to vote for Reverend Jackson, a Black man, for president. Kim was soft-spoken and authentic, and people listened intently, nodding. Every once in a while, I would hear a soft "Go on, baby," like we were in a church Easter Sunday program. Kim was coming of age in politics, and everyone who had ever seen her from the Mrs. Butterworth commercials to her nine seasons on the *Facts of Life* was proud to see her campaigning with Reverend. After Kim, Reverend would bring the message on home. "When I win, we all win," he would say, leaving the audience with a sense of hope for a better tomorrow, a better America. We would load the camper for our next stop with people still chanting, "Win, Jesse, win!"

Reverend Jackson won Michigan. No one expected it, especially not by a margin of two to one. In fact, Richard Gephardt had already congratulated Mike Dukakis on national television when the early returns came in. Kim, Jonathan and I joined the locals at the victory party to watch the returns. When the race was officially called in Jackson's favor, the vibe was euphoric. Everyone started jumping up and down and hugging each other. It was a sweet victory. Jackson won every major city in Michigan, including Detroit, where then-Mayor Coleman Young, an African American, had endorsed Mike Dukakis. The *New York Times* headlined, "Jackson Wins Easily in Michigan in Surprising Setback to Dukakis." The first paragraph read:

The Reverend Jesse Jackson dealt a blow to the Presidential candidacy of Gov. Michael S. Dukakis today, trouncing him in the popular vote and denying him the momentum he had sought in this big industrial state.

We had lost ground in Illinois, but Michigan brought Jackson neck and neck with Dukakis in the delegate count. He had 596.55 delegates, while Jackson had 584.55. Typical of me, that night I thought about Senator Simon. Had he dropped out of the Illinois contest, Jackson would have become the front-runner with the Michigan victory. I was a hopeless romantic and too ideologically pure for my own good. It was something for me to think about as I made a pathway for my future.

After Michigan, I came back to Chicago and then headed to Ohio for well over a month. When I returned to headquarters after the Ohio primaries, the campaign manager Jerry Austin informed me that Troy Deckert had been hired as the deputy national youth and student coordinator. I don't recall when Troy began volunteering for the campaign, but one day I looked up and this young energetic white guy wanted to help. He was great at crunching numbers and making calls and I immediately gave him assignments, as I had done with all the volunteers who wanted to help in my department. I liked Troy—he did great work. However, if I were going to advocate for a deputy, it would have been Mark Allen, who was equally as talented and had paid his dues in the Jackson orbit. Loyalty is everything to me. I was mad as hell I had not been consulted; after all, I was running the youth and student department. When Jerry told me I was being pulled off the road and Troy was going in my stead, I knew it was some bullshit. He was really trying to replace me without saying it, although I couldn't imagine why. There had been no discussion with me about my performance. I had submitted regular reports and, despite all the personal stuff going on with me, my department performed very well. I was blindsided, and that part was hurtful. While I had been working my ass off, Troy had been smiling in my face and lobbying for my job behind my back. In my meeting with Jerry, I forced back all my emotions. I had never really warmed up to him the way I had with his Deputy Campaign Manager Danni Palmore, a Black woman who had worked with him for years. After that meeting, I don't think I said more than five words to Jerry for the duration of the campaign.

I kept myself together long enough to walk past the executive offices and pull Tammy Fagan into the bathroom to tell her what happen. I had met Tammy through Jackson Action. She was a mentee of Reverend Barrow and a damn good organizer. She came onto the national field staff, and it was in Ohio that we became friends. I was livid and cried angry tears as I explained how those "white boys," as I called them, had double-teamed me. Tammy reminded me I was still the national youth and student coordinator. She told me to let Troy have this win, and that his deputy position didn't change a damn thing. "Don't give that white boy power over you," she said. God, we were so radical back then. She was right: My ego was bruised but the only thing that had really changed for me was that I would no longer be traveling. I dried my tears and went back to my desk. No sooner than I sat down that the ever-vigilant Hazel Thomas, the office manager, called me into her office to find out what was going on. She listened and asked questions for clarification. When I finished my dramatic interpretation of my meeting with Jerry, Hazel said, "Okay." I looked at her, waiting for more, and was mystified that her response seemed rather nonchalant. I was irritated. She took a sip of her Seven-Up. "Rae," she began, "wherever you land, you'll be alright." I sat with my arms folded across my chest thinking, *WHAT THE HELL?* This was "Mother Love," as many called her, and I wasn't feeling the love. "See," she continued, enunciating every word, "You're ba-a-ad! And can't *no one* take that away." I was stunned to learn she thought so highly of me. "Now get your attitude together and go on back out there and be great."

That was the thirty-second pep talk of my life. I went back to my desk, snatched my handbag and went into the bathroom to get rid of my teary face. I pulled myself together—yes, I did—but I was still one mad-ass Black woman. When Troy finally came over to my desk, trying to explain himself, he couldn't look at me in the face. I listened with a stoic face, but what I really wanted to do was *punch* his ass in the fucking face. Tammy rolled her eyes at him to let him know she had my back. I could have told him what I really thought about him and Jerry Austin—but I decided to pick my battles. Hazel and Tammy were right. Instead of telling his ass off, I gave him that Hazel Thomas reply, "Very well," in a tone mimicking hers—one that cut you in a few places even while she still had that lovely smile on her face. I didn't bother to tell Mrs. Jackson because I know she would have said to me, *Baby, you ain't going nowhere.* When I think about it today, I can see ever more clearly that Jerry knew he couldn't replace me; that's why he had given Troy the deputy position. But he had told me from day one, with a twist of sarcasm,you may recall, that I was not his choice, but Mrs. Jackson's. In the end, Troy and I never brainstormed together like Tyrone and I. When he was on the road organizing white college students, I was at the headquarters still running the department. We performed our jobs independently instead of as a team. I would have much preferred he worked under me, as I had for Tyrone. Instead, he reported to the campaign manager, which again proved to me that hiring Troy was an attempt to replace me.

I would never have admitted it then but being still was the very thing needed to help me get to a better place. By the time I reached Ohio, I was emotionally and physically drained. Coming to terms with HIV, keeping it a secret and maintaining a breakneck work schedule—all at the same time —took a toll. I got sick in Ohio and Dr. Cunningham had to prescribe me some medicine. Sometime after the bronchitis, I started to have severe constipation, which he attributed to stress. My anal muscles wouldn't relax, so I couldn't poop. Looking back, this was probably the onset of my irritable bowel syndrome, commonly called IBS, that went undiagnosed for years. The body keeps score, and IBS is one of those illnesses likely for adults with a high ACE score like mine. When we don't address our emotional health, it will manifest in other ways. The problem had gone away but it resurfaced in Ohio. I was miserable. Sometimes, I would go four to five days without using the bathroom.

I was tired of road life. I was tired of staying in people's houses even though my host in Columbus, Fran Frazier, was fantastic. I think that of all the places I stayed during both campaigns, her home and hospitality were the most accommodating, but my anxiety was still high. I was self-conscious and stressed out thinking about every little thing. One night at Fran's, I had a meltdown. I woke up in the middle of the night wet between my legs. I had come on my period, and it sent me into a panic. I jumped up to see if the blood had reached the sheet—and it had. I quickly stripped the bed and thanked God the blood hadn't made it to the mattress. Blood-stained sheets and mattresses are every woman and girl's nightmare. I had grown up with so much shame around my menstrual cycle. Even after all the other hurtful things around my period, Mama had told me I had better stop fucking up her sheets. But with HIV, I had more than even Mama's weight of shame. *My blood is tainted and dangerous* consumed my thoughts. It was irrational because HIV is not airborne and had died by the time it hit the sheet. On that night, however, you could not have convinced me of that. I felt as if the sum total of me was a threat. I washed the blood-stained sheet like a woman gone mad. I think now about Lady Macbeth, who, in one well-known scene, said, "Out, damned spot! Out, I say!" In an instant, the sheet I had bloodied became symbolic of the curse HIV had ushered into my life. Like Lady Macbeth, I felt doomed to hell—only, for me, it was the hell I perceived living with HIV to be versus her hell due to the horrible things she had done in the name of ambition. When I had rid the sheet of all the blood, I sat on the edge of the tub and cried. I wished there was some way to make the stain of HIV go away.

Being back in the campaign headquarters office was the salve I needed. The family atmosphere was reminiscent of my days at PUSH, and I didn't feel so alone. My feelings of isolation had started those last months at SANE it was hell-being placed on probation and being consumed by my HIV diagnosis while, at the same time, having to smile at everyone all the time. I had been afraid to take a moment to breathe while sitting at my desk because I feared I might be judged in a way that might cost me my job. In many ways, road life had a similar level of intensity. I had to perform at a high pace with all eyes on me—the girl from the national office. I was relieved to be back at the headquarters at 30 W. Washington St. with people who loved me and made me feel loved.

Each morning it was guaranteed that Maria Perez—looking fly, while draped in gold and diamonds—would be sitting at the front desk to greet me. Throughout the day, I could count on PUSH-turned-campaign volunteers for a smile, a hug and a willingness to do whatever I asked—and even the things I didn't. I remember asking Gloria Hubbard one day why she cleaned the bathrooms at the campaign office when the building had a cleaning service. She shrugged and said, "They needed cleaning right now." Gloria was one of my favorite people, as was her teenage daughter, Shawnice, who would pop in after school and hang around my desk, nagging me because she could. Betty Magness who had volunteered since the day PUSH began was guaranteed to come everyday after work. Hazel Hardaway was sweet and mild-mannered like Betty also came into the office every day after her full-time job to answer the telephones when Maria had left for the day. Esther Thompson, one of Hazel Hardaway's running buddies, was the five-foot-tall loyal gangsta who might whop your ass if the wrong thing came out of your mouth about Jesse Louis Jackson, Sr. I swear, every time she saw me, she opened her arms wide and I would bend down to hug her, surrendering into her big bosom. Jerome Jones, aka JJ, on the other hand, stood about six-foot-three and didn't say hello without opening his arms. Some evenings I lingered long after I was finished—too exhausted to make another call— just for the togetherness. I had even missed the banter with Ken Bennett and the concern in his eyes when he asked how I was doing in a way that said, *Don't bullshit me. How are you rea-l-l-y doing?* Even if I couldn't give him an honest answer, I felt better knowing he was there. We eventually had that lunch and I saw even more of the sensitive side of him. He was a good man. It was clear to both of us that we had chemistry. But it would be his stops by my desk just to ask about me that told me what we had was even more than chemistry; we had a dope-ass connection.

It was the small things like that which helped to keep me from giving up. Every single one of them was my political family and it felt very much like I imagined a biological family should be. It had been a year and two months since I learned my status and, in that whole time, I had not grieved. I kept busy focusing on work, my mother's healing, our relationship, relocating and the campaign. Now, I was grieving for myself and for the change my life had undergone in such a short period of time. Sure, Troy and Jerry conniving against me was a punch in the gut but, in the end, sitting still was everything I needed and would never have done on my own. With Jesse and Jonathan mostly on the road, I had the house to myself, and I sat with my pain and wept.

Chapter 45

❦ ⚶ ❧

HEALING DAYS

❝The Lord is near to the brokenhearted and saves the crushed in spirit.”
—Psalm 34:18

The campaign was coming to a close, and I should have been looking for a new job. However, continuing to do a good job at the one I already had and dealing with my depression at the same time were all I could handle. HIV had my emotions in a bundle of knots, but it hadn't disrupted my plans to keep building on the work in social justice I had already done. Scientists still didn't know if everyone with HIV would transition to AIDS, and that assessment reassured me I should continue my life as planned. I wanted to continue this work on a national scale, and believed I would have significantly more options in D.C. In fact, I was over Chicago and anxious to get the heck out. I had developed a profound dislike of Chicago politics and most of the politicians. It was too cutthroat for me.

What I should have been doing to secure my future played nicely in my head, but I was paralyzed by inaction. I'm just thankful that God opened a door for me that I was unable to open for myself. As dazed as I was, at least I recognized God working on my behalf as it started to unfold. One afternoon, Hazel Thomas called Tammy Fagan and me into her office, with Dr. Leon Finney Jr.. He had gotten a whiff, probably from Hazel, of the discomfort among the young people in the office who were trying to figure when their last days on the campaign would be. They wanted to know so they could plan their next moves. I knew Dr. Finney's reputation and had seen him in and out of the campaign headquarters, but I had never had an occasion to talk with him. He was legendary in Chicago community development, Chicago politics, and barbecue.

Dr. Finney had about as many accomplishments as he had critics and controversies. Nevertheless, by his death in 2020 at age eighty-two, everyone agreed he was a brilliant man and an organizer's organizer. He was mentored by the great Saul Alinsky—a political theorist and the father of modern community organizing—and he mentored others, including me. Finney could spot the potential in you before you saw it in yourself and was willing to take a chance on what he saw in you. I will never forget when I started working with him, he asked me one day about the Alinsky Rules of Organizing.

"The Alinsky who?" I asked.

"Girl, if you don't know about the great Saul Alinsky, then you ain't no serious organizer," he said. The next day he laid Alinsky's book, *Rules for Radicals: A Pragmatic Primer for Realistic Radicals* on my desk. "I want it back," he said, and walked away.

That day in Hazel's office, Tammy and I expressed our frustration. "I got this," he said. "No one is throwing you away." He said we would be part of the team that would transition to the delegate tracking office. I had never heard the term "Delegate Tracking" prior to that day. However, if it meant I would continue to work on the campaign, I was willing to learn. It would also give me more time to figure out how I was going to return to D.C.

Hazel Thomas and Leon Finney, who were both in charge of the Delegate Tracking operation up to and through the convention, picked a talented team of young African Americans for the tracking operation. Everyone on the team had worked in some aspect of the campaign during the primary season and would make their own mark in the world following the campaign. In addition to Tammy Fagan and me, there were Mark Allen, Ken Bennett, Kevin Jefferson, Melissa Holloway, and Tracie Miller. I shifted from the campaign headquarters to the delegate tracking office about a month following our meeting.

It had been fifteen months since I learned that I was HIV-positive. I had come to a level of acceptance, but I still couldn't find the center of my joy. There was a sadness that hovered over me and dominated my spirit. Ken Bennett was right when he said I always seemed sad. I was mourning the life I had before HIV. I still didn't know what other changes were ahead of me, but the ones that had already come impacted me profoundly. I knew that something had to give. I just could not find a way to untie the knots and loosen the pain. The Psalmist says that *God is near and saves the crushed in spirit* and that, I believe, is exactly what God did for me during the summer of 1988. Slowly but surely, the knots began to loosen in the least likely of places—a one-room office on the South Side of Chicago. One office, consistent work hours and a solid team working every day toward the same goal constituted a change of pace my spirit welcomed. Our assignment was nowhere near the level of intensity during the primary season. Hazel ran the day-to-day operations and set the tone. At fifty-five plus years and standing a little more than five-feet-five, she was impeccably dressed every day. She was nurturing, she didn't suffer fools or foolishness, and with one look she could reduce you to nothing or lift you up to the sky and back. I latched onto her nurturing spirit at the campaign headquarters; however, in the tracking office with a smaller team our relationship grew. I even began going to church with her on Sundays—a routine I had missed since moving to Chicago.

Some mornings, I walked to the Delegate Tracking office. a fifteen-to-twenty-minute walk from my house. It was one of the little things I found that gave me solace and comfort. I loved the beautiful parkway positioned between the South Shore and Woodlawn communities a few blocks west of Lake Michigan. I'd cut through the park, past the Jackson Park Golf Course, I admired the beautiful landscaping that surrounded the Museum of Science and Industry before crossing Stony Island Avenue at 63rd Street to head to the office. The melody of birds chirping together affirmed I needed to get on with the life in front of me.

We were tasked with calling all the delegates to the Democratic National Convention. Hazel divided the list of delegates among us with a questionnaire designed to help identify any uncommitted individual who might be willing to vote for Jackson. These calls were the first vital steps in a larger, more sophisticated and cutting-edge process of tracking delegates. Hazel had hired someone to create a computer program that could analyze the information we collected to help determine the probability of a Jackson vote.

Reverend Jackson came in second, earning 1,075 delegates to Mike Dukakis' 1,790. If not for the winner-take-all primary rule, it was estimated that Jackson would have surpassed the number of delegates that were awarded by four hundred. Jackson won almost seven million in popular votes to Dukakis's ten million, doubling the 1984 popular vote; Al Gore followed Jackson with three million votes. In total, we won ten states, three territories and ninety-two congressional districts in thirty-two states. Jackson had been arguing for a rule change in the Democratic Party that would render a more equitable distribution of the delegates. This time around Jackson had more power and was in a better bargaining position. Ron Brown, our convention campaign manager and former deputy chairman of the DNC, headed a phenomenal team that included Harold Ickes, a Democratic party icon; Ann Lewis, a former political director of the DNC;

and Eleanor Holmes Norton—now a thirty-year veteran congressional representative for D.C.—to battle the rule changes and platform inclusion. Jackson might have lost the nomination but, three weeks before the convention began, the efforts of this team helped secure a reduction of superdelegates by one-third less than ten percent and eliminated the winner-take-all primaries in Illinois, Maryland, Pennsylvania, New Jersey, West Virginia and Puerto Rico. Never again would a candidate win the primary by one percent and take all the delegates. These changes would help to make the primary season more equitable moving forward. In a 2008 article for the *Atlantic*, Ta-Nehisi Coates argued these changes also opened the door for an Obama victory in 2008.

The campaign leadership had done its part going into the convention, and I was doing my part with a team of peers on Chicago's South Side. I felt as if God had made this job in heaven with me in mind. I was also the only one on the team who had a history of making cold calls—and I was damn good at it. Immediately, I sought to establish a good rapport with each delegate to gain their confidence, at a minimum, to open the door for a larger discussion about Reverend Jackson. By the time I reached the last question, I could tell you everything there was to know about a particular delegate. Like I had done as an intern at PUSH, I dialed number after number. I stood, sat, and squatted but I never stopped calling. By the time we completed the project, I had personally called thirty percent of all the delegates to the convention.

The camaraderie among the team was wonderful. We held each other in high esteem and respected the work each of us had done until that point. We talked, laughed and bonded between calls. We socialized outside of the office and became friends. We worked hard and were fiercely loyal, even when we were mad at each other. I wouldn't have traded working with them for any amount of money. Tammy and Ken became an item and my friendship with them continued to grow. Ken and I took walks, sometimes just around the block, and talked. I would tell him bits and pieces about my childhood—not seeking sympathy but trying to make sense of it from a new lens. Maybe a part of me was testing the waters to see if I could trust him with the ultimate of my hurt: HIV. Somedays I wanted to tell him, but I just couldn't get there—not with Ken or any of them. Whatever moments of weakness I had were dismissed quickly. I had sworn myself to secrecy and I was not going to break that promise to myself.

I became especially close to Melissa Holloway and our friendship spanned across decades, until her death in 2008. She impressed me from day one. She was tall, elegant and well-dressed, and with a degree from Rutgers University. Sometimes she walked home with me, and we'd spend our time together talking about what was next and how we wanted to change the world.

It wasn't always peachy. I was sometimes a little too intense and irritating to my teammates. In my opinion, sometimes the laughing and lollygagging were way too much and way too loud, and I was not shy about telling the rest of the crew just that. I'd turn around with my hand over the phone and shush them or give someone the evil eye. When they had enough of me, they took it to Hazel. One day, she called me ever so sweetly in her *I-love-you-all-the-time* voice. When I got to her desk she calmly said, "You are making ev-er-y-bo-dy in this office mis-er-able. I want you to stop it!" In jest, I looked around the room, as if I wondered who told on me. "But Nana," I whined. "STOP IT!" she said, through clenched teeth. The room got quiet, and I walked back to my desk. I sat down, mean-mugging the entire room, turned my back and went back to calling. That's how it went in the tracking office. We worked hard, fought, made up, laughed, talked, and developed friendships that would last for a lifetime.

The only disruption in the office happened between Kevin Jefferson and me. I met Kevin in the campaign headquarters a couple months before the tracking office opened. He had come to the campaign from the East Coast by way of Joe Gardner, another

Chicago politician who ran parts of the field operations. Kevin was politically astute, a sharp dresser and self-assured. He was definitely my type, and there was an immediate attraction between us. I wasn't going to pursue it because I had too much going on to add a man to the equation. Kevin seemed to think I was playing hard to get or something and started wooing me. He began pulling out all the tricks: calling, sending flowers, and even sending me a telegram! Kevin was BRING-ING it! I was smitten with all the attention, but the flirting was at a safe distance until he came to work in the tracking office.

That first week, he moved into the house until Dr. Finney secured him other housing. By then, he had already broken me down. We didn't hook up that first night. I hadn't had sex in the house and was a little leery about being that bold. I eventually gave in, and we hooked up again and again. One night after we had sex, he told me that he was seeing someone from out of town. Of course, I was pissed. In all the months he'd been wooing me, he hadn't mentioned this fact. Now, after he had gotten me to open my legs, he called himself coming clean. I told him to go fuck off. The next morning, Kevin left the house early. I didn't think anything of it. He arrived at the office sometime after me with a woman—HIS woman. I understood then: He'd confessed because she was coming to Chicago for the weekend. My feelings were already hurt about his confession, but then he poured salt into the wound. Instead of taking her straight to the hotel—or even leaving her in the car, as far as I was concerned—he brought her into our one-room office and sat her tail down in front of me, like he and I hadn't just fucked less than twelve hours earlier. My immediate reaction was raw, unfiltered hurt. I got up from my desk, went into the bathroom and cried. Tammy knocked on the door, and I let her in. She knew what was going on and was mad as hell. In that moment, she had all the fight in herself for me that I could not muster. I think if she hadn't come in the bathroom, I would have stayed there until they left. I was so ashamed. She talked me back to my senses, as she had done that day when I learned that Troy had been hired. I cleaned my face, picked up my dignity, and went back to my desk and got back to work. Tammy was already outside letting Kevin have it.

With my desk facing the wall and my back facing the rest of the office, I was able to hide my distress from everyone except Melissa. When Kevin and Tammy came back inside, he was a little shaken. Melissa tapped me on the shoulder. "Let's talk," she said, discreetly. She knew Kevin had been wooing me but not that we had actually hooked up. When I told Melissa what transpired, she was disappointed in Kevin and had a talk with him, too. I don't know who told Hazel, but she called Kevin over to her desk. I was watching like a hawk. "Get her out of this office," Hazel said. She told him while maintaining her control, like when your mother tells you to stop embarrassing her in public but doesn't want to bring any attention to the two of you. I could see him trying to explain himself and we could hear Hazel tell him, "I- don't- care!" It was the first time she raised her voice at him. Then she said through clenched teeth, "Get her out of here—and I mean now." He walked away dejected and grabbed his suit jacket, and they left. I don't know if his girlfriend heard, and I didn't give one fuck either way. I was reveling in the feeling that my friends had my back. Feeling vindicated still didn't take away the hurt. Later that afternoon, I heard Hazel tell Dr. Finney he needed to have a talk with Kevin.

My pain turned into rage when Kevin walked back in the office to finish his workday. Looking at him all smug at his desk, all I could think about was fucking up his relationship with her. I asked Tammy to find out what hotel they were staying at during the weekend. I called his woman at the hotel and told her EVERYTHING. She told me something like she didn't believe me, and that Kevin had told *her I* was interested *in him* and blah blah the fuck blah. Not getting the reaction I wanted, I hinted I had HIV. Although Kevin and I had used condoms, I wanted to scare the fuck out of her. I learned later she was a physician and probably not easily swayed. I don't recall what kind of medicine she practiced. She probably thought I was making shit up to get a buzz.

Thank God, I thought after it was all said and done. I swear, men can make you do some stupid shit. I was hurt and so set on giving back the hurt I felt that I hadn't considered the repercussions. If it had gone differently and she had taken me seriously, especially about the HIV, my secret would have been shot to hell and back. I'm even horrified now that I tried to weaponize HIV in this way. I had done the very thing to myself I didn't want others to do to me. While there was no easy answer for me living with HIV, I definitely had a big learning curve. HIV added another layer of trauma I had to work my way through. I wouldn't realize this until after I transitioned to AIDS. Trying to deal with a new trauma on top of old ones made for a long road to recovery. That evening, when I returned to the house, I went straight to where Kevin had been sleeping and pulled my sheets off his bed and took my towels. *Motherfucker, you can sleep on the mattress for all I care.* When he came to pick up his clothes, we had it out. "I never told you that we were exclusive," was his excuse. Jonathan got wind of it and gave me that brotherly watch-your-reputation talk. I appreciated the talk because he cared, but I resented it because it reflected a double standard that holds women to a higher level of accountability than men in matters of sexual behavior. The office came back to about as normal as it could after Kevin's girlfriend went back east. I stopped talking to Kevin for almost two years. Every time we bumped into each other somewhere and he looked my way, I gave him the look that said, *Nope, don't even think about it. I still smell the stench of your shit on top of me.* After hesitating for a moment, he shrugged it off and kept it moving. Then one day it didn't matter to me anymore and we were friends again—just like that.

We arrived in Atlanta to learn the person who'd been responsible for crunching the data we'd collected hadn't done a damn thing. Hazel fired him and hired his replacement; still, we had to do the grunt work of inputting the data. It would have been our only free day before the convention began and I was livid to the point where I made everyone else miserable. I was one sight to see: pouting and pecking away with one hand, as my typing skills hadn't improved much since my days working in Congresswoman Mikulski's office. All of us were disappointed our free day had been taken, but I was the only one who reacted like I had personally been hurt. I was over-the-top mad and couldn't adapt to change. I could see myself losing control, like I was having an out-of-body experience, but I couldn't catch myself. My energy dominated the entire space. Hazel took me aside and got me together really quick. I was so ashamed of being admonished. I hated this part about me and saw it as a personality flaw—a defect. I wanted desperately to change but was clueless how to do so. It would take more incidents, shame, and self-awareness to push me to seek answers deeper than being flawed. In this case, it was the lack of control I had over my life growing up that made me want to control every aspect of my life, outside of Mama. That day it was something as simple as a new assignment when my day had already been planned that set off a trigger in me.

Once the convention began, I worked out of the trailer office and on the convention floor as a whip. Working the floor was an entirely new and different experience from being an observer, like I was in 1984. Now, I was in the thick of what felt like I had been transported to another galaxy and all my senses were activated to the next level. The convention is the culmination of the Democratic Party primary season. It's where the nominee is "christened" and deals are cut for the direction of the party. It was my job as a whip to know everything regarding the delegates. If an ant crawled on the wrong side of the floor, it was our job to know it.

I had one big moment as a whip. Some of our delegates had gotten wind of a deal that had been cut between Jackson and Dukakis and pulled some of the whips aside to see if it was true. Tammy, Melissa, and I met and headed back to the trailer to find out what was going on. Apparently, our national campaign chair—California majority whip and former mayor of San Francisco, Willie Brown—was going to put forth a motion on the convention floor immediately following the vote to accept Dukakis' nomination as the Democratic nominee by unanimous consent. We were told to go back out on the floor and inform our delegates that it was already a done deal. In other words, get over it. This was a defining moment for Jackson delegates. They told us to tell the powers that be that if things went down as they'd heard, they would stage a walkout. They believed the absence of announcing a count total meant defeat. They had worked too hard to get this far only to fold. Further, that our campaign chair would be the person making the motion felt like the ultimate betrayal.

We reported back to the trailer, and it was an all-out fight. I can't remember all the powers that be who were a part of the discussion with the floor whips, but I remember there were Ron Brown, Willie Brown, Ann Lewis, Leon Finney, and Joe Gardner. Ron told us it had already been arranged. Period. This was my first time having a conversation with Ron. I'd heard he was a political genius but, in that moment, I saw him as an arrogant, pompous ass (even if he was a political genius). Ron didn't see the point of the protest because Dukakis was going to win anyway, and that was a fact. Willie Brown co-signed what Ron had said. He was just going to do the inevitable—Dukakis was going to win, and the motion for unanimous consent would make Jackson look like a statesman. I took offense. I thought, *Why should Reverend Jackson show statesmanship when Dukakis had been nothing short of a jackass with how he handled the announcement of his vice-presidential pick, Senator Lloyd Bentsen? Here we go again—asking the Black man to behave with honor when they were not willing to do it themselves.*

For our delegates, it was the matter of principle, and they wanted a moral victory, even if it wasn't an actual one, and they planned to hold the campaign leadership accountable. Tammy, Melissa and I were the most vocal, but we were also the youngest whips, which made us the easiest to dismiss. Ron made me feel like we didn't know what we were talking about. At one point, in frustration, I said, "I'm telling y'all, they have already started organizing the walkout." And Tammy, like a bull, wouldn't let it go. Melissa was shaking her head at the pushback from leadership. Hazel, who was ear-hustling, interjected. "Leon," she said in that voice of hers that commanded attention. Everyone stopped talking and looked her way. "If Rae, Tammy and Melissa say there's going to be a walkout, you can bank on it." I breathed a deep sigh of relief. *Finally—someone talking with some sense.* She then explained that we had spent the better part of two months developing relationships with the delegates and understood their commitment, likely, more than anyone else in the room. Hazel had Leon's and Joe's attention and they started brainstorming on a compromise. Willie Brown was the one to come up with the idea that after the roll call and all the votes were in, he would announce the number of votes that Reverend Jackson received before he made the motion to accept Dukakis as the nominee by unanimous consent. The Jackson delegates agreed to the compromise but warned that if, for any reason, Willie Brown failed to implement it as agreed, they would walk out *en masse*. Willie Brown not only announced the number of Jackson votes, but he took a minute to elaborate on the campaign's journey before he moved on to the motion. In this way, the millions of viewers would see that Jackson, with 1218.5 votes, had received more votes than any other runner-up had ever received for the presidential nomination. Dukakis was able to double his vote to 2876.25, thanks in large part to the unelected superdelegates. The day before the vote, Reverend Jackson made his convention speech. I was able to find a seat on the floor near the trailer office and listen. As he neared the end of his speech, the bridge to his closing was a poem written by Daisy Rinehart. This last stanza struck at the very core of me, "Better go down in the stirring fight than drowse to death by the sheltered shore!" I knew right then and there that no matter what HIV presented me with in the future, I would not go down without a fight.

By the time the convention was over, the sadness had started to slip away. I was a little stronger than I had been the day I walked into that one-room office. It would be the time I spent with Mrs. Jackson after the convention, that would bring me back totally to myself. I started going over to the house to hang out with her every day. I think I spent more time with her that month than I had done the entire primary season. Day by day, the discord that was tangled inside of me started to unknot. She had no idea I was suffering—and no idea that her kindness and acceptance made me better and made me want to be better. We'd sit at her dining room table, surrounded by some of the most beautiful china I'd ever laid eyes on. Simply sitting among all the pretty things made me feel special. I would question her about a particular pattern of china, and I listened intently to her history lesson. I was amazed by her knowledge about everything— even something like what distinguished a Duncan Phyfe sofa from others and how she stumbled on hers while antiquing. There was never a dull moment with Mrs. Jackson. In the same setting, she'd switch to talking about politics and world affairs and not miss a beat. Then we were off to get fabric for me to make curtains and to learn how to make a duvet cover. It seemed foolish to redecorate a room I was about to leave. I had accepted a job offer with Mayor Marion Barry as a political appointee and planned to move back to D.C. at the end of the summer.

Making curtains, dusk ruffles, a duvet, and watching Ms. J crochet the most exquisite bedspread as well as listening to her opinions of the political landscape were exactly what I needed. Mrs. Jackson provided balance for those things that threatened to suck the life out of me, including HIV. Working with my hands under her guidance took me out of my head, eased my anxiety and helped set me back on course. The thing is, I had never been stuck because of Mama—I always found a tunnel and crawled out. I knew I couldn't let myself stay stuck this time because of HIV. What Mrs. Jackson gave to me was that final push toward the light, and I crawled out.

I started to live my personal life again. During the day I was across the street with Ms. J, sometimes until late in the evening. On the weekends, I hung out with Veronica. She always knew where we needed to be and when we needed to be there. She would pick me up in that beat-up car her uncle had given her, and it got us from one point to the next on the twenty-to-thirty-something social rounds. The hottest parties that summer were hosted by 601 Productions, Inc. and Veronica and I were all in. 601 Productions, Inc. was the brainchild of one of my friends from SIU, Curtis "Curt" McDaniel III. He pulled together five of his friends—Howard Brookins Jr., now a Chicago alderman; Grover Calvert; Raymond Blarney; Kirkland Townsend; and Gerald Davis—to host these parties. It was a giant step up from the college frat parties we used to attend. I loved dressing up to go dancing; I always had. It was a whole vibe. I even put myself back into the dating game and started hanging out with Curt. I had a crush on Curt before he transferred to SIU when he came down to hang out with his Alpha Phi Alpha brothers. I loved every minute of being with him. After the parties we went to Tempo, a twenty-four-hour coffeehouse in Chicago's Gold Coast—as would at least a third of those who were at the party—and we'd continue talking and lounging until the wee hours of the morning. Curt and I had fun times and a whole lot of chemistry. I'd hang out with him at his house and met his parents. I really liked Curt, but I was going to D.C. soon and decided not to tell him that I was HIV-positive.

After seventeen months, I had come to what I viewed as a compromise about disclosing my HIV status. Like I had done when I first learned my status, I demanded the use of condoms one hundred percent of the time. I had no more indecisive slip-ups in the moment of passion. I no longer went into an environment with a man where sex could happen unless I was sure I was willing to have sex and had condoms with me, even if we didn't have sex. If I had any doubts, I didn't put myself in a compromising position. I was still very much afraid of my status becoming common knowledge. Now, I started making judgment calls on the seriousness of the relationship before disclosing my status.

Curt seemed like the "forever bachelor," and I was leaving; I didn't see us getting beyond the point of casual dating. In hindsight, I was in a precarious situation that could have gone badly. If something had gone wrong and I had infected Curt, I never would have forgiven myself. Would most people have said I was selfish? Maybe, maybe not. I'm not going to debate the ethical dilemma I was in. At the time, I did the best I could with what I had. The CDC said a latex condom would prevent the transmission of HIV. I prayed to God the CDC was right because I didn't have the courage to do other than what I did at the time. Curt eventually learned I had HIV from reading *Essence*. He told me he appreciated my condom rule and was glad I never gave into his pleas to have sex without one. I was glad he was not bitter or mad at me for not disclosing. By summer's end, even with the decision to continue to keep HIV a secret, I had made it through another rough patch.

Forty-Six

MAX

" There are no perfect people.
There are no perfect heroes.
There are no perfect victims.**"**
—Don Lemon

Mrs. Jackson rang the doorbell and used her key to enter. Every once in a while, she would pop in unannounced to check on us. By the time I reached the first landing on the stairs, she was standing in the foyer. I stood on the steps, and we chatted. She said she was headed to the hospital.

"Hospital?" I asked, concerned. "What's wrong?"

"Oh, baby, nothing is wrong with me. I'm going to the hospital to sit with Max Robinson?" M-A-X R-O-B-I-N-S-O-N flashed across my mind like a neon sign on the side of the road. God—I hadn't thought about him in years.

"What's wrong with Max Robinson?" I asked, nonchalantly. Max had told me that he and the Jacksons were friends, but I didn't realize they were so close that Ms. J. would go sit with him at the hospital.

"Oh, it's just awful," she continued, "Max has AIDS." I started to sweat under my clothes. A lump clutched my throat, but I managed to get it out.

"AIDS?" I asked.

"AIDS. Of all things," she confirmed. My knees felt like they were about to buckle under me, and I sat on the step as she continued. *It didn't look good. He hadn't had a lot of visitors. She had been going to sit with him regularly.* All I could manage to get out was, "WOW."

"First, Keith—now, Max," she said, reaching for the door.

"This AIDS, baby, is a hor-ri-ble death," she concluded, before walking out the door. After she left, I tried to get up but my legs failed me.

"Max Robinson has AIDS," I mumbled, stumbling back onto the step. I stayed put until I was able to pull myself up using the banister to help keep my balance. I made it to my bedroom and sat on the floor, my back against the love seat.

"Max Robinson has AIDS," I repeated, out loud.

"Ain't that some shit?" I said, shaking my head in disbelief.

I will never forget the night I met Max. It was the Fourth of July weekend, 1983. I was living with Mama and had been an intern at Operation PUSH for two months. I woke up that Saturday morning to Mama on the telephone arguing with Grandmamma Julia, wondering when it would all stop. In the fifteen years I had observed their relationship, the competition between them had only gotten worse. Grandmamma Julia had barbecued and I, for one, was looking forward to visiting. I hadn't seen her since I'd been back in Chicago this time. Mama, on the other hand, had worked herself into a frenzy and decided she was not going over to Grandmamma's because, among other accusations, "Julia, you never come to Evanston to visit me!" Instead, Mama was going to have her own get-together and had been cooking since the day before, when she got off work. I couldn't hear what Grandmamma Julia was saying, but right before I went into the bathroom, Mama said, "I don't want to hear that shit, Julia. You always got some goddamn excuse!" Then she hung up the telephone. "Ouch!" I muttered. As badly as I felt for Grandmamma, Mama's assertion was mostly true. Grandmamma rarely came to visit Mama. But then I also knew she didn't want to be around Mama's drinking and hell-raising.

Ironically, years later, Mama would do the same thing to me Grandmamma Julia did to her. No matter how many times I invited Mama to my home, she always had an excuse. After one Easter dinner invitation, I was so irritated, I snapped, "I'm forty-one years old and you have never been to my house. You have no idea what kind of woman I am, Mama, or what kind of house I keep." I guilted her enough to get my one and only visit before her death.

I always felt like I was in the middle of Mama and Grandmamma's spats but, with age, I didn't feel like I had to take Mama's side. My only loyalty was to my own sanity. Mama was expecting her drinking buddies later that day and, like Grandmamma Julia, I didn't want any part of it. For as long as I could remember, being in their presence with Mama never turned out in my favor. On the train that morning, while headed to Operation PUSH's Saturday morning forum, I decided to keep my plans to visit Grandmamma Julia and Grandpapa Clayton.

When I arrived that afternoon, Grandmamma Julia had a spread—potato salad, fresh green beans, and spaghetti to accompany the barbecue ribs, hot sausage links and burgers. I don't know who she thought she was cooking for, but when she brought out my favorite, coconut cake, I was in heaven. Aunt Pam arrived soon after I did. I hadn't seen her in at least three years, and I was tickled pink. She was still that aunt who I very much wanted to emulate, with her glamorous lifestyle—a fabulous wardrobe, and wealthy and gorgeous men. She was alone that day and I had all her attention. I had a really great time. I ate until my stomach felt it was about to explode and talked Aunt Pam's ear off. I told her about how I had organized the buses of students for Harold Washington's mayoral campaign at SIU and was offered an internship at Operation PUSH. Pam told me to keep up the good work. When she was ready to leave, I asked if I could get a ride up to her house, which was halfway to Mama's. She said she was headed to a party and asked if I wanted to come. I couldn't believe that my cool auntie was inviting me to hang out with her. "For real?!" I asked. "Sure," she said." You'll have a good time." I was all in.

The party was held in a swanky apartment a couple blocks west of Lake Michigan in Chicago's South Shore community, close to where I was living with the Jacksons. I was astounded by the glamour. The home was as beautiful as the people and the clothes they wore—and probably their bank accounts, too. It was the type of party I would have expected Aunt Pam to attend. I, on the other hand, had attended mostly fraternity parties at the armory in South Cottage Grove with Veronica. I felt a little out of sorts in my outfit, looking like a college student Levi 501 blue jeans, an Oxford button-down shirt, brown deck shoes and my red Izod windbreaker, which I loved. I was a total contrast to Aunt Pam's fabulousness. We looked like what we were the fabulous aunt with her cute niece. Shortly after we arrived, I settled into a corner, and she went to get a glass of wine and mingle. I was captivated by the ambience and took in the scene. Jazz music was playing, and beautiful Black women dressed in pretty sundresses were chatting with fine-e-e ass Black men everywhere my eyes turned. The guests looked well-established and I could only hope that one day, when I entered the thirty-to-forty-something crowd, this would be my life.

I saw the eyes undressing me, and the obvious made me recoil. I couldn't see any man in that apartment wanting anything other than sex. Every now and then one would start a conversation with me, but I quickly shut it down. On top of the tired-ass come-ons, it was a little weird being *macked to* with my aunt in the next room. At some point, I started thinking about going home. None of the women were talking to me; I was just holding space and fading fast. I had woken to Mama and Grandmamma's arguing about six that morning. Made it to PUSH by eight, to Grandmamma Julia's by 1:00 p.m., and it had to be edging toward nine now. I figured if Aunt Pam could give me a ride as far as her North Side apartment, I could take the train the rest of the way. Just as I thought about finding her, she came to where I was and reached for her handbag that I had been watching. While touching up her lipstick, she said Max Robinson had just pulled up. I had no clue who she was talking about and, for a moment, weighed whether I wanted to look stupid and ask or remain stupid and never know. What the hell. "Who's Max Robinson?" I asked. "The news commentator," she explained, "and he— is—fin-e-e-e." *Aw, shucks,* I thought. *Aunt Pam is on the hunt.* She finished touching up her makeup and disappeared. I was left rooting for her. I was still standing in the corner next to the little table with Pam's handbag when someone came in wearing a cowboy hat. I assumed it was Max Robinson, as people cleared a path like Moses had done with the Red Sea. From my angle, I could only get a glimpse of him from the back, but I followed him moving in that cowboy hat and people clamoring to say hello until he disappeared into another part of the apartment.

After a while, I looked up and this unbelievably handsome man had zeroed in on me. My eyes moved up to his cowboy hat. *So that's Max Robinson.* I knew who he was. I had seen him on television but didn't connect his face to the name when Aunt Pam mentioned it to me. In person, he was one sight to see. I gave him a once-over, my eyes following down that silky shirt he was wearing with a denim jacket to the matching jeans that fit his long slim body to perfection, and there were those doggone cowboy boots he was wearing. I was looking at a live version of the Black Marlboro Man. *Somebody, please, pinch me back to fucking reality.* My eyes traced back up his body, and our eyes locked. He took his time as he eased his way through the crowd toward me, stopping to chat with other guests, saying hello but never changing his course and never losing eye contact with me.

"Hello," he said. "I'm Max Robinson." For a split second, I thought about Aunt Pam and what she would think about me talking to the man whose attention she had wanted to get but, apparently, I had. "I'm Rae Lewis," I said. Max started the conversation by asking me what I thought about a Black man running for president. Of all the things he could have asked, it was the one topic that had consumed the last two months of my life. I couldn't compete with the age, clothes and, probably, the education of most of the women in that room, but I could outtalk anyone about why it was time for a Black man to run for president. I ran down my Frank Watkins checklist I memorized on the subject. I could see the approval in Max's eyes. I told him I thought Reverend Jesse Louis Jackson Sr. was the best choice. He raised his glass in agreement.

"Say more," he encouraged, taking a sip of his drink, and nodding for me to carry on. I forgot all about the time and Aunt Pam. Max and I had talked a good thirty to forty-five minutes; it was all about politics, yet it was clear we were doing a dance. I'd make my point and he'd make his counterpoint, and the dance would start again. He moved into my space and asked a question, and I leaned in and gave an answer. He nodded in agreement and moved closer. His spicy-smelling cologne was sensual, and it dominated our space. Max touched my hand and I accepted it, as if my space belonged to him. I wasn't quite sure how things were going to play out, but I was intrigued by the simplicity of the dance. I was no stranger to older men, but that knowledge had come at a cost. I had been trying to put those days behind me but in talking to Max, I dismissed every ugly thing I had experienced dating older men. He had my full attention, and I was willing to let the night determine its course.

Eventually, Aunt Pam walked up to Max and me. We were engrossed in conversation, facing each other with maybe a finger's distance between us. She came up close and stood sideways. She looked first at Max and then at me in disbelief. Max and I didn't budge. *What the fuck is going on here?* was written all over her face. In an instant, I felt like that little girl who had been caught with my pants down under the porch with the little chocolate boy. Pam asked—looking at Max in a hostile manner, like she had just caught him cheating—"What do you think you're doing?" He seemed unfazed by her scrutiny and casually turned a bit toward her and said, "*WE* are talking about why a Black man should run for president." Pam looked perplexed. He had neutralized her in a little less than ten seconds. I jumped in, "Max this is my aunt, Pam Roberts. Pam, this is Max Robinson."

"Hello, nice to meet you," he said and turned back into our space, facing me. It was awkward. He clearly was not going to engage Pam and I didn't know what to say. I kept my eyes on her while she kept her eyes on Max and Max kept his eyes on me. I could see Pam's veins popping at the side of her neck. She was mad—that was clear. What was unclear was if she was mad at me for talking to Max; mad at Max because he had chosen me over all the beautiful women in the room, including her; or genuinely mad that Max was *macking to* her niece, who was half his age.

I know if I had been Pam in a similar situation with any of the young women I had mentored, I would have left no doubt for anyone that Max was out of line. One time, Mayor Marion Barry and I were chatting, and Mrs. Jackson looked over from her chair and asked the mayor, "Why are you talking to my child?" He raised his hands in surrender, and she said, "LEAVE – HER – ALONE! I mean it, Marion." And I promise you he ended that conversation. For the record, the mayor had never been inappropriate with me but Mrs. Jackson had left no doubt, if it had ever crossed his mind. My aunt, on the other hand, was behaving like a jilted lover. She reached between Max and me, grabbed her handbag and testily said to me, "I'm getting ready to leave." I looked at her apologetically because I was not trying to leave this fine-ass man. Pam slung her handbag over her shoulder. "Rae, I'm leaving," she said forcibly. "Are you coming?" Before I could open my mouth, Max said, "I will see that she gets home," still looking at me. *Damn-n-n-n.* I couldn't believe it and Pam couldn't, either. She was speechless. Before she could regain herself, Max placed his hand in mine. "Is that alright with you?" he asked.

"Yes," I said, glancing at Pam. She seemed taken aback and a little embarrassed. I felt the pings of guilt and shame in my gut.

"I'll be okay," I assured her.

"Are you sure?" she asked. For the first time, I could hear concern in her voice. Now I really felt guilty—but not enough to leave with her. Before I could respond to her question, she asked, "Is this okay with Georgia?" I looked at her like she had two heads. Whatever guilt I was feeling left my body like a ghost leaving her host. I knew Pam was trying to shame me into coming with her, but she had pulled the wrong card. What she could have done was grab my hand and say, *You came with me; you are leaving with me.* What she could have done was look Max straight in the face and tell him, *Not my niece,* but she didn't. Looking back, maybe it was a combination of her own attraction to Max and his star power that influenced her to shame me instead of him. She was too caught up in her feelings to protect me. And by the same token, I didn't think I needed to be protected. That would've been where age, wisdom and instinct kicked in like it had with Mrs. Jackson that day with Mayor Barry. If Pam had demanded that I leave with her, I would have, out of respect. Bringing Mama into the situation only pissed me off. How dare she ask about Mama's approval, of all people? I had no idea what Grandmamma Julia had told Pam about me and Mama and our jacked-up relationship. If only she knew what the last four years had been like for me, she would have asked Mama what the *hell* was wrong with *her.*

Quite frankly, I didn't give a flying fuck what Mama thought. What I wanted to say to Pam was this: *Do you know how many old-ass dicks I've sucked to put food in my belly because Mama threw me out over some bullshit? Girl, that ship sailed a long time ago.* But instead, I said, "Pam, I'm a big girl now." And just like that, she was gone. Shortly after she made her exit, Max and I left. I rested my head on the back seat of the stretch limo as we rode down Lake Shore Drive, with Max holding my hand. I took so much pride in the fact that women had been trying to catch Max's attention all night, but he had gone fishing and caught me—hook, line, and sinker. I was the least likely, and probably the most vulnerable. Max was twenty-three years my senior; I was twenty-one.

Max lived in a modest apartment in Marina City, an apartment complex that sat on the Chicago River, on the edge of downtown Chicago. He told me he had chosen this apartment because it was a block from the ABC Studios, where he could walk to work, and for the beautiful view of the Chicago skyline. He said the building was a hidden gem.

Shortly after we arrived, he opened the patio door and we stepped onto the balcony. I looked out over the skyline, and so much raced through my head. How did I end up here with *the* Max Robinson? My ego had been boosted to Mars and back, but my soul sagged. I had been here so many times with older men and it had never worked out in my favor. *What are you doing, girl?* I thought. Max moved in behind me, gently touched my waist and whispered in my ear, "You are *very* pretty and *very* smart." We went back into the living room. He made himself a drink of dark liquor and sat in the chair facing the balcony, and I sat on the end of the sofa close to the chair. We continued our conversation into the wee hours of the morning. I was enthralled. I had never held a conversation with a man that had nothing to do with sex but, at the same time, was intimate and stimulating. When we finally retired into the bedroom, we undressed down to our underwear and slipped under the sheets. He reached over and pulled me into his arms, kissed me on the forehead and said good night; we then went to sleep. The next morning, when I awoke, I was still in Max's arms. I squeezed myself away, went to the bathroom and came back to bed. I lay there watching him sleep. He was so handsome—just a perfect specimen of a man. He was brilliant and charismatic, and I felt like the luckiest girl on the planet. When he finally awoke, he pulled me into himself, and my entire body surrendered to his tenderness.

When I got home that afternoon, Aunt Pam had called Grandmamma Julia and Mama and told them that I left the party with this "old-ass man" instead of saying I left the party with Max Robinson—an old-ass famous man. It felt more like she was telling on me rather than being concerned about me. Whichever it was, it didn't matter. That ship had also sailed. I already had plans to see Max again. Mama asked, "Who is this *old-ass man* Pam was talking about?" I knew how to shut her up quickly. Her jealousy of Pam was so deep that all I needed to do was hint at Pam's failure.

"Did she tell you that she was trying to get him, too?" I asked. Mama chuckled, "I told her you were grown." By now, there was an unspoken understanding between us that I could come and go and do as I please. Mama didn't care as long as I paid my share of the bills and didn't bring men to her house. Knowing Mama as I do, she was just asking because she was nosey and needed something new to tell her friends about me. I had gambled that night going home with Max. Maybe it would end in a one-night stand but, honestly, I was so enamored with him I was willing to break that rule.

Max and I settled into an easy relationship. What I loved most about him was that he had no demands on me. He didn't come across as predatory, like some of the older men I dated in the past. He didn't want kinky sex. He didn't even want sex every time I saw him. Sex seemed secondary to the company we were to each other, and that went a long way to ease my early doubts about being with him. He would sit in a chair facing the balcony, with a drink in his hand. I sat on the sofa close to him and we talked. Max was the GOAT when it came to conversation, and I soaked up every word that came out of his mouth, like a dry sponge on a spill.

I came to know Max around the time he was in negotiations with ABC for a new contract and his separation from his wife. While he shared with me some of what was happening at ABC, I had no idea he was close to losing his job. He did say that they [the people at ABC] were trying to push him out because he dared discuss what he saw as racism at the network. He told me about his now-infamous Smith College speech on February 10, 1981, that was dubbed as "the Racism Speech" by *The Washington Post* and made headlines across the country. In the speech, Max claimed he and all the other Black journalists at ABC had been left out of the coverage of Ronald Reagan's inauguration and the release of the fifty-two U.S. hostages from Iran. ABC denied Max's claim, stating that three of four Black correspondents at the network had worked on the coverage. While this may have been true, it is also true that on one of the most important days in the country, with a three-man anchor team and hours of live coverage of the day's events—switching back and forth from Frank Reynolds, who was in Washington, to Peter Jennings, internationally—ABC had excluded Max, the third leg of the team, from the entire day of coverage. In our late-night conversations, he told me he felt targeted, used, and thrown away. This period has been described by Max's friends as him being dark and moody, drinking heavily and having blackouts—in essence, displaying erratic behavior. I could attest to the heavy drinking, but all that other stuff I had not witnessed. He was, at times, melancholy, rattling things—mostly people's expectations of him and the pressure of being *Max Robinson*. He seemed frustrated that he could never measure up, in the eyes of others. This, of course, I couldn't understand because all I saw was his greatness.

Even with flaws tagging tightly to his coattail, Max Robinson was a giant of a man. He mentored younger Black journalists and was one of the forty-four founders of the National Black Journalists Association. In 1958 at age twenty, Max was hired to read the news behind a logo scene at a local television station in Portsmouth, Virginia. As the story goes, one day he was struck by a little vanity; before going on air, he asked the camera man to remove the scene. "Some viewers were mad as hell to see a Black man," Max told me. He was fired the next day. Max's first break came in 1964 at age twenty-six, at WTOP in Washington, D.C., where he was hired as the floor director. From there, he was promoted to the news department covering fires, murders and robberies. A year later, Max went to NBC-owned WRC-TV in D.C., where he became the first African American on-air reporter. There, he won six awards and two regional Emmys. In 1969, he returned to WTOP as an on-air reporter and then midday anchor. In 1971, Max was teamed with Gordon Peterson as the co-anchor for the six o'clock and eleven o'clock news, making him the first African American anchor in the United States. He dominated the ratings and became a household name. His live coverage during the Hanafi hostage crisis in Washington, D.C. garnered him national acclaim. As a result, ABC News came calling with a new show concept of three co-anchors for *World News Tonight*. The 1978 launch featured Peter Jennings, in London; Frank Reynolds, in Washington, D.C.; and Max Robinson, in Chicago. With this position, Max made double history and became the first Black person to anchor a nationally broadcast news program and the first local anchor—Black or white—to move from local to national news.

Max and I talked about many things, some of which I will keep private because he shared them in confidence. I was fascinated by his life and admired that he was unapologetically Black. He told me people were surprised he had chosen to live in the Black community and not in a plush white community when he and his family relocated to Chicago. He hosted wonderful parties as an ode to living with his own people and it forced others—including Black people who saw themselves as superior—to come to the Black community. In fact, legend has it, Oprah met Stedman at one of Max's famous parties.

Sometimes he had already ordered food and we stayed up late talking about the plight of African American people, racism, politics and even the work I was doing at Operation PUSH. He picked my brain and engaged me intellectually. It was perfect foreplay. In a lot of ways, my evenings with Max exploring topics close to my heart were like my days at PUSH. However brazen a contradiction it might seem, those two worlds were connected and they nurtured me. At PUSH, as I've mentioned, I was in the throes of an awakening intellectually and spiritually. I had found my purpose and my senses were at full attention. Then, in my private life, I was spending time with the most magnificent man — a man who made me feel valued. The way Max engaged me — his charm, his intellect and everything else about him—made me feel like I belonged on that sofa as he confided in me, debated with me, educated me and made love to me.

I got up from my bedroom floor that day after Mrs. Jackson told me about Max, went to bed and slept my blues away. The next morning, I was literally gripped with fear of losing Mrs. Jackson. I knew there was a certain order to things for her, and Max would have been a disruption to that order. If she had gotten even a whiff of my relationship with Max, she would have accepted my HIV status but he would have caused an irreparable crack in our relationship, or so I believed.

It was painful for me to learn from Mrs. Jackson that Max had AIDS but knowing helped me prepare emotionally for his death. Had it not been for her, I wouldn't have known until after he passed. While it was rumored in some circles that he had AIDS prior to his death, he would not confirm it publicly until on his deathbed. In a *Washington Post* exposé that I read after his death, Max spoke about the speculation of his health, telling the reporter, "The curiosity has, at times, annoyed me. I'm just not going to get into the subject of what I have." Thank God Mrs. Jackson was not one to skirt the truth. On the day she told me that Max had AIDS, I was still painstakingly trying to come to terms with my own diagnosis. Whatever level of acceptance I was reaching for was interrupted. To say the least, I was left stunned and confused. I was scared shitless about my own health, and heartbroken to learn AIDS would end the story of an incredible man who had touched me deeply. In retrospect, learning Max had AIDS probably contributed to the onset of my depression at the beginning of the campaign, and that depression was compounded by the anxiety around the changes HIV was causing in my life once I moved back to Chicago.

I learned Max died from complications related to AIDS on December 20, 1988, from breaking news on television. I watched, sitting on my love seat, with tears streaming down my face. Sorrow consumed me, and I cried until I was empty. That day, I received a call from Bill McGill, checking on me. He and I were still friends and after I first learned that Max had AIDS, I didn't know where to turn. I called Bill to talk it through. The fact that Bill was checking on me about the death of another lover was more compassion than I felt I deserved. Still, I was defensive, asking him, "Why wouldn't I be okay?"

"Rae, dear heart," Bill said. "I am just checking in."

"Well, I don't know if he infected me. Maybe it wasn't him!"

Bill was trying to say to me it didn't matter if Max had infected me. That either way, Max was my friend and he [Bill] was trying to provide some solace in the face of this tragedy. I didn't want to hear it that day. To do so would have made Max's death real, which in my mind, made my death inevitable. When I hung up from Bill, I slid down from the side of my bed onto my knees. I cried and said the prayer that I had never stopped praying: *Lord, please don't let me get AIDS.*

I was so scared that day Max passed away. Scared I would die the same horrible death. Scared my relationship with Max would be discovered and the fallout from it would be just as horrible as dying from AIDS. Ironically, three decades later, I would learn from reading Kim Fields' memoir that, at the time of Max's death, she was visiting Jonathan. Reverend and Mrs. Jackson had called the family and some close friends together around the dining room table, and they shared that Max had died from AIDS. Meanwhile, I was across the street—an absolute mess. I hadn't even thought about going over to see how Mrs. Jackson was taking the news.

It was just a matter of time before Aunt Pam called to see if I had heard that Max had died from AIDS. That call came a couple of days after his death. I could only think that she was happy she had dodged that bullet. She showed nothing but concern—a testament to her. She wanted to know if I was sick and if I had been checked out. I told her I was fine. I could hear the doubt in her voice, but I stuck to the story. I told her we didn't have a lot of sex; that we mostly talked when we were together. I also told her we had used condoms, which we had—but not all the time. I felt like a foolish little girl who had stolen a cookie from the cookie jar, denying it with the crumbs still on my lips. She let it go but a few years later, when Grandmamma Julia died, she asked me again. I stuck to the same story. Six years later, when I finally went public with the *Essence* cover story, Aunt Pam told me she had always doubted I had told her the truth. Back then, I just couldn't bring myself to tell her I was infected. In part, I was ashamed I thought I beat my aunt out of a man who was now deceased from one of the deadliest sexually transmitted diseases that ever existed, and who was possibly a source of my own infection. It felt like bad karma. For many years, I thought, *That's what my fast ass gets.* Also, if I had admitted to Pam back then that I was HIV-positive, she would have told Grandmamma Julia, who would have told Mama. I was too ashamed to sit HIV at the foot of the woman who had prayed for my soul more days than not. If Mama had caught a whiff of it, she would have used it against me—as she had done time and time again—and having to cope with HIV was all I could deal with at the time.

My relationship with Max that summer was not a secret, I didn't go broadcasting it, either. I told Tyrone, who advised me to keep it to myself around PUSH. Although I met Max outside of PUSH, Tyrone didn't want people to think I was a gold digger. As I've mentioned, he was concerned about how people viewed me and, as always, I took his advice to heart. It had taken so much for me to get on the right path, and I wasn't going to jeopardize it by bragging about my relationship with Max.

While I could control the narrative on my end, I had no control over Max. He was brazen. One day I accompanied him to a barbecue at someone's home in Pill Hill, another posh South Side community of established Black people. Max was larger than life everywhere he went. We pulled up in a black stretch limousine. He was wearing that darn cowboy hat, with me at his side; we were a sight to see. When I stepped into the backyard, I saw Vergie Thompson, an older woman who had attended church at Evanston's Second Baptist and who was also active in PUSH. I wanted to crawl under a rock. After she and I spoke, you better believe she gave me that Black-auntie-side-eye, signifying, *You know you ain't got no business with this grown-ass man.* I just knew my secret was shot to hell. I kept waiting for the gossip about my relationship with Max to start but, to my knowledge, she never told. She did, however, pull me aside one day at PUSH and warned me, "Be careful." Then, after Max's death, she caught up to me one Saturday at PUSH and informed me Max had died from AIDS, adding I should get myself checked. I tried my best to keep a poker face, knowing all along I was infected and scared out of my mind.

In the nine-month span from the time I learned I was infected with HIV to the time I learned Max had AIDS, I had not considered him as a possible source of my infection. First, he wasn't on my list for the most stereotypical reason: No way a man of his stature could have HIV. Second, I couldn't see how I could have been infected so early in the pandemic when the disease was primarily a gay man's disease. Learning Max had AIDS, I now had to make sense of his diagnosis in the context of my own. No matter how painful it might have been, I had to ask myself, *Did Max infect me?* The secrecy around his AIDS diagnosis that year made it difficult even to determine some semblance of a timeline. All I could do was methodically retrace every moment I had spent with him in the summer of 1983, trying to determine if he had HIV. When I thought back to the times when we were together, Max did not look sick. Rather, from my naked eye to his naked body, he was perfect. It was an exercise in futility, mainly because there are no physical signs of HIV—only of AIDS.

After a year of secrecy and denial, Max's deathbed request was that his family use his death as an example to educate the Black community about AIDS. It came in the form of a statement through close friend and former journalist Roger Wilkins:

> During his battle with the disease, Mr. Robinson expressed the desire that his death be the occasion for emphasizing the importance, particularly to the Black community, of education about AIDS and methods for its prevention.

I thought it admirable because as much as I love Black people, there was no way in hell I would have disclosed my HIV status to be scrutinized at that time, dead or alive.

It was at this crossroads where the hard work of understanding the intersection of my HIV diagnosis with Max's AIDS diagnosis began. I read every article I could find to help me piece parts of his life together. From what I understood, Max had no idea he was infected with HIV. Like most people around this time, he only became concerned about his health in the fall of 1987, after losing a massive amount of weight in a short period of time. His physician referred him to an infectious disease doctor and, subsequently, he was diagnosed with AIDS. Max was hospitalized in December 1987. This is around the time Mrs. Jackson was going back and forth to visit Max. He was in a coma for a month and doctors didn't expect him to survive. He lived another year. I should mention that it was very common in the eighties to mid-nineties to be diagnosed with HIV and AIDS at the same time. Testing wasn't developed until 1985 and, even then, it was not widely available.

M ax's friends described him as a ladies' man with no shortage of women willing to tango. Months after his death, I stumbled upon a scathing *Vanity Fair* article about Max titled "The Light Goes Out" in, of all places, the doctor's office. The byline was so scandalous I went into the bathroom to read it for fear that someone I knew would catch me with the magazine in my hand. It read, *Alcohol, Promiscuity, AIDS — Why Did America's First Black Network Anchorman, Max Robinson, Self-Destruct?*

Clarence Page, a close friend of Max's, was quoted in the article. "He, [speaking of Max] could walk into a room, and you could just hear the panties drop." *No shit*, I thought. I couldn't debate that truth because it had been my experience. Sitting there on the toilet in that bathroom, I wondered about the other women who, besides me, got to tango with him:

> Were any of Max's other sexual partners infected?
> Was his ex-wife infected?
> Had any contact tracing been done?

There was this big perception back then that the department of health was supposed to contact a person to inform them when a sexual partner had been diagnosed with HIV; however, that was not the case. There was no uniformity across health departments. In some cities, it was completely voluntary for those who wanted a neutral source to inform sexual partners they might have been exposed to HIV. When I learned I had HIV, no health professional called from the D.C. Department of Public Health to inquire about my sexual partners. I had been left struggling to compile a list of my partners without any criteria to help me judge who may have been the likely source(s) of my infection. Dr.

Leitman had been my only help as I muddled through, building my list. I had considered only my African friend as a possible source of my infection because he met some obscure criteria of being a sexual partner who happened to live in Africa. I had no idea if he had HIV. At the time of my diagnosis, I clung to the notion he could have infected me because it was what I had available to close the door on the topic. Once I learned Max had AIDS, that door was flung open again, causing me a shitload of stress.

The *Vanity Fair* article on Max said he had made a list of his past sexual partners and called some to inform them he had AIDS. Reportedly, Max had even named three women whom he believed might have been the source of his infection.

"One, a Chicago woman," the article explained, "who briefly lived with him, now denies that she even knew Robinson." Peter Boyer wrote, "Another, a television reporter, admits that she knew him, but only as a friend." I finished reading the article and placed it in the garbage bin. It left me shaken. *Had I been on Max's list? If so, why had I never been called?* I came to somewhat of a resolution. It is likely Max had been grasping at the same straws I had been when I learned I had HIV. It is likely that Max hadn't thought about me in years, like I hadn't thought about him in years. These news stories about Max didn't get me any answers. On the contrary, they made me want to double down on my secret. The suspicions and speculation that he was bisexual hung in the air like California smog. It was a lot for me to digest. All in one breath, people painted him to be a womanizer but left just enough doubt hanging in the air about his sexuality.

It is true that, during this period, the largest percentage of men with HIV had contracted the virus from having sex with men, and that is still true today. But it is not the only truth. There were men who contracted HIV through heterosexual relationships and from using drugs intravenously. Rather than illuminate this fact, doubt and supposition were used to drive home the point of "good AIDS/bad AIDS." People used this speculation to shame men who had sex with other men.

Max understood this perfectly clear. After he learned he had AIDS, he told close friends repeatedly he was not gay and to let people know this fact after his death. Reverend Jackson told the press, "It was not homosexuality, but promiscuity." It was disheartening to me that so much emphasis had been placed on Max's sexuality rather than using his infection to illustrate HIV had no respect regarding a person's color, class or age. He was the first Black mainstream person to die from AIDS, and his death could have shed some light on the stigmas surrounding HIV/AIDS. Instead, it was made to cast a dark shadow and reinforce "bad AIDS." I agree with Arthur Ashe, who wrote in his memoir:

> *I thought this confession sad and unfortunate to worry about at the moment of one's death; whether or not one is misperceived by other people as gay or straight is a cruel additional burden to bear at a time of ultimate stress. And yet it seems to matter to the world if someone is gay or straight.*

In 1988, when Max died from AIDS-related complications, Black people constituted half the AIDS cases reported by the CDC. What we should have been doing was demanding President Ronald Reagan invest in research and education so that no more Max Robinsons would have to die from AIDS instead of trying to determine how a person became infected with HIV. This narrative that focused on Max's flaws claimed to explain his downfall rather than be an ally and friend in his last days, with whispers like, *A-ha. So, Max wasn't the man who everyone thought he was*—and that was bothersome to me. Personally, I believed then—and still do—that it is no one's business how a person became infected but the parties involved. The reality that news organizations thought speculation about his sexuality was an important enough topic to report was mind-boggling. I never questioned how Max became infected because it did not matter. What mattered was that he was infected, and I'd had sex with him.

The shame and stigma around HIV/AIDS that has festered in the Black community is an even greater sickness. In the six years from Max's death to my disclosure, I watched the drama of his death unfold like a tabloid dossier. By the time I appeared on the cover of *Essence* in 1994, Max's reputation had taken an awful hit. He had been characterized as a temperamental drunk who sometimes didn't show up for work or showed up drunk when he did. I think, in part, this was another reason I held onto the secret of the relationship. I didn't want to add to the shame already surrounding his death, so I protected him by keeping our relationship a secret. We were so embarrassed Max had died from that "gay disease," we only spoke of him in whispers. This shame created a deafening silence around his legacy that has all but written him out of history.

I believe HIV/AIDS has muzzled our collective memory—not just of Max. No one talks about the incredible fashion designer Willie Smith, whose *Willie Wear* collection generated twenty-five million dollars in sales in just short of ten years—or Alvin Ailey, Arthur Ashe and other giants in the Black community. We have even done the same thing in our families. In my years of travel, I've met so many people whose families have been torn apart by the shame and secret of HIV/AIDS.

I stumbled upon a speech given by Don Lemon, a primetime anchor at CNN, to the Hollywood Reporter Inaugural Empowerment Gala in 2019 that illuminates the point I am making about Max's forgotten legacy. Don spoke candidly, saying, "He was not only a person of color; he was a colorful person. Right. And history has neglected him because of struggles in his personal life—many of them self-inflicted." Max's legacy became a victim to a disease. One example says it all. In 2015, when Lester Holt replaced Brian Williams as the anchor for NBC Nightly News, the narrative that Lester was the first African American to anchor a national network news show was circulating. I wanted to raise my hand and say, *Hold up one doggone minute!* I was happy for Lester, especially since he anchored at WBBM Chicago-CBS during my series Living with AIDS, but I was greatly saddened that new generations had no idea that Max Robinson was the first Black anchor on national news, not Lester. I felt a sadness that Max had been reduced to the ugly stigma and shame surrounding HIV/AIDS.

It would take even more years of scientific research on HIV and AIDS to help me assess Max as a possible source of my infection. Keep in mind: When Max passed away, AIDS had only been identified by the medical community for seven years, and HIV for four years. In time, I surmised that my African friend could not have infected me. He lived in a part of West Africa where the dominant strain was HIV-2. I was infected with the HIV-1 strain of the virus, like most of the world. Most importantly, according to one of the leading HIV/AIDS researchers in my friend's native land of Guinea-Bissau, the first documented case of HIV-1 was five years after our one sexual encounter. While I have not spoken to him, I have tracked him, thanks to the internet. As of 2020, I can tell you my friend was still alive and just as fine as he was that day I met him in Moscow.

Today, as far as I know, Max is my only sexual partner who was infected with HIV when I was diagnosed in March 1987. With that said, I would come to understand that it is possible—even probable—that I was infected by Max. Contrarily, the same information that made Max a possible source of my infection also made me the unlikely source of his infection. The clinical stage, of HIV takes eight to ten years after a person is infected to develop AIDS. This is of course without any treatment or before effective antiretrovirals arrived on the scene in 1998. Full stop. I met Max in 1983, four years prior to the time he was diagnosed with AIDS.

I transitioned to AIDS between 1992-1993, ten years after my relationship with Max. Based on the timeline of disease progression, Max's AIDS diagnosis places him within the probability category of my HIV infection. And don't go COVID—crazy on me. It is a scientific fact that a person does not just get HIV and, a couple of years later, die from AIDS . I will never know for sure if Max infected me. Full stop. The only thing I can confirm for certain is that he and I had sex, and the timeline of our relationship coincides with my disease progression. I also know that, for thirty-eight years, my relationship with Max has been a monkey on my back. It is time to let her go and let the healing begin.

There is another truth that I have painfully avoided: I have often wondered what went through Max's mind that night he picked me over all those fabulous age-appropriate women at that party. I know what was going through my mind that night: This powerful man chose *ME*?!

I will never know what he thought, but he certainly knew his star power. It followed him like a shadow. He knew I was young enough to be his daughter. He also knew he had no use for me other than a casual relationship, so why even bother with someone so young? This truth has been difficult for me to admit for a number of reasons. First, Max deeply touched my life in such a short period of time, and I've held a fairy-tale view of my time spent with him. Even while writing this memoir, it wasn't until the very end (during the editing phase) that I have been willing to acknowledge Max's culpability, even though it was a legally consensual relationship. This is not to absolve me; I went in feet first. Whatever the outcome, I've lived with it and will do so until the day I die. This is what I know to be true: After I disclosed my HIV status to the world, I came to believe it is difficult to heal from what I am unwilling to face. Over the years, my transparency, while speaking and in press interviews, has even surprised me. Yet, at the same time, I've held onto Max because he represents a deep and sorrowful shame around my sex life. No matter how many times my therapist has said to me or how many times I have said to my audience, *It does not matter how many sexual partners you have; it only takes one person, one time,* this fact has not erased the judgments I placed on myself. These are judgments birthed by Mama and matured in the atmosphere of "respectability politics" in our Black churches, homes, social and political organizations, sororities, and fraternities.

I worried what people would think of me. *Uh-huh, she was a hoe right from the get-go*—and that would, in some way, absolve Max from preying on me. At some point, we must have an honest conversation in the Black community about predatory behavior of Black men. I have had to have it with myself. I wasn't always at this place of enlightenment; it took years of working on myself to understand my own biases were rooted in how I viewed my own behavior and how Black culture had shaped my worldview. A friend asked me on Facebook in a debate about Bill Cosby, "What happened to you?" What happened was that I started loving myself more than I wanted a man to love me. At some point, Black women and girls have to matter as much as Black men—especially those men we place on pedestals because of the contributions they have made to our culture. I wrote in a blog post about R. Kelly and Bishop Eddie Long that even if one of those teenaged girls wanted to be with R. Kelly, I bet she never bargained for being pissed on after sex. Do we just walk away and say she had no business with him, or do we stand up for what's right in the face of wrong? Just because white men do it does not give us a pass. Yes, Woody Allen married Soon-Yi Previn, his long-term partner Mia Farrow's adopted daughter; and Priscilla Presley's parents allowed her to date Elvis Presley when she was 14 and he was 24. However, it still does not make it right, and this argument about white men to condone what Black men do makes us look crazy. I accept my culpability in my infection because acceptance was the only way I knew to forgive myself. I might not have conquered this demon of shame, but I have battled her often. In doing so, I have fought this cycle of abuse that tries to define my worth by how many sexual partners I've had and who they were. I have fought for agency over my life in how I talk and dress, what I tweet or even how many times I curse. I am enough. There is no shame when you believe you are truly enough. Who knows? Maybe I just needed to speak my truth, say it out loud and with clarity, so I could put it to rest.

Forty-Seven

≈ ⁓

PLANS CHANGE

"The best-laid plans of mice and men often go awry."
—Robert Burns

I moved out of the Jacksons' place and moved back to D.C. about a week before I was to begin my new job. I was ready for this next phase of my life, but it was not ready for me. Everything happened so fast. At the Democratic National Convention, Mayor Marion Barry asked me what I was going to do next, and I told him that I wanted to go back to D.C. He hired me on the spot to work in his administration as a political appointee. Unfortunately, my paperwork was still being processed and it would take anywhere from three weeks to a month before I could begin my job. I hadn't saved half of what I should have the previous year. I was in a tight spot and couldn't see how I was supposed to get an apartment without a job. On top of my financial woes, I had this uneasy feeling I should be doing something else, but I didn't know what that was. I reworked every angle I could come up with and kept coming up short. *To hell with pride.* I called Mrs. Jackson to ask if I could come back to live in the house. I stayed in D.C. long enough to empty my storage, give away my furniture and send my boxes back to Chicago, marking them "RETURN TO SENDER" so I wouldn't have to pay to ship them. One week to the day I left, I was back at the house demanding that Rhoda McKinney get the hell out of my room. The week I moved out, she moved in and was sleeping in my room—and my bed—until her room was painted. I knew she was moving in, but seeing her in my room made me think she was taking my place.

"Why the hell are you in my room?" I asked Rhoda when I opened the door to find her sitting in my bed in her pajamas.

"I thought you were in D.C.," she said.

"Well, I'm back, and umm, you need to pack your shit and move to your own room," I said. Her prima-donna ass refused: "Umm—that would be a big, fat NO. Not until my room is painted," she said, all smart-alecky. At first, I thought she was joking and laughed it off, but she was dead serious. In the meantime, my luggage was sitting in the hallway. Jesse Jr. came down the stairs from his room and we all started talking over each other about why I was back and why Rhoda was in my room. I went across the street to get Mrs. Jackson to referee. As soon as she reached the second landing, Jesse Jr. asked, "Momma, why did you let that crazy girl move back in the house?"

"Now, Jesse, I told Rae that she would always have a place to live," she said.

"Whatever, Jesse," I said dismissively, walking behind Mrs. Jackson. "Can we get back to the point?"

"Ms. J., can you please tell Rhoda she has to get out of my room?"

"I'm not going anywhere until my room is ready," Rhoda said, smugly.

Jonathan came out of his room and even put in his two cents. He didn't understand why I was back. Furthermore, he said I had forfeited all my rights and should take what I could get because I was the one who had changed my mind. I lost that battle. Mrs. Jackson said fair was fair. I had given up my room by default and would have to sleep in the small room until Rhoda's room was ready.

By the middle of the week, my boxes started to arrive and I was still displaced. The paint had been sitting in the middle of Rhoda's bedroom since Sunday. I gave Jesse and Rhoda a piece of my mind, but they still wouldn't budge. They double-teamed me, and I stopped talking to them. Needless to say, there was a lot of eye-rolling and door-slamming for the rest of the week. Come Saturday morning, I woke the entire house and demanded we start painting. I told Rhoda, "If your shit ain't out of my room by tomorrow night, I'm going to put it out myself." Thank God Mrs. Jackson agreed and told them to stop being lazy and paint the room. We spent the day painting. Mrs. Jackson even helped. Sunday night, we were all in our right rooms and talking again.

Coming back to Chicago shot my plans to hell, and I was clueless about my next move. I hadn't planned to work in the mayor's office forever—just long enough to become stable. Washington, D.C., I believed, was still the best place to organize on a national level. I had a lot of soul-searching to do while living in a city where I mostly disliked the people who were my potential employers. I had to consider what type of job I could work in Chicago that would keep me on the path I had charted for my future.

Right away, Melissa Holloway, who was now Reverend Jackson's executive assistant, hired me to help sort through the hundreds of speaking requests he had received. One day, Dr. Finney was in the office and asked why I wasn't in D.C. He said I needed a real job and rattled off an address in the South Loop, on Wells Street, where I was to meet him on Monday at three. Before I could ask a single question, he was gone. When I arrived at the address, I was shocked to learn it was the Illinois Dukakis statewide campaign headquarters. *What in the world?* I thought, climbing the stairs. Dr. Finney asked me to sit in a meeting where he introduced me, nonchalantly: "This is Rae Lewis and she's going to head up the statewide youth and students." All eyes shifted to me, and I waved. I wished he'd asked me first because I wasn't so sure I wanted the job. Finney, however, rarely asked for permission. He was officially the head Black man in charge in the Illinois Dukakis campaign and no one dared challenge him, including me.

My doubts about working on the Dukakis campaign came from a couple things. I didn't want to remain locked into the student and youth category. I knew from watching the trajectory of Tyrone's career that the more jobs I took working with students and youth, the more difficult it would be to get hired for other positions. I worked hard to prove my organizing capabilities beyond youth and students during those three years in D.C. I chose to pause my career path to work on the Jackson '88 campaign because I was invested in a possible Jackson presidency. My job with Dukakis was a step backward in my mind. If I were going to work with youth and students, I preferred a lateral move as Dukakis's national, not statewide, youth and student person.

I had also developed concerns about how the team was running the campaign and if I wanted to be on that team. Two weeks after the Democratic National Convention, Dukakis followed in President Ronald Reagan's footsteps and spoke to an all-white audience at the Neshoba County Fair in Philadelphia, Mississippi, which did not sit well with me. Of course, I knew Dukakis was a liberal and a much better choice than George W. Bush, but optics are everything. It wasn't so much that he had spoken at the fair, but more that he had made a deliberate decision not to mention the three civil-rights activists—James Chaney, Andrew Goodman, and Michael Schwerner—who were murdered in 1964 during the Mississippi Summer Project voter registration campaign. It was all over the press that Dukakis had chosen to court the hate and anti-Blackness of "Reagan Democrats" over the reconciliation of the ugly past of Jim Crow. I was skeptical but, in the end, I accepted the position because I didn't want to contradict Dr. Finney. Besides, it was only a couple months out of my life.

Right off the bat, I hated the office atmosphere. The staff was almost all khaki and button-down Oxford shirt-wearing, arrogant white guys who believed they knew everything about all things. The lack of diversity and divergent ideas was astounding. They clearly had missed the Jackson memo on diversity. The United States, as Reverend Jackson put it, "was more like a quilt—many patches, many pieces, many colors, many sizes, all woven and held together by a common thread," rather than "a blanket—one piece of unbroken cloth." Likewise, a campaign, in my opinion, required a diverse staff and strategy built on that quilt analogy. I should not have been surprised that the state campaign headquarters was a microcosm of the national headquarters. Susan Estrich, Dukakis' national campaign manager, was a thirty-five-year-old white woman. While she had made history as the first woman campaign manager for a presidential candidate for one of the major parties, she surrounded herself with white men. Donna Brazile held the highest position for a Black person, deputy field director. I didn't have any contact with her during the campaign. The grapevine was alive and well, however, and I knew she was having a more difficult time than I was. She said in her memoir, *Cooking with Grease,* that she was ready to resign after the Philadelphia, Mississippi event but that the reporter Sam Donaldson talked her out of it. Finney had brought in as many Black faces as he could, but we were not the decision-makers. Most days I felt like the "Jackson girl" they tolerated. I spent as much time out of the office as I could. I had meetings on college campuses to do what I could easily have done over the telephone. Some days I worked the phone from my bedroom at home instead of going to headquarters. I didn't miss staff meetings, though. I showed my face just enough so they couldn't complain to Dr. Finney, and I ran all my plans for student and youth outreach by him. As long as he was happy with my work, I didn't have to worry about the other campaign heads.

On college campuses, I was able to turn some of Jackson's campus coordinators across the state into Dukakis campus coordinators, but none of them had the same level of enthusiasm for Dukakis that they had for Jackson. I pushed myself to think outside the box because I still had a job to do. After watching Kim Fields campaign for Reverend Jackson, I was inspired to focus on voter registration among high school seniors in Chicago Public Schools (CPS) who would be eligible to vote by Election Day. It was akin to PUSH's citizenship education program, but on steroids. I tapped into the student leadership peer program that was already in place in CPS to gain access to the high schools. With this partnership, I was able to conduct voter registration drives in over half of the high schools. I worked with Alice Tregay, a Chicago organizing legend, to place the voter registrars in the schools. We were even able to get some student leaders who were old enough to go through the training to be deputized as voter registrars for their school.

It was working on this project where I met my next boyfriend, Noble Pearce. I learned the peer program was under his purview and reached out. It was my good fortune that a citywide meeting of peer leaders was already scheduled, and Noble offered me a spot on the program and a ride. It was at the student leadership peer meeting that I was able to gain commitments to do voter registration in the schools. Noble was impressive from day one. He picked me up in his four-door silver Mercedes Benz with the vanity plate *Noble 10.* He was impeccably dressed, from a tailored suit right down to crocodile shoes. His skin was the color of rich black coffee, like my father's, and he had jet black curly hair. I think I wanted to be in love with him that very day. On our first date, I asked him his age. He asked me to guess. "About thirty-seven, thirty-eight." He led me to believe it was the latter. I had given up men who were old enough to be my father. However, with my thirties on the horizon, I thought a ten-or-eleven-year age difference was a good compromise.

I was seeing Curt off and on when I met Noble. Curt still had that "bachelor forever" vibe going on (as evident even today, as he has never married). I wanted a man who was willing to commit. Noble seemed willing to step into those shoes. On our third date, sitting at his dining room table, I told him I was HIV-positive. I would never disclose today in such a private setting, as I've heard too many horror stories about women being physically harmed. After a long discussion, he expressed his strong attraction to me and his willingness to give the relationship a chance. My comfort level with disclosing my status to Noble had a lot to do with his maturity as well as the fact that he was not in any of my circles, social or political. If he had decided not to date me, I figured my secret would still be safe. Noble and I were hot and heavy from day one. He picked me up a couple of nights a week and I would leave from his place for work, then again on the weekends.

For most of the Dukakis campaign, I was a lone ranger. I did what was expected of me, but I didn't bond with any of the campaign staff. In retrospect, I didn't enjoy working on this campaign. The momentum was off, and we never felt like a team working toward the same goal. I didn't understand the logic of some decisions. I was asked to work on the event that was planned by the national campaign headquarters. Team members had arranged for Governor Dukakis to have a multi-city live feed forum to be held on different college campuses across the country with a celebrity host moderator at each site. The program was a brilliant idea at a time before social-media technologies existed. The headquarters had already chosen the site, a predominantly white college in a suburb west of Chicago. I questioned the school they had chosen and pushed for a change of venue. I was quickly told the program was set in stone, although no one could explain why this school had been chosen. I was dumbfounded. They had chosen a commuter school in a Republican stronghold for a high-visibility event with the candidate and one of the biggest young movie stars on the planet in 1988, actor Rob Lowe. This convinced me the Dukakis team was either stuck on stupid or did not want to win. If I had planned the event this close to the election, I would have maximized Governor Dukakis' visibility among young voters more likely to vote Democratic than the ones who were more likely to vote Republican. We were past the persuasion period. I would have taken the star power of Rob Lowe and jam-packed an auditorium at one of the Chicago colleges like Chicago State University, on the South Side, or the University of Illinois-Chicago campus, then bus more students from one or two of the junior colleges. Everyone loved Rob Lowe, including me. I could tell you exactly where and with whom Julie Henderson and Lorenzo Butler—I had seen the blockbuster movie St. Elmo's Fire four years earlier. There were no Secret Service issues because Dukakis was not in Chicago physically. What did the campaign have to lose? The press would have been all over it and young voters in attendance would have talked about it up to and after Election Day. Since I was not in charge and they balked at my idea, I shut the hell up and did what I was asked: help ensure everything went smoothly the day of the program.

There were approximately a hundred students, mostly white, seated neatly in a class lecture setting. Rob never said it, but I could see him looking around the room like, *Is this it?* I thought, *Yep, this is it.* I kept Rob occupied in conversation as we waited for the program to begin. He was easy on the eyes and oh-so-charming. At some point, the conversation turned to my role in the campaign, and I explained I was a *Jessecrat* who had joined Dukakis in September. Rob started asking me questions about what it was like to work for Reverend Jackson. He told me he had missed an opportunity to meet Reverend Jackson at the '88 Democratic Convention. Before I knew it, I was telling him about the Saturday morning forum at PUSH. He was very interested, but the bigwig publicist for the Dukakis campaign poured water on the idea and I let it drop.

The program went as planned—and was as dry as I knew it would be. The only excitement came when the girls made goo-goo eyes at Rob. Afterward, Rob doubled back and asked if I really could arrange for him to meet Reverend Jackson. I told him I just needed to make a call to see if he was in town. Rob asked the publicist to follow up with me but then decided to give me his hotel information to make sure it didn't fall through the cracks. Later that evening, I confirmed with both Rob and the publicist. Rob asked if I would give him a wake-up call the next morning. It was all arranged when I told Noble about Rob and explained that I had to go to PUSH the next morning.

He had a list of objections. "Why are you the one giving Rob a wake-up call at his hotel?" he asked. "That's his publicist's job." I tried to explain that this was work, and Noble retorted, "You don't work for Rob Lowe or Jesse Jackson!" I had never seen this side of Noble and was totally caught off guard. After going back and forth with him to no avail, I shut up. He was not going to come around to my point of view and I was not changing my mind about PUSH. I should have seen this as a sign he was a control freak, but I was still in the honeymoon stage of our relationship. I dismissed it as jealousy—and a little jealousy was cute, in my opinion. Noble was correct that I had no obligation to either Reverend Jackson or Rob Lowe, but I did have an obligation to keep my word. I had arranged this visit for Rob, and I'd be damned if anything would go wrong. I believe a person is only as good as their word, and I wasn't going to jeopardize my honor over Noble's jealousy.

The next morning shortly after I arrived at PUSH, so did Rob, with a tight-jawed publicist. I ignored the publicist and ushered Rob into Reverend Jackson's office, and he stayed for the broadcast. Whether the Dukakis campaign realized it, I had orchestrated a good press opportunity with the two of them. Plus, Rob Lowe was able to give his Dukakis stump speech over the radio airwaves during the morning broadcast. Afterward, Reverend Jackson and Rob Lowe would appear on the same program in late October at Northwestern University on behalf of Dukakis.

As a Black woman coming from the Jackson camp, working for Dukakis was draining. The Dukakis campaign did not seem to care that Jackson had gotten more Black people to the polls this primary season than ever before, proving we were a committed bloc of voters. Nationally, the powers that be had a lackluster approach to Black outreach that left many of us feeling alienated. Sure, there were Jackson supporters who were less enthusiastic about Dukakis, and this lack of enthusiasm turned into apathy. Some even felt Jackson had been snubbed by Dukakis as his running mate. On top of how Black people were already feeling after the primaries, Dukakis didn't make it any easier for Black people or his staff. First, there was the Philadelphia, Mississippi event, and then Dukakis's lack of visibility in the Black community early in the campaign, which made it even harder to galvanize Black voters. The whammy for me was Dukakis' silence after the Bush campaign's infamous "Willie Horton" ad. William "Willie" Horton was a Black inmate in Massachusetts who skipped a furlough program during a weekend pass while serving life in prison. Not quite a year later, he was arrested for a home invasion during which he attacked and tied up the male homeowner, then repeatedly raped the man's fiancée. The Bush campaign and other conservative PACs locked onto this unfortunate situation and rode it like a bull until the very end. It was a simple ad with a whole lot of punch. *Which candidate for president gave weekend passes to first-degree murderers who were not eligible for parole?* the ad asked while alternating pictures of Bush and Dukakis. *Which candidate can you really trust to be tough on crime?* The punch line was a grainy photo of William with an afro and a beard. In an instant, he became a symbol of every white person's fear: the hypersexualized Black man raping a white woman. Civil rights leaders and Black elected officials called for Dukakis to denounce the ad for the race-baiting trope it was, but he just would not do it. His running mate, Sen. Lloyd Bentsen, and campaign manager Susan Estrich spoke out, but Black people wanted to hear from Dukakis I wanted to hear from Dukakis. I remember sitting in the staff meeting after Reverend Jackson and other Black leaders went to Boston to meet with Dukakis about the ad, he still would not take a stand. I felt betrayed and gutted. There was all this talk from Dukakis about not participating in gutter politics, but it seemed to be just that—all talk. In my opinion, that ship had sailed August 4, 1988, when he spoke to that all-white audience in Mississippi. This ad was just the other side of the same coin. Lee Atwater, Bush's campaign manager, declared he was going to make Willie Horton "the most famous Black man in the country," and he did just that. No one asked Dukakis to defend the crimes Horton committed, but we were asking the Democratic nominee to take a stand against race-baiting. This ad would become the defining dog-whistle moment in U.S. political history.

If working for Dukakis was an indication of the battles I would have to face in the future as a Black woman working for a white mainstream candidate, I wasn't too sure I was up for the task. I had been so focused on the ideological hurdles I had to jump to work for a political candidate, but now I learned my Blackness made my expertise less valuable than my white counterparts. It had been no different from working at SANE. Personally, I didn't know if I wanted it badly enough to fight for a place at the table and then fight again, once I was at the table, to do the job that I was hired to do. Donna finally quit about three weeks before the election, and I gained even more respect for her. Her frustrations had reached a boiling point, when she challenged the press to stop treating Bush with kid gloves. She mentioned his rumored extramarital affair, and that didn't go over very well. I, for one, was cheering for her—even if I didn't know what the future held for me.

After the election, I went back to work with Melissa in Reverend Jackson's office. I was still at a loss as to my next move. One day, out of the blue, Reverend Jackson asked me what I wanted to do with my life. In my mind, I thought, *Dude, I have no freaking idea*. However, I caught myself and gave him the easiest answer I had. "I want to go back to school and finish my degree," is what I told him. "Well, Jackie and I will do everything we can to support you," he said. His declaration of support meant the world to me, but I was grasping at straws.

Forty-Eight

NORTHEASTERN ILLINOIS UNIVERSITY

“There is but one coward on earth, and that is the coward that dare not know.”
—W. E. B. Du Bois

In February 1989, I enrolled in Northeastern Illinois University. I gravitated toward Northeastern because of Drs. Robert Starks and Conrad Worrill, who were both teaching at the university's Carruthers Center for Inner City Studies campus. Dr. Starks was a professor of political science and a political strategist who had advised both Reverend Jesse Jackson and Mayor Harold Washington. Dr. Worrill was the director of the Carruthers campus and a founding member of the National Black United Front. They both were longtime supporters of Operation PUSH, and I had often chatted with them about political theory and Black studies. Dr. Worrill invited me to the Carruthers campus and gave me a tour. I liked his program, but I wanted one that was broader in scope regarding political science and decided on the main campus.

Even though I had enrolled, but I wasn't sure if I could cut it since I had been such a failure in the past. I asked myself, *Why am I going down this road again?* In my heart, I knew I wanted a degree in political science. My ego had been a little bruised while working for Dukakis. My coworkers had no problem throwing their political science degrees in my face. It made me feel a tad inferior, even with six years of organizing experience under my belt. I had been intrigued with the intersection of political theory and political activism since the first time I chatted with Dr. Ronald Walters in 1984. Looking back, questioning myself and even telling friends I wasn't sure about college was my way of establishing a default explanation in case I failed. This was especially true after learning I had earned only twelve credit hours out of the possible forty-eight I had taken at Southern Illinois University. I did so poorly I was placed on financial aid probation, which rendered me unqualified to receive a Pell Grant to attend Northeastern. I had never heard of such a thing. I guess the federal government figured you can waste your own money, but not ours. If it had not been for Reverend Jackson obtaining some private scholarship money for me, I wouldn't have been able to attend Northeastern. So, at twenty-six years of age, here I was, starting over again.

The first quarter I took three courses: American Government, Black Studies and Mass Communication. I went to school two days a week and worked the other three for Dr. Finney as his go-to jack-of-all-trades political assistant. My tasks varied from organizing political meetings and fundraisers to typing his handwritten research papers, which I excelled in the least and hated the most. Dr. Finney had just started the Doctor of Ministry program at McCormick Theological Seminary. Coincidentally, it was the same seminary I would attend eleven years later.

I decided I would either sink or swim this time. If I couldn't cut the first quarter at Northeastern, I'd walk away. However, I wouldn't go down without a fight. I enlisted my housemate Rhoda to proof my assignments. The first time I asked her for help, she read the first page and said, "Rae, honey, I hate to tell you," continuing with a sigh, "this is bad."

"I know that my grammar may be off," I said, embarrassed, "but I think I did the assignment right. Just read it all and tell me what you think."

She asked to see the instructions for the assignment. I handed them to her and sat on her fancy love seat and painfully waited.

"O-kay. Rae, this isn't that bad," she said finally. "You just can't spell worth shit and you write how you talk."

"No shit, Sherlock." I muttered.

"Don't be a smart-ass," she said, "You asked ME for *my* help."

"O-kay-y-y, I'm sorry," I said, begging for forgiveness. She agreed to see how she could help make it better. After about ten minutes, she looked up at me and said, "Stop breathing down my neck; you're stressing me out!" Before I could respond she asked, "Can you go somewhere?" I rolled my eyes and stomped out. Rhoda finished editing the assignment and brought it to my room. She acknowledged my ideas were solid. Then, she wanted to see every assignment before I turned it in. She was irritating, though; she never just edited the assignment and gave it back. She had to explain why something was wrong. Her mini lectures on grammar were annoying but, in the end, they helped, and I really appreciated her for investing in me.

Toward the end of the quarter, my communications professor asked if he could submit my name for consideration into the University Honors Program. To be considered for the program, your first introduction to the honors committee had to come from a professor. I wanted to ask him if he was sure, but I decided to keep that question to myself. If accepted, I would receive the Honors Program Merit Tuition Award each quarter if I maintained a GPA of 3.0. Given my past academic history, I was flat-out surprised that someone believed I was capable of being in an honors program. I was approved, and I submitted an application, which was also approved. This was a FULL STOP moment for me. I had transferred in with a GPA of one point something from SIU and now I had been admitted into Northeastern's honors program. The following quarter, I enrolled as a full-time student.

One day into my second quarter, while I was sitting in the middle of my bed studying—books and notes spread all over—Jesse Jr. peeked his head into my room.

"Rae-Rae, you need to stop pretending you are in school," he said.

"Shut up, Jesse. You ain't the only one in school," I responded. He was attending Chicago Theological Seminary, working on a Master of Theology Degree.

"Anyway, I'm in the honors program. How about that?" I asked.

"Stop lying," Junior said, stepping inside. "Prove it." I got off the bed and pulled my grades out of a file and proudly handed them over.

"Damn, Rae-Rae!" he said, cheesing from ear to ear. "You ain't lying."

I rolled my eyes and put him out of my room. It felt really good to have my hard work acknowledged. SIU had been such a flop. Being accepted into the honors program helped ease all my doubts. It affirmed I was capable. I only needed to find my groove, and I did just that in my first quarter. My success was a combination of things: My classes were small, no more than fifteen to twenty-five students; I never missed a class, no matter how cold it got or how many inches of snow fell in Chicago; the lively class discussions held my interest; I stayed on top of my reading assignments; I turned in my assignments on time; and everything had to be proofread by Rhoda. (It pays to live with a journalist.)

In hindsight, I can see the recipe for my success had been there all the time, but I had too much noise in my head to pay attention. If you recall, after I was able to read at my grade level in junior high school, a whole new world opened for me. The voracious reader I am today makes it hard for me to believe I'd never read a book on my own until I was thirteen years old. Reading improved my comprehension and my ability to think critically, which became my best asset. Thank God for Mr. Murphy and Dr. Morton, at

Chute Middle School. In high school, I excelled in English classes with a heavy emphasis on literature. I had the potential, but what I needed were the right conditions to help me pull through, like I now had at Northeastern.

I continued everything I had done that first quarter and added additional tools to help. I went to the writing lab to sharpen my skills. I took detailed notes in class. I started dropping into my professors' offices to ask questions and discuss the lectures and readings. If there was something I didn't understand, I worked until I got it. Most of all, I had no distractions—no noise or major issues that could cause me to digress. I continued to live in the house and my only expenses were food and rent, the latter being a third of what a one-bedroom apartment would have cost. Mrs. Jackson's generosity took the weight of the world off me, allowing me to work part-time. I didn't have to worry about tuition, books, or a loan because I earned a full academic scholarship every quarter until I graduated.

The political science department at Northeastern had a slew of professors I believe could have taught anywhere, but they chose public education. That first quarter, my American government professor learned I had worked on the Jackson presidential campaign and asked me if I would be willing to talk about my experience. I was completely thrown off guard, but it was a privilege I dared not turn down. By the third quarter, Drs. Ellen Cannon and Valerie Simms started to take special interest in me.

Dr. Cannon lectured from the moment she stepped into the classroom and held profound discussions. She was demanding and made you earn that grade. She assigned twenty-five to thirty-page research papers and I pushed myself, choosing topics that had multiple layers. I love combing through history to gather one central idea for a paper. Dr. Simms was the chair of the department and didn't teach, but I took independent study classes with her. She was also the advisor for my senior honor's thesis. Under their tutelage, I excelled well beyond my own expectations.

Around the Jacksons' Thanksgiving and Christmas dinner tables, I joined the intellectual discourse. One time, Reverend watched, speechless, as Jesse Jr. and I debated Marxist anthropology. Junior was sitting in class with the likes of Dr. Michael Eric Dyson, but I had Drs. Ellen Cannon and Valerie Simms. Looking back, Val and Ellen simply watered the seeds that Dr. Ronald Walters had planted over the years in our talks about the discipline of political science. In fact, my two and a half years at Northeastern were a convergence of many things: All my readings, fiction and non-fiction—about race, racism and social change. I carried into every classroom my years of exposure to some of the most intellectually brilliant and provocative thinkers of my lifetime. Those conversations sitting around the Jacksons' dining room table were opportunities when the political family could come together. I sat in awe of people like Dick Gregory as he broke it down to the core, no matter what the subject. I listened to Reverend Al Sharpton dissect the current issues facing Black America at the time as we ate together. Sometimes, I never opened my mouth but took it all in. I learned to gather, analyze, and apply information toward a strategy for political action. There was a scholar in me; I just needed an environment where I could blossom. I was ready for a formal education, but I didn't know it until I was in it. My life took a turn. Class by class, I peeled the layers of doubt back so that the scholar could emerge. It is amazing what can be accomplished when you are compelled from within. To do it, I had to be honest with myself about my strengths and weaknesses. I decided what was important in my life and set parameters.

I gave school everything I had and then I pulled some more from places I didn't know I had. I didn't have a computer and Dr. Finney's accountant, Chris May, loaned me one for a while, or I went over to her house to use one. I didn't have a fancy vocabulary or writing style and, to compensate, I immersed myself in the reading material. The better I understood a topic, the better I could articulate it on paper. All my political science professors assigned a heavy reading load eight to ten books and I read every assigned book in each class every quarter. I found study partners. When Rhoda moved out of the house, I even enlisted Noble to help proof my papers.

My hardest decision was to quit working for Dr. Finney. He had no respect for my time. I couldn't do his political work all day and then spend my evenings typing his research papers when I had my own. Plus, Noble was always bitching about Dr. Finney. He blew a gasket when I went over to Finney's townhouse after hours to type a paper. I finally started to realize that what I thought was just cute jealousy was more about control. He wanted to know what I was doing when I wasn't with him, and he always had an opinion about it. The one thing I had never done was allow a man to control me, and I never would. He routinely insinuated there was something inappropriate about my relationship with Dr. Finney, even though he was completely off base. Dr. Finney was purely a mentor, but he certainly misused his authority. One day, it all came to a head when he handed me one of his papers to type close to the time I was supposed to get off. I complained. He looked me straight in the face and said, "Tell that old-ass nigga that I'm paying your bills—not him." He was way out of line, and I didn't know what to say. I took his paper and went back to my desk, but it was the last paper I ever typed for him.

Fortunately, the following week I had a new job that was a much better fit. That Saturday at PUSH, Dorothy Rivers, a Chicago businesswoman, overheard me tell someone I was looking for work and asked me to call her. Mrs. Jackson had told me more than once that you never know who's watching you. I had always admired Ms. Rivers. She was what I call, old-school dignified. She almost never missed a Saturday PUSH broadcast and had given the organization her time, money, and talents for whatever was needed. Among her many enterprises was a school for students ages six to eighteen with developmental and emotional issues, and a transitional homeless shelter. Both served African Americans and were housed in the same building on Chicago's South Side, about a ten-minute drive from my house. Two days a week, I was responsible for creating the social calendar for the students at the special education school to help build their socialization skills. Every day those students reminded me that, except by the grace of God, I could have been in their situation. We never knew what state of mind they would be in when they got off the school bus, but their resilience was remarkable. Once weekly, I tutored the children in the homeless shelter in reading, alphabets, and numbers. I saw a lot of myself in those children. Looking back, I can see the impact trauma had on their lives. They had a willingness to learn, but very short attention spans. I knew from day one they had more problems than I could solve, but I gave them what I had to give: My attention and validation during those two hours each week.

Mrs. Rivers was a godsend. This job allowed me to reduce my work hours enough so I could meet my goal of graduating in the spring of 1991. Northeastern was planning to switch from the quarter trimester system to the semester system, and I calculated that I could finish by the time the school made the change if I went year-round. I was working fewer hours than I had for Dr. Finney; however, my salary was a few hundred dollars more, and she provided me with health insurance.

October 1990, in my eighth quarter and last year of school, the president of Northeastern, Dr. Gordon Lamb, used my life as an example of excellence in his annual university address. I was exalted as an example of what could be achieved with dedication and hard work. According to Dr. Lamb, I was the epitome of a Northeastern student: A commuter who was a little older and who was starting over in higher education. I had maintained a GPA of 3.8 as a university honor student. By now, I had applied for and received nearly every academic award the university offered in addition to the honors program. I had found myself, and in the least likely of places.

It was a bittersweet moment. I had enormous pride as Dr. Lamb praised my hard work to the university community, but I was too sick to enjoy the moment. I started taking zidovudine (AZT)—the first medication approved to treat HIV—a month earlier, and the side effects sucked all the joy out of me. That July, Dr. Leitman sent me a letter explaining that the CDC had a new treatment recommendation: All infected persons with a T-cell count less than four hundred should begin taking AZT. At the time, my T-cell count was 353. I had been wondering if I would ever take the medication. AZT had been approved by the FDA in 1988, but they were still only giving it to people who had AIDS. Dr. Leitman told me it wasn't a rush, but that I needed to begin AZT within the next few months. I had not been sick. I didn't think about HIV anymore, apart from my six-month visit to NIH to see Dr. Leitman. I followed the same routine every six months. After my appointment, I had dinner with my friend Barry Saunders in D.C. and flew back home the next morning. Once I received my follow-up letter indicating my health status, I informed Veronica, Barry, Coré and Noble and I wouldn't talk about HIV again until the next six months—and neither did they. Since I wasn't "sick" I placed HIV in a box and only pulled it out when necessary. I came to learn, however, that friendships deserve to bear the full weight of the bad as well as the good, the pain as well as the pleasure. But I didn't know that then, and I was left to bear the burden of AZT on my own.

Having to take AZT placed me in a sticky situation: I hadn't told my primary care physician I had HIV. I was no longer seeing Dr. Cunningham because my insurance was with an HMO. I got regular checkups, but I had never disclosed to my regular internist. I had regular blood workups and would think that my reduced white blood counts would have set off a red flag, but that didn't happen. However, I told the gynecologist at the same HMO—I think, because he specialized in the care of women. He was also African American, and I remembered how sensitive and compassionate Dr. Cunningham had been; however, this doctor was a complete jackass. Right before he put the speculum in my vagina to examine me, he asked, "How did a pretty girl like you end up with HIV?" I wanted to crawl out of my skin and out of the room. It brought me back to the time I was diagnosed with herpes. I was so humiliated I vowed to never tell another doctor. After that, I doubled down on my secret because I didn't have AIDS so there was nothing for the HMO doctor to treat. Now that I had to take AZT, I had to disclose. At my request, Dr. Leitman sent the HMO doctor a vaguely worded letter that implied I had just learned my HIV status from the Red Cross. That way, she didn't give away the fact that I already knew my status. My primary care doctor was sympathetic, but clueless on what to do for me. This only confirmed, at least in my mind, not disclosing my status was the right decision. I know it must be difficult to believe that some doctors were still clueless on how to care for HIV patients nine years after the first documented cases of AIDS, but that was the state of affairs then. If not for the NIH study, I'm not sure how it would have panned out for me. I respected my HMO internist's honesty and her willingness to defer to Dr. Leitman's recommendations on how to treat me.

With AZT on board, my life had taken another unexpected turn. I felt like God had jokes. I resented that I had to pair my success with sorrow. AZT was a continuous cycle of ugliness. I finally understood why AIDS activists called it poison. It was brutal. I couldn't possibly see how something so bad could be good, but I was too afraid to stop. I figured being sick from AZT was better than being sick from AIDS. For about three weeks, I took six hundred milligrams of AZT a day. I was so sick I couldn't even think straight and standing straight was out of the question. Dr. Leitman said it was okay for my doctor to reduce my daily dosage to five hundred milligrams—five pills in a day. Every morning I popped the blue and white pill into my mouth and got ready for school. Halfway to Northeastern, nausea would rise like a tidal wave inside me. As soon as I arrived at school, I went straight to the cafeteria to get a ham, egg, and cheese on a croissant. Within an hour, the AZT had overpowered my breakfast. I snacked on saltine crackers and sipped water in-between classes to try and quell my nausea. By lunch, I was feeling a little better and took my second pill, chasing it with French fries and a cheeseburger. As crazy as it sounds, I thought the more grease I ate, the better I'd feel. After my last class, I headed to the library to research my senior honors thesis and it was time to take my third pill.

Heavily influenced by Dr. Simms, I chose to write my honor's thesis on Michael Harrington, the founder of the Democratic Socialists of America. For those whose understanding of socialism begins and ends with Sen. Bernie Sanders and Rep. Alexandria Ocasio-Cortez, you should take some time and read Harrington's writings. He was a political activist and theorist who was heavily influenced by Dorothy Day, the founder of the Catholic Workers Movement, and by Eugene V. Debs, a five-time presidential candidate on a third-party ticket of the Socialist Party of America and founding member of the Industrial Workers of the World. Harrington was also a professor of political science at Queens College and is best known for the book, *The Other America: Poverty in the United States.* This book illuminated what he called the "invisible poverty" in the United States. The most fascinating part for me was his theory about the cycle of poverty, how the system worked against poor people and how generations get sucked into poverty. For my thesis project, I read every book and article Harrington had ever written, and as much critical theory written about him, to determine if he had stayed true to his ideological worldview in the backdrop of a predominant two-party system; and he had.

Sitting at the reference desk in the library, I sneaked saltines to coat my stomach and got back to research. There were days on the train ride home when I was so weak all I could do was lean my head and shoulder on the train window to help hold me up. Occasionally, the movement of the train would push nausea up from my belly through my mouth onto the train floor. Vomit was everywhere and I'd look around, apologizing with my eyes and laying napkins that I kept with me on top of the vomit. In the early evening, I'd take my fourth pill. Then Noble picked me up, and the excessive eating started over again. We stopped and got carryout. My go-to meal was the wings-and-gizzards combo, fries, and mild sauce from Harold's Chicken. Before I knew it, I had blossomed from a size eight into a twelve.

On top of feeling sick all the time, fear of being found out came over me like never before. It seemed to me that those blue-and-white AZT capsules were on the news every day. I convinced myself that if someone recognized them on me, my secret would be exposed. I became hypervigilant, searching for private places to take my pills. At school, I sequestered myself in the bathroom stall or the stairwell. I found cases that didn't look like typical pillboxes to store the pills and carry them in my bag. At home, I buried the pill bottle deep inside my dresser after tearing the label and flushing it down the toilet. I never disposed the empty pill bottle in my house.

At work, Betty Ross—the school secretary with whom I had become friendly—noticed I was dragging and not my talkative self. She started asking questions I had avoided until she walked into my office and caught me with my head on my desk. I just went ahead and told her what was going on. Little did I know she had been curious about the doctor appointments in D.C. that I had to tell her about to get the time off. Betty was the best. She covered for me many times and let me cry on her shoulder every single day. During this time, I also got to know her pre-teen daughter, Lisa Sargent. Then sometime after the *Essence* cover story was released, Betty passed away from lung cancer. As a young adult, Lisa rekindled our friendship. She would have made her mother proud by choosing to work in social service, and you best believe that at every organization where she worked, she found a way to bring me in to speak. Back then, life was harder than I wanted, but God kept allies coming my way. Once home from work, I'd take a nap to sleep away the fatigue before I could study. I didn't go into a depression; instead, I compartmentalized my life as if HIV had nothing to do with school. I didn't address it emotionally. In the end, my intense focus on achieving my goal of graduating with honors helped me manage the stress of taking AZT by disconnecting it from my daily experience of school.

It didn't take long for me to have a come-to-Jesus moment with myself. I knew that if I were to finish this degree, I couldn't do it alone. I needed every single credit that school year to graduate that May. In addition to the full course load, I was applying to graduate school, and preparing to take the Graduate Records Examination (GRE) and the specialized political science competency exams. I was dragging, and my study partner—super-nosy Audrey Stone (Shulruff)—started asking questions.

I met Audrey the first quarter in my American Government class. She and I had very different personalities, and we always bumped heads during class discussions. There was another girl, too, Atha Panou. I hated them both. Audrey is Jewish and Atha is Greek, and, like me, they both had strong opinions, often framing the discussion based on their own cultures and experiences. One day Atha, who is Greek Orthodox, said something in class about celebrating Easter at a different time than other Christians. I wondered, *What the hell is she talking about?* It was also the moment I realized there was more for me to learn, and I started listening to them with an open mind. Audrey and I were both political science majors while Atha majored in criminal justice. We had a lot of crossover classes. The next quarter, Audrey had a class with me and one with Atha and, before the end of that quarter, we had become like The Three Musketeers.

Audrey and I were in so many of the same classes, we became study partners. I started to feel guilty about slacking. After almost two years of studying together, I felt I should explain or move on. I chose to explain. At lunch in the cafeteria, I told her everything. There was shock, disbelief and then a teardrop. I looked like the picture of health—a little pudgy but, for the most part, I didn't fit any image of what she had seen on television or read in a book. Intellectually, she understood anyone could get HIV, but the media was not showing people like me—just those who already had AIDS who looked like death and were mostly white men. You could count on one hand the stories told about those who were not gay white men. Most notably, there were Alison Gertz, a twenty-three-year-old woman who was a New York socialite and activist; thirteen-year-old Ryan White; and Elizabeth Glaser, the wife of actor Paul Michael Glaser (of TV's Starsky and Hutch). I was challenging every image Audrey had seen of a person living with HIV. At the same time, I confirmed what she knew to be true: Anyone could get HIV and you could not look at a person and tell that person was infected. She had many questions that I patiently answered. She expressed support for me, and she was honest right away, saying, "Rae, this is really heavy." I didn't know where she was going with that and I braced myself, wondering if this was going to be an *I support you, but…* confessional. "It's too much for me to deal with on my own. Can I talk with my sister about it?" she asked. I never saw that coming. I was so accustomed to keeping my secret I didn't know what to think. I agreed. If she needed support to back me, then why should I deny her that right? The seal of the secret had started to crack. Then Audrey suggested we tell Atha. She felt we shouldn't keep it from her because we had become good friends and we could lean on each other. I agreed to that, too. A couple of days later, Audrey and I told Atha while we all sat in the school cafeteria. She was also shocked and in disbelief. I answered all her questions. They bonded together to provide me with as much support as I needed. Graciously, they acknowledged how crippling taking AZT was for me and saw me through a lens that validated what I was going through. I hadn't known it until then, but it was exactly the kind of support I needed.

My friends who knew I had HIV prior to Atha, and Audrey were also concerned and cared about me. For sure, each supported me as much as they could, and I never doubted their loyalty. It's just that no one treated HIV like it was a big deal, especially Veronica, who was always quick to say, "Girl, you ain't going nowhere." And you can imagine how many times she has told me in these later years: "See, I told you that you weren't going anywhere." Not dying from AIDS-related complications is not the same as living with HIV. It wasn't so much the larger concerns about HIV I needed to be validated, but rather the related micro issues as they started to unfold. I think everyone was so accustomed to me forging ahead, they didn't have to feel compelled to deal with their own feelings about it, as long as I seemed good. I didn't bitch and complain about my illness but tucked it away. Living with Mama all those years conditioned me to push through the pain and become tough, and I think this unwittingly gave my friends permission to avoid asking me about HIV or even bringing it up. In retrospect, disclosing to Atha and Audrey at this juncture in my HIV journey and having them hold my hand on those days—when all I wanted to do was sleep nausea away—allowed me to be vulnerable and cared for. In the end, their support helped me to realistically process the changes I was undergoing.

Noble was another story. Every time I tried to explain the emotional and physical toll AZT was taking on me, I came off as a whiny little girl in his eyes. One day he told me, "Get over it. People take medication every day." I dismissed his insensitivity because I figured having a man who already accepted my HIV status was better than starting again. That logic was fool's gold—that is, having something that looks like gold is better than having nothing. He didn't seem so concerned about me taking AZT, but he was certainly thinking about himself. One day, out of the blue, he asked me if I douched. I wasn't sure where he was going with this line of questioning, so I hesitantly said, "I used to... I mean... I guess, but not really."

He asked, "Not even after your period?" *Boy, that was a loaded question.* We had been together two years and he had never asked about my menstrual cycle. We didn't have sex during that time of the month, so what did it matter? This questioning was way out in left field, even for Noble. He had criticized the type of panties I wore, so I traded my bikini underwear for some big-ass bloomers just to shut him up. With the douching question, I felt like he had crossed a boundary, and I needed to draw the line. "Well, all the gynie doctors I've seen in recent years say that douching is bad for you," I said with confidence.

"But you have HIV," he said.

"I don't understand," I said. This was a truly dumb and insulting road he was taking us down. I knew what he was hinting at, but I was going to make him own it. "What does that have to do with anything?" I asked, shrugging my shoulders.

"After your period, you still have blood up there," he stated, like he was an expert on my vagina. This time, I raised my hands in the air like, "So?"

"Don't you think you should get it out?" he asked, continuing, "Before we have sex?" Then he explained to me that HIV was in blood—like I had explained to him when we first began dating.

"Noble, the blood goes away on its own," I said, all testy. "Plus, we use condoms." I was annoyed as fuck. On the one hand, according to his logic, taking AZT was no big deal and I was supposed to "get over it!" Now, suddenly, he's concerned about my menstrual blood. We had never stopped taking morning baths together since the beginning, even after my cycle. He was talking some bullshit, and he knew that I knew.

"What's the point of all of this?" I finally asked. To my surprise, he didn't answer, and he dropped it. Then one night after he picked me up, he stopped at Walgreens, turned to me, and said, "I thought that maybe you wanted to get one of those disposable douches." I was hurt, but, I bit that bullet and did as he asked. This became routine with him after each menstrual cycle. For me, it was beyond humiliating; when I had had enough, I became defiant in my own surreptitious way. I would go into the bathroom, turn the water on and pretend to douche. Then I turned my back to him in bed and told him I didn't feel well. I be damned if he got some sex that night.

As the school year became even more demanding, I used studying as an excuse to avoid spending nights with him. I spent many weekends over at Audrey's studying and curled with her dog, Sheena, instead of being at Noble's curled up under him. Around midterms and finals, Audrey and I divided the exam study questions and shared our answers. The division of labor cut the workload in half. It was a huge help to me because the heavy fatigue was interfering with my ability to get everything done. We were both "A" students, so we never had to worry about the quality of our work.

The day I took the GRE. I was so sick I imagined this was what dying felt like. I dragged myself out of bed at the break of dawn, took my AZT pill for the morning and picked up breakfast on the way to the exam site to coat my stomach. After I took the first part of the exam, I took my second pill for the day and was able to go get some tea and donuts before I began part two. Thirty minutes into the exam, I was so sick I couldn't think straight enough to tell you who the president was at that moment, much less the significance of the second president of the United States, whose name I couldn't remember, either. I was more than defeated when I left that room. When I arrived back at the house, I took another pill, took off my boots, crawled into bed fully clothed and pulled the covers over my head. I knew I had done poorly—not just because of AZT but, as smart as I was, I had missed the parts of my education that could help me do well on a standardized test.

When I received the rejection letter for graduate school from the University of Illinois at Chicago, it knocked the wind out of me. I think I cried more about the rejection letter than I did about being sick from AZT. Thank God, Dr. Ellen Cannon was not having it. She made me her mission. She told me, "No, we are not accepting this," and picked up the telephone and called Dr. Richard Johnson, the chair of the political science department at UIC. That day, he was unavailable, and she left a message that went something like this: *I want to talk to you about this brilliant student of mine, Rae Lewis.* After that day, she called him every day and left messages about *one of the most promising students I had taught in her years in academia.* When they finally spoke, she said she told him, "It would be a grave mistake to reject her simply on the basis of her GRE test score." No one had ever made me their mission. Not EVER. Dr. Cannon had worked her magic. I received my letter of acceptance into the graduate program at UIC about a month later.

I finished Northeastern with only one hiccup: the professor who taught international studies. He gave me a C-minus on the first exam. I was so freaking confused. I looked over at Audrey and showed her my grade. Her mouth flopped open. As he went over the exam questions and answers, I raised my hand to state, "That's what I said." My classmates got quiet. He had a reputation of being a hard-ass sexist asshole, and no one dared challenge him. He mean-mugged me and said we could talk about it after class. However, I only got more and more irritated because I had answered all the questions correctly. After he had finished, I blurted, "I answered all of these questions correctly. I don't know why you gave me a C-minus." By that time, he was flustered. I had been muttering under my breath, "I got that one right too" as he reviewed each question on the exam.

"Because it only took you forty-five minutes to complete my exam," he said, all high and mighty with his thick accent.

Damn! Dude was timing me, I thought. I was mad as hell.

"So, what does that have to do with anything if my answers are right? And they are right," I blurted out. He said something like he could do whatever he wanted because he was a tenured professor, blah-blah-blah. Then he said, "I can almost rape the president of the university's daughter in the middle of the street in broad daylight and get away with it."

My classmates gasped and froze, waiting for my response. He had triggered me in a way even I didn't understand. All the fight was drained out of me in an instant. I gathered my things and stormed out of the classroom. By the time I made it to Dr. Simms' office across the hall, tears were streaming down my face. Still crying, I explained what happened. After I had gotten the story out, I told her about the other "little" sexist things he said in passing during his lectures. She wasn't so much surprised that he was sexist but shocked he had brought that attitude into the classroom. She assured me she would handle the matter. I don't know what she said to him, but he was correct: Nothing happened to him. He had a history of misogyny and I had been the first to file a complaint. However, students talk and that's why I had only taken this one mandatory class with him. He asked that I be removed from his class because I made his ulcer worse. I completed the class as an independent study with Dr. Simms. She said I had done "A" work, but because of the C-minus grade that he would not change, she could only give me a B. It was her compromise and the only B that I ever got in my political science studies.

I graduated cum laude, but I was .03 from magna cum laude, and I cried about that, too. I should have gotten an A in my communication leadership course, but our professor had taken a leave of absence—ironically, because he had AIDS. The substitute did not see the brilliance in my paper on the leadership style of Eugene V. Debs. Nonetheless, on May 19, 1991, I walked across that stage with three medals around my neck. I could hear Jesse Jr., Jonathan, Coré and Veronica hollering and cheering me on. Jesse Jr. was the loudest, yelling, "Way to go, Rae-Rae! You did it, girl!" After my many days of pleading, Mama had even come to the graduation—with flowers. Dr. Cotton came with Coré. Afterward, I had a graduation party at the house. It was one of the happiest days of my life.

Forty-Nine

❧

POLITICS THE CHICAGO WAY

" Well, if you pick a fight with somebody that's smaller than you
and you beat them, where's the honor in that?"
—Carol Moseley Braun

In the three years since I worked for Leon Finney, I stayed away from Chicago politics. "Good riddance" was my sentiment until my friend Kgosie Matthews, the campaign manager for Carol Moseley Braun's senatorial race, came calling. Carol announced her candidacy for the United States Senate on November 19, 1991. It was a primary run against two-term Senator Alan Dixon and personal-injury attorney Albert Hofeld, who announced his intent to run the day before Carol did. The Braun campaign was jump-started a month earlier out of her outrage around the Senate hearing of U.S. Supreme Court nominee Clarence Thomas and the Anita Hill controversy.

Carol was no different than other women across the country who were mad as hell about the way the Senate Judiciary Committee questioned Anita Hill—me included. I will never forget that Sunday, October 11, 1991. I was glued to the television. At one point, I even had the portable television on the kitchen counter and watched the hearing as I cooked. Hill, a lawyer and professor, testified that years earlier, while employed at the U.S. Department of Education and the Equal Employment Opportunity Commission, she had been sexually harassed by Thomas. According to Hill, Thomas had boasted about his sexual prowess and made unwanted sexual advances on numerous occasions. It was an eyeopener. I had at times laughed off a lewd joke or sexual innuendo but never thought about it as sexual harassment in the workplace. It was jarring, and even embarrassing, to watch fourteen white men ask a Black woman such personal questions. I was also torn, which is difficult for me to admit; while I had no love for Clarence Thomas, honestly, my thinking was that at least President Bush had appointed a Black man to replace Justice Thurgood Marshall. At the time, I knew a lot of Black people who felt the same, no matter how misguided it was. I had to believe Thomas' blackness would show up on our behalf one day. I have lived long enough to be proven wrong.

Women were outraged at the lack of sensitivity and the bravado of senators as they questioned Hill. Democrats and Republicans were equally brash. At one end, you had Republican senators trying to prove Hill to be a liar with outrageous claims; on the other hand, you had Democratic senators asking extremely personal questions, trying to prove Hill had no ulterior motive. Anita Hill became every woman who had ever been subjected to a sex joke; placed in an awkward situation as a male colleague talked about his sex life; repeatedly asked out on dates; the object of sexual advances, and even had her job threatened. Women took their rage to the polls. If male senators couldn't do the job right, we would elect women who would have our best interests—and that's exactly what happened. Women ran for office in record numbers. A year to the month of the Thomas confirmation hearing, four women won United States Senate seats. They were Carol Moseley Braun, in Illinois; Patty Murray, in Washington state; and two women from California—former San Francisco Mayor Dianne Feinstein and Barbara Boxer.

When Kgosie called me, I was surprised. I didn't know Carol; I just knew of her. Occasionally, she came by PUSH for the Saturday forum, typically during election season. I thought she was qualified enough to be a senator. She attended the University of Chicago Law School, had been a prosecutor for the U.S. attorney general and had held elected office for thirteen years. She was currently the Cook County recorder of deeds. However, I knew Kgosie and considered him as political family and a friend. He came to work at the Rainbow Coalition as the road manager for Reverend Jackson around the time I moved to D.C. in 1985.

Kgosie was born in South Africa and raised in Great Britain because of his family's involvement in the African National Congress (ANC). He attended Harvard, spoke four languages fluently, favored Armani suits—and wore his arrogance like one of his tailored suits, with no shame. Early on, Kgosie had a lot of critics and was often reduced to Reverend Jackson's valet. That was laughable. Kgosie was brilliant and way too arrogant to be anyone's valet. In fact, his pedigree was South African political royalty. His grandfather, Zachariah Keodirelang Matthews, was a member of the African National Congress and helped write the ANC Freedom Charter. Kgosie had gone through his telephone book and called some of the Jackson campaign people who knew people that knew people. I was one of those people. He offered me a job right off the bat, but I wasn't too sure because I had a pretty decent job at the Girls Scouts of Chicago. Dr. Cannon had gone through her telephone book during her lunch hour once a week to make calls to people who could get me a job or who knew people who could get me a job. I sat at her side as she asked her friends for a favor and introduced me; she then handed the phone over. She had gotten me into graduate school and was determined to get me a job, too. It was a contact of hers who passed the Girl Scout job announcement our way. The biggest draw for me was its programmatic girls-only aspect that allowed girls to flourish without the pressure of boys. I had even wanted to join the Girl Scouts when we moved to Evanston, but Mama said no. Well, I got my chance to wear that polyester uniform more often than I ever wanted.

I was helping to expand the Chicago council into disadvantaged areas. I had a healthy paycheck, benefits and a consistent work schedule that allowed me to balance school. I was taking classes in the master's program at UIC two nights a week. After my first semester, I was given a partial academic scholarship. Dr. Johnson, the chair of the political science department, told me he doubted if I would be able to keep up because my GRE scores were low, and that he had accepted me into the program to get that "crazy lady" off his back. He later admitted that Dr. Cannon was correct in her assessment of me. The following fall, I was given a full fellowship for the master's program. I was entering my fourth semester at UIC when Kgosie called me. I knew that working for a senatorial candidate and going to school would require a fine balance. The hours alone on a political campaign were a big leap from Girl Scouts. Kgosie lobbied hard. He asked me to consider coming into the campaign as Carol's traveling aide. By her side, my task was to ensure that her public appearances went smoothly, get her through the crowd, and work the room, the press, and other important people she needed to see face to face. I was to share this role with a woman, Sydney Frey (Petrizzi), who had been with Carol since the beginning of the campaign. Sydney had been struck by the feminist bug after the Thomas hearing and wanted to do something—anything. She reached out to Carol and told her if she ran for office that she would quit her six-figure job as an executive at *Mirabella* magazine, and she had kept her promise.

Unfortunately, Sydney traveling with Carol had caused some talk in the Black community. In Chicago, a white woman traveling with a Black candidate gave off this Hyde Park, University of Chicago, upper-middle-class intellectual liberal vibe that felt elitist. Not even a full two months into the campaign, Sydney was criticized for a lack of cultural respect. One example Kgosie gave me was that she wore pants into Black churches. In 1992, that was a big *How dare you!* A Black woman sharing this role was Kgosie's solution. I felt honored he had asked me. I was certainly capable, with two presidential campaigns under my belt. If I took the job, Kgosie agreed not to interfere with the two nights a week that I had class. To pull it off would require a lot of juggling. I agreed to meet with Moseley Braun. From the get-go, it all seemed like a formality more than an interview. She got right to the point: "You are certainly qualified; Kgosie speaks highly of you." She was pleasant, and I was sucked in quickly.

"What do I have to do to bring you on board?" she asked, matter-of-factly.

"I need comparable pay to my current salary," I answered. After my call with Kgosie, I had checked around to get a feel for her reputation and had received mixed results. The only consensus was that I shouldn't quit my job for less than what I was currently making. No one thought she had a chance of winning, and that if I left my good job on a chance, I should at least be paid.

"Consider it done," she said without any hesitation. *That was too easy*, I thought.

"Most importantly," I said, "When this campaign is over, good, bad or indifferent, I need you to ensure me that you will use all of your political weight to get me a new job." I paused and then continued, "with health insurance."

"Done," she said. I looked at Carol intently, trying to discern the truth in her words. I couldn't be certain. She was a hard person to read so I glanced at Kgosie, and he nodded with a vote of confidence that I could trust her. I reiterated, "If I leave my job with health insurance to come work for you Ms. Braun, you have to guarantee me that you will take care of me when this is over." She looked at Kgosie and he nodded to her. I cut my eyes toward him and, again, he gave me a reassuring look.

"You can call me the patronage queen," she said, flashing that beautiful smile of hers. "I will take care of you." She stood. I also stood and we shook hands on the deal; she then left the room. That is how political deals are made in Chicago. Former Mayor Richard J. Daley, the political boss of bosses, once said, "If a man's handshake is no good, all the [legal] paper in the world won't make it good."

Leaving Girl Scouts and giving up my health insurance was scary. I was relieved by Carol's commitment to me, but I still had to figure out a way to continue my AZT regimen on the front end without health insurance. The cost was running somewhere between eight hundred and a thousand dollars a month at the time, and I certainly couldn't afford to pay out of pocket. I had been on AZT for a little over two years. When I left my job with Ms. Rivers, I was fortunate enough to stay in the same HMO at Girl Scouts without missing a beat. I spoke with my doctor, and she prescribed me a three-month supply of AZT before I quit my job. We weren't sure if the pharmacy would fill such a large order, but we had to try. If I couldn't get the medication, I would have reconsidered working on the campaign. To our surprise, the large prescription was not questioned. This would at least hold me over until after the primary election. My logic was simple: If Carol lost, then she would help me find a new job with health insurance, as promised. If she won, I would stay on staff and renegotiate my salary so that I could purchase AZT, if need be. Either way, it seemed like a win-win situation.

With all my ducks in a row, I took the job. I wasn't so caught up in the feminist euphoria that flooded the air. Neither would I have called myself a feminist at the time— at least not as I knew it in the ten years I had worked in politics. I agreed with the basic principle of equality for women but I had issues with feminist organizations and the women involved, much like I had with the peace movement, there was very little if any intersectionality. My vagina was invited to sit at the table, but my Blackness was not welcome. Nevertheless, I was an avid reader of *Ms. Magazine* and admit to being starstruck when Gloria Steinem visited the campaign headquarters. Yet, even with the respect I had for her, white women, as best as I could tell, had not made room around the table for their Black counterparts. My motivation to work on the Moseley Braun campaign was more about Black liberation and the advancement of Black people. There had only been three Black senators prior to this time. Two—Hiram Revels and Blanche Kelso Bruce—were elected in the aftermath of the Civil War in 1870, and both represented Mississippi. It took another ninety-seven years for the next Black person—Edward Brooke, from Massachusetts—to be elected, and he had been out of office for thirteen years. A victory would be a political upset.

I arrived at the campaign office bright and early that cold Monday morning in January. I was introduced to Sydney, and we were getting acquainted while waiting for Carol's arrival. After about an hour, Gus Fordham, her driver, phoned from the car to say they were on the way. Shortly after Gus hung up the phone, Sydney received a phone call and excused herself to take it—and never returned. After about thirty minutes, it became clear to me and everyone in the office that I had been ditched. I didn't know what the heck was going on or what to think. Everyone had a lot to say, and some of it was not favorable to Carol. *What in God's name is this crazy shit?* I thought. Even if Carol had changed her mind, why would she behave like a mean girl? I was embarrassed and hurt by the public display of disrespect. Barbara Samuels—who had a couple of different roles in the campaign and was a personal friend of Carol—called Kgosie to inform him Carol had ditched me. He was headed to the office and asked me to wait.

Kgosie arrived and asked me to come into his office. Apologizing profusely, he motioned for me to take a seat.

"WHAT THE FUCK IS GOING ON, KGOSIE?" came out of my mouth, before I knew it. Still standing, he picked up the phone receiver. "I cannot believe she did this," he muttered. Sydney answered the car phone.

"Put Carol on," he demanded and placed his finger to his lips to signal for me to be quiet. "What's going on, Carol?" he asked.

"What do you mean?" she responded, like she didn't know why he was calling.

"Carol, you know what I'm talking about," he answered. Carol asked him to take her off the speaker phone. He lied and told her he was alone in the office. I saw that as a good sign. In the political family, loyalty is everything. Kgosie had my back. It took a little back-and-forth before he convinced her he was alone, then she continued.

"I changed my mind," Carol said, as easily as she had said, "Call me the patronage queen," the day she hired me.

"What do you mean? You changed your mind?" Kgosie yelled, his British accent sharp as a razor blade. "I thought that we had agreed on this?"

"NO!" Carol hollered." YOU decided. I didn't decide anything."

"Carol," he said, pleading.

"I don't want her with me!" she doubled down. They argued for over fifteen minutes. The conversation turned into a fight about who was in charge. I listened in total disbelief. She never gave him a satisfactory reason about why she changed her mind. She simply said, "I don't want her with me, I have Sydney." I remembered Carol saying. "I don't need her." I wanted to jump up and scream *FUCK YOU and your mama, too!* like we'd done on the playground in Chicago. I experienced anger, frustration and disappointment all at once. At that point I didn't know if I even wanted to vote for Carol, much less work for her, but I was between a rock and a hard place. If I walked away with no money coming in and only a three-month supply of AZT, I would be in trouble. I needed to keep this job. By the time Kgosie hung up, my stomach was churning and my head was pounding. Carol had instructed him to find me something else to do. He was obviously frustrated. At least she didn't tell him to fire me. As soon as he hung up, I asked, "What the fuck did you drag me into?" Tears welled in my eyes. "I quit my job to be fucked over?" I asked.

"This is bullshit, Kgosie, and you know it!" At that moment, I remembered how much I hated Chicago politics and politicians. It had been said that Carol was an anti-political machine elected official—which, for me, meant she was against the backroom deals and corruption that plagued Chicago politics for decades. In my opinion, her politics were just as ruthless and dirty as the machine.

Kgosie tried to convince me Carol wasn't as bad as she seemed, but that ship had sailed. I had no illusions. My official position was advance coordinator. It wouldn't have mattered what position I held; I was doomed from the beginning. I was assigned to Desiree Tate, Carol's scheduler who had also been hired by Kgosie. I didn't know Desiree prior to this campaign, but I had heard her name here and there. She had been Harold Washington's scheduler and I knew that she and Velma Wilson were good friends. Velma, who was very well-connected in Chicago, was Carol's fundraiser during the primary. I had known her since my first week back at PUSH ten years earlier. Velma was in and out of the Jacksons' home, traveled with Mrs. Jackson sometimes and helped to coordinate the PUSH galas. She was the only person I believed I could trust—and because she trusted Desiree, I would come to trust Desiree, too.

Kgosie decided I would advance some events do whatever Desiree needed me to do and accompany Carol on the important Black events. I assumed this was the compromise Carol made with Kgosie about me. My pride had been kicked in the gut, to state it mildly. I wanted to quit, but Mrs. Jackson told me to be a woman and stick it out. In her opinion, there was no point in running from difficulty. I was also friends with Carol's driver, Gus. He'd been Reverend Jackson's driver and I considered him family. He did his best to help make me feel at ease in the tense environment, but he was also between a rock and a hard place because Carol demanded loyalty. I tried my best to bounce back emotionally from one of my worst workdays ever, but Carol made my life even more difficult.

One evening, I escorted her to this big African American event at the Chicago Hilton Hotel. Gus picked me up, and we picked up Carol. She was cordial and I thought, *It may not be a bad night*. We entered the event over an hour late, and our tardiness was a bad political move. It had been rumored that when Carol showed up for a Black event, she was often late and didn't stay long. This was another reason Kgosie wanted me to travel with her. Black Chicagoans were still watching and whether her behavior was intentional or not, it needed to change if she was going to get a big Black turnout on Election Day. Bad news travels fast. By the time we arrived back at the campaign office that evening, Kgosie already knew we'd been over an hour late.

As soon as we walked into the office, he called a debriefing with the senior team to find out what went wrong. One of the major critiques of Carol's campaign was that we had no structure. Kgosie had tried to create some structure during the primary. Desiree said as much when she talked with Jeannie Morris for her book on Carol, *Behind the Smile: The Story of Carol Moseley Braun's Historic Senate Campaign;* "He tried. I mean, when we started getting paid, Kgosie saw that we never missed a paycheck, and you do miss paychecks at some campaigns. He would order food for everybody and pay from his own pocket." The truth was, when Kgosie took the helm the campaign had already started to fall apart. Carol was surrounded by well-meaning people, but none of them knew what the hell they were doing. Whatever faults Kgosie might have had, he at least made it more of a campaign than it ever had been. I firmly believe that if not for him, Carol would not have made it over the finish line. His role was complicated by the fact that he and Carol were in a relationship and, say what you will, Carol would not be controlled. She willed her agency and dared anyone to challenge her.

"What happened?" was the first thing out of Kgosie's mouth in the meeting. It was my responsibility to ensure Carol's public appearances ran smoothly, including punctuality. Kgosie looked at me. "I asked, why were you so late?" Everyone turned to me, including Carol. I felt a drop of sweat roll down my belly. In those seconds I tried to calculate the outcome. I looked at Kgosie, and the expression on his face said that my job was on the line. I told the truth.

"We arrived ahead of time, but Carol sat in the car and read a newspaper," was my response. As soon as we'd pulled up to the Hilton, Carol opened the paper and started reading. Gus pulled the car back a little so that he wasn't right in front of the driveway. I was bewildered. Both Gus and I kept Carol abreast of the time, but she was not going to budge until she was ready. After she laid the paper aside, she pulled out her pretty Guerlain face powder compact, wiped the shine off her face and touched up her lipstick; then, she was ready to go inside. Kgosie went off! Carol didn't say a word. In a split second, I understood Sydney would never have told. However, my loyalty was not to Carol per se, but to the campaign she was trying to win. That day, I assumed we were a team trying to correct mistakes that negatively affected the campaign. I was wrong, at least in Carol's view. I didn't open my mouth again. Kgosie and the rest of the staff talked about all the dumb shit Carol was doing, and how to do damage control. Carol tried to defend her action but got nowhere. She was seething. When the meeting dispersed, I went straight to Desiree's office. Carol must have been right on my heels. When I turned around, she was standing right in front of me. She walked up to me, backing me into the counter cabinets in the office. For a second, I believed she was going to hit me. I didn't move. I didn't open my mouth. Shoot, for a second, I think I even stopped breathing.

"Don't you EVER tell on me!" she said, moving up on me until we were within breathing distance from one another. I braced myself: *Oh, God.* She moved back a tad and asked, "Don't you know who I am?" My heart was pounding. I didn't know how to respond but I knew I had to say something. I started rambling off what I thought. She cut me off.

"I don't care what you thought you were doing. No one tells on me!" Tears formed in my eyes. "Don't play with me little girl. You're outmatched." She said and started to move away. "You will not win." She turned and walked out of the room. A relief came over me like when I was a little girl and Mama didn't beat me. Tears flooded my face. Desiree came into the office to find me a complete mess. I cried and explained and cried some more. After I calmed down, she and Velma convened a meeting at Desiree's house later that night and devised a plan to keep me out of Carol's way as much as possible. I believed that if not for Desiree and Velma, I would not have lasted until the end of the primary.

I never understood the source of Carol's hostility toward me. There were rumors about Kgosie dating other women, but I was not one of them. I tried to stay as far away from that mess as I could. Velma and Desiree asked me if I had ever dated Kgosie. And I told them, NEVER. I never thought about it and was never going to think about it, not in this lifetime. I recounted to them my one and only experience that remotely touched upon the subject of Kgosie and me. During Reverend Jackson's '88 campaign, we were sitting next to each other on the press bus one day, and he looked at me and asked, "How about you and me?" I laughed so hard. "Negro, please," I said. "Just wondering," he said, and laughed it off. Now, if *that* was a pass, he never made one again.

All I know for sure is that Carol has stayed with me over the years. I've tried to understand why I was so hurt—crushed, really. Maybe, in part, she triggered my deep-seated issues with rejection. Or maybe it was that she was the antithesis of the other Black women I had encountered in my first ten years around PUSH and during the campaign. Even with strong personalities, they sowed into me the good things that would help shape me into a woman. Granted, at twenty-nine, I was no longer that wide-eyed, innocent young girl who came to PUSH, but I still had the same intention: to help bring about change. I had come to help Carol make history so she could help make change and had been profoundly disappointed. I have known since I was a little girl that you treat people how you want to be treated. Carol had failed miserably.

After that night, I advanced Carol a few more times. I advanced her downstate trip to Champaign-Urbana. I even continued to use my resources. While on this trip I tapped into Martin King, a long time friend and activist who was in law school, to help me. I mostly stayed the hell out of her way. By far, these were the most stressful three months in a long time. I had a knot in my stomach every freaking day. I was juggling school, AZT side effects, the campaign, and the tension. That Carol hadn't fired me gave me a glimmer of hope she would keep her word to get me a job with health insurance when the campaign was over.

It wasn't until after the primary that I understood she wasn't going to fire me then because she and Kgosie needed whatever experience and contacts I had. During the primary, I was so knee-deep in it that I became a people-pleaser. No matter what Kgosie asked, I came through. Maybe somewhere in my subconscious I thought that by completing one more task with excellence, Carol would treat me with some decency. When Kgosie was planning Carol's first Washington, D.C. trip, no one was answering his calls. Actually, most people did not support Carol's candidacy until after she won the primary. Kgosie asked me if I could help. I went through my Rolodex. The first person I called was my good friend Carlotta Scott, who still worked for Congressman Ronald Dellums. Between the two of us and whatever little headway Kgosie and Desiree were able to make, the trip was a success. Kgosie would circle back and thank me for helping him pull it off, but it never changed how Carol treated me.

On another occasion, Velma wanted to host a fundraiser for Carol that targeted people in their twenties and thirties. She approached one of my housemates, Ray Anderson, about being the lead. I sat on the committee with other young adult movers and shakers in Chicago—Michelle Robinson (Obama), Wally Burris, Jesse Jackson Jr. and others—to host the event. We pulled off one heck of an evening at one of the most popular nightspots in Chicago, the Kaboom nightclub. Not only did we have a packed house, but we featured an impressive list of speakers, including Jesse Jackson Jr., Christopher Kennedy (son of former U. S. Senator Robert F. Kennedy), Barack Obama and J.B. Pritzker (of the Pritzker dynasty, and the current governor of Illinois).

Chaos followed the campaign up until the very end, election night, March 17, 1992. Earlier that day, I had helped Velma and Desiree decorate and rushed home to change. Veronica wanted to attend the victory party and I hitched a ride back with her. When I arrived, people had started to file into the ballroom and, before I knew it, there were wall-to-wall people. Carol was winning and people wanted to be where the action was. The crowd was growing, and so was the press, and the area in the ballroom where they had been placed became overcrowded. For a while, I was the only staff downstairs; everyone else was upstairs putting out fires. The moment I spotted Desiree in the ballroom, I told her that press had started to become anxious, and they needed to send the press secretary down. "That girl has lost her mind," Desiree told me. She explained that Celia was having a meltdown and refused to leave her room. That the press secretary was too afraid to come out of her room to handle the press was a satire unfolding before my eyes. Some of the Chicago press knew me from working with Reverend Jackson and started pulling me to the side to ask about interviews with Carol. John Davis, Jay Levine, and Carol Marin had all given me their interview requests. Other press saw them talking to me and, before I knew it, I had a stack of requests. Everyone was vying for that first interview with Carol. Desiree told me to keep accepting them until they figured out what they were going to do. After a while, I stepped out into the hallway and spied Kgosie. "The press is losing their mind, Kgosie," I said. He confirmed what Desiree had told me. "That crazy broad won't come out of her room," he said.

"What do you want me to do with these press requests?" I asked as I handed him my notes.

"Handle it for me," he responded. After I had gathered all of the requests, I went into the corner to devise a plan. I had promised John Davis, CBS News, I would do my best to see that he received the first interview, and then have Carol talk with the other big names for Chicago local news. After Carol's speech, I escorted her straight to John and then to the other interviews, making sure the local press had first dibs—and it went off without a hitch. I went home that night and thought, *This woman is very close to becoming a United States Senator.* I was happy and sad. We had been a serious mess, yet we had seen Carol through to victory. When I arrived at the campaign headquarters early the next morning, the telephones were ringing off the hook. A couple days later, there were rumors Kgosie was restructuring the campaign, which is not uncommon. Everyone was wondering if they would still have jobs, including me. Our ma-and-pa operation was coming to a close. It was time to bring in the big guns. In the end, very few people who had used their resources in the primary were kept on for the general election. I had given Carol Moseley Braun all that I had, and she had given me nothing but grief. I was willing to kiss her ass all day and night if it meant I could make a way to get my HIV medication. I didn't know if I wanted to stay on staff, but I surely expected Carol to honor her commitment to me. Kgosie and I had a meeting. He conveyed Carol's thanks for saving the night, saying, "Carol knows you covered her butt election night and appreciates it very much." He assured me that as long as he had a job, so would I. A few weeks after that meeting, Kgosie and I stood in the same spot as he terminated me. Honestly, I was surprised I had lasted that long.

"Carol doesn't want you here anymore," he said. "I've tried everything." I gave him a doubtful look. I knew it was every man and woman for himself or herself at that point. He told me he was tired of fighting with her about me. I asked about Carol's promise to me. I asked for severance pay. Kgosie told me he would try, but it was doubtful. He doubled back to me later and told me Carol said the only thing she would do for me was to accept a letter of resignation rather than say I was fired. It was ironic that I had hated Chicago politics and most of the politicians because of how they treated people; now, I was on the receiving end of what I hated most about them. For a brief moment, I thought about explaining my situation to Kgosie—that I had HIV and needed medication—but I wasn't sure if I could trust him anymore. I doubted if it would do any good, anyway. Carol had been so heartless I couldn't take any more humiliation. Instead, I went into the bathroom and cried. Carol was correct about one thing: I was outmatched. I submitted my letter of resignation on April 6, 1992. I had come into a project I believed was for me—one pregnant with possibilities. Instead, it miscarried all the potential I thought was waiting for me. I was without a job and health insurance and was running out of AZT.

The next day, I received a telephone call from Joe Gardner to inform me a reporter was trying to track me down for an interview, and he asked if he should give her my number. I said no. There was a lot of media buzz about the disorganization of Carol's campaign, about Kgosie and women, and Kgosie and Carol. I chose not to discuss the campaign publicly. Again, I was between a rock and a hard place. If I talked to the reporter, that would make me a snitch—and no one wants a snitch in private circles. Honestly, I wouldn't know what to tell except that the first soon-to-be-elected female African American senator didn't like me. Rather, I chose to say I left the campaign to complete my education. The other thing—for as much grief as Carol had given me and as much as I had come to dislike her because of it—was that she was impressive and very qualified. I didn't want to contribute to the witch hunt. If she won, she and all her brilliance—with her flaws hanging close to her coattail—would make history. That was important, at least for me. No one is perfect. I decided to take one for the Black Woman team.

Fifty

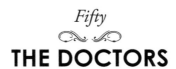

THE DOCTORS

" I retain a terrible reputation for excessive optimism.
The glories of humankind's ingenuity and inventiveness have not yet
been exhausted. The future can be bright, but only if we work to make it so.**"**
—Quentin Young, MD

I was out of work, and out of AZT. To make matters worse, I couldn't find a job for the life of me. No one would touch me with a ten-foot pole. With all the rumors about Carol and Kgosie, along with my unwillingness to talk about the inner workings of the campaign, it gave the impression I was hiding something. Others, even volunteers, talked to the media about the chaos. And people reasoned my silence meant something was wrong with me. I started to sink into a deep depression. I told everyone I was fine and tried to focus on school, but I was not speaking the truth. My spirit was broken. People told me I would bounce back, but then no one really understood how desperate I was to find a job with health insurance. All those people who wouldn't return Carol's calls during the primary whom I considered allies now wouldn't return my calls, now that she was that much closer to being a senator.

On top of all that, Noble and I were arguing all the time. One day while dropping me off at school, he and I had tense words. The light in me started to float out of my body. I had never given up to the point where I couldn't see at least a glimmer of hope at the end of a tunnel. That part scared the fuck out of me. When I got into the building, instead of going to class, I went straight to a campus phone and asked if we had a counseling service. Tears were streaming down my face by the time I was connected to the office. They told me, "Come right now." I completed all the forms and a woman counselor saw me immediately. I hadn't seen a therapist in five years—when my mother cut off her breasts. I cried and cried and cried. After almost two hours, Dr. Rebecca had gotten me together enough to go home. The receptionist told me there was a waiting list, and this was a one-time emergency appointment. The next day, they called me back, and I began seeing the same therapist two days a week to coincide with the days I had class.

I was at my wit's end finding a job. Then, as quick as the snap of a finger, my luck changed. One day, Michelle Robinson (Obama) was over to our house. We were chatting and she asked what I was doing with myself these days. "Looking for a job," I said. She told me her fiancée, Barack, was working on a voter registration campaign and needed staff; she would see if he could use me. That next week, Barack hired me to serve as the youth/student coordinator for Project Vote. I didn't want to be relegated to youth and students, but I would have organized skid row at that juncture. The pay was measly and there were no benefits, but some money coming in was better than none. I hadn't paid rent in a month. Thank God for Mrs. Jackson's benevolence, or I would have been staring at an eviction notice.

Barack Hussein Obama, who would become the 44th president of the United States, was, at the time, the coordinator of the Cook County voter registration campaign for Project Vote. We were friendly, but I mostly knew him as the love of Michelle's life.

He had taken time away from writing his memoir, *Dreams of My Father,* to run this voter registration campaign. Project Vote was a not-for-profit that focused on voter registration in mostly impoverished Black and Brown communities across the county. Now that we were in a hotly contested Senate race, the organization had landed in Chicago. We rented office space from the Community Renewal Society, another not-for-profit organization located in downtown Chicago. More than "office space," we had a strip of desks partitioned from other offices inside their suites. We had a small paid staff and most of us spent almost all our time in the field or, like me, on the phones plugging student leaders into our voter registration campaign.

Barack ran a phenomenal voter registration campaign that had a powerful punch. He was the master at community outreach, leaving no stone unturned. He was laid-back and easygoing as a supervisor; however, he was meticulous and focused. He valued my opinion but, most importantly, he wanted results. It was refreshing to be in a positive environment after three months of working on the campaign from hell. I could even appreciate Barack's dry humor. Most importantly, we moved as a team with one goal and a whole lot of purpose. Our campaign slogan, "It's A Power Thing," sent a message that we (Black people) had not given up and were willing to fight for a seat at the table. I hadn't realized how much I missed the movement atmosphere while working on the Braun and Dukakis campaigns. Project Vote gave me something to believe in again.

The registration campaign was reminiscent of Harold Washington's '83 primary campaign. Posters and buttons were everywhere. I think, in part, Carol's primary victory had re-energized Black Chicagoans and helped to fuel our work. It was as if someone had turned the switch back on. Even with all the gossip circulating about the dysfunction inside her campaign, the Black community held a lot of pride in Carol's victory. We had lost so much politically after Harold Washington's death. With all the infighting and the special election that would cost us the seventh floor (the mayor's office) we had lost faith. Her campaign gave African Americans hope again. We trained close to a thousand voter registrars throughout Cook County. Money and resources were coming from everywhere, including thousands of dollars from Soft Sheen Products, a Black-owned hair-product company in Chicago. We had radio ads and our registrars went to summer festivals, shopping malls, churches, beauty shops and barbershops—anywhere people were most likely to be. In the end, we registered approximately one hundred and fifty thousand people.

Right around the time I began working at Project Vote, I received my first discouraging report from Dr. Leitman since I had begun the NIH study five years earlier. My CD-4 T-cell count had dropped, and she recommended I get more blood work in a couple of months. If there was no improvement, I should begin taking a new medication called didanosine (DDI). At the bottom of her letter she wrote, "Please make sure you have an active health insurance policy soon! DDI is expensive."

I felt like everything came crashing down on me at once. I had been off AZT for a couple of months with no money to purchase more and, now, Dr. Leitman was talking about another medication that cost even more than AZT. A whole new set of emotions about health insurance emerged. I didn't know who to be angry with: myself for leaving the Girl Scouts, thus losing my medical insurance; Carol for reneging on her promise; or a healthcare system that was more concerned with profits over patients. The update scared the daylights out of me. Dr. Leitman had never asked me to get blood work done outside her study. I knew this had to be serious. One thing was crystal-clear to me: I needed a job with health insurance, and fast. I started making inquiries as soon as I received that letter. It was Barack who informed me that Physicians for a National Health Program (PNHP), which also shared office space in Community Renewal, was looking for a national field director.

PNHP had been advocating for a single-payer healthcare system in the United States since 1986. Rev. Jesse Jackson and a host of others advocated for universal healthcare—a public-option medical delivery system paid for with citizens' taxes. In fact, Rev. Jackson had campaigned on single-payer. The two founders of PNHP, Drs. Steffie Woolhandler and David Himmelstein, had advised Rev. Jackson on health policy for both of his campaigns. To my surprise, there was even more overlap with PNHP and my political world. Their national president, Dr. Quentin Young, was Reverend's personal physician and an adviser on healthcare reform.

When I approached Dr. Young, I learned Barack had already put in a good word for me. You never know where your blessing will come from. I had known of Dr. Young, but we had never met until now. His reputation as a human-rights activist was older than me the day we officially met, and I was thirty years old at the time. He was a co-founder of the Health and Medicine Policy Research Group in Chicago. An antiwar and civil-rights activist, he also founded the Medical Committee for Human Rights, which provided medical care to civil-rights workers during the Mississippi Freedom Summer, and he helped set up the Black Panthers' and Young Lords' community health clinics.

PNHP had expanded from Boston to Chicago six months prior to my employment. I was hired on a year-long grant to specifically help grow the organization's field operations. The paid staff consisted of me and the executive director, Ida Hollander. We had a slew of doctors who volunteered time and resources to the organization. In addition to Dr. Young, Dr. Ron Sable was the national coordinator for PNHP. An internist at Cook County Hospital, Ron was a well-known gay-rights activist in Chicago who ran for City Council. The board of directors was also very active and provided support to the staff. The board members I worked with the most were Dr. Gordon (Gordy) Schiff, an internist at Cook County Hospital; and two African American women, Dr. Linda Rae Murray—who, at the time, was the medical director at Near North Health Services and Dr. Claudia Fegan. Schiff and Fegan would later serve as PNHP National presidents.

This was an exciting time to be at PNHP. Healthcare reform was at the top of the progressive agenda in the 1992 election season, a direct impact of the '88 primary. Rev. Jackson had awakened the progressive wing of the Democratic Party about so many issues, including healthcare reform. Bill Clinton capitalized from Jackson's agenda to placate progressives by addressing healthcare reform on the campaign trail. Once elected, he established a White House Task Force on Health Care Reform chaired by Hillary Clinton. Her appointment caused a stir and brought forth the best of misogyny regarding the role of a first lady. Still, there was no single-payer advocate on the committee chaired by Clinton until Rev. Jackson insisted on the inclusion of one. He, Dr. Young and Dennis Rivera, the head of the 1199 National Health Workers Union, met with Hillary Clinton to discuss the matter. As a result, Dr. Vicente Navarro landed a spot on the task force. The entire country was talking about healthcare reform. And it was a great organizing tool. I was on the phones from day one, using lists of doctors the PNHP board members gathered. Mainly, my role was to help expand the organization's chapters and reach across the country. PNHP's overall goal was to educate doctors and other healthcare workers on the need for "a comprehensive, high quality, publicly funded healthcare program, suitable [for] and accessible to all residents of the United States." I was pitching both forums on single-payer and the formation of chapters to doctors. If Dr. Sable was going to an area, I arranged meetings and forums for him. It was constant, grueling phone work, but it kept my mind occupied on something other than my problems.

I worked almost exclusively in the office on the phone organizing. My one road trip was to the National Medical Association's (NMA) national convention held in San Francisco that year to recruit for PNHP.

This was my second trip to San Francisco, and I wondered if it would be my last. Dr.

Leitman had shaken me to the core. I walked the wharf each evening, talking to God and wondering about my future. I had asked Ida to process my health insurance as quickly as possible. Once we completed the paperwork, I learned PNHP had to purchase me an individual health plan rather than a company plan because of our staff size. I had no idea there was a difference in insurance and a different standard for approval until I was denied because I had a pre-existing condition. I was denied two more times. When I received that last denial letter from Blue Cross and Blue Shield Insurance, I cried. If I worked in a company large enough to buy into an HMO that waived pre-existing conditions, I would have been insured. Everything kept going back to Carol's broken promise to me. If she had opened a door for me into government, it would have been all I needed to get health insurance.

Dr. Leitman called again and expressed emphatically I needed to see a doctor sooner rather than later. I finally told Ida I had a pre-existing condition, but I was too embarrassed to tell her or any of the doctors I worked with at PNHP that I had HIV. I'm sure if I had any health issue other than HIV, I would not have hesitated one second about seeking help. She offered to add the premium cost of what PNHP would have paid to the insurance company to my salary but it was not enough even to get blood work up, much less expensive HIV medication. *Make it make sense.*

What finally made me give in was that my fear of dying became more powerful than my fear of being judged. Dr. Leitman had never been so adamant about anything since I had been in her study. I knew my life depended on seeing a doctor. I decided to tell Dr. Sable instead of Dr. Young. I can't really explain it. In retrospect, maybe the intersection of our political worlds gave him more value to me and I didn't want to disappoint him. It was irrational to choose one doctor over the other because I would learn they were birds of the same feather. One evening, I asked Ron if I could speak with him privately. I didn't know it at the time, but I had struck gold. I hadn't been at PNHP very long and Ron was on leave from Cook County; somehow, I missed that Ron and another doctor at County, Renslow Sherer, had opened the Sable/Sherer AIDS Clinic at Cook County Hospital nine years earlier. The way the story goes, just two years into the pandemic, Ron and Renslow's caseload of AIDS patients had grown exponentially. Dr. Gordy Schiff, who was the director of the general medicine clinic, gave them part of a hallway that they partitioned to create the clinic. To have the insight to develop a specialty clinic to treat people living with AIDS was cutting-edge in 1983. Yes, I had walked into a gold mine. Yet again, God placed me right where I needed to be, with the right people at the right time in my life.

The moment Ron stepped into my office, my palms started to moisten and I could feel the perspiration building under my top. "Ron," I said nervously, "I have HIV." When he didn't respond immediately, I started rambling. In usual form, I told him everything in one fell swoop.

"I was in a study at NIH and the doctor informed me that my T cell count has dropped, and I may need to take a medicine called DDI. Ida tried but couldn't get me health insurance," I said. After I had gotten it all out, I started to cry.

"It will be alright, Rae," he said, as he gave me a hug and held me close.

"We will take care of you." And that was the honest-to-God truth. He instructed me to call Gordy Schiff at home to speak with his wife, Dr. Mardge Cohen. That they had different last names confused me, at first. I asked him to explain who I was supposed to call again. I think that in all my years, Mardge was the first married woman I met who kept her maiden name. Gordy answered the phone and I told him Ron had asked me to call his wife.

"Mardgie, you have a call," Gordy said. After telling her Ron had asked me to call, I attempted to explain everything I told Ron. She cut me off.

"Are you saying that you have HIV?" she asked.

"Yes," I said meekly. She instructed me to come to the radiology clinic on Wednesday at one o'clock and she hung up the phone. I stared at the phone receiver still in my hand and wondered why the heck I was going to the radiology clinic when I had HIV. Also, I thought she was a little rude. But I had placed my trust in Ron, and I liked her husband, Gordy. I figured I could at least give her a chance.

I stepped into the radiology clinic and experienced a culture shock. There were wall-to-wall women of different ages, and I couldn't make heads or tails of what the hell was going on. I went to the counter and learned that I was, indeed, in the right place. All the seats were taken and, after I registered, I stood in the corner dressed in a badass black Anne Klein suit and matching black pumps with Dorje's pearls—reminiscent of my first appointment at NIH. I was beating stereotypes with the clothes on my back. It may seem superficial, but it was all I had at the time to keep me from being judged.

I took in the chaotic scene. Some, but not most, of the women looked sick. And even if they didn't have on Anne Klein suits, they were the women in our own families. Women were hugging each other, chatting and laughing like they were at some kind of meet-up. *My God, they are loud. What in the hell?* I thought. *This is a doctor's office, not a picnic.* Every now and then, a woman would shift her eyes at me trying to figure who I was, but I was not going to give any of them an opening. I just turned my head, like *Gurrrl, don't come over here trying to talk to me.* There were some children seated; I wondered if they had HIV, too. The clinic was every Wednesday at one o'clock. I had arrived that day at 12:45. My plan was to see the doctor on my lunch break and go back to work. What's that saying about best-laid plans? After about an hour of standing I finally took a seat. A chaplain assigned to the clinic arrived making rounds from client to client. She eventually made her way to me.

"Hello, I'm Judith," she announced. *Hmm—*, I wondered, meeting her eyes. I looked at that white lady to make sure I had seen a clergy collar around her neck because I didn't know an African American minister who would have introduced herself by her first name. I was curious, but not enough to have a conversation. I was stuck in my attitude. I didn't want to know these people up in here, and I didn't want them to know me. That's it and that's all. I was here to see a doctor, just like I had been in every other clinic or doctor's office I had visited over the years. However, I didn't want my tone to sound rude.

"I'm Rae," I mumbled. She caught my disinterested disposition quickly and kept on moving. She didn't push that day, but Reverend Judith Kelsey-Powell, the pastoral care minister for the clinic, would continue to speak to me. Sometimes she spoke and sat down next to me, not saying another word. I learned she was very popular, as women talked to her about nothing and everything. And that was another thing that didn't sit well with me: *Why are they telling all their doggone business?* Reverend Judith didn't force scripture on the women. In fact, I don't recall her ever opening a Bible. She never demanded a woman stop talking to let her pray, but she ministered to us from the moment she walked into that room until the last patient left. Eventually, we became friends and I learned that she and her husband, who was African American, were pastors in a United Methodist Church.

I had been there for over two hours when I heard my name called. I looked up and saw this petite woman standing about five-feet-one, with brunette hair in a cute bob, holding a file in her hand and impatiently waiting for me to answer.

"Rae Lewis," she called out again.

"That's me," I said, and jumped up.

"I'm Mardge Cohen," she said. I followed her to the examination room. I couldn't believe she was Gordy's wife because Gordy stands well over six-five. However mismatched they were in height, they were both strong advocates for everything that should be right in the world. Their love story began the first day of school at Rush University Medical

College in 1974. They married four years later and had two children, a boy and a girl, who would also become doctors. After Mardge and Gordy completed their medical residency at Cook County Hospital they stayed, and when I met them, they had been there for sixteen years. They would remain for over thirty years before retiring into their second careers.

In 1988, Dr. Cohen founded one of the first HIV clinics for women in the United States, at Cook County Hospital. When the Sable/Sherer AIDS clinic was started at Cook County, very few women were infected; however, by 1988, the number of cases among women had risen by fifty percent. At the time, Mardge was a practicing internist in the general medicine clinic at Cook County Hospital. She often tells the story of the clinic's inception. One day she was cornered by Ida Greathouse, an HIV-positive patient at the clinic. Ida was loud and aggressive, and didn't hold back a damn thing. She wanted to know how Mardge could call herself a feminist when women had been left out of the research and resources for those living with this disease. Women needed child care and had medical conditions with HIV that were different from men, and no one was doing a damn thing about it. Ida had asked her point-blank, "What are you going to do?" And Mardge heard Ida's message loud and clear either "put up or shut up." The Women and Children HIV Clinic (now the Core Center) opened its doors, under Dr. Cohen's leadership, that same year and set out to right this wrong. And just like Sable and Sherer took a hallway and turned it into an AIDS clinic, Dr. Cohen took that small radiology room one afternoon a week to treat women with HIV.

From day one, Dr. Cohen designed the clinic to serve women and their children as a family unit, which explained the children I saw in the waiting room. They would also see a woman's partner. In fact, when I first started dating my ex-husband, he came with me to the clinic to be evaluated and tested for HIV. The concept of a mother and child receiving medical care on the same day was a brilliant idea, and reduced the burden of a double appointment. Dr. Cohen has explained women are often the caregivers in the family and are willing to sacrifice their own care at the expense of others. It was common for a woman with HIV to bring her child to the clinic, but then rarely come back for her own appointment.

In that small clinic space, magic happened. We had pastoral care, internists and pediatricians. There were case managers who got women into drug rehabilitation programs and found them housing and counselors. There was a women's group that provided lunch because some women came to clinic hungry. If needed, even bus money was provided for them to go back home. No stone was left unturned at the clinic because public health officials had long understood that poverty affects health delivery outcomes. We had a gynecologist, and that also lifted the burden of two appointments. I saw Mardge and the gynecologist, Dr. Linda Powell, the same day. Most importantly, it was clear that women with HIV had more gynecological issues than women without—including me. We needed Pap smears every three to six months rather than one to two years because we had more yeast infections, vaginal dysplasia and irregular menstrual cycles. I loved Dr. Powell. She had a gentle way about her. She smelled of motherland oils and wore her dreadlocks in elaborate wraps. I had never seen a physician wear her Blackness with such boldness.

The clientele came in all colors, shapes, sizes, socioeconomic and educational backgrounds, and we each had our own set of issues that landed us with HIV. Our number-one commonality was that HIV had set up camp in our bodies and Mardge Cohen had created a space to affirm that we mattered. I would come to understand that the clinic was the balm I needed to help soothe my soul.

A curtain served as the door for the smallest examination room I had ever seen. It had a desk and a stool for Dr. Cohen, and an exam table that I had to squeeze pass to reach the chair. All the impatience I had detected on the telephone and when she called my name disappeared when I sat in the chair. She listened to my story from the top and then went about taking care of all my needs, working down the checklist one at a time.

I was overwhelmed by the boatload of information she was giving me. I was shocked but mostly ashamed about how ignorant I truly was about this disease. The surgeon general's reports I had read years ago were so out of date. Time had passed, new developments about HIV had come down the pipeline and I had avoided it all to protect my secret. I was determined to never create a reason to be questioned about HIV. Pam and Vergie had already questioned me after Max's death, and that was more than enough. The irony of being ashamed that I was positive and afraid of being judged was that I had rejected my natural curiosity and voracious appetite for information. Now, I was ashamed of being ashamed. In a matter of months, it all changed. I would come to understand that my ability to digest the information Dr. Cohen spouted would mean the difference between how long I lived and how soon I died. Dr. Cohen understood that from the get-go. That's why she spent time with me and the other women and showed tolerance for all our questions, even the ones we didn't know how to ask with efficiency. There was no HMO time clock ticking in that room, with her to usher me out within an allotted time. I would walk out only after she had taken care of my every need and answered every question. The doctors in this clinic understood that sometimes you had to work through the emotional needs before you could even get to the questions about a woman's physical needs. Case managers had to hear about our children, boyfriends and husbands as well as any little story that had triggered us before they could ask us to complete the paperwork. This is one reason I support an ACE's evaluation for every patient, like they currently do in California —under Dr. Burke-Harris' leadership. The better informed the healthcare provider is, the better they can treat a patient. Of course, I was resistant to the case managers. I was gainfully employed and didn't need anyone's welfare, and I had that take on things for months. But just like Reverend Judith wore me down, so did Sheila Cooper, the case manager who spoke to every single woman in the clinic. She sat next to me at every clinic visit, biding her time until I was willing to open up to her.

After that first appointment, I instinctively knew Dr. Mardge Cohen was a keeper. There was something about her that I couldn't pinpoint, but it drew me in. Dr. Cohen was a no-nonsense, tough-love kind of woman; however, just under the veneer, she made you feel you mattered. That day, she prescribed me two HIV medications: 300 mg of AZT, and DDI. She also prescribed fluconazole to prevent fungal infections, both vaginal and oral; and acyclovir to prevent herpes and cytomegalovirus (CMV) of the eye, which caused blindness in people living with AIDS. I hadn't had a herpes outbreak in years, until about six months prior to this visit. I couldn't understand why, after eight years, I had an outbreak every other month, and why they were more painful beyond any I had ever experienced. Despite the pain, I would let the herpes run its course because I couldn't pay for a doctor. Dr. Cohen explained that the herpes virus had become more active because HIV had compromised my immune system. Likewise, it was the reason I had recurrent yeast infections. I didn't even know there were medications to prevent herpes and yeast infections. She also prescribed amitriptyline for depression and HIV-related peripheral neuropathy. Apparently, the tingling I felt from time to time in my feet and legs was also related to my failing immune system. I hadn't mentioned depression, but I guess the crying spells that day was a clear indication. The more she explained, the more I wanted to know. On the way out of the clinic, I slipped a few HIV magazines into my handbag: *Test Positive Aware*, *AIDS Treatment News* and *The Gay Men Health Crisis*. It was the second proactive decision I had made about my life with HIV since Max died; the other one was disclosing my status to Ron, and that landed me at the clinic.

After I left Mardge, I went upstairs to the Fantus Clinic to get lab work. Gee, I hadn't been up there since I was pregnant with Randy's child. The wait was even longer in the lab than I had remembered. I learned, from eavesdropping on the women's conversations in the clinic, it was because no one wanted to draw blood for people with HIV. You better believe I raised hell when I learned the reason. It was my opinion that if a lab technician didn't want to be exposed to people with HIV, that person should get another job. If a tech didn't believe the science that a latex glove would prevent the transmission of HIV, that person didn't deserve to work in that setting. I was unwavering. Slowly but surely, the AIDS activist in me was beginning to rise.

Once I completed my labs, I went to the pharmacy and waited some more. Dr. Cohen had already warned me to drop the prescription off before I went to get labs. When I got back on the bus to head home, it was eight o'clock that night. I had spent eight hours at County and a little over four of them was the wait to fill my prescription—and that was a quick day. The wait was typically five to eight hours. I wanted to go home and come back the next day after work, but the clerk told me the hospital had a rule: You had to pick up your medicine the same day you dropped it off or it was canceled at midnight. The sheer volume of prescriptions dictated such a policy and was another example of how broken the health system was in the United States. County was the only place in Chicago where a person with no health insurance, HIV or not, could see a doctor and receive medications at no charge. Quentin Young had also been the chairman of medicine at Cook County Hospital for nine years and was a strong advocate of the Cook County system. He writes in his book, *Everybody In, Nobody Out: Memoirs of a Rebel Without a Pause*, "I am convinced that until we, as a nation, have a system of universal health care, including everyone — everybody in, nobody out — until we provide that, we as a society must provide care through a system like County." No lies or half-truths were detected because I was proof of the value of Cook County on the one hand, and the failure of the health delivery system in the United States, on the other.

It would take two more presidents after Clinton and eighteen years to pass the Patient Protection and Affordable Care Act that President Barack Obama signed into law March 13, 2010. It was a full-circle moment that the same Barack who hired me to work at Project Vote—which opened a door to doctors I could trust to take care of me—would become the U.S. president to eliminate pre-existing conditions that became the primary reason I could not buy health insurance after my employment with Carol Moseley Braun. Still, the Affordable Care Act would sadly fall short of a public option and gain a friend like Quentin as a critic: "There are sixteen million to twenty million poor people in this country who will not be covered by the Affordable Care Act." On the bright side, Young explained in an interview with Phil Kadner of the *Southtown Star*: "At least under this plan, millions of Americans who had no insurance will get insurance, people with pre-existing conditions can now buy insurance, and children are covered longer under their parents' plans."

On my way home I stopped at The Village, a 24-hour grocery store near my new apartment, to purchase a few groceries. I had ended my four-year residency with the Jacksons a week before my appointment at the clinic. Therapy had been helping to keep me from totally falling apart, but I was hanging on by a thread. My therapist thought that it was time to create a space for myself—one where I could breathe freely and cry openly. I hadn't had a depressive episode like this since after I was diagnosed with HIV. It began with all the madness at the Braun campaign and stayed with me due to being unemployed and uninsurable, thanks to my failing health. And then, there was Noble.

He and I were growing further apart and spending less time together. Looking back, I think I had become bitter. I had hoped Noble would marry me after graduation. Yes, even with his control issues, I wanted to marry him. I didn't want to be alone with HIV.

Instead, he started disappearing, and that is always a sign of a cheater. I became a crazy lady, calling him all hours of the night to no avail and no answer, and showing up at his apartment early mornings to see if he had slept in the bed and if his face towel was dry or wet. I was losing my mind and dignity trying to hold onto him, but it was discovering his real age and the aftermath that caused me to accept it was over.

One day I was standing by his dresser in the bedroom, and I looked down; his driver's license renewal was staring back at me. At first, I didn't know exactly what I was looking at. Something was just off. His birthday was correct, but the year threw me for a loop. I started counting on my fingers, then found a calculator. Noble was almost twenty years older than me. I was stunned! He had been lying to me all those years. The moment he walked back into the apartment, I confronted him. At first, he tried to claim the weight of the lie was on me, because I was the one who had assumed he was only ten years older than me, and that he simply didn't correct me. I looked at him like he was crazy. "Noble," I said to him, "I have been celebrating your birthday every year and you never once corrected me." He knew he was wrong, but he kept trying to flip it. He resorted to the same bullshit I'd had with Bill McGill about snooping. I resented his accusation. In the four years we'd been dating, I had plenty of opportunities to snoop but I respected his privacy. It had been a hard lesson after Bill. In the course of our heated discussion, Noble slapped me so hard the sting reverberated. I grabbed my face, stunned, and I looked at him for a few seconds and went to the bathroom, still holding my face. When I removed my hand, his handprint was painted across my face in red. I didn't walk away that day, but I knew we were done. Mama had beat my ass, and I promised myself I was never going to allow a man to beat me. I only needed time to allow my heart to accept what I knew intellectually.

He helped me move into my new one-bedroom apartment in Hyde Park the day of Barack and Michelle's wedding. After I moved into my apartment, I would see him less and less until we were no longer a couple. I had just enough time to pop into the hair salon on the ground level of my building, dress and head to the church. Rev. Jeremiah Wright, the pastor of Trinity United Methodist Church of Christ, had married my girlfriend Leslie Priest and her husband Mike, and I knew he performed a beautiful wedding ceremony. I was not disappointed. When Barack became President Obama and Michelle became the first lady, I could hardly believe I'd had a window seat to their courtship and marriage, but I had. I felt a sense of pride knowing they were the same couple with whom I had laughed and cracked jokes with at Cornell McClellan's gym, Naturally Fit, but indeed they were. I didn't always agree with President Obama's policies and, yes, I have a list, just like I have for Clinton and the Bushes. Friend or not, I would never sacrifice my ideological worldview, but I have never forgotten he and Michelle had been central to that next phase of my life. That night at their wedding reception, I danced and laughed as if I didn't have a care in the world. I was so skilled at hiding my pain.

That coming Wednesday, I was going to have my first appointment with Dr. Cohen. I had no idea what was waiting for me. I was scared out of my wits. I had assumed the urgency with which Dr. Leitman pushed me about seeing a doctor had to mean my situation was serious, and it was. I had placed five different medications on top of my counter. After I put away the groceries, I was so exhausted physically and emotionally from the day all I wanted was to go to bed. I was thinking I could start taking the medications in the morning. However, on second thought, I could hear Dr. Cohen telling me to begin taking the medications right away. Plus, I had bemoaned that I couldn't get AZT for five months, and now I needed to make good on this blessing. That night would set another pattern; I would follow Dr. Cohen's instructions, no matter how agonizing they might be.

DDI, was the size of a Susan B. Anthony silver dollar—honest to God. I had to take two twice a day. That night I crushed the pills with a glass and mixed them in apple juice. Dr. Cohen had explained that DDI was a chewable pill that could also be taken with water or a non-acidic juice. I took a tiny sip because the smell was already awful. I actually thought I was drinking piss. My first impulse was to pour it down the drain, but I talked myself off that ledge. Dr. Cohen had also been very clear I was to follow the instructions and not make any changes without talking to her first. I quickly forced the mixture down and chased it with water. The aftertaste was awful. I finished taking the rest of the medication and brushed my teeth and tongue to get the taste out of my mouth, but the DDI and toothpaste combination made me nauseated.

If I thought AZT was a monster, well, DDI was the devil—or maybe it was a combination of the two. The next morning, when my alarm went off at six, I was sick to my stomach and felt drugged, like I had taken a Tylenol with codeine in it or something else that strong. My body had to totally readjust to AZT, plus I had the side effects of DDI kicking my tail. I forced myself out of the bed and vomited on the way to the bathroom. I left it right there on my pretty, cream-colored carpet, used the bathroom and laid back across the bed. I just needed a few more minutes, then I would get ready for work. I woke up three hours later. I should have been walking through the door at PNHP, instead, I called in and took the day off. When I finally was able to function, I paged Dr. Cohen. She explained amitriptyline was the culprit that had drugged me and made me sleep. She reduced the dosage of amitriptyline from seventy-five milligrams to twenty-five and I was to work my way back up, but I could never tolerate it and she switched me to Desipramine. There was no way she could adjust the HIV medication; I just had to stick it out until my body adjusted, *if* it adjusted. This became our pattern. We were a team. She was the pilot, and I was the co-pilot. I did everything she asked, and she made the adjustments when I expressed distress.

The next day I called off work again. I needed to take some time to digest the radical change my life had taken overnight. By midday, I walked down 53rd Street, the business strip that still anchors the Hyde Park community. My first stop was the health food store to purchase a marbleized green granite pestle and mortar. If I had to grind DDI twice a day, at least I would do it in something pretty. We were experiencing an "Indian summer" that day and I perused the stores that lined the street to clear my head. When I reached Artwerk, an Black art gallery owned by an African American man named Joe Clark, I stopped in my tracks. I had never purchased a piece from him because they were expensive. Even the prints were outside my budget. Then this color-pencil drawing of a Black lady looking over her naked shoulder captured my attention. I went into the shop and was mesmerized by the detail. She had individual microbraids that looked so real. The blue butterfly perched at the bottom of her torso was simply beautiful. Joe approached me and started pitching the sale. I thought he had lost his mind when he told me the painting cost one thousand and five hundred dollars and that was a "steal of a deal," he explained. "Too deep for my shallow pockets," I told him. I continued to browse around but kept going back to the painting, and each time Joe would pitch the sale all over again with a new angle. He told me the artist W.M. Christian was very ill and needed the money, and that was why the price was so low. I gave him my don't-bullshit-the-bullshitter look. When he said I could pay for it in installments, which was to me the same as layaway, he had a deal. About a month later, I brought her home. My rationalization for the purchase was that I was creating a sacred space for myself, like my therapist suggested. What I didn't know then was that I really was creating a sacred space that would add to my emotional and mental well-being through some very dark patches for the rest of my life.

About nine years after I brought that painting home, I discovered a tiny AIDS ribbon wrapped around the bottom of one of her braids. So many questions fluttered my mind. *How had I missed this little detail all these years? Had the artist passed away from*

AIDS-related complications? I would never get answers, but I don't believe in coincidences. I believe God gives us everything we need when we need it, sometimes through the most unlikely things.

After I gave Mr. Clark a deposit on the painting, I picked up fresh flowers and a vase, and that would become a weekly ritual, reminding me that everything and everybody dies and everything and everybody once lived. Still today, each fresh batch of flowers fills me with gratitude for the life I am still living, no matter the condition of my physical health.

Those two days were the beginning of a whole new life for me, but I didn't understand it then or even a week later. I just kept doing everything that felt right to me. Dr. Cohen felt right to me, and I was correct. In time, she would become "Mardge," my friend. The painting felt right, and it would give birth to the collector in me. As I traveled around the world speaking about HIV/AIDS, I would bring home more art that spoke to my soul. Over the years my collection that would comfort me at the most vulnerable stages of my journey.

When I returned home from my walk, I arranged the flowers in the vase, made me a cup of tea and read the HIV/AIDS magazines I slipped into my purse on the way out of the clinic the day before.

Fifty-One

≈ ✦ ≈

DYING TO LIVE

" Yea, though I walk through the valley of the shadow of death, I will fear no evil: for thou art with me; thy rod and thy staff they comfort me. "
—Psalm 23:4 (KJV)

It was a cold January day, sitting in that cramped corner in Dr. Cohen's office, that I was finally learning the T-cell game—and it was a mindfuck that would take me on a rollercoaster ride for the next four years. I had been taking DDI and AZT for a few months, and my T-cell count had gone up by a whopping ten points. *Thank God,* I thought. Dr. Cohen had a lot of good news that day. The CDC had officially changed the criteria for an AIDS diagnosis to include a T-cell count of two hundred or below; and opportunistic infections specific to women, such as chronic yeast infections, vaginal dysplasia, cervical cancer, pelvic inflammatory disease, pulmonary tuberculosis, and recurrent pneumonia.

Prior to this time, doctors had correlated a lower T-cell count with more illnesses for people with HIV, but T cells had not been included in the definition of AIDS until this change. The first criteria of AIDS were based on infections that had been identified mostly in men who had developed and died from AIDS-related complications. For example, Max Robinson and rapper Eazy-E were both diagnosed with AIDS because they had *Pneumocystis carinii* pneumonia (PCP). Arthur Ashe was diagnosed with AIDS because he had toxoplasmosis, a parasite on the brain. These opportunistic infections that determined AIDS were very unlikely to occur for people with healthy immune systems. It is also true that people with a failing immune system may have a difficult time fighting more common illnesses like bronchitis, which was the case for me when I started seeing Dr. Cunningham in 1988. However, it was that established list of opportunistic infections that defined AIDS.

As the landscape of AIDS changed, it became clear among those specifically working with women that disease progression in HIV looked different for women. Advocates had been pushing the medical and AIDS communities for years on the specific issues facing women and HIV. Still, there had been reluctance to address HIV in women beyond mother-to-child transmission. If a woman was pregnant with HIV the attention was directed toward the child, who was seen as a victim of the mother's wayward behavior. Women weren't permitted in drug studies unless they were on birth control or willing to terminate the pregnancy. It was as if a woman had no importance of her own outside her child. The racism, sexism and misogyny embedded in U.S. culture was apparent in the scientific and medical communities.

In Victoria Noe's book, *Fag Hags, Divas and Moms,* she documents the battle straight women had to fight to gain a platform for women and people of color living with HIV/AIDS. Even within ACT UP, Noe says there was a fight within the organization about focusing on women's issues. Nevertheless, the women's caucus prevailed, and, by the early nineties, the group took to the streets on behalf of women and people of color living with HIV/AIDS. At a protest at NIH on May 21, 1990, protesters demanded that women and people of color be added to HIV studies. Then, in October 1990, ACT UP descended on the CDC in Atlanta and in D.C. on the same day demanding the expansion of the AIDS definition to include women. Even at Cook County Hospital the administration would not admit women to the AIDS ward but scattered them throughout the hospital because there was no bathroom to accommodate them and no money to make the adjustment. In April 1990, ACT UP staged a protest in front of Cook County Hospital. I saw the news report on television. The protesters lined the street in front of County with fifteen mattresses to represent the fifteen empty beds in the AIDS ward that could create a section for women. Within twenty-four hours, County found the thousand dollars to make the adjustments.

I had no idea what planet my brain had been on. I had watched all the news reports on ACT UP and other advocacy groups with a cautious eye—never looking too close for fear someone would notice and assume I had HIV. I remember one time while I was at NIH for my study appointment, ACT UP took over parts of the campus. Protesters were standing on the top of buildings, rolling signs down the sides. They were all over the place, blocking doors and the sidewalks. It was wild, even for radical me. *These crazy people mean business,* I thought. It was bizarre how disconnected I was from activism around HIV/AIDS. I gave a silent *Rah! Rah!* cheer and kept walking to the metro.

Around this time, U.S. Rep. Ted Weiss, chairman of the House Committee on Government Operations' Human Resources Subcommittee, held hearings on the disparities of women and HIV/AIDS. Forty percent of people living with HIV in New York were women. Testimony was given that Social Security weighed heavily on CDC's narrow AIDS criteria to determine disability benefit rulings that women often had to appeal. Some died before being approved. It was argued that a man with Kaposi's sarcoma—another opportunistic infection characterized as a skin cancer that causes purple lesions—would be approved for Social Security disability insurance over a woman whose immune system had been severely damaged by HIV. Frankly, an oral yeast infection in a man with AIDS carried more weight than a woman with a vaginal yeast infection with AIDS. The discrimination was blatant.

Even after the change in definition, it was an uphill battle for women and Social Security benefits. When I first applied for disability, I was flat-out denied although I had a T-cell count below one hundred. I filed an appeal. The appeal representative at the Social Security Administration was a blind man. He patiently listened, with a sober face, regarding how AIDS had changed my life: the pill load, the fatigue, the feeling of pins and needles in my legs and feet all day, the night sweats, diarrhea, and weight loss. When I finished, he said, "I don't know what's wrong with these people up here. You should have never been denied." I won that appeal.

Women had been ignored too long in the AIDS pandemic. I often wondered if, in part, it was because the majority of cases were among Black and Brown women. There— I've said it. Misogyny is one thing, but the addition of racism has followed Black women around medical care for decades, from the stealing of Henrietta Lacks' cancer cells that created a medical revolution to Fannie Lou Hamer's unapproved hysterectomy. Even in 2021, Black and Brown women are often diagnosed late in HIV disease progression and die quicker than men.   In the early nineties, HIV testing among women hardly occurred. For those who were socioeconomically disadvantaged, access to HIV testing was nonexistent unless they ended up in a clinic or hospital exhibiting symptoms of advanced AIDS. Even if a woman requested an HIV antibody test from her physician, it was more common for a doctor to rundown an embarrassing list of questions or dismiss the request altogether because she didn't meet some stereotype about HIV, when the physician could've just ordered the darn test. I have said it before: I thank God for the blood drive where I learned I was infected with HIV because the medical community had absolutely failed women. As 1995, when AIDS was the number-one killer of Black women ages 25-44, doctors were still hesitant to test them. When I first started promoting HIV testing at speaking engagements, women would tell me their physicians told them they didn't need an HIV test. I told them to tell the doctor everyone needs an HIV antibody test, including the doctor. The best anecdote I can give is the time I conducted a weeklong series of HIV/AIDS sensitivity trainings for the administrative staff at a large HMO. The director of human resources, an African American woman, balked when I said doctors discourage women from being tested, especially if a woman was from a high educational or socioeconomic background. Unbeknownst to me, the director went to the doctor's office that week while I was still conducting the workshops to see if I was exaggerating. I was shocked when she reported what she had done. She said the first thing out of her doctor's mouth was that she did not need to be tested for HIV because she was "not that kind of woman." Mind you, she was single, in her forties and dating.

Needless to say, these new changes from the CDC were very much welcomed and considered a step in the right direction. It had taken five years after that day Ida had cornered Dr. Cohen in the general medicine clinic in 1988 for the CDC to make this change. Thank God for Ida Greathouse and other advocates who had been on the front lines for infected women. Dr. Cohen had a right to be excited about these new changes and so did I, once I understood the full scope of them and what they meant for me and other women.

Learning about the changes to the definition of AIDS, it immediately occurred to me that I didn't know the old definition of AIDS, and that was a little disconcerting, to say the least. I had to face the fact that I had not asked Dr. Leitman the important questions over the years. All I ever wanted to know was whether I had transitioned to AIDS, rather than what constituted an AIDS diagnosis. When Dr. Leitman called about switching my medication in June 1992, it was no different; I had asked through tears if I had AIDS. "No," she reassured me. "You do not have AIDS," and that was good enough for me. She said, "This T-cell drop just means that the HIV virus is active." She recommended I switch to DDI because AZT may no longer be effective alone.

At the time, my T-cell count was 134; now, it was 144. Dr. Cohen was happy, saying, "This is a good thing." But it hit me like a paintball in my face. In a matter of seconds, my good news of ten more T cells had turned into bad news. It knocked the fucking wind out of me. In a roundabout way, Dr. Cohen was telling me I had AIDS. I didn't know how to respond except to ask for clarity. "I got AIDS?"

She nodded, adding, "But nothing has changed, Rae." It was her answer and encouragement wrapped in one neat bow. I gave her a side-eye to signify, *Who are you trying to convince—me or you?* We talked it through as always and, surprisingly, after the initial shock, I was fine. When I left Mardge that day, I didn't freak out. I had AIDS, but my fat ass wasn't even close to dying. At least, that's what I told myself to cope. I compartmentalized AIDS, just like I had with HIV. In the same way I kept saying, *At least I don't have AIDS*; now I was saying, *At least I'm not sick.* Nothing had really changed, but everything had changed. Technically I had AIDS, but no one on the planet would have guessed as much. Thank God my secret was still safe. I was optimistic: My T-cell count was up by ten, and I was still a size twelve from eating all that carryout with Noble and the emotional eating I did on my own. I still didn't look sick. My skin was super-clear; I didn't have blotches, like I had seen with other people with AIDS. Also, my hair was thick and healthy, not thinning like the hair of some of the women in the clinic. I didn't feel sick unless you want to count the side effects from AZT and DDI—nausea, fatigue, peripheral neuropathy, headaches, diarrhea, and vomiting. DDI also caused pancreatitis. Thank God I never got that one.

No matter how I tried to avoid the big fat elephant in the room, I was sick, even if I dismissed it. I had already began to show signs of a compromised immune system a year earlier when my T-cell count first dropped. The aggressive herpes and chronic yeast infections were clear indicators, but I didn't know this was the beginning of what AIDS looked like for me. At the time, my doctors didn't know how to treat HIV. Remember that the internist at the HMO deferred to Dr. Leitman on issues around HIV, but Dr. Leitman was not my primary physician, and her NIH study did not provide medical care. I knew something was off. That's why I told the gynecologist at the HMO about the recurrent yeast infections and that I had HIV, and he missed an opportunity to get me additional help. By then, Fluconazole had been approved for systemic candidiasis for people infected with HIV. I wanted him to help fix my vagina but all he could think about was how it (and I) came to be broken. I am almost certain that my Black male doctor would never have responded to a white woman the way he responded to me. It was misogyny at best, and borderline medical malpractice at worst. I need to double down on this point. If I did not know I was infected or had I not begun care with Dr. Cohen when I did, I would have continued down this path until I was so ill, my health could not be dismissed by the medical establishment—which is how most Black and Brown people learned they had HIV. This is the clearest example why testing is as important as a doctor who knows how to treat HIV. I had been embarrassed that I ended up at County but, standing at death's door, it was the best place for me—and being there saved my life.

I continued to tell myself nothing had changed. Therefore, my goals had not changed. I currently had two classes to take; to complete my master's degree in political science. I also had to write my thesis paper, and I was considering a comparative analysis between the 1984 and 1988 Jackson presidential campaigns. After graduation, my plan was to go straight into a Ph.D. program.

I had come a long way in that year since the Moseley Braun campaign. My therapist had gotten me to a good place. It was a lot of painful emotional work, but I was at peace. I trusted her and mostly dealt with these new health developments in therapy. She had been on the mark about me moving into my own space. I settled into a routine of my own and, best of all, I didn't have to argue with housemates over stupid shit. After Rhoda moved out, Karen Warfield, who had known the Jacksons since childhood, moved in. Her father was the executive director of PUSH in the seventies. She didn't stay long and moved out of town after she got this big job. Ray Anderson moved in after Karen. He had gone to high school with Jonathan at Whitney Young and was close to the Jacksons, like me. He stayed until he moved to D.C. to travel with Reverend Jackson. Living with twenty-something men involved more testosterone than I could deal with. One day, Noble and Ray got into an argument because Ray asked me if I would sew a button on his shirt. Ray was standing in my open doorway with his shirt in his hand. Noble was sitting on the love seat and quickly stood up; before I could say anything, he jumped in.

"You don't ask my woman to sew a goddamn thing," Noble said. Things unfolded quickly and before I knew it, Noble and Ray were arguing. Ray was trying to explain he didn't mean any harm and that he viewed me as a sister. Jonathan stepped out of his bedroom. Ray and Jonathan were ready to whip Noble's ass. We still laugh about it but, at the time, I was a nervous wreck. If Noble had not been there, I would have sewed the button but not before telling Ray his request was sexist as hell. That was our way, and I felt that Noble was out of line. Of course, he and I argued about it afterward. I was glad I moved for so many reasons. I wasn't so dependent on Noble to take me to run errands anymore, and that was a freedom I cherished. In the Hyde Park community, I was within walking distance of the Hyde Park Co-op, my favorite grocery store; Walgreens; bookstores; and restaurants. I could walk through my apartment naked if I wanted to. I enjoyed decorating. I purchased my first bookshelves and a beautiful cream sofa with deep cushions that I plunged into on Saturdays to read. I made beautiful lace curtains, and, on a clear day, I could see Lake Michigan. I felt mostly on track.

Work at PNHP was good. When I first began, I didn't know what to expect, but I really liked working with these doctors. I had never met doctors so passionate about healthcare reform or other social justice issues. And it was a new and welcome lens through which to see physicians. I had viewed the medical profession as a career choice to become wealthy. However, these doctors were advocating for change that would place people over profit and were unwavering in their mission. Quentin summed up our work—at the ripe age of eighty-seven, no less: "Healthcare is a human right, and I don't understand why people in this country still refuse to accept that. In every other nation, that's how they look at it." Working at PNHP felt right within my soul.

I had taken this job out of desperation for health insurance and, at first, I felt as if some of my friends had passed me by. Melissa Holloway ran for city council in Jersey City and won. She was earning a reputation as an elected official who used unorthodox political thinking to get things done for her constituents. Unfortunately, ten years later, Melissa would have a stroke and pass away. Her legacy however, had already been cemented when she secured a 150-million-dollar rehabilitation project for her ward. In 2009, two of the new buildings were named after her. At the time she took office, though, I was in my feelings *woe is me*. Melissa was out there slaying dragons, and I was working in the national headquarters of an organization that had a two-person staff. Even though I had a big title—national field director—with a lot of responsibility and good pay, I wondered if the grass was greener on the other political side. Kevin Jefferson called just as I began working for PNHP, saying the Clinton-Gore campaign was looking to hire more Jackson people on the advance team and the job was mine, if I wanted it. The promise was that any of us who came on board would go to the White House or work in the administration if they won. Sure enough, Kevin was now working in the Clinton White House, as were Minyon Moore, Leah Daughtry, Donna Brazile, and my good friend Craig Kirby. I turned the offer down because there was no way in hell I was going to go work on a campaign and forfeit health insurance again. At the time, I had just sent my first health insurance application, and it had not yet been denied. But in the end, it was denied, and I couldn't help but think I had turned down a job of the lifetime and still didn't have health insurance.

At some point, I managed to stop thinking about what everyone else was doing and focused on my job. Plus, in my pity-party comparisons, it never occurred to me that I would have had to give up graduate school if I had taken a job for the Clinton-Gore campaign. Working at PNHP felt as if God had placed me in the center of advocacy work that addressed my own personal crisis. Maybe my commitment to PNHP came from my own experience. I hadn't thought much about health insurance until I was faced with having none. I was the epitome of the health-insurance problem in the United States. My situation was not a theoretical paradigm written in health-reform reports. I was a living, breathing crisis and, like so many others without health insurance, I ended up at the hospital that continues to bear the brunt of the uninsured and underinsured. On top of that, there was nothing like working with Dr. Young. I loved his ability to unpack a topic all the way to the bottom of the box. My God, he was brilliant and passionate. I looked forward to every visit he made to the office, even if it meant I didn't get much work done. Once he got started talking, there was no stopping him. He gave me hope, even not knowing I was infected. His optimism was a thing to be admired and I pulled what I needed when the glass seemed half empty—only to see it was also half full.

Quentin was very proud of the work I did regarding HIV/AIDS and thought it was extremely important. After my *Nightline* television special "Rae's Story" aired in March 1996, Reverend Jackson wanted to have a special tribute to me at the Saturday morning forum and Quentin was asked to speak. For Reverend Jackson to honor me at PUSH during the Saturday morning forum, where it had all begun, was better than receiving an

Emmy Award. In the end, to have all my mentors on that stage together in recognition of my work meant the world to me.

Quentin was a tsunami, while Ron Sable was a little more laid-back—just as brilliant and passionate, but more like a cool breeze on an island. When he came into the office, he checked to see how I was holding up. I reflect on his compassion and think how blessed I was to have him in my life. He was careful not to violate my privacy. What I liked about him the most was that his expectations of me never changed, despite my diagnosis. He always had ideas he wanted me to execute. AIDS or not, his expectations were high. What I didn't know at the time was that Ron was also infected with HIV and would pass away a year later from AIDS-related complications.

Dr. Cohen was determined to make an AIDS activist out of me. She always had something going on and I always politely declined until she just wouldn't let me off the hook. She was working to bring a study on women and HIV to Chicago and asked me and some other women if we would sign a letter seeking congressional support for the study. The letter would be sent to U.S. Sens. Paul Simon and Carol Moseley Braun, who represented Illinois. I thought it was a worthwhile project and agreed to sign, provided the letter would not reveal I had HIV. After that, she had me—hook, line, and sinker. She asked if I would serve on the Community Advisory Board (CAB) for the study, explaining that my years of experience in the NIH study could be helpful. She had a point, but I was undecided until I was assured no one's HIV status would be disclosed. In fact, there was one woman on the board who went by a pseudonym because she had young children and had not disclosed her status. I said yes, again.

The Women's Interagency HIV Study (WIHS)—pronounced "wise"—created a partnership between the patient and the investigators from day one. That participants were able to have input into the design of the study was a powerful incentive to be in it. We felt like we mattered. The first CAB was composed of a diverse group of infected women of different races, educational backgrounds, and socioeconomic statuses. Just like in the clinic, we had women who had been infected from heterosexual relationships and those who were infected through intravenous drug use. We didn't always agree, but we agreed to disagree because the goal was greater than any one individual.

It was exciting to be on the cutting edge of a groundbreaking study on women and HIV. I couldn't believe I had been committed to the NIH study for seven years and they had missed an opportunity to learn specifically about me as a woman with HIV. There wasn't anything wrong with the NIH study per se; it was the knowledge that I had no value to research as a woman and that rubbed me the wrong way. In all those visits, I did not receive a single gynecological exam. The exclusion of women in HIV studies was defenseless neglect. It's mind-blowing to me that the fire alarm had never been pulled, given the alarming rate women were dying from AIDS toward the mid-to-late eighties and into the nineties. Epidemiologically, the HIV/AIDS paradigm had shifted; however, there continued to be a lack of recognition in the scientific community of the need to expand studies from MSM (men who have sex with men) to include women. The proposed WIHS study had a male study counterpart at NIH for the previous ten years. That alone had spoke volumes about the neglect of women.

Dr. Cohen wrote and secured the grant for the WIHS study in Chicago. She was a groundbreaker and a flamethrower, for real. It was unprecedented for NIH to make a grant to a physician at a public hospital like Cook County. Typically, grants of this nature were reserved for plush academic medical centers with healthy budgets, such as teaching hospitals like Rush Presbyterian, which was up the street from Cook County. Dr. Cohen argued that public institutions like Cook County—which provided the medical care for up to eighty percent of the infected women in the city—should not be pushed aside for plush medical centers that conducted studies but were not willing to provide medical care for those in the study. In my opinion, it was like we were guinea pigs or something. Dr. Cohen retained the role as lead investigator for the study even after she retired from Cook County.

The study began enrolling HIV-infected women and those at a higher risk for infection in October 1994 at four medical centers in Chicago: Cook County, Rush Presbyterian, Northwestern, and the University of Illinois. In addition to Chicago, the original study sites were New York, California, Hawaii and Washington, D.C. I enrolled in the study and began my visits every six months, not missing an appointment in twenty-nine years. At each visit, I receive a physical examination that includes skin and oral; examination of the breasts and lymph nodes; a gynecological exam that includes a Pap test; and, if needed, a follow-up colposcopy and biopsy to investigate cervical cancer; a cervicovaginal swab; blood work; and tests that include hair, saliva, and a urinalysis. There was also a dental aspect to the study led by the wonderful Dr. Mario Alves of the University of Illinois Dental School-Chicago. Come to find out, those living with HIV/AIDS have more gum disease and a host of dental issues than non infected persons.

Over the years, the WIHS study would change, as women lived longer with the disease and as investigators learned more about the disease in women. For example, they added menopause and lipodystrophy to help understand the fat redistribution that began to appear the longer women lived with HIV. Like many other women, I would have to face both these issues in the years to come. WIHS would eventually expand to more states and medical centers, but the Chicago site would be the highest performing one in the study. In 2019, WIHS marked twenty-five years, making it the oldest study of women and HIV in the United States. To date, WIHS has published some of the most important research on women and HIV/AIDS.

Remarkably those first three months or so after my AIDS diagnosis, I kept it together. I was busy with work, school, and CAB. AIDS, somehow, seem doable. I started to think, just maybe, I wouldn't die. I had Dr. Cohen in my corner, and she was willing to fight to keep me and the other women in the clinic alive. When I say "fight," I mean it: She has been known to get in a person's face—another doctor, a case manager, a nurse and even her patients. One such patient and I often tell Mardge Cohen stories when we bump into each other in the clinic. A recovering addict, she told me once that Mardge pushed her against the wall one day and asked, "When the fuck are you going to get it together? You want to die? Is that what you want?" Mind you, the woman is at least five-nine. She said, laughing, "I was high as a kite that day, but Dr. Cohen scared the fuck out of me." Mardge was clearly about saving lives against the odds, and she was willing to go the extra mile. She had surely influenced my one-hundred-eighty-degree turn. In a scared-straight kind of way, I knew that I had to get it together. I doubled up on my reading and began scouring the bookstores in Hyde Park like a hungry animal. I wanted all the latest news about HIV/AIDS. I subscribed to *AIDS Treatment News* and the *Gay Men Health Crisis Journal* because they were more difficult to come by, unlike the *Test Positive Aware* magazine that was always in the clinic. Other magazines also started popping up in clinic, like *POZ-Positively Aware*. I would add those monthly journals to my Saturday leisure reading.

Mardge was doing her part, and I was going to do mine. We had a partnership based on mutual respect for what we each brought to the table. She knew the science and I knew my body, and we brought what we had, and it became the recipe for my survival. Because antiretrovirals were at best mediocre back then, survival meant preventing, diagnosing, and treating an opportunistic infection as quickly as possible. I didn't take anything for granted and Mardge didn't want me to. If there was something out of the ordinary, I was to let her know sooner, not later. I always had diarrhea because of the medications, but sometimes I had more than what was typical. In those times, she wanted me to come and get my poop tested. It could have been some parasite that was causing the diarrhea instead of the medication. HIV had depleted the protection of my immune system and that was the crux of the problem.

The first thing I did was change parts of my diet. I boiled my drinking water or purchased sterilized bottled water because there is a parasite in tap water called cryptosporidium. I stopped eating my eggs over easy, tasting my cookie dough and cake batter because raw eggs contain salmonella. I ate my red meat well-done to ensure I wasn't exposed to *E. coli.* I stopped eating at buffet restaurants because of bacteria, limited my leftovers to two days and checked all the expiration dates on food. I don't know if it made a difference, but at least I felt proactive. I took all the medications Dr. Cohen prescribed. I had two categories of medication I took back then: HIV medications (antiretrovirals) and medications to prevent opportunistic infections. In addition, I took Fluconazole to prevent yeast, both vaginal and oral; acyclovir to prevent vaginal herpes, CMV and herpes zoster. Dr. Cohen also added Rifabutin to prevent *Mycobacterium avium complex* (MAC). To prevent I took Bactrim, but woke up one morning with a hot, burning red rash all over my face and down my chest and back. Dr. Cohen switched me to Dapsone. Eventually, I would take all the medications available to treat and prevent PCP. They would fail me, and I would have PCP three times, with two hospitalizations. I was watching myself deteriorate and it scared me. I was trying to live but, in my heart, I knew that I was living to die. I was not going down without a fight, and Dr. Cohen had on her boxing gloves every day. She fought for me when I couldn't fight for myself.

I started alternative therapies to complement my medical therapies. For example, I had massage therapies like shiatsu that were supposed to boost my immune system. I joined a gym not far from PNHP and started working out. I ran across Louise Hay's book, *You Can Heal Your Life,* and *The AIDS Book: Creating a Positive Approach,* in Borders bookstore. I was already familiar with New Thought teachings in a small way, and I really liked her positive thinking message. I even purchased some of Hay's tapes. I never believed I could heal myself but, hey, tools to help keep you focused on the positive never hurt anyone.

When I look back, I realize I had adopted a multifaceted approach to taking care of myself. I read my Bible, and Hay only confirmed for me what Proverbs 18:21 says: "Life and death are in the power of the tongue." Also, there's Proverbs 23:7: "For as he thinks, so is he." So, I continue to do both to this day. Hay's tapes helped clear my head, especially at night. My pastor, Reverend Clay Evans said prayer changes things, and he was right. I had known that since giving my life to Christ, and a reminder each Sunday kept me on my knees. I prayed for a miracle because sometimes in darkness you forget there ever was any light. In the meantime, I took my medication, worked out, went to therapy, and did whatever other positive things I could to keep me from slipping into the darkness.

It didn't matter what Dr. Cohen and I did; AIDS never changed its course. My T-cell count would bounce back by ten and drop by thirty. Waiting on a new T-cell count was awful. It was like waiting on Mama to decide if she was going to beat me naked or with my clothes on. Either way, I was going to get that beating.

By that spring, I had other AIDS-related opportunistic infections. One night I woke in a night sweat; my gown and sheet were soaked. It scared the daylights out of me. I wondered if I was dying. I felt around my body, and everything seemed okay. I got up, took a shower, got a fresh sheet and blanket, and laid on the sofa. The next morning, I paged Dr. Cohen. She told me night sweats were common. They were not going to kill me, but they were certainly a pain in the ass. In the scheme of things, the night sweats were a signal that my body was not working properly. Waking at all times of the night to change my gown added to the fatigue I had already begun to experience. Some mornings, even if I hadn't woken in the middle of the night, I didn't want to get out of bed. After work, going to the gym seemed like more of an effort than it was worth. Some days I pushed myself, and my usual sixty minutes on the treadmill felt like I had a box of books on my back. I knew that fatigue was common among people living with AIDS, and my determination to fight it was to no avail. No matter how much sleep I got, it never seemed like enough.

For a while, I kept up appearances, hanging out with the girls on the weekends when all I really wanted to do was sleep. My school routine was disrupted. Sitting through a class after work and then getting back on public transportation was more than a notion. Instead of reading on the way home, I focused on staying awake. Therapy was on school nights right before class and, sometimes after therapy, I would go home and go to bed instead of class. My statistics class kicked my ass; I had no other choice but to take a grade of incomplete. This was my second incomplete and the overachiever in me judged me without mercy. I felt like I was losing control. I was not keeping up. Even at work I was dragging.

When I first started losing weight, I didn't think anything of it. I had been going to the gym at least three times a week with Mary Cummings, a woman I had befriended at the Community Renewal Society. One day at lunch Mary said, "How come you losing all the weight?" I rolled my eyes, "Girl, please—my fat ass?" She looked doubtful but it hadn't occurred to me that my weight had anything to do with my health, especially since I was in the gym on a regular basis. I was either in denial or I liked being smaller. It may have been a little bit of both. I mean, I was calling myself fat at a size twelve. In reality, I had an opportunistic illness called wasting syndrome. Just like the night sweats were a deficiency in the immune system, wasting syndrome affected the metabolic function. Wasting is the involuntary loss of weight and muscle mass.

The fact that my weight loss was connected to HIV became real when Dr. Cohen prescribed the appetite stimulant Megace. The first thing I asked was whether there were any side effects, and it is still the first question I ask when I am prescribed a new medication. I have to prepare myself psychologically. The most noticeable side effect of Megace was dry mouth. I already had dry mouth from taking Desipramine and I figured one more medication with the same side effect couldn't hurt. I chewed gum all the time to counteract the dry mouth. One time Noble said to me, "A lady doesn't chew gum." "Really?" I asked and started chewing my gum like a cow chewing its cud. That was another reason he had to go. I was so sick of his passive/aggressive crap that was counterproductive to my physical and emotional health. No matter how he tried to demean AIDS, it was staring us both in the face. The next time we were having sex and he wanted oral sex, I whispered, all sexy, "Oh, baby—my mouth is too dry."

By the time my job ended at PNHP, I was a size eight. Mary asked if I was sure I was okay. "Yeah, girl," I said. "I guess the gym is paying off." I owned a lot of oversized, loose-fitting type of clothes, so I thought people believe this was how they were supposed to fit. I would buy one size down every once in a while, but, after my job ended, I didn't have a lot of extra money to spend on clothes, so I continued to wear what I had. I thought I was making it work. I don't know who I was trying to fool. People noticed, and I was amazed at how easy it was for me to lie and how quickly people accepted it at face value. It says a lot about how we view size. I must have been told a thousand times, "Girl, you're looking good." When I was asked how I had gotten so small I spurted a half-truth: "I took my tail to the gym."

Nothing Dr. Cohen did for me warded off the weight loss. She added Ensure, and I hated the taste of that with a passion. After I tried other nutritional drinks that I still didn't like, Mardge allowed me to switch to milkshakes, which didn't work either. Also contributing to the weight loss was the fact that I never got hungry. I would go all day without eating or thinking about eating. I was being hit from every angle. My white-girl ass became no ass, my Black-girl hips disappeared into thin air and my size 36-C bra was too big. These were the first visual signs that I had AIDS.

By June 1993, I was on six medications to treat or prevent opportunistic infections, plus the HIV antiretrovirals. Dr. Cohen took me off AZT and, for a while, I was only on DDI. I didn't know whether to be happy or sad. The side effects were mostly the same but, emotionally, AZT was an easier drug to take. Grinding DDI was drudgery a painful reminder of AIDS in a different way. AZT just made me sick, but the fact that DDI required more than popping a pill in my mouth and that it was downright nasty added to the psychological impact of taking this drug. I tried once to chew it, and it was what I imagined chewing chalk was like. The giant pills turned to white paste, and it seemed like I chewed forever. It smelled and tasted worse when I mixed it with water. I went through every brand of apple juice I could lay my hands on, and it never got better. I still don't drink apple juice today because of DDI.

In the morning, I'd put it in a carryout cup and drag it out until I was on the train headed for work. If I tried to drink it in one swoop, it came right back up all over my clothes. God, I hated taking it more than I detested the side effects. One day I overheard the women in the clinic talking about mixing it with Kool-Aid. I turned around and asked, "Kool-Aid—for real?" It was the first time I engaged the women in conversation in the three months I had been in the clinic. Everyone chimed in with her recommended flavor. I settled on grape and reported back that it actually was better than mixing with apple juice. I think that was the day I truly became one of them.

My CD-4 T cells were still wavering—ten up and then twenty down; that was more scary and frustrating because I didn't have a good take on what it meant for me. Dr. Cohen eventually took me off DDI. Good freaking riddance! So far, I had been on AZT alone. Then it was DDI with AZT, and then DDI alone. She replaced DDI with another HIV medication called Zalcitabine (ddC) combined with AZT—yes, again. Studies showed combining the two increased CD-4 T cells dramatically and sustained them over time. Zalcitabine was approved a year before DDI, but Dr. Cohen had chosen to go with the newer drug first. The side effects were headaches, more nausea and more peripheral neuropathy. I still don't know how I managed to wear three-inch heels to work every day with what felt like pins and needles sticking in the bottom of my feet, but I did. I figured a way to cope with every side effect. After ddC, I took D4T (Zerit) and AZT, which had the same side effects of ddC, except ddC also caused pancreatitis. I'll say it again: Thank God I never had that. After D4T I stayed on AZT and added another new medication, 3TC. The side effects were more of the same: headaches, fatigue, and diarrhea. The side effects kept coming, along with the changes in my body and the medications. These medications that fought the HIV virus were toxic and could kill you before AIDS, but I didn't let myself go down that road because I would have surely died from AIDS-related complications. I didn't know it at the time but switching my HIV antiretroviral medication would become the pattern over the next three years. As antiretrovirals were approved by the FDA and became available at Cook County, Dr. Cohen would switch the combination and I kept up. Ultimately, I would take most of the first generation of all the HIV medications from 1989 through 2007. For the record, I have taken a total of seventeen HIV medications: AZT; Emtriva; Epivir (3TC); Viread (Tenofovir); Videx (DDI); Zalcitabine (ddC); Zerit (d4t); Ziagen; Sustiva; Crixivan, which was six pills a day twice a day and for which I had to drink 72 ounces of water a day or I would get kidney stones; Kaletra; Ritonavir (Novir); which was 12 pills a day, twice a day; Prezista; Viracept; Isentress; Tivicay; and Fuzeon, which is an injectable medication in the stomach, done twice a day. The side effects of Fuzeon were painful nodules in the injection site, as small as a dime and as large as the bottom of a soda bottle. I cried every day for a year, but I never missed a dose. Dr. Cohen and I were fighting against the timeline of death, not just a disease.

Fifty-Two

❧ ✦ ❧

LETTING GO

❝
And you will know the truth, and the truth shall set you free."
—John 8:32

A sadness swept over me that I had never experienced before or since. I could be standing in the line at the grocery store and tears would start running down my face. Neither the antidepressant I was taking nor the therapy I had twice a week was able to curb the sorrow that bellowed from my gut. My T-cell count had dropped below 100, and death was calling me to her resting place. I just couldn't understand why God had left me. These words of the prophet Jeremiah weighed heavily on my heart:

Is there no balm in Gilead?
Is there no physician there?
Why then is not the health of the daughter of my people been restored?
What travesty have I committed that God has turned away from me? I thought.

Sure, I had made missteps—blunders, even. God had saved me so many times, but I still could not get it right. *Maybe God is tired of me,* I thought. Then I would pick up my Bible and turn to Romans 8:31-39 and read the apostle Paul's words, that "nothing could separate me from the love of God," and I found reassurance in the word of God. I had done the best I could with what I had. I fought so damn hard for myself—now what? I couldn't believe God had carried me this far just to call it quits. I never thought HIV was some sort of punishment. Rather I believed that my missteps had caused my infection. I understood none of the circumstances that landed me with HIV could be undone. That was water under the bridge, no matter how many times I played it in my head. At some point, I simply pushed those thoughts away so I could cope. God had carried me through miles and miles of missteps and now, at the most important part of my life, God was silent.

At church, I could see the Holy Spirit moving in the clapping of hands, the stomping of feet and the swaying of bodies. Each Sunday, I would return to God's house hoping that She would return to me, but She continued to pass by me. God had never felt absent from me until now. Even when I'd been at my worst, I saw a flicker of light—a path out of the tunnel—but this time I could see nothing. Everything had turned dark. Death was knocking at my door. My body was wasting away, and all the life had been zapped out of me. I was a living, breathing shell and I was just plain tired.

Tired of the pain I had never been able to avoid in my thirty years of living.

Tired of always having to fight.

Tired of taking pills.

Tired of smiling and pretending.

Tired of feeling sick from medicine that was supposed to make me better.

Like Fannie Lou Hamer, I was even tired of being sick and tired.

Even at the bottom of the pit I never stopped praying and seeking God's face. I didn't know how or when God was going to show up, but my history with Her told me She always shows. I held full-fledged conversations with God. I quoted all that scripture I had learned over the years, throwing God's word back in Her face. I couldn't figure what purpose my dying would serve for God. I had done what I believed I was supposed to do. I had been on the front lines, demanding justice in an unjust world. There was no redemption in death, and no salvation—not for me, and certainly not for others to see.

One Sunday after church, I started to think that maybe God wanted something from me. I thought, *Maybe I need to come clean. Maybe it was time to face the demon my cousin Eleanor had said was inside of me twelve years earlier, when she caught her son between my legs.* I had avoided the topic of men and sex with God because I was too ashamed to speak about it, even to myself—and certainly not to God. Grandmamma Julia used to say, "You can fool yourself, but you can never fool God. You can run, but you cannot hide." Now, that was God's honest truth. That morning in church, I cried through most of Reverend Evans' sermon. I had gone up to the altar call for prayer but lamented more than I prayed. Replaying the church service over in my head, it occurred to me I was mad at God when I should have been mad at myself. *God did not do this to you. You did it to yourself. You cannot keep running from the truth Rae,* I told myself. I looked up to heaven and asked, "Come clean. Is that what you want from me, God—to lay my transgressions at your altar?"

I grabbed a journal and started with my uncle. I still couldn't remember what he did to me—just how dirty I had felt that day he hugged me in our living room in Evanston. Does the little chocolate boy that Mama would never let me forget count?

Certainly, Junior, Aunt Betty and her girlfriend counted, even though they had forced me. James counted, for sure, because he was the person I'd chosen to lose my virginity to, at thirteen. There was also Robert, in the halls of ETHS; there was Mickey; but then, I didn't want to do it; there was L.D., whom I'd foolishly agreed to have sex with. Randy was a no-brainer, but at least I loved him with all my heart and had given myself to him out of that love. *If it's done in love, doesn't it count for something?* I pondered my relationship with Randy, and then I laid my head on the pillow and started to cry. I fell asleep and woke up in pitch blackness. It occurred to me I hadn't eaten that day. Dr. Cohen would not be happy. I got up and made a grilled cheese sandwich and a cup of chamomile tea. I sat at my table with fresh cut Alstroemerias in the vase I had purchased at the artisan store in Hyde Park. The vase was art, too—the beautiful blown glass, in a kaleidoscope of blues, comforted me every time I sat at my table. I continued to ponder and analyze every man and woman who ever touched me. There were names I could no longer remember but faces and situations I had never been able to blot out of my head— like on the boat with my friend and the friends he invited to have sex with me. There were the failed relationships, all the men I loved and those whom I wanted to love me; they played over and over again in my head. When I finished, I got up from my simple mahogany antique table—a perfect fit for my modest kitchen—and slipped under my pretty white ruffled duvet cover. "Now what?" I asked God, and drifted to sleep.

I started therapy with my confession that week. Now that I had admitted to myself and to God that I had had sex with more men than I would have ever admitted to anyone other than my therapist, for fear of being judged, I needed to process it all. What did it really mean? Why could men have as many sexual partners as they wanted without any consequences? A man could just have sex for sake of the sex, but why is a woman left to defend her sexual prowess? Even today, it's alright for a man to say he wants to *fuck a wet-ass pussy,* but a woman cannot talk or sing about her own vagina on her own terms. Here I was, trying to figure out if I was redeemable. Did the context or circumstance matter? Was I as horrible as society would have claimed me to be? Did I deserve to have AIDS? Why hadn't I been able to fix myself? God knows I wanted to, and tried, but I just couldn't seem to get it right. Somewhere in the recesses of my mind, I was really trying to find a way to turn death around. My sex life had become my bargaining chip with God.

If it meant a chance to survive, I would have shouted those names from the top of Sears Tower.

"If I hadn't been this sexual person, I wouldn't have AIDS," is how I started the conversation. "I've been having sex my whole life," I said, as if it was a proven fact. The puzzled look on Dr. Rebecca's face turned pensive. Before I could go any further, she said, "Rae, tell me how does a six-year-old have sex?" I didn't know how to respond. I could feel the moisture of nerves build under my wire bra. This was my chance for absolution, and I didn't understand why she was changing the narrative. *Explain it, Rae,* I told myself.

"See, I just know," I said. "Like when Mama caught me under the porch on top of that boy." I explained to her that it was the same thing my Uncle Michael's friend wanted to do with me after school, so Uncle Michael and I had to have done it, too.

"Rae, you were just a child," she said with the compassion of Mother Teresa on the streets of Calcutta and Princess Diana sitting in an AIDS clinic holding the hand of a dying man, wrapped up in one. I continued my explanation. I wanted to come clean, and she was confusing me. A tear dropped. "But I came home every day for lunch to LET (I said with an emphasis) Junior have sex with me," I said.

"Rae, a ten-year-old cannot have sex," she said. Before I could open my mouth again, she repeated, "Rae, you were a child." She waited a bit, then continued, "You were not having sex. You were molested."

One tear had turned into many, swimming down my face. I couldn't speak. She was correct. I had come home to feed Mr. Tom, and Junior seized that chore as his opportunity. It was not of my making or doing, but I had internalized his violation of me as me being *fast.*

"You did not cause this to happen to you; it was done to you," she said. I remembered those books on adult children of alcoholics that I had read years ago. I hadn't looked at them since Bill, but I dug them out of my blue trunk. I had underlined this sentence: "Some survivors of incest believe they can only obtain love and affection through sex." I can see I was reaching for some kind of explanation, even back then, but there was still a disconnect. In my mind it was still hard to grasp incest as rape and sexual molestation. I believed sexual violence had more to do with stranger danger, like the man who raped me coming home from Grandmamma Julia's church when I was eighteen. Betty allowing her friend to have sex with me felt more like rape and violence than it had felt with Betty, even though they had both done the same thing to me. I felt the same about Junior. I knew it was wrong, but I didn't know the wrong began and ended with him. Charles grabbing my breast and pushing me in the corner had felt more like violence than my "special" relationship with Junior even though Junior—whom I knew and loved as my big brother—had raped me, destroying me physically and emotionally. It was nothing but violence, with me going back to school with blood and semen in my vagina.

It was such a profound revelation for me that, even weeks later, I cried every time I thought about it. All those years, I believed I had been a *fast* little girl. Instead, I had been violated in the worst ways possible by the people I trusted the most. Maybe it wasn't God's forgiveness that I needed, but my own. I had been so hard on myself all these years. It was a relief to shed the burden of what they had done to me. We spent many more days processing the sexual violence that had happened to me, all by the age of eleven. All these years I had held on to the secret of my abuse, thereby protecting my abusers. I let it all go—every sick detail that I could remember. I sang it like the hallelujah chorus. These revelations opened a path for me to heal. What I understood after those sessions was that I had been sexualized at a very young age—not just by the sexual abuse, but also by Mama, who made me believe I was *fast.* The sexual grooming that I experienced was akin to training a child to play a sport or learn the violin. I can see how I claimed their sickness for my own. The work had only just begun. Coming to terms with sexual abuse was one thing, but I still didn't understand how it had impacted my sexual behavior.

I continued to be hard on myself in therapy sessions. Beyond the abuse, I asked my therapist, "Why had I not been able to stop myself all those other times?" That was the hundred-thousand-dollar question I could not answer. It would take many more years of unpacking the trauma. Rape, violence, rejection, manipulation, name-calling, and shaming shaped how I viewed womanhood, sex, and love. And it certainly affected my decision-making. In time, I was even able to see clearly how sex became an energy in my life. Thank God I have lived long enough to do the work that would bring me closer to the person I was meant to be, rather than the person my ugly childhood shaped me to be.

Keeping the secret of having HIV occupied way too much space in my life. I was mentally and emotionally exhausted. I had thought a lot about disclosing lately because the isolation was doing more damage than good.

I had gone to the women's group at the clinic for support, and got the culture shock of my life. You would've thought I was raised in a middle-class sheltered home the way I reacted, instead of Georgia Lee's hell raising, drinking, and cursing. They talked a little too freely for me, and I sure as hell wasn't going to tell these women my story. I came home and went to bed to sleep it off. In time, I would feel more at ease and would shoot the breeze with the women as we waited to see the doctor. But still I had no friends with HIV. Then one day, a woman walked up to me in clinic.

"Don't I know you?" she asked. I shook my head; I didn't want to hurt her feelings.

"Naw, I don't think so," I finally said.

"What school did you go to?" she asked. I wanted to say none of your goddamn business.

"Evanston Township," I said. She shook her head.

"I know you," she repeated. I shook my head and shrugged. She stopped talking to think about it. I was trying to be nice to this woman, but she was being a little too nosy for my liking. Well, I'll admit that I am a bit of a snob—one who curses worse than a sailor but a snob, nonetheless. I was not in denial: I knew I was one of them, but I wasn't trying to let them know all my business. Loose lips sink ships, and I had worked too darn hard to let gossip sink my dreams.

"I know you from PUSH," she finally said. She had piqued my interest, but I couldn't remember ever seeing this woman at PUSH. In any case, she was getting a little too close for comfort. I never answered her. "You may know my sister," she said, "Jan Camps."

B-I-N-G-O! Of course, I knew Jan; she was one of Mrs. Jackson's other play daughters. Jan had been in and out of the Jacksons' home, hanging around since the first day I landed at PUSH. She saw the recognition in my eyes.

"My name is Gail—Jan's my little sister," she said. I grabbed her hand and moved us to a private corner outside the radiology clinic. The first thing that came out of my mouth was, "Don't no one at PUSH know I have AIDS." Come to find out, Gail and I were in the same boat, as she hadn't disclosed her HIV status either. We exchanged telephone numbers and forged a friendship. Gail was the first person with whom I could really talk freely about HIV, and it didn't seem like I was complaining. She introduced me to another woman who had HIV and a history at PUSH. The three of us got together, and it was like we were a secret pack. Gail and I talked often on the phone and shared our secrets of trauma and how it had landed us with HIV. Her health was as bad as mine, but we were a comfort to each other.

With my health on a continuous downward spiral, it was becoming way more difficult to peddle the lie. I had always been an honest person, and I started to dislike who I'd become.

One day, just like that—poof! I decided it was time to let the secret go. At least I needed to prepare people for what seemed inevitable. I called Dr. Cotton and asked to see her; she agreed right away. Coré was still living in another state. Dr. Cotton had moved to the northern suburbs, and I took the commuter train an hour each way to her house. She picked me up at the train station and we went back to her house to talk. She listened as I cried through my shame. After I was done, Dr. Cotton counseled and reassured me; then, she prayed. On the train ride home, I felt as if I had received absolution. If only I could have been as gracious with myself as she was with me.

After I told Dr. Cotton, I talked to Veronica about our other friends, and we decided to tell Leslie Priest and Sharon Williams together. Outside of Veronica and Coré, they were my oldest girlfriends; I had met them through Veronica in 1981. This was also true of our girlfriend Becky Smith, who I told at dinner one night. She and I would go to the movies and have dinner afterward; it was our thing to do together. They all were shocked and couldn't believe Veronica and I had been keeping my secret for years and had not brought them into my circle of care.

Leslie, the mother hen of our group, kicked into gear. When she learned I had been going back to Cook County Hospital on the bus late at night to pick up my medicine after being at the clinic all afternoon, she was not having it.

"Veronica doesn't take you to pick up your medicine?" she asked. I could hear the indictment in her voice, and I tried to smooth it over. Veronica was still a flight attendant and was mostly flying, and she didn't drive in inclement weather—which meant if it was raining or snowing, I was shit out of luck.

"She is always on a trip," I said, "but then you know how Ronnie got all these rules. She doesn't drive in the rain or the snow so, honestly, I just don't ask." The next thing I knew, Veronica was calling me to see why I had told Leslie she didn't take me to pick up my medicine. Lord, it became a thing. As soon as I picked up the phone, she asked, "Why would you tell Leslie I don't take you to pick up your medicine?" I tried to explain I wasn't talking about her but about my routine, and that Leslie had asked. We then had a three-way call. "Leslie, will you pleassse explain to Ronnie that I was not talking about her," I said. Then they started arguing about Veronica living around the corner and not taking me back to pick up my meds. Veronica was mad at me that I had told Leslie and mad at Leslie for trying to run her life. That was how it went until I got married and my husband picked up my medication.

After I told Leslie, Sharon and Becky, the dominoes fell one by one. When I went to my NIH study appointment, Barry and I had dinner at The Wharf with Keith Jennings and Greg Moore, and I told them together. Next to Tyrone, they were two of my oldest political friends. I went up to the Capital Hill and told Carlotta Scott—we cried ugly tears. I decided to tell my play brother from high school—Tory Johnson, who now lived in D.C.—on that same visit.

Tory was a member of PAGE and the life of the party. He became closest to Coré and, right along with her, I adopted him as my little play brother. He never said he was gay, but as time passed it became an unspoken reality. Coré and I talked about me talking to him to make sure he was keeping himself safe. AIDS was the number-one killer of Black men between the ages of 25-44 at the time. I will never forget that day. We met at a swanky restaurant in D.C.'s newly remodeled Grand Central Station. Tory always loved clothes that were more flamboyant than not. That day, he surprised the heck out of me. Living in D.C. and working at a law firm, he had morphed into Beltway attire. He was wearing a light-colored seersucker suit that complimented his tall slim body, paired with a crisply starched blue shirt and a bow tie. He was cleaner than the board of health, right down to his wingtip shoes.

"Why are you telling me to be safe? Because I'm gay?" was the first thing that came out of his mouth. "You should be telling our other friends." Tory knew how to read a person from cover to cover—LOL! And he let me know he did not appreciate my sisterly advice one bit. I let him get it all out. He was going on and on. I grabbed his hand.

"Tory, I have AIDS," I shot back at him. "I just don't want you to end up like me." He was stunned and, for a brief moment, I saw the pain and empathy in his eyes. He still wouldn't let his guard down. I assured him I was not stereotyping. I knew not all gay men would end up with HIV, but that D.C. had more Black men with HIV than any place in the country was something that should not be ignored. He was sorry for me and assured me he was using condoms and had no plans to ever get HIV. I reported back to Coré, and I let it go. Not quite two months after *Essence* magazine hit the newsstand, Tory's sister Doria Johnson called. Tory was very ill—he had AIDS. Apparently, he kept his illness a secret from everyone. Coré and I dropped everything and went to D.C., it was too late. All we could do was say our good-bye's. Tory passed a week later. I was determined more than ever, to beat back the stigma associated with HIV/AIDS with all of my heart and soul.

I kept going down the list. I told Hazel Thomas (Nana). That was hard on me and her. She gave me another one of her pep talks and we went about as usual: talking every day, her picking me up on Sundays for church, and her giving me advice about everything under the sun, whether I wanted to hear it or not. Some Sundays, when tears streamed down my face, she would pull me into her and whisper, "You're going to be alright, baby."

I stood in my kitchen looking out of my lace curtains and told my mother, Dorje, on the phone. Her guilt and mine were enough to fill a football stadium. It was such a clear day that I could see Lake Michigan six blocks away. I pondered: *Wouldn't it be nice if life were this clear?*

"I'm so sorry that I wasn't a better mother," she said. That was water under the bridge. None of it could be taken back—not even the sex that had caused my fate.

I knew it was only a matter of time before that dam broke and I absolutely needed to preempt the gossip. I have no recollection of why I decided to tell Reverend Jackson first. One afternoon, I was sitting at the dining room table, chatting with Mrs. Jackson, when Reverend walked past us and into the kitchen. Something said, *Do it now.* I went to the kitchen and Reverend was drinking a glass of water by the sink. He looked up when I walked in.

"Hey, baby," he said to me. I went over and gave him a hug, then stepped back on the other side of the kitchen island. Keeping the secret from the Jacksons had been painful for me and added another layer of stress. Without a doubt, I can say it was the most irrational decision I had made about my diagnosis. None of them had ever given me reason to think I'd be rejected. I had witnessed their compassion and the sorrow they felt about Keith. I witnessed firsthand the way PUSH came together for Reverend Barrow and her husband, and we knew even less about AIDS in 1983 than we did in 1987 when I learned I was infected. I knew Reverend Jackson had been one of the few outspoken leaders, Black or white, who prioritized HIV/AIDS. I had insurmountable guilt about keeping my secret from them. Honestly, I was a nervous wreck thinking the family would feel betrayed in some way. I feared I would lose the admiration of Reverend Jackson and his wife.

"Rev, I need to talk to you; it's serious," I said. He looked puzzled,

"You pregnant?" he asked jokingly.

"No, I'm not pregnant." I said, thinking, *Boy, I wish that was my problem.* Before I lost my nerve I blurted, "I have AIDS." The expression on his face turned serious, and it felt like a hundred million years before he opened his mouth.

"You mean you have HIV?" he asked for clarification. Years later, in an interview for a feature article on me in *O, The Oprah Magazine*, Reverend Jackson explained he didn't know what having AIDS meant for me. He said, "At the time, it was a death sentence for most people." His sentiment was felt by all families. There was hope in HIV, but none in AIDS.

"No, Rev," I responded, "I have full-blown AIDS." I started talking fast, like I do when I'm nervous. I was rambling on, trying to fill in the last seven years of my life in about six minutes. He listened until he had enough. Reverend had never been one for other people's monologues and, true to his nature, he stopped me.

"Rae, stop," he said in a commanding tone. I shut all the way up. My nerves felt like I was about to pee in my pants.

"None of that matters." he said. "I loved you before you had AIDS, and I love you with AIDS." I was flat-out done; you could have buried me that day. This man, who I had admired so much, proved everything I ever believed about him to be true. Yes, he might have been flawed, but his capacity for compassion and empathy were gifts from God and he never shied away from it—not in the minor way like with me and Keith, or in a major way like working for voting rights, economic parity, and healthcare and all the other issues that he has fought for in his life of ministry.

"If there is anything I can do," he said, "you let me know." He walked over to me and grabbed my hands. "Let's pray." After he prayed, he asked me if I told Mrs. Jackson. I told him I was too afraid.

"Let's do it together," he said. Mrs. Jackson was sitting in the same spot at the dining room table where I had left her. When we walked into the room, she looked up.

"Jackie, Rae has something to tell you." She looked up from under her reading glasses that I always joked with her about and sat up straight. "Go on," he urged.

"I have AIDS," I said. She looked at me and positioned her head sideways like, *What in God's name did you just say?*

"You have AIDS?" she asked rhetorically, trying to wrap her brain around what I had just told her.

"Yes."

Reverend stood next to me as Ms. J processed what I had told her.

"You… have… AIDS?" she asked again, slowly, and methodically. I nodded yes.

"You mean, YOU have AIDS?"

Reverend Jackson came to our rescue, saying, "Jackie, I told Rae that she has our full support."

"Oh, absolutely," she said with emphasis. Reverend left the room and I sat across from her in my spot at the table. She turned to me and repeated, "Girl, you… got… AIDS?"

I didn't leave the dining room table with Mrs. Jackson until well after ten that night. Every thirty minutes or so, she looked at me and said, "Baby, you got AIDS." We have talked about this day over the years, and she explained that it was as if I had knocked the wind out of her, like, *Are you telling me you are getting ready to die on me?*

I told Jesse Jr. and his now ex-wife Sandra together and the rest of the family was told by Mrs. Jackson. Jesse Jr. would call often, "Rae-Rae, how you holding up girl? You know if you need anything, I'm right here," he said. And I did know. He had been floating the idea of running for Congress and I hoped I would be alive to witness that day. Mrs. Jackson thought I should move into their home so that they could take care of me. I quickly vetoed it. I needed my independence. I figured we could cross that bridge when I could no longer take care of myself.

Gossip in my political circle spread faster than a California wildfire. Surprisingly, I didn't care. It felt like tons of bricks had been lifted off my shoulders. I hadn't realized, the toll the secret had taken on me—how much power I had given it over me. I realized people were going to talk, and that some of it would be malicious. I also realized some of my friends just needed to process what they had learned. It got crazy for a minute. My close male friends' girlfriends wanted to know if they'd had sex with me. If we are to be completely honest about it, there is always just a little doubt that a man and a woman can honestly have a platonic relationship. Men who had wanted to get with me, and who I had rejected, checked in with me. *Girl, you really got AIDS.* Mostly, though, I received gobs of moral support. People stepped up. Even PUSH friends gathered around me. Reverend Derrick Anderson, who traveled with Reverend didn't let a week go by without checking on me.

My friend Barry Saunders was the big difference for me, despite his own health challenges. He had been diagnosed with cancer of the mouth. He had approximately seventy percent of his tongue removed and had continued to push through. He was my inspiration. Doctors had told him he would never talk or eat again, and he defied the science. We talked every day and sometimes his tail would hop on an airplane, even after I was married just to see me face to face. "Girl, I just wanted to lay eyes on you," is all he'd say, and that night he would be back on his way to D.C. He'd drop me a check in the mail if I hadn't had a speaking engagement. Rather than saying, "It will get better," he said, "Here's some grocery money." This is the way it was between us until his death in 2001.

After Barry passed away, my friend Keith Jennings promised he would fill the void Barry left, and he did just that until his death in 2021. He didn't hop on a plane to cold-ass Chicago like Barry, but he made sure I had food on my table and "a little extra for bubble gum" is how he put it. He was the one friend out of my political circle who worked internationally, and he checked on me from Kenya, South Africa, Mozambique, Ethiopia, Ghana, Indonesia, Paris or wherever the heck he was. There was never a week when I did not hear his voice.

I never regretted my decision to disclose. I just wished I had the courage to have done it earlier. But then, 1993 was vastly different from 1987, when I learned I had HIV. We knew more about HIV than we had then. The scientific community was slaying dragons. There were five HIV medications, with more effective ones on the horizon. The world-famous NBA player Earvin "Magic" Johnson had gone public with his HIV status right around the time I started to experience a decline in my health. I had seen, with trepidation and hope, that things were getting better. If nothing else, he certainly made HIV a topic at the Thanksgiving dinner table in a way that hadn't been done before—at least not in the African American community. Progress had been made, but we still had many more miles to go. There was no cure for AIDS or any life-saving medication; because of this, death was considered inevitable. I was praying for a miracle in everything that Dr. Cohen had me doing but, emotionally, I was preparing for the inevitable: death.

I had told all the important people in my life I had AIDS—except Mama. Shoot: It had been almost two years since Grandmamma Julia's death, and I was still barely speaking to Mama. I did what I considered my daughterly duty: I called every other week and went out to Evanston every two months or so. I never stayed longer than an hour. I had decided I could not force Mama to treat me with respect, but I could certainly protect myself from her madness. Grandmamma Julia's death was the line I drew in the sand.

Grandmamma Julia passed a week after Thanksgiving, in December 1991. A few days before Thanksgiving, she and Mama had that same crazy argument about whose house to have dinner and yada-yada-yada. I didn't even give it a second thought. I went over to Grandmamma's. I had been dropping over more often, running errands, going to the laundry mat—things like that. Noble and I had taken her to have a medical procedure a few months earlier. Well, he dropped us off and picked us up. The night Grandmamma Julia died, Mama called to inform me what happened, and she demanded I drop everything and get over to Grandmamma's house to make sure no one took anything. I was studying for finals, but dropped everything—not for Mama, but out of concern for Grandpapa Clayton. I couldn't make heads or tails out of what Mama was saying. I kept asking about Grandpapa Clayton and she kept saying, "He killed my momma." When I arrived, Grandpapa was walking around in shock. He had come out of his bedroom into the dining room where Grandmamma was sitting in her favorite chair that sat in the dining room, right outside her bedroom door. He had tried to wake her and couldn't. He called his young adult cousins who, like me, came over to the house to help out every now and then. They in turn called Mama who then called me. By the time I arrived, Grandmamma's body had already been picked up by the coroner's office.

The moment I walked in, Grandpapa Clayton explained through tears, "Julia wouldn't wake up." He and Grandmamma had been married for over thirty years. I didn't know how to console him. Mama walked in about an hour later, hollering at him.

"You motherfucker! You KILLED MY mama!"

"You a motherfucking lie," he retorted, his words slurring through the tears. I had to hand it to him: Grief-stricken and all, he fought back as best he could. Mama came up on Grandpapa, and he tried to block her. However, before he could get his hands up good, she hit him on the head.

"MAMA, STOP!" I hollered, jumping out of the chair to defend Grandpapa. "LEAVE GRANDPAPA ALONE," I screamed at her.

"Bitch! Who the fuck you think you talking to?!"

"Mama, just leave him alone," I said, deflated. She stood in the middle of the floor between the dining room and living room, with a cigarette hanging out the side of her mouth and her hand on her hip. I shook my head and led Grandpapa to his bedroom and told him to lie down. When I walked back into the dining room, Mama demanded I find Grandmamma Julia's insurance papers. "I know she left all of this to me!" Mama said. I methodically went through Grandmamma Julia's dresser, but could find only one insurance policy, which would go to cover her burial. Mama started pacing the floor.

"You ain't found them yet?" she wailed. I hadn't and started looking through the bags and boxes that were in her closet; still, I had no luck. Mama started pulling Grandmamma Julia's clothes out of her closet, piling them on the bed.

"Bitch, you better find it," she demanded. "I know she left me something!" I smelled a rat, and so did Mama. I couldn't find any of Grandmamma Julia's fine jewelry or her minks. I didn't know if Grandpapa's cousins had cleaned her out, and I didn't try to figure it out. Mama complained, "I know them low-down dirty motherfuckers took my mama's stuff," but that was as far as she took it. Mama's false sense of entitlement made me sick to my stomach. The only relief I had that night was the bathroom, where I would go wet my face and take a breather. I was so sick from AZT; I couldn't even think straight. Grandpapa slept a long time, thank God, while Mama raged at me like a maniac to find those papers. It reminded me of that time she made me stay up and watch for Tobie to come home—except I wasn't eleven years old anymore. I was a grown-ass twenty-eight-year-old woman. I had never cursed at Mama, but I wanted so badly to tell her to *shut the fuck up*. She had called a friend to come over and, at the break of dawn, they began loading Grandmamma's clothes into her car. I watched, not lifting a finger to help.

"What you doing with Julia's things?" Grandpapa protested.

"This is my motherfucking mama," she said. God, I hurt for Grandpapa, but short of calling the police on Mama, I didn't know what to do. Once the car was loaded to the max, her friend drove the car to Mama's. I was so happy when Aunt Pam walked through that darn door. She had taken a redeye from Los Angeles, where she had joined her other two sisters who had already been living there. It took her all of two minutes to assess the scene. She told Mama, "Georgia Lee, you are not going to disrespect my father."

"I can take my mama's clothes if I want," Mama, protesting like a child. Pam made herself clear that Grandmamma's personal belongings were all Mama could take until she could figure the next steps.

At the funeral, Mama laid all over Grandmamma Julia in the casket. "My Mama-a-a-a gone. I ain't got nobody," she wailed. I was so embarrassed for Grandmamma's reputation with all her gospel-singing friends there, Mama smelled like a fifth of whatever she was drinking. After the burial, things went from bad to worse. I rode back from the burial with Aunt Pam and her sisters because I had had enough of Mama cursing me. We stopped for carryout to bring back to Grandmamma's. Mama got to the house but didn't eat or stay long. I knew she was expecting me to ride back to Evanston with her, but I be damned if I would. I was physically and emotionally drained. I hadn't even had a chance to mourn because of Mama. I told Mama I was tired and that after I finished eating, I was going home to go to bed. Of course, in her mind, I had chosen Aunt Pam over her. At that point, I didn't give two flying fucks about her feelings. Before Mama left, Pam explained to her that she was taking the rental car back and needed Grandmamma's car to run errands. I put my head down. I didn't want any part of it. Mama didn't respond; she just put on her coat and walked out the door. Before I left to go home, Pam called Mama and left her a message that if the car wasn't in front of the house by six that evening, she was going to report it stolen. Mama was already looking for a lawyer to take the house from Grandpapa. I had the deed to the house and Grandpapa's and Grandmamma's names were on it. I tried to explain to Mama that, according to Illinois law, the house belonged to Grandpapa. "Lawyers will take your money, Mama, but you cannot win," I told her about fifty times in the week that passed since Grandmamma Julia's death and burial.

"Bitch, you don't know what the fuck you talking about. You so goddamn smart; you think you know everything," Mama said.

Later that day, I hadn't been home a good fifteen minutes before Mama called to give me a piece of her mind. As soon as I answered the phone, "Bitch! You low-down, dirty bitch! You don't mean me no good!" I couldn't get a word in. "After all I've done for you. Bitch, I will come down there and blow your motherfucking brains out," she said. I hung up the telephone. After that madness, it had taken a good six months for me to call her again. So, hell to the motherfucking no! I had no plans to tell Mama I had AIDS. I just couldn't imagine how telling her could benefit me. I was under no illusion she would ever have my best interests at heart. After how she treated Grandpapa, I didn't know what to think about her, so I thought about her very little after that. In retrospect, if it had not been for the *Essence* cover story, I would have waited even longer to tell her. The way I felt then, I'd probably had to have been near death before I uttered a word to her. However, since I was going to tell the world, I thought she deserved at least to hear it from me. That was more grace than she ever showed me.

D r. Cannon was the final person who I felt should hear from me that I was dying. She had invested so much in me. I called, and she suggested we catch up at dinner. "Oh no-o-o, Rae," she said. I could see the pain in her eyes as her lip quivered just a tad. No one ever said to me I would beat AIDS except Veronica, because you couldn't beat AIDS in 1993. Instead, they either gave me that I-feel-sorry-for-you look, gave me a hug of empathy, or attempted to make life better for me until I died. Dr. Cannon's remedy was to treat me monthly to the finest restaurants in Chicago. The only one I can remember is the infamous Pump Room, in Chicago's Gold Coast. We would dress up, have an exquisite meal and make small talk. And we always avoided the sticky conversation about AIDS. These monthly dinners were extended to me in the same way Sandra Jackson would splurge on me when I tagged along with her while shopping. She and I had become good friends. I had been the one to get the house together and decorate for she and Jesse Jr.'s last-minute decision to have their wedding at the house. These little gestures went a long way to lift my spirit.

I always wanted to visit Paris and one of the airlines had a special from Chicago to Paris, and I called Mrs. Jackson, who frequented Paris, to see if it was a good deal. The trip became her gift to me. She invited Sandra to join us, which was perfect in my eyes. We stayed at one of those boutique hotels off the Champs-Elysées, and it was a three-minute walk to the *crème de la crème* of Paris. It was every bit of wonderful as I imagined.

Sandra and I had so much fun touring the city—including the Louvre and shopping. On other days, Mrs. Jackson walked with us on the Champs-Elysées, where we window-shopped the most exquisite stores and perused Galeries Lafayette, a grand department store consisting of many stores.

The best parts of the trip for me were the architecture and the food. There is nothing in this world as divine as a warm croissant in the morning, warm crepes in the afternoon and an exquisite dinner to cap the day. Sandra and I took turns each morning going out to the street cart to pick up warm croissants; in the evening, Mrs. Jackson took us to the finest restaurants. Looking back, I'm sure it was the combination of Paris food and those dinners with Dr. Cannon that fostered the beginning of my love of food. Those late-night dinners in Paris were the best and the worst of the trip for me. After site-seeing all day, by Chicago's dinnertime, I was ready to have a meal and relax. By Paris' dinnertime—sometime after eight in the evening—I was ready to go to bed. Therein lay the problem. My body failed me almost immediately and I never adjusted to the seven-hour time difference. Our second night, my menstrual cycle started, and I was hurting. I didn't want to eat; I wanted to sleep. I told Sandra to relay to Mrs. Jackson I was taking a pass on dinner. First off, you don't relay anything to Mrs. Jackson, but I just couldn't face her. When I saw her coming through our room door with Sandra on her heels, I knew I was in trouble.

"Get your selfish ass up out of that bed and get dressed for dinner," she said. I didn't open my mouth. I got up out of that bed and got dressed for dinner. We went to an Italian restaurant that, to this day, offered the best Italian food I have ever had. When I finally lay my head on the pillow that night, I was thankful for that experience but, God, I was hurt. Mrs. Jackson had told me on that trip, "You've got to keep fighting, Rae, in order to win." I knew she was hurt, too. I believe she took my not going to dinner as a sign I was giving up. She had been so accustomed to me hanging with her, often until late in the night. AIDS was changing our relationship and she was fighting back. I wanted to console her, but I did not know how to explain what I did not truly understand. I only knew something had changed profoundly, and my body was making that clearer each day. I couldn't keep the pace like I had in the past, or even do the things I was accustomed to doing. It was a painful paradox: Letting go of the secret was a form of liberation but then, I was in another kind of prison watching the people I cared about the most watch me deteriorate. Back from Paris, my menstrual cycle lasted another twenty-one days.

Fifty-Three
❧ ❧
THE WOUNDED HEALER

"The main question is not 'How can we hide our wounds?' so we don't have to be embarrassed, but 'How can we put our woundedness in the service of others?'"
—Henri J. M. Nouwen

Purpose had been the one thing that kept me going most of my life. Now, between life and death, I did not know what was going to become of the life I created. The loss of all the hard work scared me more than dying. Six months into my AIDS diagnosis, my health had changed so drastically I had a serious existential crisis. What was I supposed to do with myself until I died? How does one plan a life with no expectation to live?

The prognosis of death was playing out in real time. In six months, my T-cell count had dropped from 166 to around 89. Waiting on my T-cell results every three months was pure torture, especially if they had gone down from previous labs. If I had a rise in T cells, no matter how small, it gave me hope for another day. But when they dropped, it was like watching my ice cream tumble off the cone just as my tongue touched it. The lower they dropped, the closer to death medical science claimed me to be—and I concurred. Death by AIDS was a foregone conclusion to every top doctor in the country except Dr. Cohen. She never, ever, told me I was dying. Instead, she continued to work against the clock. I leaned on her pushing through to help get me through because my resilience was dwindling with each new change my body underwent. My body had turned on me, and I was lost. After all I had gone through in my thirty-one years of life, I couldn't understand why God would get me this far and then just drop the ball. BAM! Your time is up.

In the meantime, I still needed to pay my rent and put food on the table. The grant that secured my job at PNHP ended. I reached out to friends who knew people who knew people. The Boyz from the Hood Foundation came by way of my good friend Dwayne Kyles and his business partner Calvin Hollis. I met them both while planning the debate party for Carol Moseley Braun's campaign. At the time, they owned the Clique nightclub and had graciously donated their space for the debate party. Dwayne, the son of infamous civil rights activist Reverend Billy Kyles, and I bonded right away. I had known his father since I first started at PUSH but didn't meet Dwayne until Hazel Thomas introduced us the night the planning committee convened. One night after a planning committee meeting, Dwayne offered me a lift home and we have been friends ever since. After I left PNHP, he thought I would be perfect to coordinate community outreach for the organization and introduced me to the executive director, Benjamin Garrett.

The Boyz from the Hood Foundation was a great concept in an era when celebrity philanthropy was not as prolific as it is today. It was the brainchild of NBA players Kendall Gill, Marcus Liberty, Nick Anderson, Tim Hardaway, and Calvin Hollins, from the Clique. One day they were reflecting on their own humble beginnings—living in the inner city—in single-family homes and decided to find a way to give back. They hadn't made it on their own and wanted to return the good that had helped make them successful men. They brought together other NBA players like Charles Oakley, Craig Hodges, and Byron Irvin, along with other athletes such as Mickey Pruitt, from the NFL;

boxer Mike Tyson; and John Davis, a Chicago on-air news personality. When I joined the team as the project coordinator, the organization hadn't been established a full year. I was hired to arrange a weeklong series of community activities to culminate with *The Slam Jam,* a celebrity basketball game.

It was a lot of work in a short period of time. I had to find contacts out of thin air to make the programming for the week happen. As usual, I did what I do best: I picked up that damn telephone and got to work. I pushed back my anxiety about my future and jumped in feet first—actually, feet *and* legs that felt like they were on fire every day, all day, from the AIDS-related peripheral neuropathy and the HIV medicine. There was no way around peripheral neuropathy for me; it felt like pins were sticking me in my legs and feet with different levels of intensity. I continued to take Desipramine, one of the old-school antidepressants that also treats nerve pain off and on for about seven years, with only mild relief. I woke up groggy and with a dry mouth every morning. By mid-morning, the grogginess had worn off, but the dry mouth lasted twenty-four-seven.

My health had become intrusive, and I could no longer place AIDS in a box. I had to accept my new reality, but it didn't mean I had to give in to it. My diva behind was on public transportation in heels and in the office every day. To make my mornings easier, I got some box braids like the ones Janet Jackson wore in the movie *Poetic Justice,* so I didn't have to worry about combing my hair in the morning. That gave me an extra thirty minutes to lie in bed, listen to a little gospel music and center myself. I was now taking twenty-three pills a day, and I didn't dare miss one dose. It was very clear they were helping to keep me alive, no matter how they made me feel. It was a painful tradeoff. The tenacity I had developed over the years was second nature to me; I did what I had to do. I had developed a reputation as one damn good organizer, and I approached every project with dedication and hard work.

I worked past 7:00 p.m. most nights, headed home and crashed. My social life sunk to an all-time low. I didn't feel like pretending I was good when I was struggling physically and emotionally. My perception of my girlfriends around this time was that they needed me to be okay, like with Mrs. Jackson in Paris. Whether it was true or not, I felt I had to present Rae as she used to be. I couldn't show any weakness or signs of dying. I would pop into the PUSH Saturday morning forum when I could drag myself out of bed, and I still went to church on Sundays with Hazel. Beyond that, I was like the walking dead on the inside. God still felt absent to me, and I agonized over it. People I didn't have to pretend with noticed my sadness. My new hairstylist, Deidra Cayolloe told me so. Before the braids, I started getting my hair done regularly at the salon OMS, which was on the ground level of my building. Deidra also lived in the building, and I bumped into her often. I hadn't told her about having AIDS for fear she would no longer service me but once I started speaking in the high schools, I knew word would get back. When I finally disclosed, Deidra told me she thought something was wrong with me and she had mentioned to her sister Linda that I seemed sad all the time. A testament to her, she remained my stylist for almost two decades and she became my friend.

Around this time, I bumped into Ken Bennett, and he could always read me like a book. I was walking down the street and stepped into his girlfriend Lisa's—now, his wife—hair salon to say hello. Ken was there and saw the sadness written all over my face. He stepped out with me to find out what was going on and how he could help. We went to the restaurant next door, the Tiki Room and I told him I had AIDS. My T-cell count had just taken another hit and God it hurt. Ken assured me that I would always have his support and he has been true to his word.

In the midst of my work at the Boyz from the Hood Foundation, another project landed in my lap. One day, while sitting around the dining room table at the Jacksons, National Black Expo CEO, Reverend Bernard Taylor asked if I would work the event.

I needed to stack my coins as the young people say today and I said yes. The Black Expo was originally organized by Operation PUSH in 1969, and it ran through to 1979. Reverend Jackson had given Taylor his blessing to reestablish the expo a few years earlier and it became a huge success. July 1993 was the fourth expo under Taylor, and there would be over two hundred thousand attendees during the weekend.

Reverend Taylor looked over to me and asked what I was doing the next weekend.

"Why don't you come work the expo for me? I have the perfect spot for you."

"Bernard Taylor, I don't want any funny business with our Little Rae," Mrs. Jackson interjected jokingly. I smiled. Reverend Taylor then explained he wanted me to coordinate ground transportation and be responsible for the celebrities' movements on the days they were supposed to speak. I worked all week at the foundation and started working with the expo that Thursday until late that night. I made it to the McCormick Center exhibition hall an hour before the ribbon-cutting with Mayor Daley and the other dignitaries that Friday morning. I had a breakneck schedule and worked closely with Cheryl Porter, who was in charge of security at the expo. Our drivers were brothers from the Nation of Islam. We were an awesome team. I don't think Cheryl and I got more than three hours of sleep over those three days. There were flight delays, talent changing their flights, and at the end of the day they wanted to venture out for Chicago's nightlife, and we had to accommodate them. I carried my walkie-talkie to bed with me every night.

We had some great panelists on the workshops that weekend. Thomas Ford, who played Tommy on the television show *Martin*, couldn't believe I didn't know who he was and had never watched the show. Richard Brooks, who played assistant district attorney Paul Robinette on *Law and Order* was also on the panel, and I was a huge fan and told him so. My work with celebrities was so different from today, when everyone pops out a phone for a picture and then pretends to be friends with the celebrity. I was hired to help with their participation in whatever event it was and I stuck to my assignment. From my early Jackson days, Rob Lowe was the only celebrity I took a picture with, and gospel artist Tramaine Hawkins was the only talent who rendered me speechless when I was first introduced to her. I couldn't get a word out of my mouth those first fifteen seconds. Her 1983 album, *Determined,* had gotten me through a storm, a hurricane, a tsunami, and a tornado, and just being in her presence blessed me.

Jada Pinkett was the other big name at the expo that year and she impacted me in an unexpected way. *Menace II Society* had just been released, and she was on a panel with other Black actors. Her stardom was on the rise, and everyone was clamoring to get to her. After the panel discussion I escorted Jada inside the exhibit hall, where she would be autographing her photographs and T-shirts. I had my hands full, to say the least. She even gave me an autographed long, fitted T-shirt dress as a thank-you gift for taking care of her that day. You better believe I was on my A game that weekend, regarding work and my personal appearance. I prided myself on being put together well, and AIDS was not going to change that fact. No matter what I looked like on the outside or how well I performed my duties, emotionally, I was crumbling and burrowing in shame. At one point Jada commented on how pretty I was, and I thought, *If she only knew how ugly AIDS made me feel on the inside, what would she really think of me?*

That Monday, I was back in the office working on the Boyz from the Hood Project. With the event a few weeks away, I was working a lot of hours. In fact, we all were burning the midnight oil: Ben Garrett, who was overseeing the operation and raising money; Dawn Hendricks, who was working on securing the talent for the Slam Jam; and me, working on the community outreach. We kicked off the weeklong community outreach at La Rabida Children's Hospital on Chicago's South Side by the lakefront. La Rabida is a hospital that treats children with complex and chronic health issues regardless of race or the parents' ability to pay. At the time, most of the children were Black and Brown. It was amazing watching these six-foot-plus NBA players with the children. We gave the hospital a twenty-thousand-dollar donation. The players spoke at day camps in low-income communities throughout the week, and we culminated with a big event with young people on the West Side of Chicago. It was sponsored by long-term Chicago financier Jonathan Rodgers, and Cirilo McSween, one of the African American McDonald's owners in the city, provided the food. We had a star-studded Slam Jam at halftime, with singer Brian McKnight. We had pulled it off, and I could put a check mark beside another successful project under my belt.

When the project was over, I was right where I started, trying to figure out my next move. I had been in conversations off and on for about two years with Vanessa Kirsch about an organization she was trying to launch, Public Allies. My friend Greg Moore had introduced us and thought I would be a perfect fit, and so did I. Our first meeting was in D.C. during one of my NIH visits. I placed my name in the bucket as the director of the organization. I wanted this job badly. I had paid my dues organizing young people, and the thought of helping to develop future leaders struck a chord with me. I had been mentored at PUSH and I could see the potential. Vanessa wanted to do for other young people what had been done for me at PUSH. It was a wonderful concept to take young adults with potential and help develop them for service.

Finally, the day came when Vanessa offered me the position as the executive director. I was sitting at my small antique table in the kitchen. It was one of the happiest—and saddest—days of my career. The only catch was I would also be responsible for fundraising; in fact, I would have to raise a good portion of my salary. Raising funds had never been an area for which I'd been tasked. However, I knew how, and I had the contacts. I had even trained the leadership of nonprofits on fund development. I wanted the job, but I had to be honest with myself: I just couldn't see how I would be able to run a startup organization, raise my salary, and manage my health. I really wanted Vanessa to succeed. I wanted Public Allies to succeed. I wanted other young people to follow in my footsteps and reach their full potential in a safe space, like I had done. I turned the job down. When I hung up from talking with Vanessa, I cried. It was the first definitive loss I had to face because of AIDS, and I mourned for my life in service that I had always known. The next thing I knew, my friend Michelle Obama was running the organization. I was happy Vanessa had found someone passionate about developing young leaders for service. Michelle would help to put Public Allies on the map. She would also honor me at a Public Allies event, recognizing my long history working in student/youth advocacy.

With my fading health, working short term projects was easiest because all that was required of me was helping organizations meet their goal. I started re-creating myself by marketing my skills on my own terms as a consultant. I was never going to get health insurance, so a stable job no longer mattered. What mattered was making enough money to live and being able to take care of my health. I purchased some stationery and business cards and went on the hunt for my next short-term project. One Saturday after PUSH, I was over at the Jacksons and Joe Gardner offered me a ride home. We sat in his car and talked.

"I guess you heard that I have AIDS, Joe?" I asked.

"I heard the rumor, but I didn't know if it was true until I'd heard it from you."

"Well, it's true." I told him. We talked about my health, and he asked if I could handle working on a campaign. I shifted and turned toward him. "I'm going to run for mayor and I'm pulling my team together. I would like you to be my field director." I was absolutely stunned. This was a big job with big responsibilities, and I was humbled that he thought I was capable. But I didn't want to tarnish his name.

"What about AIDS?" I asked.

"I don't care about that," he said. He explained he had watched me grow into an incredible organizer and thought I deserved the opportunity as much as he believed I could get the job done. I was blown away. I had worked so hard to be sought after. I had turned down the Clinton campaign and Public Allies. AIDS had already cost me so much. I wasn't going to let it cost me another thing. I accepted his offer. I always liked Joe. He started as a community organizer in Chicago. He was the vice-president of programs at PUSH and worked under Dr. Finney as the deputy director for the Woodlawn Organization. He ran for commissioner of the Metropolitan Water Reclamation District in 1988 and won. Our paths crossed often but it was the 1988 presidential campaign where I really got to know him. He had been a loyal soldier for progressive politics in Chicago. There had been talk he could be the Black person to beat Daley and the machine. Although he had not officially announced his candidacy, I joined the staff immediately. We had a lot of ground to cover if Joe was going to run a strong campaign.

I should have been in the office doing what I did best: working the phones and managing the folks we had in the field. Instead, here I was in an auditorium full of high school students. *What the hell am I doing here, getting ready to speak?* I asked myself as I watched the teachers escort their classes into the large room. The noise level was extremely high, only adding to my jitters. I had been bamboozled, not by one person, but by two.

Anthony, whom I bumped into occasionally at events, was the volunteer coordinator at Test Positive Network, a local HIV/AIDS organization in Chicago. He asked if I would be willing to speak at Bowen High School.

"Hell to the naw," I quickly spurted.

"Who told you that I wanted to speak about having AIDS?" I asked him. No one had, but he learned through the grapevine I had HIV and thought I might be willing to put my activist skills to work for HIV/AIDS. "You're barking up the wrong tree," I said, in no uncertain terms.

I had never considered myself a public speaker and I had no intention of becoming one now. The work I was doing around HIV was more than enough. In addition to my participation on WIHS' advisory committee, Reverend Judith had talked me into accepting a position on the board of directors of the Pastoral Care AIDS Network. It was an ecumenical network that helped educate pastors on the topics around HIV/AIDS. In the beginning the only person who knew I was HIV-positive was the executive director, Carol Reese. Now that I had become gossip, it seemed to me that everyone and their momma—except mine—knew I had AIDS. "You all have tons of volunteers over there," I told him. He explained the teacher specifically asked for a speaker who was living with HIV but was not gay or an IV-drug user. She had been down that road before and the students couldn't relate or connect with the speaker. He thought I might be perfect. Anthony convinced me to at least call the teacher, Willa Johnson, who was also the peer education coordinator at Bowen High School. I called with the intention of telling her no; however, her sincerity touched me, and I said yes.

Willa had a difficult time settling the students down and after she introduced me, they continued to talk instead of listen. A couple of the young men asked me for my telephone number. Everyone started laughing. At least they weren't hostile like the boys at that private school where I had spoken in 1984 for the Jackson campaign.

"Awww, you got jokes huh?" I asked jokingly.

"Naw, you just fin-n-n-eee," he said, rubbing his chin like he was macking.

"I'm serious, though. How about that number?" The laughter started up again. I barely got through with the basics of HIV when a girl said, "We know that stuff already."

"Alright, Ms. Smarty Pants," I said walking over to the girl. "Give me your hand."

"So can a person give you HIV by touching you?" I asked.

"Nope," the girl said, and gave me her hand. I had their attention now.

"What if I cut myself and all my blood came running out over your arms. Can you get HIV now?"

"Naw-w-w," she said, but with a little less confidence. "You're right," I told her.

Someone else said, "I don't know about that—if you bled *all* over her arm?"

"Yes," I confirmed and explained to him that HIV could not penetrate skin. Rather, it needed a way to get in, like a cut or broken skin. I could see the heads nodding. I knew I had their attention. I continued to hold her hand and made a smooth transition to sex, explaining how a woman becomes infected while having sex. "You see," I said, "when the penis enters the vagina…." and, at that point, there were a few giggles. I told them, "If you're too immature to learn how you contract HIV, then you are too immature to have sex."

"Aww, SNAP!" someone hollered.

"I'm just sayin'," I said, shrugging my shoulders. Now, I had their full attention. Then I explained how a guy is infected from vaginal sex. When I moved on to anal sex, I had a little protest.

"Ain't nobody doing that faggot shit," a male student said. The impulse was to give him a lecture on homophobia, but I was asked to come educate these young people about HIV and I was not going to get sidetracked. I had them right where I wanted them: at the place where they were open to new ideas. I didn't want to lose the momentum.

"That ain't a nice thing to say," I said, walking over to him. "What if you have anal with a girl?" I asked. He started smiling.

"You can still get HIV," I said. That smile disappeared.

"A butthole is a butthole, whether it is male or female," I said. Someone yelled, "Sho' you right," and the room roared with laughter. I explained why the easiest form of HIV transmission was anal sex. That it had nothing to do with being gay, but how you have sex. I had made the point without being judgmental and you could see the light bulbs going off.

I had no idea where all of this was coming from, but I was intuitive, and my answers were spot-on. I shocked my own self that day. I would come to understand that as unorthodox as I was, God was moving through me every time I stood in front of an audience. No matter how large or small—whether it was a higher-level school like Stanford University; Hyde Park Career Academy, a high school on the South Side of Chicago—or at Bowen High School that day; I was a vessel.

"What about if I use my finger?" a guy asked. I walked over to him.

"Give me your hand." I requested. He stretched his hand out and laid it in mine, then rubbed my other one over the top. "Soft…" he said, smiling.

"Okay, Prince Charming, if you have this finger right here," I said, taking his middle finger and pointing it up, continuing, "in a girl's coochie, and if she has HIV—the HIV is in all of her vaginal secretions, and you got all her wet stuff on your finger and if it has a cut on it—yes, you could possibly contract HIV." He snatched his hand back and all the young men looked at their fingers.

"Okay. Can you look at a person and tell if they have HIV or AIDS?" I asked.

"No!" came loud, and in unison.

"Are you sure?" I followed. "I mean are you really sure that there is NO way to tell if a person has AIDS? Come on. Be honest. No judgment." They were thinking but no one dared say what he or she really believed. A girl finally spoke up, with an attitude: "We told you, no!" Heads nodded in agreement. I had them right where I wanted them.

"Okay, so no one is surprised that I have AIDS," I said. The room exploded with disbelief, shock, stunned faces and mumbling. I calmly and slowly repeated myself, "I have AIDS." A young man spoke up, saying, "You mean you got AIDS right now? No joke?"

"No joke. I got AIDS—right now."

"You too fine to have AIDS," another guy hollered. There were mumbles of agreement.

"But you just told me that you couldn't look at a person and tell if they had AIDS.

So, what does being cute have to do with anything?" I asked.

"Yeah, but that was different. I mean, you're not gay," he replied. I pushed them to think. I asked, "What does being gay have to do with whether you can tell if someone has AIDS?" A young man explained how he had seen gay men on television with AIDS, and how they were skin and bones. Others had that image in their heads also, but they were afraid to say so for fear they were stereotyping people with HIV. They had learned the sound bite that you cannot look at a person and tell if they had HIV, but the reality was they had only seen one image of HIV/AIDS, and it was mostly white gay men. Ms. Johnson had been on point in her assessment. Students fired their questions at me back-to-back, and I surprised myself by how transparent I was. I told them to keep asking, and that no question was too personal, silly, or stupid.

"How did you get it?"

"Unprotected sex," I fired back.

"How did you find out?"

"I donated blood," I answered.

"How long you got to live?"

"By the time your freshman class graduates, I will be dead," I said directly. They got quiet again, and someone changed the topic.

"What do you do for a living?"

"I'm a political organizer," and then explained.

"Wow, that's great," someone said. That eased the tension for a moment, but then someone asked, "How many pills do you take?"

"I take twenty-three pills a day."

"Straight?" a guy said. And someone followed up immediately, "Damn, that's deep."

"Correct," I said. "AIDS is deep." A girl asked, "What did your momma say when you told her?"

"I haven't."

"Damn-n! You ain't even told your momma?" someone asked.

"My mama told me that I was never gonna be shit. I'm not trying to hear 'I told you so.'" I saw a girl in front of me whose eyes were watering.

"I know what you mean," she said. I walked over to her and squeezed her hand, and silently mouthed to her, "You're going to be okay." She smiled. Then someone blurted, "You know who gave it to you?" "No." I said, because I was not ready to discuss Max. Neither Mrs. Jackson nor Reverend had asked me who infected me, and I saw no reason to throw gasoline on the fire. It would take more therapy and more confidence. The room grew quiet. Another one asked, cautiously, "Well, if you don't know who gave it to you... was you—I mean—getting down like that?" I was clever and responded quickly.

"As fine as I am, don't you think I've been taking applications for my stuff?" I asked. Laughter filled the room. Then I explained the cycle of dating: "You meet a guy and ya think he's the best thing since sliced bread. Then the bread molds." I paused and asked, "And what do you do with moldy bread?"

"Throw it out!" the girls yelled loudly.

"Correct," I said. And then, you cry about it. Talk to your girlfriends about it. Try to figure how you hooked up with his crazy ass in the first place, and then you move on to the next Mr. Right. And the cycle keeps going until you get married. Let's say you start having sex when you are thirteen, like I did, and I'm not married yet. Say you start having sex at sixteen and you don't get married until you are twenty-six. That's ten years of dating. The younger you start having sex, the more sexual partners you accumulate—even if you never had a one-night stand or only had sex with guys in a committed relationship." I could see the expressions of deep thought on the faces of the girls. "Once the relationship is over, you can't take back the sex; it's too late," I said.

"You got a point," a girl responded.

"If I could've, would've, should've don't mean a damn thing in the real world," I said, continuing, "This is the only life you got. Grandmamma used to say: You make your bed hard; you lay in it."

The final question came from a girl: "Do you still have sex?"

"Yes," I said. "Finding someone to have sex with you is the easiest thing you will ever do in your entire life. Men think with their little head—not their big one." The girls laughed loudly, and the guys protested. The bell rang and students came up to me to ask more questions. The next group of students entered, and I followed the same pattern. I finished with that group. When the last group of students for the day came in, I noticed there were two male students still sitting in the same spots. They had been up front to talk to me in between groups, but this was the first time I had noticed they were sitting through the other sessions. I looked around the room and spotted others from my previous two sessions. I asked Ms. Johnson why they were making some students stay. She told me they were skipping class to hear me speak again. I thought about it on the bus ride home. I wondered what I could possibly have said that was important enough to make them skip class.

I couldn't stop thinking about that day. The next set of workshops was two days later. As I dressed that morning, I had a bounce within me I had not had in a year. Shirley Caesar was singing a song from her new CD; *He's Working it Out for You* in the background. I felt connected to God in a way I hadn't in months. I started crying uncontrollably.

When I entered the room at Bowen High School that morning students were lined up along the walls. Those who had heard me speak two days earlier wanted to hear me again and those who weren't scheduled had decided to skip class to see the lady with AIDS for themselves. Between sessions students crowded me with more questions, hugs, and tears. In their embraces they told me their dark secrets—of family members with HIV; their own sexual escapades; and childhood sexual, emotional, and physical abuse. I had struck a chord. It was as if they had been waiting for an adult to give them room to address these forbidden topics.

Some of the faculty disapproved of my candor, and that remained a pattern. Whether I was speaking at a school or for Jack and Jill, adults were uncomfortable. Because of my potty mouth, it was also assumed I was not educated. The young people would holler when I said I had graduated from college *cum laude* or that I was in graduate school on an academic fellowship. Inevitably, some adult in the room would try to assert his or her moral superiority with a question. It always went something like this, and that day at Bowen was no different: "Can you explain to them that there is no such thing as safe sex because condoms break?" I had never forgotten the day back at that private school in Maryland. I made myself a promise never to go into a situation in which I had not immersed myself in the topic. I had done my homework. I talked about condom studies and how durable condoms were, and my own experience with condoms. In all the years of sex, even to date, I've had maybe three condoms break.

"If you could do it over again, would you have waited and started having sex later?" was another common adult question. I made myself clear, there are no do-overs. If I could do it over again, I would ask God for new parents so that my starting point in life would be different. I had been birthed in chaos; on that much I was very clear, and it became the narrative of my life. I never pushed the idea that they would end up like me, or that I regretted my life. I did, however, want them to learn from my missteps. I came to understand I was the bearer of knowledge, and they would take what parts of my life they needed for themselves. Some of them asked me more about surviving my childhood than about AIDS.

That day at Bowen, as a teacher was pushing her agenda, a young man said, "Aw, shut the fuck up! You don't know what it's like to live with AIDS! Ya'll think ya'll know everything." The students smirked and nodded their heads in agreement. Once at a Jack and Jill National Convention when I was just getting ready to enter seminary, a mother said under her breath, "She will never make it in anyone's seminary." As is the way of life, I spoke at the convention three years later right after I graduated, and the young person who introduced me reflected about the smart comment a mother had made about me three years earlier.

As time went on, I developed a rule I strictly followed: When I was speaking to a teen audience, the adults could not ask questions. I now know that I had a unique gift to reach young people and I was not going to allow interference. It was akin to people walking in and out of church when the preacher is delivering a sermon. Reverend Evans would say all the time that walking while he was preaching will kill the spirit, and I agree. I didn't know any of this at that first speaking engagement; I simply felt God moving in my life in a way I had never known. At the end of that second day at Bowen, a Latina girl came up to me and said, "Ms. Lewis, I know you said you weren't a public speaker, but you shouldn't stop because God is using you." I thanked that baby and gave her a hug.

In the days that followed, I thought about the students and what had transpired. They had such an impact on me, I couldn't let them go. I told the story of those two days to my friends, trying to make sense out of what I was feeling. It really was a no-brainer, but I still let my brain get in the way. I could feel God pushing me in the direction I was to go, but I still had doubts. I was a doubting Thomas. I was not a speaker.

Politics and social-justice work had been my life for the last ten years, and it had become painfully clear I couldn't keep up the pace. I realized I was having difficulty getting up and moving in the mornings, and those late-night meetings were killing me. I didn't know if I could cut it or at what cost. I asked myself if I wanted to die on this political hill. Now I wondered if God had a different plan. The more I thought about those young people at Bowen, the less focused I became on my campaign job. I began seeking more advice. Noble came over to visit and I talked to him about it. In the past, I had never talked to him about my career choices but being a principal, I thought he might have a relevant perspective. Boy, did he burst my bubble.

"Why would you tell all your personal business to kids?" he asked. I tried to explain it wasn't like that, but it was exactly like that. I had told them some of the most intimate parts of my life that I would have never dared to address prior to that day. He made me feel stupid. He told me students didn't take those lectures seriously, anyway. I started to doubt myself even more, but he had been wrong. Those students had taken me seriously. In fact, they couldn't stop thinking about me, like I hadn't been able to stop thinking about them. They decided they wanted to write me letters; here's one:

> Dear Rae Lewis,
> Hi. How have you been? Healthy, I hope. People say that I'm sort of a funny boy, well right now I don't feel so much like laughing. Rae, sometimes when I go to one of them places where some adults is talking about AIDS, I always ask if they have AIDS and they say no. When I heard you say you had AIDS, I turned my head with my mouth opened like some fool for like an half an hour. All I could do is pay attention to every word you said. Anyway all I want to say is I hope you keep healthy cause that's the only way you'll survive.
> Sincerely your friend,
> Eduardo

Ms. Johnson called for my address because the students had written me letters. When I received the manila envelope and pulled out the hundreds of letters, I was in total disbelief. Never in my wildest imagination had I expected so many. I made a cup of tea, sat on the sofa, read, and cried, and read and cried some more. God was knocking me on my head, and I was still dragging my feet. How many more signs did I need to move forward in faith?

It occurred to me that Noble's advice was more about him than about me. We had dated for almost five years and my HIV status had been a well-kept secret. By speaking, I was not only exposing myself to critique but exposing our relationship to his peers. I tell people all the time: Be careful who you ask to validate what God has called you to do. I was talking to Nana about Noble's advice one day and she said, "Noble don't know what he's talking about. I don't know why you keep talking to these insignificant people."

"But Nana…" and, before I could finish, she said, "See that's the problem. You're thinking when you should be acting." She told me she knew the person I needed to talk to and asked if she could call me right back. Five minutes later she called and told me to be at her condo at 3:00 p.m. When I arrived, there was a man who looked familiar but who I did not know sitting in the living room.

"Rae, this is Reverend James Bevel and I asked him over to counsel with you on this endeavor you are considering."

"Bevel, this is my precious goddaughter, Rae, and she is a BAD Mama Jama," Nana said. She went on to sing my praises about how I had organized youth and students for the Jackson campaigns and on and on. Reverend Bevel stood up and offered me his hand.

I had heard so many stories about him when I worked at PUSH. He was a master strategist who had been one of Dr. Martin Luther King Jr.'s lieutenants. He was the ex-husband of Diane Nash, one of the founders of the SNCC. "Well, daughter, let's talk," he said, motioning for me to sit. Jeez! Sitting with this legend, I was nervous. I started sweating underneath my clothes. I began by telling him what an honor it was to meet him, but he stopped me.

"I didn't come over here to hear about me. I came to hear about you," he said. Now, I was totally thrown off. All I could think of to say was, "I have AIDS." Then I sighed like I had the weight of the world on me. Before I could say another word, he asked, "And what are you going to do about it?" I tried to explain the work I had been doing and he asked, "What does that have to do with what God wants you to do now?" He continued, "You see, Martin [speaking of Dr. King] didn't stay stuck; he started with public accommodations and the boycott on Montgomery, then moved on to voting rights and then poverty." Bevel was so profound. And he asked me a question I will never forget: "Do you think God is a one-track God?" It went like that for over two hours. He counseled me and every now and then Nana interjected with, "See, Bevel? I told Rae." And another round of the discussion started. He made it clear that having AIDS was bigger than just me.

"Our people are dying from this disease," he continued. "What are you going to do; just die, too?" When he had exhausted every angle, he said, "Let's pray." We stood and held hands, and he prayed. As he was putting on his coat, he said to me, "This is your Esther moment. Now, what are YOU, going to do?"

I went home and replayed our conversation in my head. I had known since that day at Second Baptist that God was calling me to do work that was bigger than me. As I've mentioned, I had always assumed that social-justice work was it, but now maybe that work had been preparation for the work I would ultimately do. I stopped all the moaning about dying and began praying for direction and clarity. I asked God, "What do you want me to do with the rest of my life on Earth?" I prayed constantly on the bus and walking down the street. Sometimes I had full conversations with God. I know people must have thought I was crazy, walking and talking to myself, but I didn't care; I needed answers. Reverend Bevel believed this was my Esther moment. I would have never described it that way—not then, at least, but I could see his point. Again, I was not a public speaker and, before I made a fool out of myself, I wanted to know this was what I was supposed to do. I stayed in God's face. One night, I prayed the same prayer over and over until I fell to sleep: "Please God, show me your will for my life." When I woke up the next morning, I felt the presence of God. Tears of joy streamed down my face. I bolted up and started pacing the floor. God was speaking to my spirit and all my confusion had been wiped away. *Thank you, Jesus. Yes God. Yes, to your will. Speak Lord! Yes, to your will—hallelujah!* I praised God until all my tears were gone and my mouth was dry. I had more clarity than I'd had in years. AIDS would not be about my sufferings, but about how God intended to use me to help others. I called Joe at his office and asked to meet with him. I put on my newly released Yolanda Adams cassette, *Save the World* and I replayed "The Battle Is the Lord's" a few more times before I left to meet Joe. We had lunch in the eatery of the Saks building a block from his office.

I told him about my experience at Bowen a few weeks before. He thought it was wonderful I'd been willing to expose myself in that way to educate young African American people. I told him I was sure that God wanted me to speak about my life and that I wanted to focus my attention there. "That's great, Rae. I have absolutely no objection," he said. I realized he had missed what I was trying to say. He thought I was asking for permission to speak while working on the campaign.

"Joe," I told him. "I love working for you, and I'm honored that you have trusted me with such a valuable position, but I'm resigning." I had never seen Joe speechless until that moment.

"Well, if that's what you want to do," he said with a shred of doubt. And it *was* what I wanted to do. "I can see you have given this a lot of thought. Where do you speak next?" he asked. I explained that I didn't have any more speaking engagements but was sure this was the direction my life was supposed to take. I told him I felt incredibly strong about my decision. Despite the fact, I didn't have a brochure or any idea how to go about seeking another engagement. He looked at me like I had two heads.

"What are you going to do for money?" he asked. I hadn't even thought about that. I knew God had a plan and that was all I was sure of that day. I couldn't see how it was going to work out, but I knew it would. After experiencing God that morning, I was not going to back out. To bring God's plan to fruition, I had to be willing to step out on faith. The Bible says, "Faith is the substance of things hoped for and the evidence of things unseen."

"I don't know, Joe," I responded. "I haven't gotten that far." He gave me two months' severance pay with the hope it would help until I figured things out. "It's the least I can do, Rae." When I got to the office to pack up my desk, the check was waiting. I have never forgotten it was Joe who hired me knowing that I had AIDS. And I have never forgotten he believed in me and invested in what looked like a pipe dream when he didn't have to.

Soon after I resigned, Ms. Johnson called from Bowen and asked for an invoice for the two days. I had volunteered my time, but apparently the Chicago Public Schools had money for these types of workshops. "Other people get paid," she said, "and so should you." With that, she invited me to speak at a conference for teachers that coordinated the peer programs in the Chicago public high schools. She believed if these teachers had an opportunity to hear me speak, they would also bring me in to conduct HIV/AIDS workshops at their schools. The conference was going to be held at a hotel in the western suburbs of Chicago. I still didn't know how to drive and to ask someone to take me an hour both ways for fifteen minutes was a whole lot. That Saturday was reunion day at PUSH, and I bumped into Cheryl Porter from the Black Expo. She had heard I had AIDS and asked if she could help. I didn't waste any time in asking if she would take me to the event. I moved forward preparing a brochure to distribute to teachers at the conference. Tyrone allowed me to use the equipment at his church to produce and print them. Everyone was proud and provided fuel to my engine. I even borrowed a binding machine from Dr. Finney's office.

I had no idea what I was going to say to the teachers, but I only had fifteen minutes to say it. I had to quickly gain their attention. "I have AIDS," is how I started off, and it would be my trademark for the next twenty-seven years. I have no clue what I said after that; I just know that, after I finished speaking, over half of the teachers expressed interest in bringing me to speak in their schools. Some even booked me on the spot for the coming semester. Cheryl, who worked nights volunteered to drive and accompany me to speaking engagements. God had indeed worked it out.

Fifty-Four
UNTIL DEATH DO US PART

> " Be careful what you ask for; you just might get it."
> —Aesop fable

The sadness I felt seeped out of me like air from a balloon. I became a new person overnight. Accepting the call from God lifted the burden of death. I was at peace. Of course, I hurt. The emotional pain and physical toll AIDS had on me were seemingly insurmountable. There was no way around the disease and no way to fight it. It just was. Dying with a purpose took away the agony of wanting the life I made for myself. I started to live in the present. No more bemoaning what was and what was never going to be. I had accepted death, but I was going to *live* until I died. That mindset was apparent in all my actions. For Christmas, I gave my friends gifts that meant something to me so they could have a part of me. I gave Leslie my beautiful porcelain teapot I hand-carried from Moscow in 1985. Leslie gave it back this year, and it now graces one of my bookshelves. I gave Veronica the dress I wore to my grandfather's funeral for her little girl, if she ever had a little girl. She sent it back to me when I had my first goddaughter. It has been framed as art to add to my collection as an ode to Little Rae, who survived every damn thing that came her way. Cheryl had a nine-year-old daughter, Latoya Renae, and I gave her almost all the teddy bears I had collected since 1984. I purchased my first on the campaign trail in Atlanta and had been collecting them ever since. Even Mrs. Jackson had indulged me with a bear or two. God knows what happened to that collection, but Latoya hit me up about eighteen years ago. She said, "Tee, I have mad skills and I want to help you." She has been my executive assistant since that day.

I was still trying to finish graduate school. I didn't want the completion of my master's degree to be another thing AIDS would take from me. I didn't know what I would do with this degree, but I would at least have the satisfaction of completing the master's program at UIC. It would prove harder than I could ever imagine. My ability to get things done was replaced by fatigue. No matter how much sleep I got, it was never enough. Simply reading was exhausting. My incompletes were increasing and hanging over my head like a guillotine.

I was already booked to speak at a couple of high schools after the holiday break. Then, my former housemate Ray Anderson—who was planning a fundraiser to help with the famine in Somalia and who wanted to recognize my work concerning HIV—offered to create space for me to speak at his event. He had pulled together an ad hoc committee of other like-minded young adults to work on this fundraiser, from which the proceeds would go to Africare. I was also on the committee but had stopped going to meetings. "Imani for Somalia" was an even larger fundraiser than the one for Carol Moseley Braun the previous year. I was humbled Ray wanted to honor me but speaking to my peers was an entirely different thing from talking to a group of high school students. Ray said this was a perfect audience to reach about HIV prevention. I thought the timing was lousy. "Who wants to hear about HIV on New Year's, when the after-party is sex?" I asked Ray.

"That's the point," he said. "Maybe we will save a life that night." I couldn't argue with him on that, and I agreed to speak.

You couldn't have paid me a million dollars to believe I had become a speaker. I used to be in awe of Sister Souljah's speaking ability. She was so gifted, and I couldn't get a word out of my mouth without it sounding like mumbo-jumbo. I would have mapped what I was going to say in my head; however, when it came to delivery, I couldn't get it out of my mouth. Writing it down was no better. I would get so nervous that I would skip over some of the points I wanted to make. I felt like Moses in Exodus when he told God, "But Lord, I am telling you, I am not a good speaker." Then the Lord told Moses, *Look, man, I made the mouth to speak, the eyes to see and the ears to hear* (my words). "I am the Lord. So go. I will be with you when you speak. I will give you the words to say." Despite my doubts, just like Moses, I put my faith in God and went through every door God opened.

Veronica offered to buy me a new dress for the fundraiser, and we went to Marshall Field's. I found the perfect dress. It was a rich, dark purple, knee-length velvet sheath that had a dip in the back and with purple chiffon draping. The last set of clothes I purchased had been a size eight. I knew I was steadily losing weight, but I didn't give it a lot of thought. I had been taking the Megace to stimulate my appetite and drinking the milkshakes, as instructed. I had to have still been in denial. I picked up a size eight and thought, *Well, maybe I should take the size ten, just in case.* I tried on the ten and quickly went to the eight. Veronica was in and out of the dressing room. I darted out and picked up a size six; it was also loose. I sat on the little bench inside the dressing room in disbelief. I had been lying to everyone about my weight loss; it turned out I had been lying to myself the most. I had avoided the topic subconsciously. I had seen many images of white men with AIDS who were skin and bones, and there was something about being visually connected to those men that scared me. Veronica came into the dressing room. "Why in the world do you have so many of the same dresses?"

"Ronnie, I can't believe how small I've gotten," I said with a sigh. She wanted to know what size I had on. "It's a six, and it's too big," I whined.

"Stop being a drama queen, Rae," she said. "Stand up and let me see." I did as she'd requested. Then she asked me to turn around. "Yeah, it's a little big here," she assessed, reaching for the extra space under the arms. "I'll see if they have a four." She came back and handed me the four. I put it on and she said, "That look's great on you." I looked at her, like, *Give me a break.*

"Rae, do you know how many women wish they were a size four?" I rolled my eyes at her and changed back into my own clothes. Ronnie was right, though. I had been one of those women who was on and off fad diets and working my body in the gym until I hurt. When we got into the car, she knew I was in my feelings. She began her little pep talk. "Rae, so what? You're a size four. You are not dead, and you are not going to die. Well, one day you're going to die—we are all going to die. You just ain't going nowhere anytime soon. I wish you would get that through your thick skull." Veronica was a pain in the ass, but I was deeply appreciative of our years of friendship.

After my meltdown in Marshall Field's, I went through my closet to see what didn't fit and what I could get away with, even if it was too big. Being such a shopaholic, I literally had piles of clothes on my living room floor; I even had clothes with the tags still on them. Mama had rubbed off on me, for real. Her love for clothes had become my love for clothes. The clothes she purchased me made me feel loved, and the clothes I bought fed that empty space inside of me. It had only gotten worse over the years. The more money I made, the more clothes I purchased. After I tried on every piece of clothing, I started giving away the ones that were way too big for me. I had been giving Shawnice Hubbard from PUSH clothes since she was a pre-teen, and she always got first dibs. I didn't have money to purchase new clothes in those early days, so I went to resale shops — I still do — and purchased other people's clothes so that I had something that fit.

My first big wardrobe overhaul came by way of a woman named Phyllis Milliken-Schopp in the spring of 1994. She was a stylist and salesperson at the Ann Taylor clothing store in Water Tower Place. By now I was rapidly making my way to a size two. Phyllis was introduced to me by a mutual friend. While I had an eye for clothes, I didn't know how to address the shifts in weight. It was emotionally draining and overwhelming. She held my hand through that process and never let it go as my weight continued to fluctuate over the years. She kept me abreast of sales and when I would arrive to Ann Taylor, she had clothes already pulled for me to try on. She even got me a gig speaking to employees at the store. As a result, the store manager offered to loan me clothes for the CBS news series. Phyllis dressed me every night I sat anchor for the CBS series, and Deidra had my hair looking fly.

Ray's event was a huge success. The place was packed with the twenty-something/thirty-something crowd of Black Chicagoans. Everyone looked fabulous, and so did Veronica and me. When I started to speak, it was difficult to get people to quiet down. I felt a little nervous perspiration under my dress. *Why did I let Ray talk me into this? These people want to party, not hear about HIV.* I started talking anyway.

"I have AIDS," I said. People started shushing so I could be heard. "I know you don't see AIDS when you look at me, but it's real. You don't see the twenty-one-day menstrual cycles, the fatigue, the diarrhea, the twenty-three pills a day, but it's real." After I had their attention, I talked about condom use and HIV testing. Then I was done. People who knew me but had not heard the rumor rushed up to me. A couple of men who had hit on me that night came up to me and asked, "You really have AIDS?" I wanted to say, *No, dummy. I just told over a thousand people I have AIDS for fun.* I had empathy for their stupidity. No one wanted to believe that anyone in *their* world could have HIV/AIDS. I made it too close and too personal; it rocked their world and everything they believed about the disease. At midnight, the music was cut, and we were asked to join hands to pray. I love how Black people can transport the church to any place at any time. My heart was filled with so much gratitude. It had been a year since I had officially transitioned to AIDS. When I added the months after my T-cell count had dropped to 134 and the other medical conditions that signaled a failing immune system, I had survived the first eighteen-month death sentence that characterized full-blown AIDS. I re-upped on my commitment to do God's work for as long as I had breath in my body. *Use me, Lord, until you use me up* was my prayer of supplication.

By early spring, the idea of consultant work had been overshadowed by speaking engagements. My name and telephone number were being passed around Chicago Public Schools like a joint at a house party. Everyone had heard about me and wanted to bring me to their school: Teachers, principals and even students who had been told about me from their peers called to see if I could come to speak at their high schools. I was still utilizing Tyrone's church office equipment to put together my speaking packets, and that's where I met my future husband: Kenneth "Kenny" Thornton Jr.

Kenny was a member of Tyrone's church and one of his roommates. He was in and out of the office when I was around, and we were cordial. On one of those days, he noticed me looking through the want ads to find jobs to complete my unemployment papers and offered to help. Later that week, he dropped off an employment listing. I don't think he stayed more than ten minutes. I hadn't given any romantic thought to Kenny, but he was on it. The next day, he left me a phone message asking if I would go to the movies with him. I was a little hesitant because I was already spending time with another of Tyrone's friends, a minister visiting Chicago, but we really hadn't gone anywhere. Kenny was handsome, standing six-foot-three with a medium build and teakwood-brown skin. He wasn't as polished as I preferred my men. Nonetheless, there was something appealing about him. *What could it hurt?* I agreed to go out with him. What Kenny lacked in style and intellectual banter, he made up for in kindness and charm. A week later, we made it to the bedroom. The sex was good—I mean, rea-l-l-y good—and he had no problem whatsoever with me having HIV or with using a condom. I was already speaking, so he clearly had no concern about what people thought of him dating a woman with AIDS. The following week, we were in a full-fledged relationship. Veronica wasn't impressed. I remember the first time she met him; he wore a jacket that had seen better years.

"You know, he looks like a country bumpkin with that raggedy-ass jacket on," she said. My bougie friend was right, but Kenny was laying it on just right and I dismissed the ways we were mismatched. One night, about a month into the relationship and after some electrifying sex, we were in bed talking about marriage. He confessed he had been married when he was younger, and had a daughter from that marriage who was about eight that lived in Texas now. I had already met his toddler son, who he got every other weekend. He had also told me about his oldest daughter, who was in middle school. I did the math: three children, three different mothers, one marriage under his belt— and he was three years older than me. The first two children were at least three years apart, and the youngest, even more. I rationalized that a lot can happen in three years. Circumstances change. Shit happens! Who was I to judge Kenny? And, I had HIV. I told him about wasting four years of my life with Noble and how he had gotten married—yes, married—six months after we ended our relationship. Noble had the nerve to tell me he was lonely. I asked his old ass, "What the hell do you think I am? Over here with AIDS, by myself, after waiting on you to marry me?" I had wasted all that time, and I figured I would probably never get married.

"If our relationship continues to grow like this in the next six months, I could marry you," Kenny said, from out of nowhere. I didn't think marriage would be possible with AIDS. I hadn't had any issues with casual dating, and it surprised me that men were willing to have sex with me infected, without a commitment. I thought about all those years I stuck with Noble because I was afraid of rejection. Getting someone to have sex with me was the easiest thing of all. But what came out of my mouth shocked me. "Me, too," I said, following with, "Why wait? Why don't we plan to get married in six months?"

"Okay, let's do it." Kenny quickly agreed. And, just like that, I was officially engaged to be married. We decided to keep it under wraps, at least for a while. We told Tyrone and I told Veronica. "Rae, he doesn't even have a job," was Veronica's response and I couldn't argue with that. Kenny had started taking me to my speaking engagements when Cheryl wasn't available, and he was looking for a job. There were so many red flags, but I forged ahead, and so did Kenny, cementing his place in my life. He was attentive to my every need. He rubbed my hands and feet to help ease the nerve pain from the peripheral neuropathy. He ran me bubble baths, washed me, and put lotion on my body. Oh, yeah—he was a keeper. It could have been a thousand red flags dropping on my head like hail, but I was going to weather this storm. One evening, while dropping me off at school, he told me he was going to drop off a birthday card to his daughter. I had never heard her name before. I went completely off the rail. We spent hours talking about our lives and, in all our talks, he had failed to mention this daughter. "How the fuck do you have another daughter that you have never told me about?" He had four children by four different women, and that didn't sit well with me. I seriously thought about putting on the brakes but, God, he was so good to me.

I finally told Nana about Kenny. She thought I was rushing into the marriage, and she adamantly disapproved of us living together. Kenny had already moved into my apartment so we could save money. Around the same time, Nana informed me she had submitted my name to receive this community service award, and I had been chosen. The

Expo for Today's Black Women was under the leadership of a local Black businesswoman, Mary Green, and sponsored by Chicago radio station V-103. Nana was on the advisory board and told me it had been effortless persuading the committee to choose me. AIDS was such a new topic in the African American community, and I was one of the very few Black women who was speaking out. The award was to be given at a black-tie banquet the night before the opening of the expo. I used the money from my previous speaking engagement to buy a new dress. I found the perfect little number in the Lillie Rubin boutique. It was a simple sleeveless, ankle-length sheath dress—gray silk with sequined triangles and a front split that came up to my knee. It was fabulous, and I was fabulous in it. I went to Marshall Field's and purchased Kenny a tie to match my dress and a shirt for his black suit.

The night of the event everyone who was somebody in Black Chicago was there. The house was packed, and people were primped and wearing the best of their Sunday best. Veronica, Cheryl, Leslie, and Gail came to support me. Tyrone was there but, then again, he was among Chicago's social elite. When I was introduced, I think most of the audience somehow missed that I had AIDS, and only got the part where I was educating young people about HIV/AIDS. Standing at the podium, I looked out across the banquet hall at Chicago's best and brightest in the African American community—and all I could see was a room of potential HIV cases. I thought about the men who had been hitting on me all night, even with Kenny prominently on my arm. Some of them even had dates. Black people were now disproportionately impacted by HIV, and we were living a free and cavalier life—as if this disease had nothing to do with us. I thought about the men who were willing to have sex with me in the months before I met Kenny and didn't give two cents about HIV or a commitment. I knew if we Black people didn't get it together and begin to take HIV seriously we, as a community, were headed for trouble.

"You know, Black people, we are in denial." I started. "Men have been hitting on me all night. Not only do I have HIV, but I also have full-blown AIDS, and you would never know it if I did not tell you." There was complete silence. I went on to talk about how AIDS was ravaging my body and had changed my life. I begged them to get tested and use condoms. I thanked them for the award but told them, "This award cannot save my life." I received a standing ovation. As I proceeded off the stage, Susan Taylor, the editor-in-chief of *Essence* magazine and the keynote speaker for the evening, grabbed my arm as I passed her. "Can I do a story on you?"

"Yes," I answered, I then walked down the stairs and went back to my seat. Kenny and I had been sitting at the table with Ms. Taylor's husband, Khephra Burns, and some of the Essence staff. They were blown away, right along with the rest of the audience. No one at the table realized I had AIDS until it came out of my mouth. Just like at the high schools, my physical appearance conflicted with everything they understood about AIDS. That would be evident over and over again. Physically, I challenged the paradigm of AIDS, whether I was a size twelve or a four. People did not see AIDS when they looked at me, and how I looked became some kind of scared-straight movement. Those working in HIV/AIDS had been trying for years to dispel stereotypes that it was not a white gay male and IV-drug user disease. The messages they had been trying to convey were that anyone can get HIV. The images of people whom we had seen those first twelve years of HIV/AIDS showed individuals who looked sick and despondent. When the event was over, they rushed Susan out of the room, and I never got the chance to give her my telephone number; neither did anyone ask for mine. I mentioned it to Mary Green, but Susan hadn't mentioned our conversation. *Oh, well,* I thought, and dismissed it.

A couple weeks later, I was taking a bubble bath in the middle of the day when the phone rang. "Hello, may I speak to Rae Lewis?" asked this smooth voice on the line.

"This is she," I said.

"Hi Rae. This is Susan Taylor." I was so shocked the phone slipped out of my wet hand, and I caught it just as it was about to hit the water. I jumped out of the tub, grabbed my robe, and sat on the floor in front of the sofa. She told me she and her team discussed me and decided they wanted to put me on the cover of their magazine. For a second, I was speechless. I had to let this marinate. *The* Susan Taylor of *the Essence magazine* wants to put *me,* Rae Lewis—who had been born to drug addicted parents, discarded, and rejected—on the cover of her magazine. The scripture, *The rejected stone became the cornerstone....* came to mind. This was the most surreal moment of my life.

"Ms. Taylor, I'm so honored," I said to her. Within a split second, that scripture was replaced with doubt. I started with a little speech:

> *I know there isn't a Black woman in America that wouldn't want to be on the cover of your magazine, but you know nothing about me. You heard me speak for five minutes. Why would you put me on the cover of your magazine?*

"Rae, I believe that you have a story to tell, and I want to tell it," she said. There was nothing more to say, except yes.

Once I was headed for the magazine cover, Nana, even with doubts about my upcoming nuptials, asked if there was something she could do to help us. Kenny needed a job. We had been dating now for almost three months and mostly living off my speaking engagements and his unemployment check. I asked if she could check around for him. Karen Nash—the best friend of Nana's daughter, Ann—came through and hired Kenny to work on a temporary project.

Opposition to me marrying Kenny was swift. Everyone wanted me to be happy but questioned the short time I had known him. There were two exceptions: Coré and Barry. They pretty much said, *If you are happy, so am I.* Nana and Ms. J started receiving unsolicited intel on Kenny. I don't know how I could have been so naive. He had already told me he and his ex-wife had been members of Fellowship Missionary Baptist Church and married by Reverend Evans. Ms. J and Nana had attended Fellowship for almost as many years as there had been a church. Well, apparently, everyone knew the story of Kenny and his ex-wife, or so it seemed to me. They were lining up with the intel. Ms. J and Nana were not pleased with what they were told. I was getting an earful from two women I admired and respected deeply. I didn't know how to address the gossip. Basically, the rumor was that Kenny wasn't taking care of the children he had, so how was he going to take care of me? He hadn't done shit with his life, and I was both his meal ticket and his claim to fame. I dismissed the claim-to-fame analysis because we were engaged before I was asked to be on the cover of *Essence.* I had, however, already been interviewed for an article on Black women and HIV/AIDS for *Ebony* magazine when I met Kenny. That article appeared in the April 1994 issue—around the same time our engagement became public. John Johnson, the founder of *Ebony* and *Jet* magazines, was very proud his publication was the first to feature me. The *Ebony* article received mild buzz on my end. However, it was probably clear to everyone except me that the cover of *Essence* was about to change my life. What was clear to me in 1994 is that AIDS was a death sentence. Since Kenny was willing to support me through this horrific journey, well, I would support him. That was my sentiment. I might have looked like a picture of health, but my T cells were hovering between 60-80. I was not getting better. Dr. Cohen was working against the clock, which was ticking loud and clear. I had started to depend on Kenny more each day. We had long talks about our relationship and about his role in my life. He believed God had sent him to take care of me. I thought how gracious it was of God to send me someone at this time in my life. Nothing else really mattered to me. I had my ministry educating and challenging stereotypes around who and how one becomes infected with HIV and Kenny had his ministry—me. It was a twisted way to view our relationship, and neither of us put on the breaks.

All I needed was a little truth to dismiss the whole truth. Kenny confirmed he was behind in child support. *Of course, he was; he was unemployed,* I thought. The hard part came when the mothers aired their grievances. I can see how it was all a little disconcerting that Kenny was going on with his new life when there was still unfinished business in the life before he met me. The youngest child's mother asked for an agreement of financial support in writing; otherwise, she would cause a stink. One mother called and left a message on *my* telephone asking if Kenny planned to invite their daughter to the wedding; he did not. The issue that knocked me flat on my ass was that the ex-wife was still the wife. When Kenny told me, I almost lost my freaking mind. Our wedding invitations had just been mailed and I felt like a complete fool. In all our thousand and one conversations, I absolutely didn't understand how he could not have told me he and his wife were not divorced.

She made herself perfectly clear: *I am not giving you a divorce until I am certain that you are going to take care of your daughter.* I was not mad at her; I was mad at the situation. I put on my hiking boots and kept on climbing through the shit. I was going to marry this man. Period. He worked out arrangements for the children whose mothers were demanding child support and, frankly, I agreed with the mothers. I asked Kenny, "How the hell are we going to be around here talking about you taking care of me, and you're not even taking care of your children?" I don't think Kenny was a *de facto* father but in over his head. He should have—how can I say this diplomatically? —kept his male anatomy in his pants instead of making babies he couldn't take care of. I know he loved his children. It's just that life throws you curveballs. If a man doesn't have Nick Cannon kind of money, then one child will certainly fall by the wayside for another, especially when you have four. After we married and the money for speaking engagements came in, I stepped up, over and beyond, not just because it was the right thing to do. I'd be damned if I'd be the woman attached to a derelict father.

Kenny and I slipped and had sex without a condom. I was scared but mildly reassured he was probably not infected because it is more difficult for women to transmit HIV through vaginal sex. In 1994, only about eight percent of the men infected in the U.S. got HIV from heterosexual sex. Kenny took a series of HIV antibody tests at the clinic over a couple of months, and they all came back negative. That was a sigh of relief and we both became diligent about ensuring his safety. What we hadn't considered was there might be a baby in the oven. I woke up one morning with a familiar feeling. I was pregnant. I got off birth control pills after I was diagnosed with vaginal dysplasia. I had a D&C to remove the cells but decided to take a break from the pill since I was using condoms. This was one heck of a dilemma. There was about a thirty-percent chance I would transmit HIV to my child. I had always felt that even five percent was too much of a risk. Today, with all the medical advances in HIV, if an infected woman takes a specific antiretroviral regime during the first trimester of pregnancy, the risk of infecting her child is zero. The AIDS community has argued for years that HIV testing should become a standard part of prenatal care. That was not the case in 1994, and Dr. Cohen was more concerned about my health. She flat-out told me that if I was able to carry this baby to term, of which she was doubtful, it might kill me. Kenny and I went back and forth. He was committed to raising our child after my death. This would be my last chance to have a child, and I knew it. Years earlier, I decided not to have a child because I wasn't sure I could raise one alone. I was still adamant about how a child should be raised because of my horrible childhood, and Kenny's track record left me uncertain about leaving a child behind. I had a consultation to abort but was still wavering. Dr. Cohen had been right about my health. Shortly after the consult, I started spotting and my health became the determining factor. Dr. Cohen got the procedure pushed up.

This abortion was harder on me than the one I'd had almost fifteen years earlier. Laying on that table, I wept for the child I would never have. I screamed like a madwoman.

I screamed at the doctor for the physical pain I was feeling. I screamed at AIDS for the havoc it was causing in my life. I screamed so long and loudly, Dr. Linda Powell came into the room. I could hear her asking the physician conducting the procedure had she read my chart and seen that I had AIDS. I cannot remember her response. Dr. Powell took my hand into hers, and the warmth of her touch comforted me. The doctor conducting the procedure changed her disposition. With Dr. Powell at my side, I became a human being and the physician conducting the procedure began talking me through it. I have never forgotten Dr. Powell and what she did for me that day. She did more than comfort me; she gave me my dignity back.

Recovery was slow and I bled longer than what was normal, but I had to keep it moving. Speaking had started to dwindle because we were coming to the end of the school year, but I still had to pay for a wedding. I pulled myself together enough to get the last few gigs in before school shut down for the summer.

The planning of the wedding got crazy. At first, Mrs. Jackson offered to pay for the wedding reception. She had even taken me to one of her seamstresses, Gloria Winston, to design and make the dress. We were going to be married in the small chapel at Operation PUSH. I loved that chapel. The reception was going to be in the community hall at PUSH, so we didn't have to worry about the cost of renting a facility. Then one sunny Sunday afternoon in the Jacksons' yard, Mrs. Jackson and I had a falling-out about plates, of all things. I'm sure it was so much more than plates, but I never stopped to consider the real reason. She pulled her financial support and didn't come to the wedding. We wouldn't talk for almost a year. Then one Saturday I was at PUSH and Reverend Jackson asked me, "Have you spoken to Jackie?" I had not and he encouraged me to do so, "She's at the house, why don't you go to see her," he said. I went over that day and we started just like old times.

Nana continued asking me, "Baby, are you sure you *know* him?"

"They just mad," I replied, which was my scripted response. I was tired of hearing it and stopped calling. Nana didn't push it; she just let me be. She had also promised to help pay for the wedding but held onto the money until that day. I had taken Kenny to meet Mama. She always knew how to count the money and told me he was just in it for what he could get. She also passed on the wedding. Kenny's parents attended, as did his siblings. In the month leading up to the wedding, rumors were buzzing like flies on shit. People speculated that Kenny must have HIV; otherwise, why would he marry a woman with AIDS? I had to fight that rumor down. Some even dared to say they didn't understand why I would want to get married since I was dying—as if to say, I didn't deserve to have love these last years, months, or days of my life. It became me and Kenny against the world, and it became a more powerful bond than love.

Barry Saunders agreed to walk me down the aisle. I think I cried on his shoulder the most. He held my hand through the entire process. He'd ask, "You need me to come to Chicago and kick some ass?" I asked Coré and Veronica to stand with me. That became a thing, too. Veronica was not happy Coré was going to walk down the aisle ahead of her. She felt like Coré had been away at college, then law school and now, was off becoming famous singing with a grammy award winning R&B group, she had been there all the time, through thick and thin. It was true that my friendship with Coré after high school was mostly through the phone because of distance, but she had always supported me. Maybe I felt closer to Coré because she and I had spent a lot of time together those first two years they moved to Evanston. Dr. Cotton had allowed me to tag along in those early years of our friendship. It meant something special to me.

After the wedding, Veronica stopped talking to me for years until, one day, we were friends again. Coré bowed out of the friendship around fifteen years ago—just walked away. Life is a strange thing, is all I can say. We had a junior flower girl, Toi Richardson, who was one of the young ladies I met while speaking at Hyde Park Career Academy. Tyrone was Kenny's best man.

Reverend Jackson married us on August 27, 1994. The little chapel at PUSH had people standing around the walls. There were so many people, they had to open the extension into the foyer. I believe some came to legitimately support me, while others came to see if I was going to go through with it. As I entered the door, I heard someone whisper, "Does he have AIDS and they're just not telling?" I shrugged it off. Coré sang me down the aisle to "You Are So Beautiful." There wasn't a dry eye in the place. Even Reverend Jackson was crying.

After the reception, Kenny started moving some of our things into a new apartment. We were at least three months behind in the rent and dodging an eviction notice for the rent and my first poodle, Imani, which was prohibited in the lease. None of that mattered. Kenny had made a commitment to stay to the very end, and I didn't give two cents or have a care about anything else.

Fifty-Five

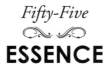

ESSENCE

> **"** Change—releasing the known and embracing
> the new—is the encompassing theme of our lives.**"**
> —Susan Taylor

The day I received my copy of *Essence* magazine, I ripped open the envelope, pulled it out and sat on my sofa, shuffling through the pages to see the center picture in color. I had seen the galleys before publication, so I wasn't surprised by the pictures they chose; I just hadn't seen the inside center picture in color. I didn't hate the center picture, but it certainly wasn't my favorite. It had been a twelve-hour photo shoot. Kip Meyer took over seven hundred photographs of me that day. My vanity was working overtime; I had seen a few of the other shots, and I thought they were better choices for the center than the one Essence ultimately chose.

Essence flew Kenny and me to New York for the photo shoot that June. I was a little self-conscious because I was still carrying the extra weight from the pregnancy. They had asked me for my size, and I told them a four. That Black dress that graced the cover was too small and was open in the upper back for the entire shoot. The morning we arrived at the studio the beauty and cover director, Mikki Taylor, met us. Mikki walked me through all the beautiful evening gowns chosen for the holiday cover issue, which I would grace. I was awed and speechless. She then introduced me to renowned makeup artist Roxanna Floyd, who gave my skin a look. Then, I was taken to the set. My eyes shimmered with tears as Mikki explained the team had placed over a thousand red ribbons, which had become the symbol for HIV/AIDS awareness, on a board for the backdrop. It was magical, and it stirred me deeply. It felt right, like a confirmation I was supposed to be here doing this thing at this time in my life. Even the fact that the entire photo shoot would take place with me sitting on the hard-ass floor didn't change that opinion.

It was a long day of fashion-shoot magic. Back-to-back make-up, hair, wardrobe changes, pictures, and more pictures—all to capture those two photos that would be in the magazine. The team was awesome. Roxanna beat my face to the nines and back, giving me a very different and distant look for each stunning gown Mikki chose for each set. MAC Cosmetics had just launched its AIDS Fund VIVA GLAM lipstick line for which one hundred percent of the funds goes to AIDS research. According to a 2019 article in POZ Magazine, VIVA GLAM has raised 500 million dollars, and has delivered close to ten thousand grants to eighteen hundred organizations over the years. The first VIVA GLAM lip color featured the incomparable RuPaul, and I was honored to wear that brownish-blue-red lip color in the center picture of the magazine. Of course, back then I had no idea VIVA GLAM would become iconic and help so many living with HIV/AIDS, but I continued to support it every year. I had no say and voiced no opinions for once — when I didn't like it (like those bangs in the center photo). I had never worn bangs in my life, a subtle side swoop, but not a bang. They were the experts and they asked me to trust them, and I did because the photos were for the coveted *Essence* magazine, every Black woman's bible on lifestyle and fashion. But I surely had a few *I'm losing control of me* moments. I came away thinking supermodels are worth every damn dime because this work was grueling. When Kenny and I got back to the hotel, it was close to 10 p.m. I was dog-tired. Roxanna had made me look like a supermodel. I didn't want to wash my face but before I walked out of the studio, she handed me some make-up remover and told me not to sleep in the make-up. My eyebrows had never looked so perfect. By the time I took the make-up off, I was shocked to see Roxanna plucked most of my brows and penciled them back in. I was a mad-ass Black woman. LOL.

I looked out of my hotel window at the bright lights in Times Square and I knew in my gut—like I had the day after I dropped the article in the mail—that this was huge. I just didn't realize it would change my life. I would also come to understand the importance of the center picture. It was a serious, in-your-face photo that asked, *Here I am, now what are you going to do about HIV/AIDS?*

A few weeks after I initially spoke with Ms. Taylor and agreed to the cover story, Linda Villarosa, the health editor at Essence, called to talk to me about what the magazine was looking for in the article. Essence wanted a first-person, intimate portrait of my life with AIDS. Linda then followed up with examples of past features. I spent countless hours pouring my guts out on paper. I wrote the article on a white legal pad and went to Tyrone's church to type it. I asked Nana to go over the grammar. The day I dropped it in the mail, I felt like I had given up a part of me I would never be able to regain. I cried like a baby. I didn't understand what I had just done by being so transparent, but I knew it was significant.

Linda called and told me it was a good start, but they wanted a writer to jazz it up. Teresa Wiltz, a freelance writer, came to my apartment; we talked for a couple of hours. She, in turn, gave the article the edge it needed. I read the final version and was pleased. Teresa tweaked it but did not change the tone or the salient points about my story. I read the article again, and I called Teresa to thank her. She hadn't seen the magazine yet and asked me to read the cover line to her: "Facing AIDS: I'm young, I'm educated, I'm drug-free, and I'm dying of AIDS, by Rae Lewis-Thornton." I read it with so much pride. Teresa asked for clarification if her name was on the front cover with mine, and it wasn't. I could hear the surprise and then, the irritation in her voice after learning she had not been given front-page credit. At the end of the article, Essence did write "as told to Teresa Wiltz." I didn't know what was appropriate, but I viewed Teresa as the editor of my article. I respected her as a journalist, and I felt bad she was not pleased. The National Black Journalists Association awarded us both with a second-place journalism award for Outstanding coverage of the Black Condition – *Facing AIDS*. I was happy she had been officially recognized.

Seeing the byline on the cover "And I'm dying of AIDS," for the first time shocked me. "My GOD," I moaned. "I really am dying." When I first wrote the article, my T cells were 66. By the time the article was published, the count had gone up to 84. This declaration of my death made it real. It would also cause bitter critiques from the AIDS community; even women in the clinic wanted to know why I would allow Essence to say I was dying. I didn't allow Essence to do anything, as I had no approval rights to the feature. The contract gave me ownership to the story and pictures on the back end. While I was shocked by the byline, I would tell critics in the AIDS community, "Don't make me lie because you can't handle *my* truth."

Clinically, my body had failed me and all I had was a prayer, a will to live and a doctor who would never stop fighting for me. All that yapping was bullshit, and I told them just that. My biggest critic at the clinic was Gigi Nicks, who was a powerful AIDS activist in her own right. She was also Dr. Cohen's patient and a member of CAB. She walked up to me in the hall over at the WIHS administrative office one day, saying, "The problem I have with the article is that you are giving the impression that WE are all dying, and I'm NOT dying from AIDS; I'm living with AIDS." For a moment, I was stunned.

Who does this woman think she is? I was so proud of the article. How dare she rain on my parade? "You don't speak for all of us," she continued, and that was a fact. I came back to myself within seconds and told her as much.

"The article is on *ME*, Gigi," I told her defensively. "MY LIFE!" I said, hitting my chest with my finger. We both turned and walked away. She stopped speaking to me like, forever. If we were in clinic together, we'd nod an acknowledgment and never say a word to each other. Then, oh, about a decade later, she sat next to me in clinic and started a conversation about the harder she and I worked to educate women, the younger the women were who we would see in the clinic. We deliberated the question, *When is this cycle ever going to stop?* That day, we made peace over all the new faces in the clinic and would remain friends until she had a heart attack, and died at her desk while at work in the clinic. I understood the AIDS community wanted to provide hope, and my declaration had seemed to strip it all away. It wasn't my choice for a byline, but it was effective as a scared-straight moment Black women needed.

Even the Essence staff was divided about me gracing the cover. You have to remember: *Essence* covers had been reserved for supermodels and entertainers. Ms. Taylor's proposal to put a woman on the cover whose name had no monetary value, with a dreadful story about living with AIDS, could not have been an easy sell—and for the upbeat and glamorous holiday issue, no less. Ms. Taylor prevailed, and I would love to have been a fly on the wall as she fought for my story. About six months after the story ran, I bumped into Ed Lewis, the founder of *Essence*, while shopping in Bloomingdales in Washington, D.C. He told me about the controversy—even that he was hesitant, but Susan Taylor was adamant. Thank God for Susan's leadership. In his memoir, *The Man from Essence,* Lewis writes about my feature: "Essence's December 1994 cover was its gutsiest ever, and became the highest newsstand seller in the history of the magazine." Ironically, they made a mint off my cover story—but that month I was so broke I couldn't pay my rent.

Kenny lost his job about a month after the wedding, and there hadn't been a lot of requests for me to speak that fall. He was looking, with no success. A couple months into the new year, he got a job at a hospital in the western suburbs as a transport person. I tried hard not to doubt God, believing it would get better. In the meantime, Mardge arranged for our rent to be paid by the Housing Opportunity for People with AIDS. While Kenny and I were the perfect public couple, in private we were experiencing tension. Our marriage hadn't made the six-month mark and we were already in trouble. Besides the finances, we would get into contentious arguments over stupid shit where he always had to show me, he was a Man, with a capital M. On Thanksgiving, I learned the mother of one of his children would be at his mother's house. I didn't want to walk into that situation to be scrutinized. We argued bitterly, he got all up in my face. It was threatening. I tried my best to hold my own and not show any weakness. He left me at home and went to his mother's. She made him come back to get me. Of course, she did. My cover story was all the talk, and his family wanted to assess me up close.

I should have known that fight was the beginning of the end, but I was determined to make the marriage work. I had defied my friends and mentors for Kenny; now I believed I had to save face and stick it out. However, what really made me stay was my health. I was so afraid of dying alone. I hadn't heard a peep from Mama. I knew Mrs. Jackson would have made sure I was taken care of, but I didn't want her to see me this vulnerable. Kenny was willing, and I thought his baggage was the tradeoff I would have to make.

I developed nationwide celebrity status in a matter of weeks after *Essence* hit the newsstands. Perception is everything, but it never tells the full story. Contrary to what people believed, by medical standards I was dying, just like *Essence* announced to the world. The death angel set up camp and was waiting for its chance to grab me. Yes, I was fighting hard to live, but my poor medical condition could not be ignored. Most people looked at me and saw a supermodel figure, but all I could see was death. My fatigue was so bad it was a struggle just to get out of bed in the morning. If I had a speaking engagement, the most I could do was pull myself together. Even then Kenny ran the bathwater and plugged the curling iron so I could stay in bed for as long as I could. I'd go to speak with Kenny at my side and come straight home and go back to bed. I was even more dependent on him.

Besides Kenny, Toi Richardson, the young lady who was the junior bridesmaid in my wedding, was at the house every day after school, and she would eventually stay on the weekends as well. As mentioned, I met Toi speaking at her school, Hyde Park Career Academy. High school students continued to love me while the faculty thought I was way over the top. The emotions were often running so high at my speaking engagements that I started giving select students my telephone number. The next day after speaking at Hyde Park, I received a call from another student, Davita Britton. She said her friend Toi wouldn't stop crying and asked if I would I speak to her. I talked to Toi and invited her to church with me and Kenny.

I called Toi's grandmother, who was her primary guardian, to get permission for her to come to church with us and the rest is history, as the saying goes. By the time of the wedding, she was calling me Mommie and the other girls I had met around this time were calling me "Tee Tee." They were *my girls*: Toi, Jénale King, Davita and Jamilla Butler were students at Hyde Park. Tiashia Green was a pre-teen who came by way of Davita. Jermella (Jay) Ruther attended Senn High School; LaShonda Flowers attended Currie High School. Then I met Ericka Summers, a student at Northern Illinois University that February right after the article published. These girls would be the core of my support system and in and out of my house for years. Some of them lived with me at different stages of their lives. I even gave some of their friends shelter, like Masoe Owens. I had definitely gotten the hospitality bug from Mama. I understood what a difficult home life could look like. I knew all about the need to have a safe place to rest your head at night at critical transitions in life. I wanted my home to be that refuge. My last child — yes, I call them my children would come two decades later. She was Tiara Williams, who I met when speaking at her college, Eastern Illinois University. She was a freshman who began following me on Twitter. She'd check in with me and ask if I was alright or needed anything. I invited her to dinner when school was out for the summer and, again, the rest is history. She was glued to me when she wasn't in school. We talked every day. Right after she finished graduate school, she had a daughter, Jo'Rya Peeples. She is my precious Goddaughter and the center of my heart. In 2020, Tira dropped dead in her bathroom. Just like that, all her dreams of opening a senior-citizen home and launching her nail-polish line vanished. God sent these girls to me, and I am forever grateful for the roles they played in different ways and at different stages of my life.

My life was changing before my eyes. By the middle of December, the phone was ringing off the hook with requests for speaking engagements from across the country, as well as for television and radio interviews. My first television interview came a couple of weeks after *Essence* was released through Cheryl Burton, a reporter who now anchors at ABC-7 Chicago news. She recommended me for the series, *Someone You Should Know*, with Chicago's legend, Harry Porterfield. NBC News came calling next. After the story aired, the station came back and wanted to do a series, but CBS WBBM-Chicago had already signed a deal with me.

It was Reverend Barrow who opened the door for me at CBS. She had been in a meeting with executives at CBS and asked, as she put it, "Have you all seen my baby on the cover of *Essence* magazine?" The assistant news director, an African American named Kathy Williams, had seen the article and was interested in meeting me. The meeting marked the beginning of what would become an awesome project. I was asked to return with a proposal in a few days.

All of these incredible things were happening, and my health was failing quickly. I had already began experiencing symptoms of PCP but dismissed them because I had not missed one dose of Dapsone, the medication I was taking to prevent the illness. It was only through sheer determination that I was able to sit up and write the proposal. My shortness of breath felt like someone had grabbed my airway and held tight. My coughing was intense, and my chest and head ached. I would wake up in the middle of the night gasping for breath. I knew I had to tell Mardge, but I couldn't afford to miss the next meeting. That morning, it took every bit of strength I could muster. Kenny helped to bathe and lotion me; after that, I slowly dressed. It took almost two hours because I had to take breaks after each task. Kenny put a chair in front of the full-length mirror that hung on the door in the hall so I could curl my hair and apply my make-up, because I didn't have the strength to stand. AIDS had not changed my belief that first impressions are lasting ones. I was determined not to let it interfere. When I stepped out of my house, I was dressed in a perfectly tailored suit and my make-up was applied to perfection. I was wearing three-inch heels even though each step I took seemed to cut off my windpipe.

Holt Owen, a communications consultant who arranged the meetings for Reverend Barrow, accompanied me to CBS for the second time. In the three-hour meeting, I pitched my plan as if I was a picture of health. I talked slowly so no one noticed that my breathing was impaired. The plan was good. I chose topics that I believed were most important to people with HIV. Each topic would stand alone, and I would allow TV cameras to come into the most personal areas of my life. I believed and argued that my news reports would help dispel some of the myths and misconceptions people had about HIV/AIDS as well as the people infected and affected by it. When the meeting was over, I gave a sigh of relief. I excused myself to go to the ladies' room, but I was really calling Mardge. She asked me to meet her at the clinic. When Holt and I got in his car, he was elated, believing the meeting had gone extremely well. As he pulled out of the garage, I asked him to take me to County Hospital.

"Why are you going there?" he asked.

"Holt, I'm sick and my doctor wants me to come in," I responded.

"Sick?" he asked, baffled. "But you just had a great meeting and didn't appear sick." I filled him in on the past week and the fact that my temperature was 102 when I left home that morning. He couldn't believe it.

"How did you pull that off?" he asked.

"That's what I do Holt, that's what I do," I said.

I was diagnosed that day with my first major opportunistic infection, *Pneumocystis carini* pneumonia (PCP)—a parasite that sits on the lungs and inhibits one's ability to breathe. At the time, PCP was the number-one AIDS related infection, killing 54 percent of all people with AIDS. Mardge believed we caught PCP early and decided to treat me as an outpatient. I was grateful because I didn't want to be hospitalized. We tried Bactrim again but after two days, my entire body felt as if my skin was burning. My chest looked like it had been burned. It was either go into the hospital to have Pentamidine treatments for twenty-one days or take a medication called Atovaquone for twenty-one days. It resembled bright yellow paint in color and consistency and left a nasty taste in my month and a film on my tongue. As always, I took it as prescribed because the alternative was death.

Later that evening, I received a call from Kathy Williams with an offer. I was overjoyed, but then I dropped the bomb. "Kathy," I said, "I'm sick and not sure when I will be able to start."

"What do you mean you are sick? You were fine earlier in our office," she said. Then I explained to her I was actually very sick and hanging on by a prayer during the entire meeting. She was just as amazed as Holt had been earlier, and she was still committed.

I continued to bare stark contradictions. I experienced extreme highs professionally but extreme lows personally, physically, and emotionally; but it didn't matter. Essence had catapulted me onto the national platform, and I grabbed it by the horns and never let go. All the years of waiting, hoping, and praying to do the work I believed God had call me to do had finally arrived. God had used Susan Taylor and Essence to get me to the place I was meant to be. All my other work had been the training ground, preparing me to walk into my light.

My goal was to speak to as many people as possible about my life before I died. That mission has never been far from my heart. I understood early that AIDS was the catalyst that got me through the door. It was the reason I was booked to speak. My intention, however, was to be God's vessel to enrich the lives of God's people. I would often tell the program organizers they had brought me to speak for one reason and God had brought me for another. It would be the same for every newspaper article, magazine feature, television and radio show that followed. I never knew what revelation God would give me to give to my audience, but I embraced my ministry with my heart and soul.

AFTERWORD

WHEW! What a life I've lived! I thank God each and every day that I not only survived, but I thrived in spite of what I went through. Can you believe it's been twenty-eight years since I appeared on the cover of *Essence* magazine?! So much happened in my life after that cover story. Many of you heard me speak; read an article; saw me on a television show; heard me on the radio; read my blog, *Diva Living with AIDS*, followed me on social media; joined my book club, *RLTReads,* and purchased my handmade bracelets and knitted accessories *RLT Collection* – and I am evermore thankful. I've said from the beginning that I cannot do it alone and that is a fact. For sure, so much on my life since *Essence* played out on the national stage, but some things did not. So, I thought that I would end this book by giving you a brief update on some of the people in this memoir–good or bad–like the closing credits at the end of a movie.

The Toblers

Tobie passed away unexpectedly during the campaign in March 1988. My ex-boyfriend Bill McGill came to Chicago to preach the eulogy for us. Then I was back on the road, keeping a breakneck schedule. Kathy and I would talk periodically, as would Ethel and me. I mostly stayed away because I just couldn't bring myself to tell them I had HIV. I didn't invite any of them to the wedding because I had kept this secret from them. We lived in such different worlds that they never got a whiff of my status until the *Essence* cover story. Kathy called. It was a difficult conversation. Her starting point: how did I end up with HIV? What happened? The conversation felt like an indictment of me, or maybe it was my own self-judgment. I tried to explain my dating and sex life to my big sister, but I was still trying to connect the dots of my childhood sexual abuse to my current life. "Kathy, you have no idea what life was like for me after you left, and when we moved to Evanston," I said. I was attempting to explain to her how hard everything had been for me when, out of nowhere, I blurted, "Junior molested me."

"No," she said emphatically.

"He did, Kathy and he wasn't the only person," I sighed. "Life was hard for me, and I did the best I could."

"Are you trying to say that Junior *molested* you?" she asked. "Yes, he did," I said, with such sorrow and clarity. There was silence, and then Kathy hung up the telephone. It would be the last time I would speak to any of them. Over the years, I've wanted to reach out but how do you explain what you don't even understand? That would take more years of therapy. None of them reached out to me, so I didn't reach out to them. But they have stayed in my heart. That can never be taken away.

Randy

About a decade after the night Randy put me in a chokehold, we reunited. I was sitting on the bus and looked up, Randy was standing in the middle of the bus wearing a McDonald's manager uniform, smiling from ear to ear and taking me all in. We exchanged numbers and he called that night. The next day he came over. He was living with his sister, whose house was close to my apartment. That first day, I told him I had AIDS. It was around the time I was going through a dark period, and I told him I didn't know how much longer I had to live. Tears rolled down his face as I explained what was happening to my body–the pill load, the side effects, the weight loss, the fatigue, and the pins and needles that had set up camp in my legs. He apologized for everything he did to me. Randy understood the impact he had had on the trajectory of my life, and he asked for my forgiveness, which I granted. What was so interesting is that he had a better grip on how I ended up at this place with HIV than I. We started spending more time together. He would come over and make me his specialty: neck bones with white potatoes. One Saturday morning he came over and made us breakfast. He asked if he could make love to me. I wanted him but didn't have any condoms. He didn't care and asked if he could pleasure me. I gave in to his kisses and when his tongue reached my clitoris, I surrendered. He took his time as he had done so many years ago. Orgasm after orgasm, he methodically twirled his tongue, licking me. When he was satisfied that I was satisfied, he sat up. I reached for his belt buckle, and he grabbed my hand and shook his head, no. "I don't want anything from you," he said, with tears in his eyes, "I just want to take care of you." We both knew what he meant. "I will always love you, girl. You will always be mine," he said at the door, just before he walked out of my apartment later that evening. The next day he was supposed to come over and cook dinner. When I called, his sister answered the phone. "Rae," she said, "Randy is dead." She'd found him that morning in his bedroom. He'd died from a brain aneurysm. My girlfriend Leslie went with me to his funeral.

Emmy Award Winning New Series: *Living with AIDS*
At WBBM, I was partnered with a wonderful team. Mary Ann Childers, a longtime reporter, and anchor at WBBM was the executive producer. Edie Turovitz-Kasten, who I worked with the closest was the writer/producer; John Leonits was the cameraman, and Carolyn Broquet edited the series. I learned through the grapevine that some employees were concerned about working with a person with AIDS, but management made it very clear they were equal opportunity employers. Bob McGann, the general manager, had given this project his full support and everyone had fallen in line by the time I arrived. Overall, people were extremely kind and went out of their way to make me feel like a part of the team. The cameras followed me to speaking engagements and at home. Sometimes they were intrusive on our private space. Kenny never complained, and I knew it was worth the sacrifice. Even some of my friends agreed to be a part of the stories: Audrey, Atha, and Coré appeared in the report on friendships; Dr. Quentin Young appeared in the report on AIDS in the Workplace; and they interviewed Dr. Cohen about my health.

The night the reports aired; local HIV/AIDS organizations manned the phone bank. They answered questions and made referrals to people seeking information about HIV and AIDS. The phone bank was flooded with so many calls that some nights the hours were extended. Chicagoans tuned in every week for eight weeks to see how my life unfolded. People told me they laughed, cried, and became better informed about HIV/AIDS. The reports had such a positive impact on the perceptions of people living with AIDS. People with HIV would stop me and say, "Thank you for giving us a face," or "Thank you for making us human." I was knocked off my feet with jubilation when the series received two nominations by the Chicago/Midwest chapter of the National Academy of Television of Arts and Sciences for an Emmy Award. The first nomination was for an Outstanding Feature Series Hard News. The nomination qualified the entire team for an Emmy. John was also nominated for a separate Emmy for Outstanding Achievement for Individual Excellence for Non-Performers, Camera/ News. We were stacked against anchor-reporter Lester Holt from our Chicago affiliate and who currently hosts national evening and weekend news for NBC. He had not one, but two series nominated: "Dreamland" and "Back to Iraq."

The night of the Emmys—October 21, 1995—I wore a black and gold evening gown with an empire waist that was black velvet at the top. I purchased it from a resale shop in Memphis with my girlfriend Mary Cummings, who had moved there from Chicago. We were in the last category of the evening. I sat with anticipation and when the host, Charles Perez announced the winner and I heard "Living," I started screaming. Kenny thought I had lost my mind, but I knew that our series was the only one with "Living" in the title. I ran to the stage; Edie followed. It was the most magical moment of my life. We hugged and cried. Robert Feder of the *Chicago Sun-Times* called it the "emotional high point of the evening," and Steven Nidetz of the *Chicago Tribune* said it was "the most touching moment." I had never been prouder of myself. Later that week, someone asked if I told Mama. I had not. I couldn't see any good coming from informing her of my news. This was a great accomplishment, and I couldn't trust her not to ruin it. In the months that followed the series, I received two additional awards: the prestigious 1996 *Cardinal Bernardin Professional Communications Award*, for Outstanding Series and the *Illinois Associated Press Broadcasters Association* award, for which I won second place for Best Continuing Series. Jonathan Rodgers, the CEO of *TV One* was vice president of CBS at the time and approached me about syndicating the reports. To take them nationally would have done so much good toward conquering the stigmas associated with HIV and AIDS. However, as soon as we began working out the deal, it was squashed when Westinghouse Electric Corporation purchased CBS and bought Jonathan out of his contract.

Rev. Otis Anderson
One night after I was off-air, I walked into the call center and someone said, "I have a man on the telephone who says he's your pastor." At the time, I was still at Tyrone's church and couldn't imagine who it was. It was Rev. Anderson. Lord, I hadn't seen him in over two decades. I took the phone receiver. "Is this my Rae Rae?" was the first thing out of his mouth. I could feel him smiling through the phone. "I am so proud of you, and I know your grandmother would be, too," he said. The following Sunday, I was at his church speaking. I had always known in my heart that this man of God was a gift from God to me when I was a child; now, it had been confirmed at the age of thirty-two.

Cousin Eleanor
Another night, a volunteer handed me a message from a lady claiming to be my cousin. I couldn't even stretch my imagination to figure out who the heck it could be. It was Eleanor, of all people. I hadn't thought about her or Kenneth in years. I sat in one of the chairs and called her back.

The first thing I asked was, "How is Aunt Lula Mae?" She said Aunt Lula Mae had passed away. It hadn't occurred to me, Aunt Lula Mae had to have been in her early nineties. I was hurt that I didn't have a chance to say goodbye. I asked why no one reached out to me, and she gave me some excuse about Aunt Lula Mae not wanting a big fuss when she died. She said that there was no funeral because she had donated her body to science and blah, blah, blah. In that moment, I felt my biggest regret for having sex with Kenneth. I had no one to blame but myself. Shame had kept me away from Aunt Lula Mae. After Eleanor and I talked about Aunt Lula Mae, she reminded me she had foreseen the direction my life was headed. It was no surprise to her I ended up with HIV. It sounded to me that she actually took pride in having warned me about my *sex sickness*. I felt like that nineteen-year-old girl who needed to go get some hair oil all over again. She made it a point to tell me Kenneth was married. *Good for him,* I thought. *I'm glad he could go on with his life while I still felt the residual effects of our illicit hookups.* She even had the nerve to say, "You're still family, though, and you don't have to die alone." Not once did she acknowledge the work that I was doing. I had taken a bad situation and turned it into something good, and I resented that all she could see in me was bad. She went on and on about her own righteousness and my lack thereof. *Good Lord,* I thought. *It has been almost twelve freaking years, and now it is time to move on!* At some point, I stopped listening and began looking through the other phone messages. I finally cut her off, saying I had to get off the station's telephone. After we hung up, I thought about Rev. Anderson's call. What a stark difference between two people claiming to do God's work. I thought of Eleanor as the kind of minister who would make you stop going to church. I tore her telephone number into tiny little pieces, and I kept it moving.

Cousin Kenneth

Four decades after the last time I saw Kenneth, he reached out to me through social media. At first, I didn't know how to respond. He had let all those years pass and hadn't bothered to check on me. Eventually, I gave in. I told him about his mother's telephone call. He was surprised. He said she never mentioned me and that he had no idea she knew how to reach me. By then, both his mother and her sister Ann had passed. No point in being mad at the dead; let the dead bury the dead.

After his first call, I fell apart in therapy. I hadn't realized until then that those emotions of shame, regret, and anger were still inside of me, and they triggered a meltdown. The next time we talked I told him I believed he threw my ass under the bus in some sick game with his mother and let me take all the blame. If he had any regret, he didn't express it. Instead, he talked about how his mother tried to run his life. In another conversation, we talked about my childhood sexual abuse, which seemed to explain my behavior to him. Still, we never discussed his own actions or his culpability in the situation. During another one of our phone conversations, he told me my behavior provided an easy way out for the family so that they didn't have to address why I had been thrown away and left with Mama all those years in the first place. *No shit, Sherlock!* He continued to be on-again, off-again in my life. It felt like talking to him was some sort of secret he kept from the rest of the family. Ann's daughters never reached out. I refused to be in some kind of clandestine relationship with him, so I stopped responding to his *whenever I'm in the mood to talk to her* conversations. I worked it out in therapy and left him to deal with his own shit. I resolved that as long as I worked through my shit, I'm good. My healing cannot be predicated on the culpability and healing of others.

Rae

AIDS didn't kill me, but not for lack of trying. In February 1996—a year and two months from my first bout of pneumocystis pneumonia (PCP)—it crept up on me again like a thief in the night. About a week before I was scheduled to speak in Iowa while on a two-day city tour, I started having difficulty breathing. Mardge ordered an X-ray that came back normal, but it was clear my breathing was impaired. She wanted me to have a bronchoscopy, the next level of diagnostic testing but Cook County Hospital was an antiquated dungeon, and I didn't want to stay there. Mardge called a colleague, Dr. Steven Fox, at Illinois Masonic Hospital and he agreed to admit me for the procedure. I was adamant I wouldn't be hospitalized for the test until after we came back from Iowa.

The first night in Des Moines, I awoke in a panic. It felt as if someone had grabbed hold of my windpipe and wouldn't let it go. I called Bill McGill, who had moved there and was also doing HIV work in the community. He arranged for me to see a physician who treated HIV patients the next morning. That X-ray was also normal, but the doctor insisted on giving me a pentamidine breathing treatment. I spoke that night at Drake University; then, we drove the next day to Waterloo. I had a reception that evening, and I spoke at two local high schools the next day. I was so sick at one point that I sat on the auditorium stairs to conduct the question-and-answer session.

When I arrived back in Chicago and made it to the hospital, my breathing was so impaired the staff had to give me oxygen in the admitting office. I was scared. I had heard many stories about people who had died from PCP. After three days in the hospital, I was back at home and back on Atovaquone; two weeks after that, I was back on the road. Four months later Mardge asked Dr. Fox to admit me again. It seemed as if this parasite was determined to kill me. My T-cell count was 11. I was so thin that when I looked in the mirror, I saw death staring at me. I needed to either stay in the hospital and receive the standard course of pentamidine treatments or go back on Bactrim because Atovaquone and Dapsone had not prevented PCP in my case. Kenny was by my side every moment attending to my every need. Mardge Cohen, however, was not prepared to let me die without a fight. This time she and Dr. Fox worked a scheme to desensitize me to Bactrim by giving me low dosages over a period of days. It worked for the most part: I didn't have a rash this time, but I was constantly itching. I knew it was do-or-die and I did not miss a dose. Recovery this time around was slow. My T-cell count dropped to an all-time low of 8. I spent more days at home in bed in the two months that followed than I did on the road speaking.

The HIV medicines on the market were limited in their ability to work against this virus. There was a new class of medications being developed called protease inhibitors, but I had decided early on that I would not participate in drug trials. I came to that conclusion because the HIV medications approved by the FDA were extremely toxic. I couldn't imagine how much more toxic this new class of drugs would be. Dr. Cohen supported my decision, but it left her with few treatment options. We were always in the waiting game for the next drug to be better than the last drug. We also had to wait until Cook County Hospital received whatever the new drug was because at that time Medicare did not pay for medication, and I was solely dependent on Cook County Hospital. Yet again, I thought about what I had sacrificed to work for Carol Moseley Braun.

Abbott Laboratories' Ritonavir arrived, and I started taking it right away. It was twenty-two pills a day in addition to my other medications. The adverse side effects far exceeded anything I had ever experienced. The fatigue was so debilitating there were days I was too weak to lift my body. I had severe gastric problems that included nausea, vomiting, and diarrhea. At least with AZT and DDI there was a brief period where the queasy feeling wore off before I had to take my next dose; however, with Ritonavir, I never got a break. Mardge prescribed medications to help with the side effects, but then those medications had side effects as well. The quality of my life had deteriorated to an all-time low. I continued to speak and travel, hanging on by a thread. Mardge continued to encourage me, but I was losing faith in it all.

One morning I woke at 5:00 a.m. leaving a trail of vomit from the bed to the toilet. I sat on the floor and leaned into the toilet as the vomit violently came from my body. Kenny kneeled and provided comfort with his hand resting on my back. After what seemed like forever, the only thing coming up was air. While I was brushing my teeth, I could feel a loose substance seeping out of my behind. When diarrhea ceased, I lay back in bed and Imani curled up into my stomach, which seemed to help ease my pain. I slept for about an hour and was awakened by another disturbance in my stomach. I was too weak to run, and poop rushed down my leg as I made my way to the bathroom. The pattern remained the same all morning. I curled into a fetal position on the cold tiles in the bathroom; tears streaming down my face, and I moaned to God, "Help me." When it passed, Kenny came in and ran me a bath. He placed me in the tub and with each stroke of his hand, I started to feel human again. After he finished cleaning me, I mustered up enough strength to phone Mardge.

"I quit," I announced. "The quality of my life is more important to me than how long I live." I was prepared to die. Mardge put on her boxing gloves and came out swinging.

"Rae you cannot stop taking this medicine," she insisted. I had no more hope and no illusions that I would be spared from a horrible death at the hands of AIDS. I had watched with anxiety as my T cells and weight went up and down like a rollercoaster. I had fought a good fight, but I was tired. In six years, I had been a trooper and taken more combinations of HIV medicines than I thought humanly possible. I had done what I was supposed to do when I was supposed to do it, and nothing had saved me from this miserable-ass life living with AIDS. I was currently on thirty-one pills a day and I couldn't see how this new drug would make a difference. I had no more chutzpah!

"No!" She started screaming at me. I could hear the desperation in her voice that said, *If you stop taking this medication, you are going to die.*

"You can't do this!" she hollered, "You have to give me some time!"

I protested, "But Mardge"

"No," she cut me off. "You can't do this! You have to give me time."

Then, abruptly, her temperament changed from frustration to anger. She coldly asked, "What do you want to do Rae? Die?" She had never told me I was dying, and this was the closest she had come to it in the years she had been treating me. No, I didn't really want to die; but I was prepared to die. I had beaten the odds so far, and now I had accepted death as my fate because AIDS was the undisputed grave-filler. A part of me hoped that, somehow, death would pass me by. I had no more fight that day, but Mardge had enough for both of us. I surrendered to her request.

Dr. Mardge Cohen

Mardge would remain my doctor until she and her husband retired from Cook County Hospital in 2006. When she left, I cried for over a month. (I still don't do well with change.) Renslow Sherer was now treating patients at the University of Chicago Hospital and offered to see me there. Mardge wanted me to start seeing Dr. Audrey French, her co-collaborator in the WIHS study. She had assumed Mardge's position as director of research for the CORE Center. By this time, the Women and Children HIV Clinic had moved into the 23-million-dollar Ruth M. Rothstein CORE Center and Cook County Hospital was now a brand-new building that sat behind the old building. It had been renamed the John H. Stroger Hospital. Both Ruth Rothstein and John Stroger were strong advocates of delivering health care in an environment of dignity. They both helped to make these two new facilities a reality. They were both my friends.

I begrudgingly went to Dr. French. It was at another turning point in my health and I was having a lot of issues. My impulse was to compare her to Mardge and second-guess her advice. I even called Mardge a couple of times to confirm if what Dr. French told me was correct. Mardge stopped returning my calls, THANK GOD, or I would have never trusted Dr. French. I can honestly say, she saw me through some rough patches and earned my trust and respect. I remain with the CORE Center in part because of her, and in part because they provide some of the best care in the country for people living with HIV. It is my diamond in the rough all of them: Dr. Jorelle Alexandra, my dentist and director of oral health for the Cook County system; my dermatologist, Dr. Joerg Albrecht; and my favorite nurses, Ms. Kim, and Mannie Sotomayor. There are still other long-term survivors around who started with me back when we used Radiology in the old Cook County building, like Rowena Thomas.

Eleven years after the WIHS study began and, coincidentally, eleven years after the Rwandan genocide, Dr. Cohen opened an HIV clinic and began a research project identical to WIHS, in Rwanda. She and Kathleen Weber, the administrator of WIHS were approached by some women at the International AIDS Conference in South Africa about helping the women who had been raped and infected during the genocide. WE-ACTx, Women's Equality in Access to Care and Treatment for HIV in Rwanda is going strong seventeen years later. Today, Mardge and Gordy are on their second careers. In addition the WIHS and WE-ACTx, Mardge treats patients part-time at a homeless clinic in Boston. Gordy would later serve as the President of PNHP. He is currently the safety director for the Harvard Medical School, associate director of Brigham Women's Center for Patient Safety Research and Practice, and associate professor of medicine at Harvard Medical School. A lot of titles, right? But Gordy deserves every one of them. They could be called the power couple of public health.

Physical Trauma of AIDS

My emotional attachment to clothes was compounded by my physical sickness from AIDS. As my health deteriorated, I continued to drop weight. I went from a size four to a two and, eventually, a size two was too big for me. I refused to buy a zero. In 1996, when I received the Cardinal Joseph Louis Bernardin Communications Award for my CBS series, the suit I was wearing was a size two and noticeably too big. I was stressed out that morning not being able to find something in my closet to fit me well for the occasion. When the photos of me receiving the award arrived, I was horrified at what I saw.

Of all the opportunistic illnesses, Wasting Syndrome caused some of the most severe emotional distress for me because, with the naked eye, it was a reminder that AIDS had affected my body and it was taking a part of me away without my permission. The emotional wear and tear of the physical changes and the financial burden AIDS has caused over the years have been tremendous. It is my reality. I have gone through more sizes and clothes than three people. Just by sheer volume, there was no way to hold on to clothes I could no longer fit. Outside of friends I can't remember everyone to whom I have given clothes. I donated to women's homeless shelters, other women's programs, and Dress for Success. I even took bags of clothes to the CORE Center and asked Sheila Cooper to distribute them. Then the buying would start all over again. Sure, some of it was vanity. I had a reputation as a well-dressed woman, and I'd be damned if I would let AIDS take that away from me. Once I started to get better, I believed that the shifting of my weight had been resolved, but it hadn't. When new medications came around in 1998 and my health improved, I went back up to a size six, then an eight. I needed all new clothes because no matter how hard you try; you cannot fit a size-eight body into a size-two garment. By 2000, my T-cell count was 227, a stark contrast to my lowest of 8. My viral load was 13,851 a long way from its peak of 440,000. I was happy to be alive. But in time I became ambivalent about the trade-offs I had to make for my life. My weight had continued to increase; now, I was 146 pounds. A couple of months after I signed the final divorce papers, I noticed another shift in my body fat. It seemed to happen overnight. The fat shift distorted my entire body, making me large at the top and small at the bottom. The fat was lodged in my stomach, back, and chin. In the front, I looked six months pregnant. There was so much fat deposited under my face I developed a triple chin. Like many others, from the back, I developed a hump that people nicknamed "buffalo hump," and it only added more emotional agony. In contrast, my bottom was emaciated. My buttocks sunk in overnight, and my hips seemed to disappear. It wasn't just that I could no longer fit any of my clothes. The problem was complicated because I had gone from a perfect size six to three different sizes. Across my breast I was a size fourteen to sixteen, my waist was a size ten and my hips were a size two. Even buying new clothes was emotionally exhausting. Phyllis, at Ann Taylor tried to be encouraging, but nothing comforted me from this distortion of my body image.

I brought it to Mardge's attention, and she basically told me to get over it. "You are healthy. Who cares that you're fat?" was her response. That might have been true if I didn't look like SpongeBob SquarePants. About a year later, I appeared on a *Nightline* special for the twentieth anniversary of AIDS "Plague: AIDS at 20." It was a live show with host Ted Koppel; Dr. Anthony Fauci; AIDS activist Martin Delaney, founder of Project Inform; and me. I will never forget that night. When we met in the green room, Koppel was so shocked by my fat redistribution that he asked Dr. Fauci what was happening. *Nightline* had featured me two other times and Koppel had seen tons of footage of me, and he was dumbfounded by the change in my appearance. I thought the conversation had dropped, and we moved on. However, Koppel asked Dr. Fauci about my fat right off the bat when we went live. I wanted to crawl under the chair, honest to God. After the segment ended, Dr. Cohen called and said it was time to figure this out. She added lipodystrophy to the WIHS study; I wasn't the only woman complaining.

Eventually, the medical community coined the term "HIV lipodystrophy." It was a side effect of long-term use of some of the HIV medications. Lipodystrophy is an abnormal metabolism of fat creating fat pads in some areas and the loss of fat (lipoatrophy) causing thinning in other areas of the body. Researchers later determined lipodystrophy caused diabetes and a weakening of the cardiovascular system, and at one point, they even thought I might have diabetes. Even worse, they had no idea what to do about it. There were reports people with HIV were having the humps in the back surgically removed only for them to return. I became quite depressed and started isolating myself. My self-esteem was hit as if a bulldozer had slammed into it.

One evening, Usef Jackson, Rev. Jackson's youngest son introduced me to Cornell McClellan, a trainer and owner of the boutique gym Naturally Fit. Cornell is most famous today for Michelle Obama's arms. She and Barack begin working out with Cornell about a year after I began. Usef is always joking about how we all took his trainer.

"I'm fat. Can you help me?" I asked.

"Of course, I can," Cornell said confidently.

"I'm real-l-ly high maintenance," I said. "Will that be a problem for you?"

"Believe me, I'm used to high maintenance," he chuckled.

At that first consultation, Cornell was emphatic that he could help me, but I had to "make a lifestyle change." He laid down the law. There would be cardio five to six days a week, for an hour each; weight-training at least twice a week; and a radical change, not just in my diet, but when and how I ate. Hallelujah, he was a genius! I approached this plan like I had others. I declared war on this fat, and I set out to win. All I needed was for someone to tell me it was possible. In the gym, I became the undisputed cardio queen! The medical community wouldn't have a remedy for the fat until after Cornell and I had already succeeded. They would eventually make the same recommendations as Cornell had, weight-resistance training and cardio. I never returned to a size six to my upper body, but I was comfortable with how we had reshaped the fat so that I didn't appear so disproportionate. While I was happy with my results, I would learn I could never stop working out because any weight gain meant fat redistribution.

While we were successful with the reconfiguration of my body, my face was still very much distorted, and I still had the hump in my upper back. The physical changes that I could do nothing about has definitely had an impact on my self-esteem. About eight years ago, I went from a size ten to a 2X across my back. That's when I started CrossFit. Around this time, Dr. French believed I would be a candidate to receive Sculptra injections for HIV facial lipoatrophy to help the fat loss in my face. The fillers build collagen over time. The pharmaceutical company made the fillers available for compassionate use because they were too expensive for most people living with HIV.

Dr. Joerg Albrecht the medical dermatologist at Stroger and CORE gave me the Sculptra injections in my cheeks. Still, even with injections, the deformity of fat under my chin was so extreme he continued to ponder what could be done. On the day of my last Sculptra injections he decided he would perform liposuction on my chin, which is typically done by a cosmetic surgeon rather than a medical dermatologist as a compassionate procedure rather than one for profit. It was such a success, he put together a presentation for other doctors that specialized in medical dermatology to consider liposuction as a medical solution for extreme cases of HIV lipodystrophy. In early 2022, he performed liposuction on my back and removed the hump. I cannot tell you how profoundly I had been affected by the removal of this hump; to stand straight and not look like I'm hunched over. Thank God for physicians like Dr. Albrecht who understands the importance of treating the whole person.

Kenny

"AIDS had not killed me; Kenny was not going to kill me either," was the explanation I gave to my audiences when they asked why I divorced my husband. My response resonated with most of them, and they'd laugh and let me move on to the next topic. This answer was the easiest way out, but it also bears truth. The other truth, I was content to have Kenny with me until the final hour and he was equally content in the role as the dutiful husband. For the record, when a marriage is based on such an asinine idea it is already in trouble. Kenny and I both had planned for death, but God's plan for my life was bigger than I could have ever imagined. Those first couple of years, I think we bonded over my health in spite of the ongoing friction that is, until I didn't die. By that third year our marriage sunk to an all-time low and I'm never the one to wallow in the shit. I filed for a divorce on September 24, 1998, four years, one month and two days from the day we were married. The divorce was final May 1999. Kenny was escorted out of the apartment by four police officers and two sheriffs on September 4, 1998, two days after I filed for an order of protection. A month later, in compliance with the order of protection he was escorted to the apartment by two police officers to pick up his clothes that I had already packed. That day would be the last time I laid eyes on him.

Mama

Mama was Mama and that did not change not even on her deathbed. In December 2000, right before Christmas, I called to check on her and she said, "Baby, I got a hole in the front of my mouth, and it hurts." She explained she had gone to the doctor, and he sent her to the dentist, and she was waiting on her appointment. What she was describing didn't add up. She even said she hadn't been drinking because it was too painful. Mama was too sick to drink, and that meant it was serious. I intervened. I found her old doctor and made an appointment. Ten years prior, she had been diagnosed with cancer of the mouth. The surgery was successful, but they told her she could never smoke again. It was during one of those times she and I were on the outs. About a year later, she resumed her smoking routine of a couple of packs each day. When I inquired about it, her response was, "You got to die from something." I was afraid cancer had come back. A few weeks later, I took Mama to her doctor's appointment and my suspicions were confirmed. She had a tumor on her tongue that reached down to her voice box. How ironic that the weapon Mama had used to cause me so much pain for all those years was the very thing that was causing her pain now. After the surgery to remove the tumor, Mama was in the hospital for about three weeks. I was there every day. She was released into short-term nursing care until she was able to swallow again. I continued to be diligent, and Mama seemed to be appreciative –until her voice came back and she turned on me like Dr. Jekyll into Mr. Hyde. Barely able to talk, she cursed and fussed as usual, about everything and nothing. She never gave an inch, and one time I almost told her to shove it where the sun refused to shine. All that driving ran the mileage up on my car. I was at the end of my lease and asked if I could use her car for one week until my new one arrived. She agreed, but when it was time to pick it up, she told me she had given it to her boss. His car needed repair, and she explained that he had no way to get to work. I was simply beside myself.

"Mama," I said through tears, "I asked you for one thing, and you couldn't even keep your word on that."

"Well, he's been good to me," she said. I wanted to say, *Where the hell was he all those days you were laid up in the hospital, unable to talk?* But I didn't. I just shook it off.

The tumor came back six months later. I was in seminary by then and was juggling Mama, a full-time class load required to keep my scholarship, and my speaking engagements. I transferred her medical care from Evanston to the University of Chicago Hospital by my house because they were conducting cutting-edge experimental treatment for this type of cancer. In the beginning, I handled all the transporting myself. I drove those thirty miles back to Evanston, picked her up, drove her to chemotherapy, sat with her all day, and then drove her, and myself, back home. When it became too much, I ordered hospital transport for the morning. I would then meet her at the hospital and sit with her during chemotherapy between classes. When she was done each night, I drove her back to Evanston, got her settled in, and drove myself home.

In spite of our tumultuous relationship, she still had a hold on me. She would always be Mama – good and bad. I believed if God continued to love me in spite of myself, I could extend a hand to Georgia Lee who could never get out of her own way. By now, she was a helpless woman who had withered away from years of alcohol abuse and the hardships of working-class life. She was sixty-seven but looked at least ten years older. I felt sorry for her more than anything, yet she could still pull my strings like a puppet master.

She received chemotherapy and then second-time radiation, which is very risky, at best–but it was her choice. I was there every step of the way, talking to the doctors and then translating the information to her in a way she could understand. One time, I got smart with the doctor, who tried to tell me I was incorrect about the study. I said to him it was time to move on from chemotherapy.

"You don't know that," the doctor said.

"Excuse me…" I said with all of my Black-girl attitude. "How DARE you tell me what I don't know."

"Baby," I heard Mama's hoarse voice trying to intervene, "the doctor knows what he's doing."

"Mama, I know what I'm talking about." She shut up.

"I know," I said, turning to the physician, "because I read the damn study."

"You read the study?" he questioned.

"From front to back," I said, all smug. I thought about all the poor uneducated people who had came through those doors and stayed in a study longer than they should have because of doctors like him. Mama never interfered again and relied on me to translate.

I wanted to move Mama in with me, but she insisted on staying at her own apartment. She had been helping raise her friend Gertrude's great grand kids. Their mother had also moved in. I agreed because of my breakneck schedule. Mama's husband was in the early stages of Alzheimer's, and I had to draw the line. She put him in a nursing home and her pastor assumed responsibility for him.

One day while visiting her in the hospital, she started cursing me in her hoarse voice. I said, "Mama, I'm leaving." I got up from the chair and walked out in tears. It hurt to leave her there alone, but I had to establish boundaries. I could no longer permit her to abuse me. I was back the next day and that's how it went. On another occasion, she lit into me again.

"Bitch, you ain't never meant me no good," she said. I was the only somebody taking care of her, and I had had enough.

"Mama, you have cursed me for the last time," I said coldly and got up from my chair.

"I'm sick of your shit!" I told her, and said, "I'm not coming back." Before I reached the door, I heard her scraggly voice speaking at the top of her lungs, "Don't go!" I was startled. The fear I felt from her sent chills up my spine. I translated that to mean, *Don't let me die by myself*. I stopped and turned to her.

"I love you!" she declared. "You all I got." This was the first time she ever told me she loved me. I was overwhelmed, but it had come way too late.

"Mama, I love you, too, but your love hurts," I said and walked out with tears in my eyes. When I got to school for my class, I sat on a bench to get myself together. Here I am, a grown-ass woman, and I had that ugly face of tears and snot. One of my classmates, Rev. Dr. Jeanne Porter, stopped in her tracks and asked if she could help. She sat with me and listened, and then she prayed for me.

When I arrived the next day, Mama's smile welcomed me into her room. I felt like the war was over. We had gone back and forth like the British and French but, in the end, we had both stood our ground and emerged tall in our own way without sacrificing the essence of who we were. I knew she would never change – not even now at death's door. I also knew she would never say she was sorry, nor did I ask her to apologize. I just needed her to accept what had taken me years to learn: I was God's wonderful creation who deserved to be respected.

In the weeks preceding her death, Mama was afraid to be left alone. I had admitted her into a hospital in Evanston closer to her friends. I drove there every morning and stayed until she had fallen asleep. Most nights it was between one and three in the morning because she was afraid to go to sleep. Finally, the doctors told me there was nothing else they could do for her, and she agreed to stop taking any type of medication.

The doctors told me that one day Mama's windpipe would just shut down. The day I brought her home it was hot as hell in Chicago. With only the window unit air conditioning it felt like a sauna in her apartment. I got her settled and went home to pack and pick up my dogs. When I arrived back at Mama's, she was drenched in sweat and thirsty. I leaned over and whispered, "Mama, I'm back." She nodded her approval. I dried her off, gave her some water, and sat on the sofa in front of the hospital bed. I knitted and monitored Mama for the rest of the evening. I wiped her sweat and reassured her I was still there. Sometimes she would open her eyes and nod. Around midnight, I decided I would admit her to hospice care as soon as possible because she was too sick to remain in her apartment. I began making calls to see if it could be arranged and continued my routine of wiping her face and reassuring her for the next three hours. The last time I leaned over and reassured Mama, she smiled and gave me a nod. I sat back down, but within minutes she was gone. I had kept my promise; she had not died alone.

I laid her to rest July 30, 2002, in a beautiful burgundy and pink St. John knit that I had worn to her house once. She'd said she wanted one like it. I was planning to buy one for her, but she became sick. Mine was a size four and had been way too small for her then, but it fit her now. On the day of the funeral, a friend who knew what my life with Mama was like asked, "How could you do all of this?" I knew what she was asking, and I told her, "I did this because of who I am, and who I say I am to God. My faith is not predicated on what people do or don't do to me."

Charles

I have no idea what happened to this man. But I am still following the lead on the rumor that he died from AIDS. I want to know how deep the deception really went with his psycho ass.

Dorje

Rae,

I'm writing to tell you that I hate you and all niggers. You are a bitch and I wish to hell I had had an abortion rather than having you and your sleazy father in my life. Fuck you! I tried and all you did was play games.
Bye
Dorje

There is no preparation on earth for a letter like this from your mother. NONE! Someone should have told my mother that much. After Dorje came down from whatever mental break that prompted her to write this letter and actually put it in the mail, she called. The phone rang; I looked over and the caller ID read "private," and I looked at the clock. It was 4:00 a.m.

"Not at this hour," I said to myself. "Whoever it is can talk to me when I get up." I went back to sleep. Before I left that morning for the knit shop, I checked my voicemail. Dorje's crackling voice came over the waves. She said, "Hi, Rae. I was recently raped by a Black man, and I went off the deep end and sent you a bad letter. I hope that you can forgive me." I checked my mail, and the letter was in the box. It had taken her the time it took for the letter to get from Buffalo to Chicago in the U.S. Mail to call. I went on to my car. I was not going to change my plans to go to the knit shop because she had sent me a "bad" letter. Plus, if it was that bad, I was going to need all the knit therapy I could get that day.

Dorje never got help for her mental illness and it had been a rollercoaster. Some days she was bright and cheery, and we could talk for a good hour, catching up. Other days, she was dark and dreary. Now, this. I read the letter out loud. I was stunned. This letter had been intended to hurt me, and it achieved its mission. My first reaction was, *If you had protected me like a mother should, then maybe I would have never been raped and I wouldn't be so damaged and having this crisis right now.*

"What if she had been raped by a white man?" I wondered out loud. "Would she have sent a letter similar to this?" The fact that my mother had played the race card was hurtful. White people always know how to reduce a Black person to the *nigger* they believe us to be. I never saw that one coming: maybe from my grandmother, but never from my mother.

This letter came at another crazy time in my life. I had just entered the PhD program at the Lutheran School of Theology at Chicago when suddenly I started to sink into a deep depression. Dr. Greg, my therapist, and I had just started working on the difficult issues around my childhood sexual abuse. I had touched on the subject years before with Dr. Rebecca, but it had been too painful to continue. Now, for the first time, I was talking about what had been done to me, in detail. I was overwhelmed with all that my childhood had been taken from me. I mourned for Little Rae. If I hadn't had the knit shop, I probably would have never gotten out of bed. "Get up girl and get to the knit shop," I would tell myself. If I could get out of the house and to the knit shop, I would make it through that day. Some days I would go to the knit shop with no money and no projects. Betty, the owner could see the light shine in my face when the new yarn arrived, but I hadn't been speaking since the winter and I couldn't buy penny candy, and the new exclusive yarn was out of the question. After a while she made sure my supply never ran dry. Betty would slip the yarn, already in a bag, by my purse and say, "Take this home with you, Dolly."

It was the worst time for Dorje to flip out on me. She had done it before, on 9/11. When I finished speaking that morning at Savannah State University, I learned all the planes had been grounded. That evening I called, looking for comfort from my mother;

all she could talk about was whether my cousin Juli, who lived in New York, was okay. We weren't a good five minutes into the conversation when she said, "I don't want to talk to you!" and hung up the phone. I was stranded for a week and rented a car to drive back to Chicago. A few weeks after 9/11, I found the knit shop. It was serendipity. Knitting was a salve for my soul. I think it was a long time coming, and it was an extension of Mrs. Jackson's introduction to working with my hands. The shop, We'll Keep You In Stitches, was on Oak Street off the Magnificent Mile. They carried some of the finest yarns I had ever touched in my life. It was owned by two women in their seventies who were full of life. Sisters-in-law Betty Goldstein and Renana (Ronnie) Lavin had been in business together for over thirty years. When I walked in, everyone stopped knitting to see who'd come in. "They told me down the street at Bravco that you can teach me how to knit," I said. Ronnie pulled a chair next to her and said, "Have a sit." Ronnie taught me the knitting basics, and over the years, Betty sharpened my skills. I had been going to the shop for almost three years when I got Dorje's letter.

When I arrived at the knit shop that day with the letter in tow, I settled in my spot next to Betty and showed it to her. "She's one sick cookie," Betty said. "You need to leave her alone." My therapist said the same thing. Dorje was like a wounded animal, hurting everything in its path. The only way to not get hurt was to move out of her way. I walked away cold. About four years later in February 2008, I received a MySpace message from Michael. "Did you know that your mother is in the hospital dying?" As typical, Michael was straight to the point. My mother was very ill. He said she had wanted to reach me but didn't know how. Like I had done a couple of decades before, I dropped everything and flew to Buffalo. The day I walked into Dorje's hospital room she looked up and said, "You are so beautiful," like she had said the first day we met at the Denver Airport. She was very sick but coherent. We talked; I caught her up on my life and explained how I found her. She said I didn't have to come; that she didn't deserve me; and blah, blah, blah. I sat with her well into the evening. The next morning when I arrived, Dorje had started to die. It was as if she had been waiting on me. Her organs were shutting down one by one. The hospital was at its wit's end. My grandmother Florence had visited her, but every time they reached out to her about my mother's care, they told me she said, and I quote, "I don't want anything to do with it." Picture a Black woman trying to convince a slew of white doctors concerned about HIPAA that I was the decision-maker if my grandmother had washed her hands of my mother. What convinced them to work with me was when they talked about her mental health and mentioned she'd been raped, and the rapist had cut off her breasts.

"Who told you that stupid shit?" came out of my mouth with a quickness. (LOL!)

"Your mother," a doctor said to me, all testy.

"That's not true. Look," I said, "My mother sat in her living room and cut off her breasts years ago." Their eyes bulged. One doctor's hand went up to her mouth. Then it was my turn to be shocked.

I had narrated to the part where I was explaining that my mother hadn't used drugs in years when a doctor said, "She's on methadone." I saw black. One of the doctors grabbed me before I hit the floor. My mother had been using drugs again but at some point, decided to get clean again. Her social worker at the methadone clinic said she never missed an appointment. The doctors and I decided it was time to trust each other. My mother was dying, and decisions had to be made. I sat with her well into the evening. The next morning, I went to her apartment to pack it up. It was a nice building, but she was literally living in squalor. In her filthy studio apartment were a bed, no sheets, no dishes, and very few clothes. I sat on the side of her bed and cried. After I got myself together, I broke her lease; donated her clothes; and brought all her papers; especially those related to Buddhism, back to Chicago. When I arrived at the hospital later that day, I learned that my grandmother had just left. I believe that was

God's intervention. I was never to see her face to face. She hadn't called so she obviously didn't want me there. I called my cousin Juli – the daughter of my mother's sister when I returned home. She was shocked that our grandmother hadn't told her my mother was dying. My grandmother was just going to let her daughter die just like that and no one would have closure. Before I left, I arranged for Dorje to go into hospice care and asked the social worker to call me if anything changed in her condition. My mother passed away at 7:25 p.m. on March 3, 2008 the day before she was to be transferred to hospice and two days after I left. The hospital called and told me they had informed my grandmother of my mother's death, and she told them, "I don't care what you do with her body." I immediately claimed her body and arranged for a crematorium to take care of her remains. My mother was a devout Buddhist in life, and I would ensure she would be one in death. I held a Buddhist ceremony in Chicago; Michael held one in Boston and scattered some of her ashes at her favorite retreat center. My grandmother told my cousin that I was interfering. She and I talked again, and I recounted what the hospital told me. I guess my grandmother felt some remorse, but it was too late.

In that same conversation with Juli she said to me, "My mother is no better off than your mother." In that moment, I remembered my conversation when my mother had already explained to me that my grandmother raised Juli because Toni Rae was not capable at the time. I don't remember exactly what happened, but something she had done during her pregnancy caused a medical condition that stunted Juli's physical growth, specifically, her height. Now, Juli was implying her mother had a dysfunctional life just as my mother had, and I was sure there had been unnamed trauma in their home. In that same conversation, Juli advised, "Be glad we both made it out." I reached out to Juli again via email, but she never responded.

When my grandmother passed away seven years later at the ripe old age of ninety-seven, a law firm reached out to me about her will. They wanted me to sign a waiver disavowing any rights to the will. Apparently, it's a formality in New York for anyone who might have a claim to a will they are not mentioned in. I was shocked because my mother always told me that I was in the will. I would learn my grandmother changed her will the same day my mother passed. The new will indicated if my mother preceded my grandmother in death, her portion of the will would be divided between my aunt and her two children: Juli and her brother, Christopher. I was completely left out of my grandmother's obituary. My grandmother had managed to reject me, even in death.

Where Do I Go From Here?

I want to rest my mind, body, and spirit for at least a little while. When I'm not out speaking about my story and the ways trauma affected my life, I want to knit, bead, and read all the books I neglected while writing this memoir.

Quit? Never! It's just not in my make-up. I watch Reverend Jesse Jackson, still pushing through with Parkinson's and I ask Ms. J, "When is Reverend going to SAT DOWN?" but she and I both know the answer; like Reverend, God called me to ministry, and I will continue to minister in some form until I die. Full Stop. Other than lecturing and writing, I would love to open a wellness center, *Healing Hands* for crafting and wellness. Another book? Absolutely! But something about my lessons on healing. I've also thought about a fictional book using Mama as my protagonist, and one on my family and the impact of migration. God, I have lots of ideas.

Personally, I want to become financially stable, which is something I just haven't been able to do since the 2008 recession and the loss of the original book deal. It's been up and down and crazy. I want a simpler life. A small house someplace that I can call my own. I want it surrounded by trees and nature so that I can go out and listen to the birds chirping while having my morning tea. I want my red room and a room of books, and all my art displayed throughout my little home; these few things are the center of where I find peace. I want to get to know my family who I just learned about through working on my ancestry. I had a breakthrough in the fall of 2021 and found cousins from my paternal grandfather's side of the family, and God, some of us look alike. I want to meet everyone from the Dixon-Lewis-Perkins-Bowden line. So far, I've talked to a good many, have met some and follow them on social media. Most of them are fourth and fifth generations, but I have even found some second and third cousins. I talk to Kerry Davis, the first of the cousins from this family line who I met, and Ericka Smith, my twin, who is just a shade darker than me, most every week. I have even spoken to third cousins on Dorje's side: the Sengers, Koesters, and Skolyons; probably ones she never knew she had. She has a half-sister that I've found, too, whose son I've spoken to via text. Maybe I'll get to meet them one day too. I still have to figure out the life and extended family of my paternal grandmother Jane Clara. I'm getting so good at this ancestry thing; I might open a business.

I am so very happy to be alive. What I know for sure is this: when I wake up in the morning, I am still a part of God's earthly plan, and the first two things out of my mouth are "Thank you, Lord," and "How can I be of service today?" When my earthly plan is over, my prayer is that those who witnessed my life will be able to say, Well done, good and faithful servant; well done.

ACKNOWLEDGMENTS

I thank God I have lived to tell this story. Full Stop.

I could not have completed this book without my editor, Vivian Feggans. I am forever indebted to her for giving this project her talent, time, and her soul for almost three years. Your ability to keep my voice intact and push me is remarkable. On this journey, we became friends. I thank Vivian's daughter, Jocelyn Saunders for introducing us. A big thank you to my final proofreader, Andrew Davis who helped Vivian and I put the finishing touches to the manuscript. Thank you, Tracy Baim, for the recommendation. My beta readers were wonderful; Cathleen Myers, Judy Jordan, Randolph Sturrup, and Dwana De La Carna. Thank you for your time, commitment, encouragement, and feedback. Relana Johnson, has been my ride and die book designer for ten years. First in 2008 she designed the cover and interior of my second book, *The Politics of Respectability* in short of just two weeks. The cover design of this book is nothing short of amazing. Thank you for your time, expertise, and patience, never complaining about my requests in the layout of this book.

To my sister-friend and forever Soror Sheryl Lee Ralph—Thank You for two decades of friendship, your support of this body of work and your fidelity to the work of HIV/AIDS.

A big thank you to my photographer, Kirsten Miccoli, for your time, talent, and studio. You gave Relana something to work with. My glam team-Tia Dantzler, celebrity make-up artist. From the first day that you "beat my face" in my kitchen in 2010 to the *Essence* photo shoot in 2014, to this fabulous look for my book cover, I thank you for your time and talent; Trayce Madre, it's been a 10-year journey of hair growth and wonderful looks for photo shoots; thank you; Brandon Frein and Arlene Matthews, extraordinary stylist of *Kit This*. Whenever I call, you show up with the baddest wardrobe and best ideas—Thank you! A big thanks to Nikia Jefferson for the introduction eight years ago. Thanks to Bloomingdales's, Magnificent Mile, for providing the wardrobe.

A special thank you for the people who helped me on this journey. Kenneth Bennett, 28 years of friendship. You came through for me in the most unexpected way and I am eternally grateful. Thanks to my biggest cheerleaders on this journey; Luther Burke, love you to the moon and back, Reverend Peter Matthews, your friendship is the calm to my chaos. Mrs. Jacqueline Jackson, the wisest woman I know. Terri Garvin, for being you. Veronica Slater, my friend forever, for providing me with a year of travel to research and work on this book. My social media supporters: You all know who you are. Thank you for your retweets and reposts, the encouragement, and the money you dropped into my cashapp when my speaking engagements dried up during COVID. Your donations afforded me food on my table so I could keep writing. Thanks to everyone who contributed to my Bali Writing Retreat.

As promised, the patrons of this book get a special mention: Kindra and Donna Robinson, Reverend Peter Matthews, Dr. Frantonia Pollins, Reverend Leslie Sanders, Vivian Feggans and A Literary Collective of Black Women (LCBW of Charlottesville, Virginia), Consuella Brown, Dr. Monica Vernette Gray, and Terri Garvin, Esq.

In advance, I'm thanking everyone who purchased this book.

READING RECOMMENDATIONS

Health/HIV-AIDS

And The Band Played On
(Shilts, Randy. New York: St. Martin's Griffin, 1988)

Believing in Magic
(Johnson, Cookie, and Denene Millner. New York: Howard Books, 2017)

Fag Hags, Divas and Moms: The Legacy of Straight Women in the AIDS Community
(Noe, Victoria. Chicago, IL: King Company Publishing, 2019)

From the Crack House to the White House: Turning Obstacles into Opportunities.
(Stokes, Denise. Morrow, GA: Life's Work Publishing, 2012)

Inflamed: Deep Medicine and the Anatomy of Injustice
(Marya, Rupa, and Raj Patel. New York: Farrar, Straus and Giroux, 2021)

Remaking A Life: How Women Living with HIV/AIDS Confront Inequality.
(Watkins-Hayes, Celeste. Oakland, CA: University of California Press, 2019)

The Immortal Life of Henrietta Lacks
(Skloot, Rebecca. Crown Publishing, 2010)

Trauma/Healing

Adult Children of Alcoholics
(Woititz, Janet Geringer. Deerfield Beach, FL: Health Communications, 2000)

After the Rain: Gentle Reminders for Healing, Courage, and Self-Love
(Elle, Alexandra. Chronicle Books, 2020)

Baffled by Love: Stories of the Lasting Impact of Childhood Trauma Inflicted by Loved Ones (Kahn, Laurie. Berkeley, CA: She Writes Press, 2017)

Born for Love: Why Empathy Is Essential: And Endangered.
(Szalavitz, Maia, and Bruce D. Perry. New York: William Morrow, 2011)

Childhood Disrupted: How Your Biography Becomes Your Biology, and How You Can Heal. (Nakazawa, Donna Jackson. Pocket Books, 2016)

Homecoming: Overcome Fear and Trauma To Reclaim Your Whole Authentic Self
(Bryant, Thema, TarcherPerigee, 2022)

My Grandmother's Hands: Racialized Trauma and the Pathway to Mending Our Hearts and Bodies (Menakem Resmaa Central Recovery Press, 2017)

The Body is Not An Apology: The Power of Radical Self-Love
(Taylor, Sonya Renee. Berret-Koehler Publishers, Inc., 2021)

The Body Keeps the Score – Brain, Mind and Body in the Healing of Trauma
(A., Van der Kolk Bessel. New York, NY: Penguin Books, 2015)

The Book of Awakening: Having the Life You Want by Being Present to the Life You Have
(Nepo, Mark. Conari Press, 2011)

The Boy Who Was Raised as a Dog: and Other Stories from a Child Psychiatrist's Notebook: What Traumatized Children Can Teach Us about Loss, Love, and Healing.
(Perry, Bruce D., and Maia Szalavitz. New York: Basic Books, 2017)

The Deepest Well–Healing the Long-Term Effects of Childhood Adversity
(Harris, Nadine Burke. Pan Macmillan, 2020)

Together the Healing Power of Human Connection in a Sometimes Lonely World.
(Murthy, Vivek H. New York, New York: Harper Wave, an imprint of HarperCollins, 2020)

Unbound: My Story Of Liberation And The Birth of The Me Too Movement
(Burke, Tarana. The Oprah Books, Flatiron Books, New York: 2021)

What Happened to You? Conversations on Trauma, Resilience, and Healing.
(Perry, Bruce D., and Oprah Winfrey. New York: Flatiron Books, 2021)

Political

Keeping Hope Alive: Sermons and Speeches of Rev. Jesse L. Jackson, Sr.
(Jackson, Jesse L. Rev., and Grace Ji-Sun Kim. Maryknoll, NY: Orbis Books, 2020)

I Am Somebody: Why Jesse Jackson Matters
(Masciotra, David. London: I B Tauris, 2021)

Rules for Radicals: A Practical Primer for Realistic Radicals
(Alinsky, Saul D. New York: Random House, 1972)

Speaking Truth To Power
(Hill, Anita. New York, NY: Anchor Books, 1998)

Socialism: Past and Future
(Harrington, Michael. Arcade Publishing, 2020)

The Other America: Poverty in the United States
(Harrington, Michael. New York, NY: Macmillan, 1969)

Everybody In, Nobody Out: Memoirs of a Rebel Without a Pause.
(Young, Quentin. Friday Harbor, WA: Copernicus Healthcare, 2013)

Except for Palestine: The Limits of Progressive Politics.
(Hill, Marc Lamont, and Mitchell Plitnick. New York: The New Press, 2021)

A Testament of Hope: The Essential Writings and Speeches of Martin Luther King, Jr.
(King, Martin Luther Rev., and James Melvin Washington. San Francisco: HarperSanFrancisco, 1991)

APPENDIX

FIGURE 1: Adverse Childhood Experience (ACE) Questionnaire for Adults
The Adverse Childhood Experiences (ACE) Study links childhood abuse and household dysfunction to poor health and social outcomes over the span of one's life.

Instructions: From the list below, place a checkmark next to each experience you had prior to your 18th birthday. Add up the number and enter total at the bottom.

While you were growing up, during your first 18 years of life:
1. Did a parent or other adults in the household often ... Swear at you, insult you, put you down, or humiliate you? **Or** Act in a way that made you afraid that you might be physically hurt? YES   NO   If yes enter 1_____

2. Did a parent or other adult in the household often ... Push, grab, slap, or throw something at you? **Or** Ever hit you so hard that you had marks or were injured? YES   NO   If yes enter 1 _____

3. Did an adult or person at least 5 years older than you ever... Touch or fondle you or have you touch their body in a sexual way? **Or** Try to or actually have oral, anal, or vaginal sex with you? YES   NO   If yes enter 1_____

4. Did you often feel that ... No one in your family loved you or thought you were important or special? **Or** Your family didn't look out for each other, feel close to each other, or support each other? YES   NO   If yes enter 1 _____

5. Did you often feel that ... You didn't have enough to eat, had to wear dirty clothes, and had no one to protect you? **Or** Your parents were too drunk or high to take care of you or take you to the doctor if you needed it? YES   NO   If yes enter 1_____

6. Were your parents ever separated or divorced? YES   NO   If yes enter 1_____

7. Was your mother or stepmother: Often pushed, grabbed, slapped, or had something thrown at her? **Or** Sometimes or often kicked, bitten, hit with a fist, or hit with something hard? **Or** Ever repeatedly hit over at least a few minutes or threatened with a gun or knife? YES   NO   If yes enter 1 _____

8. Did you live with anyone who was a problem drinker or alcoholic or who used street drugs? YES   NO   If yes enter 1 _____

9. Was a household member depressed or mentally ill or did a household member attempt suicide? YES   NO   If yes enter 1_____

10. Did a household member go to prison? YES   NO   If yes enter 1_____

Now add up your "Yes" answers: _____This is your ACE Score.

Figure 1. ACE Questionnaire

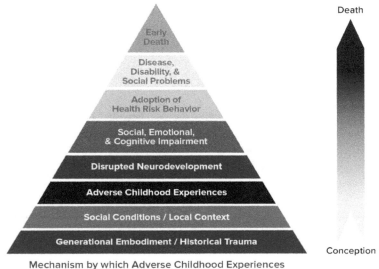

Mechanism by which Adverse Childhood Experiences
Influence Health and Well-being Throughout the Lifespan

Figure 2. ACE Pyramid

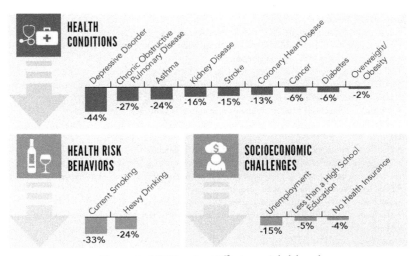

Figure 3. ACE Lasting Effects on Adulthood

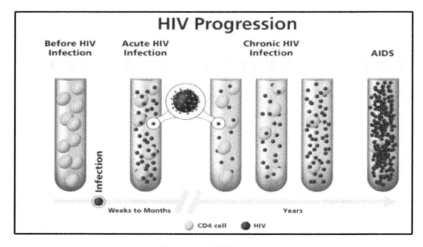

Figure 4. HIV Progression*

Acute HIV Infection
- Develops 2-4 weeks after infection
- May get flu-like symptoms (body aches, headache, rash, swollen glands
- Seroconversion-HIV replicates CD-4 cells, also known as T cells
- HIV multiplies rapidly and spreads throughout the body 7-24 days
- Reaches its peak at a million replications
- HIV levels are very high which increases the risk of infecting others
- Can stop the replication if start post-exposure treatment with 72 hours of infection

Chronic HIV Infection
- Also called Asymptomatic HIV and Clinical Latency
- HIV continues to multiply at low levels in the body, as it multiplies, it destroys CD4 T cells
- May not have any HIV related symptoms
- Without treatment HIV advances to AIDS in 10 years on average after initial expo-sure
- With treatment a person can stay in this stage for serval decades. (CDC recom-mendation is to start treatment immediately)
- With an undetectable viral load, a person cannot transmit HIV through sex

AIDS
- 200 T cell count or lower and/or an Opportunistic Infection
- Symptoms: significant weight loss, persistent fever of 100, night sweats, severe fa-tigue, rash-es, coughing and breathing problems, memory problems, chronic oral and vaginal Candidiasis
- HIV has severely damaged your immune system
- The body cannot fight off Opportunistic Infections (See Figure 5)
- The body cannot fight off other infections and cancers that occur with a weakened immune system
- Can easily transmit HIV
- AIDS survival around 3 years with no treatment

*Sources: NIH, CDC, Avert

BIBLIOGRAPHY

"Adverse Childhood Experiences (ACEs)." *Centers for Disease Control and Prevention*, November 5, 2019. https://www.cdc.gov/vitalsigns/aces/index.html

Altman, Lawrence K. "Cost of Treating AIDS Patients is Soaring." *The New York Times*, July 23, 1992, sec. B.

Apple, R. W. "Jackson Wins Easily In Michigan In Surprising Setback to Dukakis." *The New York Times*, March 27, 1988, sec. 1.

Ashe, Arthur, and Arnold Rampersad. *Days of Grace: A Memoir*. Bath, England: Chivers Press, 1994.

"AZT's Inhuman Cost." (Opinion piece) *The New York Times*, August 28, 1989, sec. A.

Barnes, Bart. "Pioneering Anchorman Max Robinson Dies." *The Washington Post*, December 21, 1988.

Berry, Jeff. "One-on-One: Mardge Cohen." For the HIV/AIDS Workforce. *TheBodyPro*, April 1, 2006. https://www.thebodypro.com/article/one-on-one-mardge-cohen

Blumenthal, Sidney. "Willie Horton the Making of an Election Issue." *The Washington Post*, October 28, 1988.

Boyer, Peter J. "The Light Goes Out." *Vanity Fair*, June 1989.

Brazile, Donna. *Cooking with Grease: Stirring the Pots in American Politics*. New York: Simon & Schuster, 2005.

Carmody, John. "Max Robinson and 'The Racism' Speech." *The Washington Post*, February 10, 1981.

Clemente, Frank, and Frank Watkins. *Keep Hope Alive: Jesse Jackson's 1988 Presidential Campaign*. Washington, D.C., and Boston: Keep Hope Alive Political Action Committee and South End Press, 1989.

Clendinen, Dudley. "Thousands In Civil Rights March Jeered By Crowd In Georgia Town." *The New York Times*, January 25, 1987, sec. 1.

Coates, Ta-Nehisi. "The Tragedy of Jesse Jackson." *The Atlantic*, July 14, 2008.

Crooks, Natasha, and Akilah Wise. "What We Risk When We Fail to Protect Black Girls." *Rewire News*, February 25, 2019. https://rewirenewsgroup.com/article/2019/02/25/what-we-risk-when-we-fail-to-protect-black-girls/

Cuniberti, Betty. "Max Robinson's Silent Struggle With AIDS." *The Los Angeles Times*, December 22, 1988.

Esposito, Stefano, and Rachel Hinton. "Rev. Leon Finney, Longtime Power Player in City Politics, Dead at 82." *The Chicago Sun Times*, September 4, 2020.

Fauci, Anthony S., and H. Clifford Lane. "Four Decades of HIV/AIDS – Much Accomplished, Much to Do." *New England Journal of Medicine*, vol 383, no. 1 (2020): 1–4. https://doi.org/10.1056/nejmp191675

Felitti, Vincent J., Robert F. Anda, Dale Nordenberg, David F. Williamson, Alison M. Spitz, Valerie Edwards, Mary P. Koss, and James S. Marks. Reprint, "Relationship of Childhood Abuse and Household Dysfunction to Many of the Leading Causes of Death in Adults: The Adverse Childhood Experiences (ACE) Study." 10.1016/s0749-3797(98)00017-8

Fields, Kim. *Blessed Life: My Joyful Journey from Tootie to Today*. FaithWords, 2017.

Gallo, Robert C., and Luc Montagnier. "The Discovery of HIV as the Cause of AIDS." *New England Journal of Medicine* 349, no. 24 (2003): 2283–85. https://doi.org/10.1056/nejmp03819

Glass, Andrew. "House Overrides Reagan Apartheid Veto, Sept 29, 1986." *POLITICO*, September 29, 2017. https://www.politico.com/story/2017/09/29/house-overrides-reagan-apartheid-veto-sept-29-1986-243169

Gould, Robert E. "Reassuring News About AIDS: A Doctor Tells Why You May Not Be At Risk." *Cosmopolitan*, January 1988.

Hall, Carla. "The Rise, and Dizzying Fall, of Max Robinson." *The Washington Post*. May 26, 1988.

Harris, Nadine Burke. "How Childhood Trauma Affects Health Across a Lifetime." TED-ED. 2014. https://ed.ted.com/lessons/eczPoVp6

Harris, Nadine Burke. *The Deepest Well*. Boston: Pan Macmillan, 2020.

Higginbotham, Brooks Evelyn. *Righteous Discontent: The Women's Movement in the Black Baptist Church 1880-1920*. Cambridge, MA; Harvard University Press, 1993

Hilts, Philip J. "AIDS Definition Excludes Women, Congress Told." *The New York Times*, June 7, 1991, sec. A.

Hinton, Garfield. "Buffalo CORE." *Buffalo-Rochester Edition Buffalo New York Challenger*, December 18, 1963, Vol 2 edition, sec. No 32.

Hinton, Garfield. "Funderburg Tells of Police Whipping at Special Hearing." *Buffalo New York Challenger News Weekly*, September 2, 1963, Vol 2 edition, sec. No 19.

Hinton, Rachel, and Stefano Esposito. "Rev. Leon Finney, Longtime Power Player in City Politics, Dead at 82." *The Chicago Sun-Times*, September 4, 2020.

Holson, Laura M. "Max Robinson, A Largely Forgotten Trailblazer for Black Anchors." *The New York Times*, June 19, 2015.

Huck, Janet. "Breaking a Silence: 'Starsky' Star, Wife Share Their Family's Painful Battle Against AIDS." *The Los Angeles Times*, August 25, 1989. https://www.latimes.com/archives/la-xpm-1989-08-25-vw-1121-story.html

Hussain, Rummana. "Oscar Chute; Integrated Evanston School." *The Chicago Tribune*, January 11, 2001. https://www.chicagotribune.com/news/ct-xpm-2001-01-11-0101110186-story.html.

Ifill, Gwen. "Dukakis' Relationship With Black Voters Under Debate." *The Washington Post*, April 25, 1988.

Interlandi, Jeneen. "Why Doesn't the United States Have Universal Health Care? The Answer Has Everything to Do With Race." *The New York Times Magazine*, August 14, 2019.

Isabel, Wilkerson. "The 1992 Campaign: Woman the News; Storming Senate 'Club': Carol Elizabeth Moseley Braun." *The New York Times*, March 19, 1992, sec. A.

Jackson, Jesse L, and Grace Ji-Sun Kim. *Keeping Hope Alive: Sermons and Speeches of Rev. Jesse L. Jackson, Sr.* Maryknoll, NY: Orbis Books, 2020.

"Jesse Jackson is a Serious Candidate for Presidency." *The Nation*, April 16, 1988.

Jones, Feminista. "[TALK LIKE SEX] Deconstructing 'Ho'." *Ebony*, January 9, 2014. https://www.ebony.com/love-relationships/talk-like-sex-deconstructing-ho-333/.

Kadner, Phil. "Even Reformers Don't Like Obamacare: A Conversation With Dr. Quentin Young." *South Star*, October 17, 2013.

Kahn, Laurie. *Baffled by Love: Stories of the Lasting Impact of Childhood Trauma Inflicted by Loved Ones.* Berkeley, CA: She Writes Press, 2017.

Kilkenny, Katie. "CNN's Don Lemon Urges Hollywood to 'Resist the Easy Path' at Hollywood Reporter's Inaugural Empowerment Gala." *The Hollywood Reporter*, April 30, 2019. https://www.hollywoodreporter.com/news/general-news/don-lemon-urges-hollywood-resist-easy-path-at-hollywood-reporter-gala-1205866/.

King, J. L., and Karen Hunter. *On The Down Low: A Journey Into The Lives of "Straight" Black Men Who Sleep With Men.* New York: Harlem Moon, 2005.

Koch, Edward I. "Senator Helms's Callousness Toward AIDS Victims." *The New York Times*, November 7, 1987, sec. 1.

Lambert, Bruce. "Alison L. Gertz Whose Infection Alerted Many to AIDS, Dies at 26." *The New York Times*, August 9, 1992, sec. 1.

Lambert, Bruce. "Clara Hale, Founder of Home For Addicts' Babies Dies." *The New York Times*, December 19, 1992, sec. 1.

Lauerman, Connie. "Vital Signs." *The Chicago Tribune*, August 16, 1994, sec. 5.

Lewis-Thornton, Rae. "Facing AIDS." *Essence*, December 1994.

"Limit Voted on AIDS Funds." *The New York Times*, October 15, 1987, sec. B, p. 44.

Love, Keith. "Jackson Wins by 2 to 1 in Michigan: He Also Leads Dukakis in Delegates in State; Gephardt Is Distant Third." *The New York Times*, March 27, 1988.

McNulty, Timothy J, and Cheryl Devall. "Jackson: Republicans Sending Racial Signals." *The Chicago Tribune*, October 24, 1988.

MMWR Recommendation and Reports. John W. Ward, Laurence Slutsker, Ruth L. Berkelman, Harold W. Jaffe, and James W. Buehler, 41, 1993. *Revised Classification System for HIV Infection and Expanded Surveillance Case Definition for AIDS Among Adolescents and Adults* (1992).

Morris, Jeannie. *Behind the Smile: A Story of Carol Moseley Braun's Historic Senate Campaign.* Chicago, IL: Midway, 2015.

Mort, Jo-Ann. "Unlike Mike." *Democracy – A Journal of Ideas*, May 14, 2020. https://democracyjournal/org/arguments/unlike-mike

Naftali, Tim. "Ronald Reagan's Long-Hidden Racist Conversation with Richard Nixon." *The Atlantic*, July 30, 2019.

Nakazawa, Donna Jackson. *Childhood Disrupted: How Your Biography Becomes Your Biology, and How You Can Heal.* New York, NY: Atria Paperback, 2016.

Navarro, Vicente. "The Birth and Death of Single-Payer in the Democratic Party." *Jacobin*, May 5, 2020. http://jacobinmag.com/2020/05/jesse-jackson-presidential-campagin-democratic-party.

Noe, Victoria. *Fag Hags, Divas and Moms: The Legacy of Straight Women in the AIDS Community.* Chicago, IL: King Company Publishing, 2019.

Office of the Surgeon General, and C. Everett Koop. "Statement by C. Everett Koop, MD, Surgeon General, US Public Health Service." *Surgeon General's Report on Acquired Immune Deficiency Syndrome*, October 22,1986.

Oreskes, Michael. "Chicago's Mayor Endorses Jackson." *The New York Times*, September 9, 1987, sec. A.

Overbea, Luix. "Network TV's Only Black Anchor Man Says News Distorts US Image." *The Christian Science Monitor*, July 27, 1981.

Pear, Robert. "AMA Rules That Doctors Are Obligated To Treat AIDS." *The New York Times*, November 13, 1987.

Perry, Bruce Duncan, and Maia Szalavitz. *The Boy Who Was Raised As A Dog: And Other Stories From A Child Psychiatrist's Notebook: What Traumatized Children Can Teach Us About Loss, Love, and Healing*. New York, NY: Basic Books, 2017.

Perry, Bruce Duncan, and Oprah Winfrey. *What Happened To You? Conversations On Trauma, Resilience, And Healing*. New York: Flatiron Books, 2021.

Peterson, Bill. "Simon Defeats Jackson In Illinois Vote." *The Washington Post*, March 16, 1988.

Reynolds, Gretchen. "Vote of Confidence." *Chicago Magazine*, January 1993.

Riding, Alan. "Scandal Over Tainted Blood Widens in France." *The New York Times*, February 13, 1994, sec. 1.

Rosenbaum, David E. "Jackson Makes Formal Bid for Presidency." *The New York Times*, October 11, 36AD, sec. 1.

Rosenbaum, David E. "Disparity Between Jackson's Vote And Delegate Count Vexes Party." *The New York Times*, May 20, 1984.

Rosenthal, Andrew. "Foes Accuse Bush Campaign Of Inflaming Racial Tension." *The New York Times*, October 24, 1988, sec. A.

Schwartz, Maralee. "Jackson Picks Party Insiders For Atlanta." *The Washington Post*, May 15, 1988.

Schwartz, Tony. "Robinson of ABC News Quoted as Saying Network Discriminates." *The New York Times*, February 11, 1981, sec. C.

Straube, Trenton. "MAC AIDS Fund Kicks Off Its 25th Year With Big Transformations." *POZ*, April 19, 2019.

Sullivan, Al. "A New Beginning for Ward F." *Hudson Reporter*, April 29, 2018. https://hudsonreporter.com/2018/04/29/a-new-beginning-for-ward-f/.

Sullivan, Joseph F. "Dukakis Said to Ignore Black Vote." *The New York Times*, October 30, 1988.

Supin, Jeanne. "The Long Shadow – Bruce Perry on the Lingering Effects of Childhood Trauma." *The Sun Magazine*, November 2016.

Taylor, Paul. "Jackson's Winning Ways Transform Candidate, Voters." *The Washington Post*, March 15, 1988.

Teicher, Martin H., Jacqueline A. Samson, Ann Polcari, and Cynthia E. McGreenery. "Sticks, Stones, and Hurtful Words: Relative Effects of Various Forms of Childhood Maltreatment." *American Journal of Psychiatry*, 163, no. 6 (June 6, 2006): 993–1000. https://doi.org/10.1176/ajp.2006.163.6.993.

Terry, Don. "Sometimes I Wished They Had Killed Me." *The Chicago Tribune*, May 22, 2005.

Tumulty, Karen. "Doubts Raised on Turnout of Black Voters." *The Los Angeles Times*, October 22, 1988.

Walsh, Edward. "Dukakis Skirts Civil Rights In South." *The Washington Post*, August 5, 1988.

Walters, Ronald W. *Black Presidential Politics In America: A Strategic Approach*. Albany, New York: State University of New York Press, 1988.

Whetstone, Muriel L. "The Increasing Threat To Black Women." *Ebony*, April 1994.

Winfrey, Oprah. "Treating Childhood Trauma." *60 Minutes*. CBS, March 11, 2018.

Woititz, Janet G. *Adult Children of Alcoholics*. Deerfield, FL: Health Communications Inc., 2010.

Wolke, Dieter, William E. Copeland, Adrian Angold, and E. Jane Costello. "Impact of Bullying in Childhood on Adult Health, Wealth, Crime, and Social Outcomes." *Psychological Science* 24, no. 10, October 19, 2013: 1958–70. https://doi.org/10.1177/0956797613481608.

Young, Quentin. *Everybody In, Nobody Out: Memoirs of a Rebel Without a Pause*. Friday Harbor, WA: Copernicus Healthcare, 2013.

CPSIA information can be obtained
at www.ICGtesting.com
Printed in the USA
BVHW091921090522
636577BV00008B/18/J